Cerebral Small Vessel Disease

Cerebral Small Vessel Disease

Edited by

Leonardo Pantoni, MD, PhD

Staff Neurologist

Stroke Unit and Neurology Azienda Ospedaliero Universitaria Careggi, Florence, Italy

Philip B. Gorelick, MD, MPH

Professor of Translational Science and Molecular Medicine

Michigan State University College of Human Medicine;

Medical Director, Hauenstein Neuroscience Center

Mercy Health at Saint Mary's, Grand Rapids, MI, USA

CAMBRIDGE
UNIVERSITY PRESS

CAMBRIDGE
UNIVERSITY PRESS

University Printing House, Cambridge CB2 8BS, United Kingdom

Cambridge University Press is part of the University of Cambridge.

It furthers the University's mission by disseminating knowledge in the pursuit of education, learning and research at the highest international levels of excellence.

www.cambridge.org
Information on this title: www.cambridge.org/9781107031661

First published 2014

Printed in Spain by Grafos SA, Arte sobre papel

A catalogue record for this publication is available from the British Library

Library of Congress Cataloguing in Publication Data
Cerebral small vessel disease / edited by Leonardo Pantoni, Philip B. Gorelick.
p. ; cm.
Includes bibliographical references and index.
ISBN 978-1-107-03166-1 (Hardback)
I. Pantoni, L., editor of compilation. II. Gorelick, Philip B., editor of compilation.
[DNLM: 1. Cerebral Small Vessel Diseases. WL 355]
QM455
612.8′2–dc23 2014002055

ISBN 978-1-107-03166-1 Hardback

To Franca, Veronica, Valeria, and Viola.
Leonardo Pantoni, MD, PhD

In honor of M. Rosita Schiller, RSM, PhD, and all who work quietly and substantially behind the scenes to improve health and mankind.
Philip B. Gorelick, MD, MPH

Contents

Section 3 – Clinical aspects of cerebral small vessel disease

Section 4 – Therapeutic aspects: prevention, future directions, and possibilities

Contributors

Rosanna Abbate, MD
Department of Medical and Surgical Critical Care, Artherothrombotic Diseases Center, University of Florence, Florence, Italy

Charlotte L. Allan, BA, MBChB, MRCPsych
Department of Psychiatry, University of Oxford, and Department of Psychiatry, Warneford Hospital, Oxford, UK

Johannes Attems, MD
Institute for Ageing and Health, Newcastle University Campus for Ageing and Vitality, Newcastle upon Tyne, UK

Richard I. Aviv, MBChB, MRCP, FRCR
Sunnybrook Health Sciences Centre and University of Toronto, Toronto, ON, Canada

Hansjoerg Baezner, PhD
UniversitätsMedizin Mannheim, University of Heidelberg, Germany

Oscar R. Benavente, MD, FRCP
Brain Research Centre, University of British Columbia, BC, Canada

Maria Bjerke, PhD
Institute of Neuroscience and Physiology, Sahlgrenska Academy, University of Gothenburg, Gothenburg, Sweden

Sandra E. Black, MD, FRCPC, FRSC
Sunnybrook Health Sciences Centre and University of Toronto, Toronto, ON, Canada

Christian Blahak, MD, PhD
UniversitätsMedizin Mannheim, University of Heidelberg, Germany

Mark I. Boulos, MD, FRCP (C), CSCN (EEG), MSc
Department of Neurology, Sunnybrook Health Sciences Centre and University of Toronto, Toronto, ON, Canada

Margherita Cavalieri, PhD
Division of Neurogeriatrics, Medical University of Graz, Graz, Austria

Hugues Chabriat, MD, PhD
Lariboisière Hospital, Universite Paris Diderot, Sorbonne Paris Cité, UMR-S1161 INSERM, Paris; Centre de référence pour les maladies vasculaires rares du cerveau et de l'oeil (CERVCO), France

Christopher Chen, MD
Memory, Aging and Cognition Centre, National University Health Services, Singapore

Martin Dichgans, MD, PhD
Institute for Stroke and Dementia Research, Ludwig–Maximillians University Munich, Munich, Germany

Maria Teresa Dotti, MD
Department of Medicine, Surgery and Neurosciences, University of Siena, Italy

Klaus P. Ebmeier, MD
Department of Psychiatry, Warneford Hospital, Oxford, UK

Elisabet Englund, MD, PhD
Department of Pathology, Lund University, and Regional Laboratories, Skåne, Lund, Sweden

Christian Enzinger, MD, PhD
Division of Neuroradiology, Department of Neurology, Medical University of Graz, Graz, Austria

Margaret Esiri, DM, FRCPath
Department of Neuropathology, University of Oxford, Oxford, UK

Franz Fazekas, MD
Department of Neurology, Medical University of Graz, Graz, Austria

Antonio Federico, MD
Department of Medicine, Surgery, and Neurosciences, University of Siena, Italy

José M. Ferro, MD, PhD
Department of Neurosciences, Hospital de Santa Maria, University of Lisbon, Instituto de Medicina Molecular, Lisbon, Portugal

Thalia Field, MD, FRCP
University of British Columbia, Vancouver, BC, Canada

Wiesje M. van der Flier, PhD
Alzheimer Center of the VU University Medical Center, Amsterdam, the Netherlands

Philip B. Gorelick, MD, MPH
Michigan State University College of Human Medicine and Hauenstein Neuroscience Center, Mercy Health at Saint Mary's, Grand Rapids, MI, USA

Steven Greenberg, MD, PhD
Massachusetts General Hospital, Boston, MA, USA

Atticus H. Hainsworth, PhD
Stroke and Dementia Research Centre, St George's University of London, London, UK

Brian T. Hawkins, PhD
Division of Hematology, University of Washington School of Medicine, Seattle, WA, USA

Michael G. Hennerici, MD
Department of Neurology, UniversitätsMedizin Mannheim, University of Heidelberg, Germany

Domenico Inzitari, MD
NEUROFARBA Department, Neuroscience Section, University of Florence, Florence, Italy

Hatsue Ishibashi-Ueda, MD, PhD
Department of Pathology, National Cerebral and Cardiovascular Center, Osaka, Japan

Yoshikane Izawa, MD, PhD
Division of Hematology, University of Washington School of Medicine, Seattle, WA, USA

Kurt A. Jellinger, MD, PhD
Institute of Clinical Neurology, Vienna, Austria

Anne Joutel, MD, PhD
INSERM U740, Paris, and Universite Paris Diderot, Paris, France

Eric Jouvent, MD, PhD
Lariboisière Hospital, Department of Neurology, Paris, and Universite Paris Diderot, Sorbonne Paris Cité, UMR-S1161 INSERM, Paris, France

Raj Kalaria, PhD, FRCPath
Institute for Ageing and Health, NIHR Biomedical Research Building, Newcastle University, Campus for Ageing and Vitality, Newcastle upon Tyne, UK

Edward G. Lakatta, MD
Laboratory of Cardiovascular Science and Cardiovascular Function Section, National Institute on Aging, National Institutes of Health, Baltimore, MD, USA

Jennifer Linn, MD
Department of Neuroradiology, University Hospital Munich, Munich, Germany

Marisa Loitfelder, PhD
MUG Research Units, Division of Neurogeriatrics, Medical University of Graz, Graz, Austria

Sofia Madureira, MSc
Department of Neurosciences, Instituto de Medicina Molecular, Faculdade de Medicina de Lisboa, Lisbon, Portugal

Hugh S. Markus, DM, FRCP
Department of Clinical Neurosciences, University of Cambridge, Cambridge, UK

Ranjith K. Menon, MD
Vascular Neurology, Division of Adult Neurology, Sunnybrook Health Sciences Centre, and University of Toronto, Toronto, ON, Canada

Vincent Mok, MD
Division of Neurology, Department of Medicine and Therapeutics, Prince of Wales Hospital, Chinese University of Hong Kong, Hong Kong Special Administrative Region, China

Makoto Nakajima, MD
University of British Columbia, Vancouver, BC, Canada

David Nyenhuis, PhD
Department of Translational Science and Molecular Medicine, College of Human Medicine, Michigan State University; and Hauenstein Neuroscience Center, Saint Mary's Health Care, Grand Rapids, MI, USA

Jun Ogata, MD, PhD
Hirakata General Hospital for Developmental Disorders, Osaka, Japan

Christian Opherk, MD, PhD
Department of Neurology and Institute for Stroke and Dementia Research, Ludwig–Maximillians University Munich, Munich, Germany

Leonardo Pantoni, MD, PhD
Stroke Unit and Neurology, Azienda Ospedaliero Universitaria Careggi, Florence, Italy

Francesca Pescini, MD, PhD
NEUROFARBA Department, Neuroscience Section, University of Florence, Florence, Italy

Anna Poggesi, MD, PhD
NEUROFARBA Department, Neuroscience Section, University of Florence, Florence, Italy

Sharon Reutens, MD
School of Psychiatry, University of New South Wales, Sydney, Australia

Stefan Ropele, MD, PhD
Department of Neurology, Medical University of Graz, Graz, Austria

Perminder S. Sachdev, MD, PhD
Centre for Healthy Brain Ageing; School of Psychiatry, Faculty of Medicine, University of New South Wales, Sydney, Australia

Reinhold Schmidt, MD
Medical University of Graz, Graz, Austria

Angelo Scuteri, MD, PhD
Scuola Specializzazione in Geriatria, Universita' Tor Vergata, Rome, Italy

Glenn T. Stebbins, PhD
Translational Imaging Core Facility, Rush University Medical Center, Chicago, IL, USA

Richard H. Swartz, MD, PhD
Sunnybrook Health Sciences Centre and University of Toronto, Toronto, ON, Canada

Ana Verdelho, MD, PhD
Department of Neurosciences, Hospital de Santa Maria, University of Lisbon, Lisbon, Portugal

Anand Viswanathan, MD, PhD
Partners Telestroke Program, Department of Neurology, Massachusetts General Hospital, Boston, MA, USA

Anders Wallin, MD, PhD
Institute of Neuroscience and Physiology, Sahlgrenska Academy, University of Gothenburg, Gothenburg, Sweden

Joanna M. Wardlaw, MD, FRCR
Division of Neuroimaging Sciences, Centre for Clinical Brain Sciences, University of Edinburgh, Edinburgh, UK

Hiromichi Yamanishi, MD, PhD
Hirakata General Hospital for Development Disorders, Osaka, Japan

Gregory J. del Zoppo, MD
Department of Hematology and Department of Neurology, University of Washington School of Medicine, Seattle, WA, USA

Preface

The brain is supplied by a network of blood vessels, both large and small. The large arteries have been the focus of extensive past study by virtue of the ease of imaging them and carrying out neuropathologic evaluation. In relation to cerebrovascular disease, the large arteries of the brain are subject to atherosclerosis similar to that of other large systemic arteries of the body. On the other hand, the smaller cerebral arteries of the brain have received less attention until more recently, when modern brain imaging advances allowed the detection of the consequences of small artery disease such as small deep infarcts, white matter disease (i.e., leukoaraiosis), cerebral microhemorrhages, and prominent perivascular spaces associated with vascular ectasia. The deeply seated small arteries and veins, moreover, have been more difficult to study directly, and less has been known about the underlying neuropathology in those afflicted. However, there has been an explosion of recent interest in small vessel disease of the brain, and a considerable body of new information about it and its importance in aging have emerged. Thus, we have devoted this treatise to this topic. With more clinical, neuropathologic, and epidemiologic studies available, we felt that it was appropriate to launch this book and share important insights with the readers.

The evolution of our understanding of vascular cognitive impairment and the role of vascular risk factors in disrupting cognitive vitality as we age has been a focus of study over the years by the editors of this book, who have concluded, as others have, that small vessel disease of the brain is the most important cause of vascular cognitive impairment. The occasion of this text provided us the opportunity to bring together international leaders in the field of small vessel disease of the brain and have them provide succinct reviews of topics germane to the field, spanning from classification, neuropathology, and basic aspects of small vessel disease of the brain, to hereditary disorders, neuroimaging and laboratory aspects to clinical manifestations, and, finally, treatment and prevention. The readers will find that hereditary models of small vessel disease of the brain hold an important place in our understanding of pathophysiology, and the neurovascular unit provides a potential final common pathway whereby small vessel changes lead to brain complications and loss of cognitive vitality and other functional outcomes.

The current literature is burgeoning with information about small vessel disease of the brain. However, there have been few attempts to organize this massive scientific knowledge base in a logical and understandable manner. *Cerebral Small Vessel Disease* links the reader to the many aspects of this disorder in an integrated and digestible presentation.

We have designed the book for both clinicians and researchers. We reach out to practicing physicians and other care providers, epidemiologists, medical students, residents (especially those interested in neurology and geriatrics), geriatricians, radiologists, pathologists, and those with public health backgrounds. The fundamental prerequisite for reading the text is an interest in the aging brain, how vascular factors and processes affect the brain, and how we might treat and prevent vascular injury to the brain. Vascular factors not only influence our risk of vascular cognitive impairment but also of Alzheimer's disease. Therefore, what we have to say in the text may be applicable to Alzheimer's disease.

The text serves as a quick topical reference for the practicing physician or care provider who needs an answer about a patient in relation to treatment and prevention. In addition, it provides a more detailed understanding of underlying mechanisms and consequences of small vessel disease of the brain. Therefore, both the clinician and researcher may benefit from exploring the text.

We wish to thank all of our patients and research collaborators throughout the years who have shared with us insights and stimulated our own thinking as we strive to better understand small vessel disease of the brain. Hopefully, the readers will be armed to provide even better care for their patients, with a better understanding of cerebral small vessel disease, and be motivated to develop an emboldened research agenda to better the health of many with or at risk of this affliction.

Chapter 1

Definition and classification of small vessel diseases

Leonardo Pantoni

Introduction

Cerebral small vessel disease (SVD) has become a popular and very widely used term today. As a reflection of this trend, the present book is entirely dedicated to this issue that has recently gained a central interest for clinicians, radiologists, pathologists, and many researchers in the fields of stroke, dementia, and aging.

In this chapter, I will briefly outline key definitions and concepts related to SVD, and also briefly report on new directions in the field. For a detailed discussion of the topic, readers can refer to a review [1] and a position paper recently published [2].

Definition of cerebral SVDs and nosologic issues

Before defining the pathologic processes affecting the small vessels of the brain, the definition itself of these vessels is needed. Generally speaking, a small vessel could be defined as any vascular structure that is not "large." Obviously, this is quite simplistic, and a more precise definition should be provided. Of note, a survey performed some years ago reported that the agreement among neuropathologists on the definition of a small vessel was not high [3]. About half of the pathologists agreed on the definition of a small vessel being one that was less than 500 μm in diameter and located deeper than in the cortex. Other reported definitions with lower agreement were "vessels with a diameter less than 50 μm" and "all the vessels within the brain parenchyma plus the vessels with a diameter less than 500 μm in the leptomeningeal space." Also, use of the term as synonym of arteriole was mentioned [3]. Many investigators use the term "small vessel" in almost exclusive reference to the arterial tree, likely because pathologic processes of the arterial component are better known than those of the other components (capillaries and small veins). Our current definition of small vessels refers to all the vascular structures (small arteries, arterioles, capillaries, venules, and small veins) that are located in the brain parenchyma or in the subarachnoid space. The general assumption behind this concept is that the diseases that affect the small vessels are at least in part different from those that affect the large vessels. This is obviously only partially true as some pathologic processes damage both large and small vessels. This is the case, for example, for diabetes and some inflammatory diseases (e.g., vasculitis). On the other hand, some other diseases, such as cerebral amyloid angiopathy, particularly affect the small vessels. The second assumption that leads to a distinction between pathologic processes of the small and large vessels is that the pathophysiology and the consequences on the brain parenchyma are different. Usually, the parenchymal consequences of SVD are less acute with the exception of lacunar infarcts, and tend to accumulate over time and may result in disability.

In addition to some inconsistencies in the definition of small vessels, another problem in the field of SVD is that current standard neuroimaging techniques used in practice do not allow the visualization of small vessels and, therefore, a direct understanding of their structural consequences. As a result, SVD is a term used today to describe the pathologic consequences of SVD on the brain parenchyma rather than the underlying diseases of the vessels. One of the consequent problems with this current view is that it tends to cause a uniform pathogenic interpretation of the brain lesions and, therefore, people to refer to

Cerebral Small Vessel Disease, ed. Leonardo Pantoni and Philip B. Gorelick. Published by Cambridge University Press.

"a disease" (see, e.g., Wardlaw et al. [4]). This approach can be somewhat misleading; for example, a small lacunar infarct can be caused by arteriolosclerosis due to aging and hypertension, but also to vasculitis or an infectious process that affects the small penetrating arteries and arterioles, and therefore is better referred to as a syndrome. Thus, just looking at the single neuroimaging lesion cannot be sufficient to make a comprehensive diagnosis.

One final concept to keep in mind when approaching SVD is that the parenchymal lesions can be of different nature, either ischemic or hemorrhagic. Hitherto, the view has been focused much more on the nonhemorrhagic brain lesions with scarce attention to the hemorrhagic ones. Our previous classification of brain lesions due to SVD recognized two types of ischemic (white matter lesions, lacunar infarcts) and two types of hemorrhagic (large hemorrhages, microbleeds) lesions [1]. Recently, the number of lesions attributable to SVD, and therefore classifiable as such, has expanded [2].

Etiologic classification of cerebral SVD

A possible etiologic classification of SVD is reported in Table 1.1 [1]. Some of the reported diseases are systemic, while others are particularly confined to the brain. As stated elsewhere [1], the relative frequency of these diseases is different, and the first two types are by far more commonly encountered in clinical practice than the latter ones.

Table 1.1 Etiologic classification of cerebral SVDs

Type 1. Arteriolosclerosis (or age and vascular risk factors-related SVD)
Type 2. Cerebral amyloid angiopathy (sporadic and hereditary)
Type 3. Inherited or genetic SVD (distinct from cerebral amyloid angiopathy; e.g., CADASIL, CARASIL, Fabry's disease, SVD due to *COL4A1* mutations, etc.)
Type 4. Inflammatory and immunomediated SVD (systemic and cerebral vasculitis, central nervous system vasculitis secondary to infections)
Type 5. Venous collagenosis
Type 6. Other SVD (e.g., post-radiation angiopathy and nonamyloid microvessel degeneration in Alzheimer's disease)

Modified from Pantoni [1].
CADASIL, cerebral autosomal dominant arteriopathy with subcortical ischemic strokes and leukoencephalopathy; CARASIL, cerebral autosomal recessive arteriopathy with subcortical ischemic strokes and leukoencephalopathy; SVD, small vessel disease.

New developments in the field of the definition of SVD

Because at present SVD is mainly a neuroimaging-defined concept, it is expected that, parallel to the development of neuroimaging techniques, the definitions of SVD will continue to evolve and change accordingly. This has been indeed the case over the last few years. In 2011, a call for a collaborative effort focused on an appraisal of the different types of SVD and their definition was launched by the Centres of Excellence in Neurodegeneration (COEN) and the Canadian Institutes of Health Research (CIHR), and an ad-hoc International Working Group was established [5]. The Working Group met twice in 2012, and the collaborative efforts ended in the assemblage of a consensus paper that is now published [2]. The paper reports on a unified approach to the neuroimaging standards for research in SVD under the acronym STRIVE (STandards for ReportIng Vascular changes on nEuroimaging). The work done by the collaborative group is reflected in a series of major conclusions. The first one was that the number of SVD lesion subtypes was broadened to include six types of neuroimaging lesions: (1) recent small subcortical infarcts; (2) lacunes of presumed vascular origin; (3) white matter hyperintensity of presumed vascular origin; (4) perivascular spaces; (5) cerebral microbleeds; and (6) brain atrophy. Perhaps, the inclusion of this latter type lesion was the most advanced change, and was determined by recent data on the association between subcortical lesions and brain atrophy [6]. The second conclusion was the establishment of a common language about terms and definitions for SVD features visible on magnetic resonance imaging (MRI). A third was the suggestion of minimum standards for image acquisition and analysis. The fourth conclusion was an agreement on standards for scientific reporting of changes related to SVD on neuroimaging. In addition, emerging imaging methods for detection and quantification of preclinical manifestations of SVD were also reviewed. This methodological paper represents the basis for relevant future projects and research in the field of SVD.

References

1. Pantoni L. Cerebral small vessel disease: from pathogenesis and clinical characteristics to therapeutic challenges. *Lancet Neurol* 2010;9:689–701.

2. Wardlaw JM, Smith EE, Biessels GJ, et al. Neuroimaging standards for research into small vessel disease and its contribution to ageing and neurodegeneration. *Lancet Neurol* 2013;12:822–838.

3. Pantoni L, Sarti C, Alafuzoff I, et al. Postmortem examination of vascular lesions in cognitive impairment: a survey among neuropathological services. *Stroke* 2006;37: 1005–1009.

4. Wardlaw JM, Smith C, Dichgans M. Mechanisms of sporadic cerebral small vessel disease: insights from neuroimaging. *Lancet Neurol* 2013;12:483–97. Erratum in *Lancet Neurol* 2013;12:532.

5. Editorial. A united approach to vascular disease and neurodegeneration. *Lancet Neurol* 2012;11:293.

6. Appelman AP, Exalto LG, van der Graaf Y, et al. White matter lesions and brain atrophy: more than shared risk factors? A systematic review. *Cerebrovasc Dis* 2009;28:227–242.

Chapter 2

Pathology of cerebral small vessel disease

Jun Ogata, Hiromichi Yamanishi, and Hatsue Ishibashi-Ueda

Introduction

The term small vessel disease (SVD) refers to brain parenchymal injury associated with distal leptomeningeal and intracerebral vessel pathology. From a viewpoint that knowledge of vascular pathology is mandatory for understanding the pathophysiology of brain parenchymal injury and establishing preventive and therapeutic strategies, the principal vessel histopathology of the most common forms of SVD is reviewed. The authors describe pathologic aspects of vascular changes in the brain associated with hypertension and other vascular risk factors (henceforth referred to as hypertensive vasculopathy) and those of sporadic cerebral amyloid angiopathy (CAA). Hereditary forms of SVD are not specifically discussed in this review, including familial CAA and cerebral autosomal dominant arteriopathy with subcortical infarcts and leukoencephalopathy (CADASIL). The different underlying mechanisms of SVD development are briefly discussed.

Materials and methods

This review is based on postmortem pathologic materials and surgical specimens in the National Cerebral and Cardiovascular Center, Osaka, Japan, from 1977 onward, and data reported in the literature. Pathologic examination was performed as described previously [1, 2]. Immunohistochemical staining for β-amyloid (Aβ) was performed with a monoclonal antibody against human β/A4 protein (DAKO) at a concentration of 1 : 100.

Hypertensive vasculopathy

Hypertensive vasculopathy takes place as follows, separately or in various combinations.

Fibrinoid necrosis appears in small arteries and arterioles in the brain, kidneys, and other organs, predominantly in patients with poorly controlled, severe hypertension. It often appears in cases with intracerebral hemorrhage. Fibrinoid material deposits segmentally and commonly occupies a portion of the vessel. The vessel wall has deposits of an eosinophilic, amorphous, or finely granular material, called fibrinoid, which appears red with Masson trichrome and blue with phosphotungstic acid hematoxylin (PTAH). Fibrinoid consists of exudated plasma protein (fibrin and fibrinogen) and necrotic smooth muscle cells (SMCs) on electron microscopic and immunohistochemical examination. Rod- or polygonal-shaped masses with high electron density are the most characteristic finding. The fibrinoid structures have two types of periodic striation of 11 and 22 nm. Mural or occlusive thrombus formation, aneurysmal dilatation, or leakage of blood components through the disintegrated wall often appears consequently [3–5]. With time, this acute vascular change loses the red tint with Masson trichrome and takes on a glassy acellular hyalinous appearance (Figure 2.1).

Microaneurysm was originally described by Charcôt and Bouchard in 1868 and is currently referred to as a Charcôt–Bouchard aneurysm. C. Miller Fisher [6, 7] described microaneurysms in hypertensive patients with small strokes or massive brain hemorrhage. Microaneurysms (also referred to as miliary saccular aneurysms) (300–1100 μm in diameter) involve intracerebral arteries (40–160 μm in diameter) and often arise at bifurcations. The wall of the aneurysm lacks even a trace of muscle or elastic tissue, and sometimes shows fibrinoid necrosis. Thrombi usually line the inner surface of the wall. The aneurysm is often surrounded by red blood cells or hemosiderin-laden

Cerebral Small Vessel Disease, ed. Leonardo Pantoni and Philip B. Gorelick. Published by Cambridge University Press.

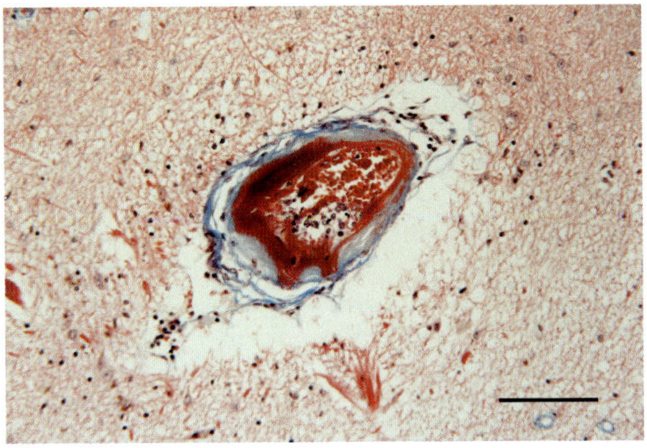

Figure 2.1 A lenticulostriate artery with an area stained red (fibrinoid necrosis and thrombus) and areas stained light blue (hyalinosis). Masson trichrome (MT). Bar = 100 μm.

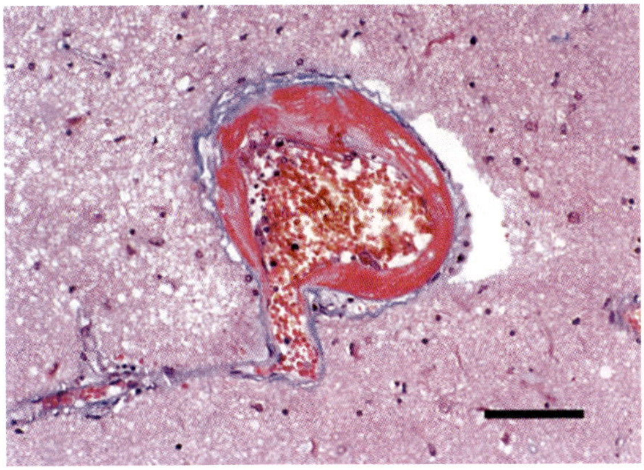

Figure 2.2 A microaneurysm with mural thrombus arising from a lenticulostriate artery. Masson trichrome (MT). Bar = 100 μm.

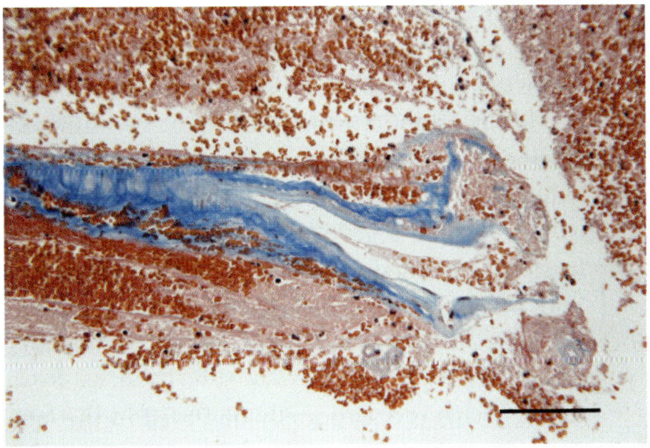

Figure 2.3 A ruptured small artery with arteriosclerosis at the hilus of the cerebellar nuclei in a massive cerebellar hemorrhage. Masson trichrome (MT). Bar = 100 μm.

macrophages, indicating both recent and old extravasation. Microaneurysms are usually found in the areas where hemorrhage is common (Figure 2.2). Bleeding globes (also referred as pseudoaneurysms) consist of masses of red blood cells and platelets (0.3–1.0 cm in diameter) that are enveloped in concentric rings of fibrin emanating from a break in the artery (100–200 μm in diameter). The bleeding globes are found in the presence of massive hemorrhages.

It remains under debate whether rupture of a microaneurysm secondary to fibrinoid necrosis of the vessel wall or weakening of the arterial wall by arteriosclerosis is primarily responsible for intracerebral hemorrhages (Figure 2.3). Takebayashi and Kaneko [8] collected lenticulostriate arteries at surgical evacuation of intracerebral hemorrhage and at autopsy, and examined them by electron microscopy to verify the mechanism of arterial rupture. Severe arteriosclerosis with medial degeneration at or near bifurcations of the artery was observed in 46 of 48 ruptured arteries, whereas rupture from a microaneurysm was observed in only two specimens. Wakai et al. [9, 10] examined complete serial sections of bleeding globes found at the wall of hematomas, following surgical evacuation of massive lobar or cerebellar hemorrhages. They confirmed that bleeding globes encompass rupture of microaneurysms in cases with and without hypertension, and in a case with CAA.

Hyalinosis appears as a light eosinophilic amorphous wall in intracerebral small arteries of hypertensive patients. This term is used because the area stains lighter with hematoxylin and eosin than areas containing fibrinoid and light blue with Masson trichrome. Hyalinosis can be differentiated from fibrinoid by its distinguishing stain to Masson trichrome and PTAH. Electron microscopic examination shows that hyalinization involves degenerated collagen and SMCs and unspecified amorphous structures [4, 5]. Hyalinization does not cause intracerebral hemorrhage, but it is regarded as a common finding in hypertensive subjects. Fibrinoid necrosis may precede hyalinosis, because hyalinosis is a prevalent finding compared to fibrinoid necrosis (Figures 2.1, 2.4). Short-lived fibrinoid necrosis may alter to a stable hyalinosis. No study, however, has proven this process [5].

Fibrohyalinosis is the term applied to the perforating arteries with thickened hyalinized wall that contain areas of fibrosis.

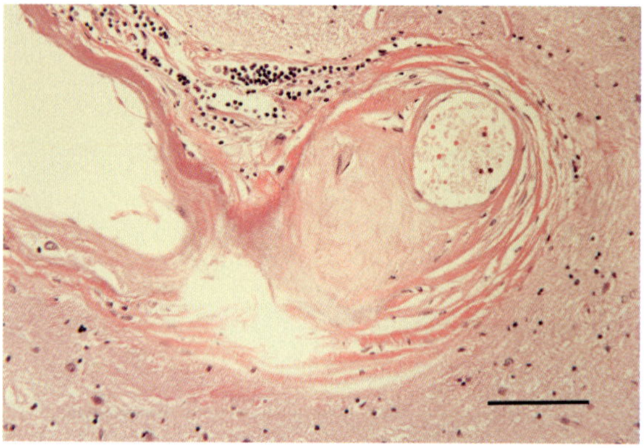

Figure 2.4 A lenticulostriate artery narrowed with hyalinous material (segmental arterial disorganization). Hematoxylin and eosin (H&E). Bar = 100 μm.

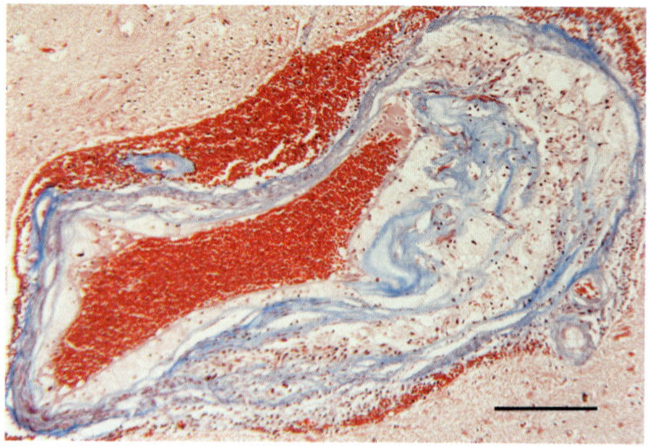

Figure 2.5 Microatheroma of a lenticulostriate artery close to the base of the brain. This artery appears vulnerable to thrombosis. Masson trichrome (MT). Bar = 100 μm.

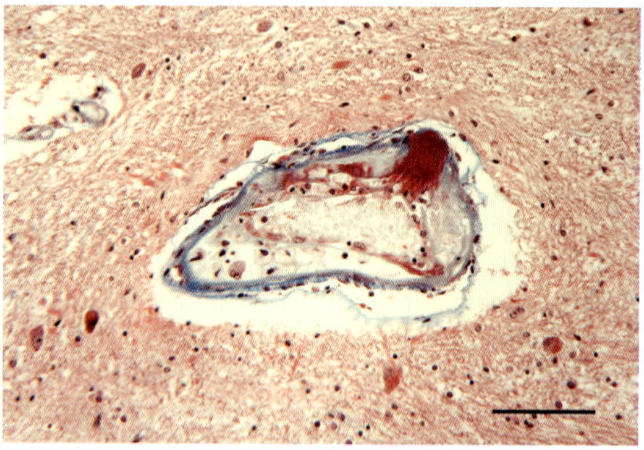

Figure 2.6 Lipohyalinosis of a lenticulostriate artery close to the base of the brain. Note areas stained light blue (hyalinosis), an area stained red (fibrinoid necrosis), and macrophage infiltration of the arterial wall. Masson trichrome (MT). Bar = 100 μm.

Microatheroma encompasses atherosclerotic changes consisting of subintimal proliferation of fibroblasts and lipid-laden macrophages, and deposition of cholesterol crystals in the penetrating arteries close to the surface of the brain. This is occasionally seen in patients with chronic hypertension. Though microatheroma that looks vulnerable to thrombosis [11] is occasionally encountered (Figure 2.5), we have not experienced a microatheroma responsible for recent occlusion.

Lipohyalinosis is a term introduced by Fisher [6] to describe a destructive vascular process with deposition of hyaline and fat-laden macrophages in the wall of the penetrating arteries. Fisher described lipohyalinosis as preferentially appearing in the regions that frequently show hypertensive hemorrhages and lacunar infarcts. Our own observations indicate that lipohyalinosis appears at the penetrating arteries in the basal ganglia and thalamus as well as the cerebral cortex close to the brain surface, in contrast to fibrinoid necrosis and hyalinosis situated deep in the brain. A lipohyalinotic artery wall may be admixed with fibrinoid and/or fibrosis (Figure 2.6). In the areas where lipohyalinosis is detected, we also find microatheroma. We regard lipohyalinosis as a pathologic feature combined with both hypertensive arteriolar and atherosclerotic arterial changes. We have not encountered a lipohyalinotic artery responsible for a recent occlusive event.

Atherosclerosis is occasionally observed in the leptomeningeal portion of the penetrating arteries at the base of the brain and in the distal convexity leptomeningeal arteries in cases with chronic hypertension. "Capsular infarct" associated with atherosclerosis was designated by Fisher [12] for infarcts larger than lacunes that mainly involve the internal capsule. The segment of a single lenticulostriate artery immediately distal to the orifice of the middle cerebral artery up to the middle of the basal ganglia is involved, and the vessels are 300–800 μm in diameter. The underlying arterial changes are composed of atheromatous plaques with severe stenosis, some of which are associated with superimposed thrombi. The arterial lesions within the brain parenchyma can be referred to as microatheroma. An intracerebral artery involved in Fisher's capsular infarct [12] was exceptionally occluded by a hemorrhagic lipohyalinotic lesion.

"Intracranial branch atheromatous disease" was designated by Caplan [13] for pontine infarcts caused by atherosclerotic occlusive lesions at the mouth of a single artery branching from the basilar artery [14]

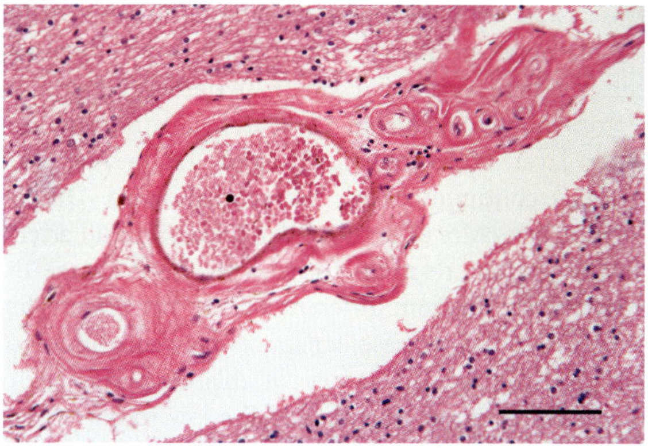

Figure 2.7 Vascular bundle formation in a dilated perivascular space in the parietal deep white matter in an 83-year-old man with nonamyloid subcortical vascular dementia. Hematoxylin and eosin (H&E). Bar = 100 μm.

and other infarcts associated with the same mechanism in the major cerebral arteries. This infarct characteristically abuts the basal surface, while lacunes are ordinarily caused by vascular lesions deep within the parenchyma [15]. Therefore, this type of infarct is not included among the SVD.

Segmental arterial disorganization is a nonspecific term introduced by Fisher [6, 16] to describe a variety of focal vascular changes, mostly old, that have the common feature of loss of arterial architecture that leads to stenosis or occlusion of the lumen. Connective tissue often entirely replaces the vessel eventually (Figure 2.4).

Microangioarchitectural changes of the cerebral arteries have been analyzed by using high resolution microradiography of brain specimens treated with intra-arterial injection of barium, scanning electron microscopy of corrosion casts of the arteries, and alkaline phosphatase-stained thick celloidin sections. Arteriolar tortuosity in the cortical branches, as well as in the medullary arteries of the white matter, is more common in the elderly [17, 18]. Paraffin sections occasionally show large periarterial spaces in the white matter containing tortuous or intertwining arteries in the elderly (Figure 2.7) [17]. These appear to be a contributing factor to impaired cerebral perfusion, especially in the white matter, but the relationship between the arterial changes and tissue damage is not clear [17, 18].

Arterial lesions related to lacunar infarcts were meticulously studied by Fisher [15]. Fisher defined lacunar infarcts as ischemic infarcts of restricted size, less than 15 mm at their greatest diameter, in the deeper parts of the brain. They are commonly observed in the chronic healing stage, forming irregular cavities principally in the basal ganglia, thalamus, and basis pontis. They predominantly occur in patients with hypertension and/or diabetes mellitus. Fisher [16] in 1969 investigated the arterial lesions causing lacunar infarcts from four patients with histories of hypertension and small strokes. In 45 of 50 consecutive lacunar infarcts, the artery supplying the territory of the infarct was occluded. Most of the vascular lesions showed segmental arterial disorganization occluding a single artery. Fisher [6] found two lacunar infarcts in the subcortical white matter due to thrombotic occlusion of the asymmetric fusiform miliary aneurysm of penetrating arteries running in the cerebral cortex, but he did not make a systematic study of lacunar infarcts in the subcortical white matter [15].

Challa et al. [19] in 1990 used the alkaline phosphatase technique of microvascular staining and high resolution microradiography to make three-dimensional observations in a study of 31 lacunar infarcts from 15 hypertensive subjects. Their study supported Fisher's conclusion that SVD was the cause of lacunar infarcts, but with one major difference. Variable narrowing due to intimal hyperplasia or atherosclerosis was demonstrated in the vast majority of the lacunar infarcts in the basal ganglia and thalamus. These lacunar infarcts were from patients who predominantly had well-controlled hypertension with current antihypertensive regimens that were not available before the 1960s, while 36 of the 50 lacunar infarcts studied by Fisher were from a single patient, who probably had more severe hypertensive SVD. Challa et al. [19] also observed a high incidence of lacunar infarcts in the deep white matter. The susceptibility of deep white matter to lacunar infarcts could derive from the characteristic angioarchitecture, including the long, penetrating medullary arteries, which show segmental or extensive narrowing of the lumen.

Cerebral medullary artery lesions in serial sections were investigated by Tanoi et al. [20] to identify arterial changes characteristic of Binswanger's encephalopathy (BE). They analyzed leptomeningeal and intracerebral arteries of BE autopsy specimens by reconstructing serial sections of individual arteries from the penetrating site at the cortical surface to the distal portion in the deep white matter. The results were compared with those from hypertensive

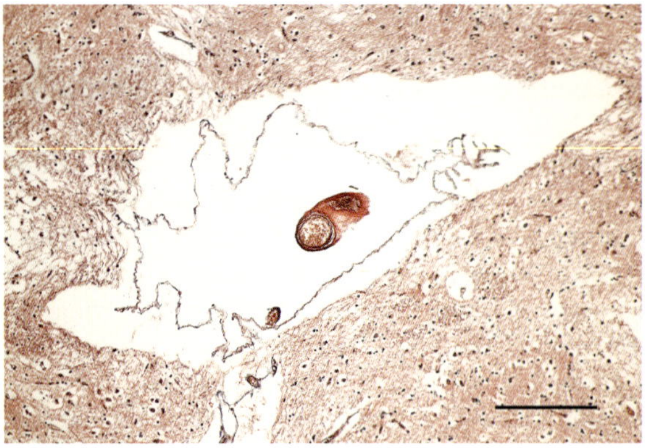

Figure 2.8 A dilated perivascular space in the basal ganglia. A membranous structure exists between the patent small artery and the brain parenchyma. No gliosis in the surrounding brain parenchyma. Watanabe's reticulum fiber silver stain. Bar = 200 μm.

intracerebral hemorrhage (HH) and normotensive (NT) specimens. There was nonspecific but significantly more widespread intimal fibrosis with or without atheroma, as well as segmental loss of the SMCs, which was sometimes associated with intimal plasma exudation or microaneurysm. Intimal fibrosis of the leptomeningeal arteries was significantly more widespread in BE than HH and NT. The media of the leptomeningeal and intracerebral arteries was significantly thicker in BE than in HH. In NT specimens the intracerebral arteries tended to be thinner in medial thickness than the leptomeningeal arteries. They regarded dysfunction of blood flow regulation, secondary to increased intimal fibrosis, and loss of medial SMCs to be the essential mechanism for diffuse myelin loss of the subcortical white matter in BE.

Dilatation of perivascular spaces, which commonly appear in the basal ganglia, are lined by a simple membranous structure but are not surrounded by gliosis (Figure 2.8), while cavities associated with lacunar infarcts are surrounded by gliosis [21]. Pollock et al. [21] analyzed the difference in structures of perivascular spaces in the basal ganglia and cerebral cortex. They found that those in the basal ganglia dilate to form dilated perivascular spaces and, rarely, accumulate Aβ in Alzheimer's disease (AD); however, in the cortex lacunar infarcts are rare but amyloid angiopathy is common. The arteries in the basal ganglia are surrounded by two distinct coats of leptomeninges separated by a perivascular space, which is continuous with the perivascular space around arteries in the subarachnoid space. The inner layer of leptomeninges closely invests the adventitia of the vessel wall, and the outer layer is continuous with the pia mater on the surface of brain. In the cerebral cortex, there is only a single periarterial layer of leptomeninges. Veins in the basal ganglia have no outer layer of leptomeninges and the perivascular space is continuous with the subpial space. Differences in structure of perivascular spaces around arteries may reflect relative efficacies in the drainage of interstitial fluid from different sites in the brain. The structure of the perivascular spaces may contribute to the relative high frequency of dilated perivascular spaces in the basal ganglia, and the low frequency of amyloid angiopathy at this site in AD. Regarding the pathogenesis of the dilatation of the perivascular spaces, Pollock et al. [21] suggested abnormality of the arterial permeability, allowing fluid to leak out and overload the perivascular space to form dilated perivascular spaces, and fibrosis and obstruction of perivascular spaces along the length of arteries increasing the impedance of fluid drainage pathways, among others.

Cerebral amyloid angiopathy (CAA)

CAA denotes progressive amyloid deposition in the vessels of the central nervous system (CNS). Sporadic CAA commonly seen in the elderly and AD patients shows Aβ peptide deposition within the intracortical and distal leptomeningeal blood vessel walls, and secondary vascular changes [22–25].

The incidence and severity of CAA increase with age and in association with AD pathology. CAA appears first in the intracortical and distal leptomeningeal vessels of the neocortex. The posterior portion of the cerebrum is involved more frequently and heavily than the anterior portion. The allocortex and cerebellum are involved next. The medial aspects of the temporal lobes, hippocampus, basal ganglia, and thalamus are rarely involved, and the brainstem is usually not involved. CAA is not associated with hypertension, arteriosclerosis, or amyloidosis of other organs [22–26].

Aβ accumulates in the wall of arterioles, small arteries, and medium-sized arteries, and rarely occurs in the veins and capillaries in the cerebral cortex and leptomeninges. CAA appears to be widespread, but in a patchy or segmental fashion. The large branches of the circle of Willis are not involved. In advanced CAA, staining with hematoxylin and eosin reveals acellular thickening in small artery walls. Under

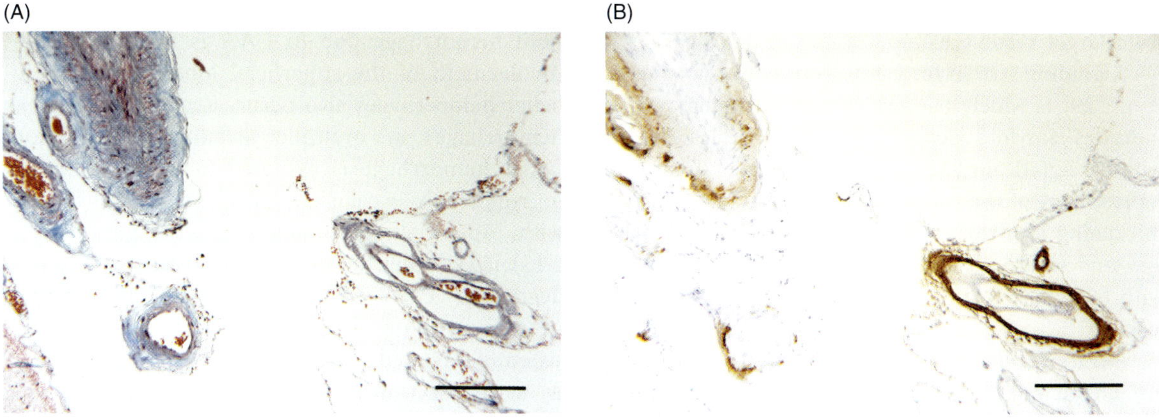

Figure 2.9 Leptomeningeal arteries of the parietal lobe show β-amyloid (Aβ) positions in the abluminal media and adventitia, and double-barrel formation. (A) Masson trichrome (MT); (B) immunostain. Bar = 200 μm. (A) is an adjacent section to (B) immunostained with an antibody against β/A4.

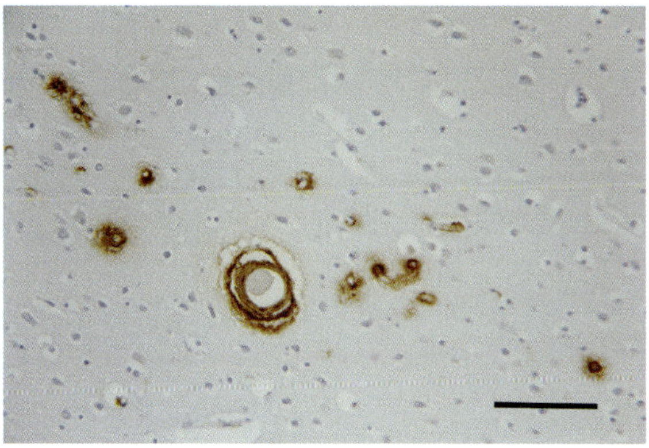

Figure 2.10 β-Amyloid depositions and dyshoric changes of capillaries and larger vessels in the parietal lobe. Immunostain. Bar = 100 μm.

polarized light, thin sections of vessels stained with Congo red show apple-green birefringence in the walls. Vessels affected by Aβ and senile plaques stain positive with anti-Aβ antibody. The deposition of Aβ begins from the abluminal side of the media as well as in the adventitia (Figure 2.9A,B). The medial smooth muscle layer is infiltrated and substituted with Aβ, which reaches to the intima. Vascular endothelial cells are preserved [22–25].

A hypothesis on the pathogenesis of CAA by Weller and his co-workers [27] has advocated that Aβ is deposited in periarterial interstitial fluid drainage pathways of the brain in AD and that this contributes significantly to CAA. Weller et al. [27] examined the evidence for this hypothesis. There is firm evidence in humans for drainage of interstitial fluid from the brain to cervical lymph nodes along periarterial spaces. Biochemical study of brains without AD revealed a pool of soluble Aβ in the cortex. Histology and immunocytochemistry of brains with AD showed that Aβ accumulates five times more frequently around arteries than around veins, with selective involvement of smaller arteries. Initial deposits of Aβ occur at the periphery of arteries. These observations support the hypothesis.

The vessels involved with Aβ show secondary changes, such as fibrinoid necrosis, loss of medial SMCs, microaneurysm, thrombus formation, fibrohyalinous wall thickening, luminal stenosis, amyloid depositions in the surrounding neuropil (referred to as dyshoric changes), inflammatory cell infiltration at the vessel wall and around the vessel, and perivascular blood pigment deposition. The vessels affected by CAA show thickening or thinning of the tunica media, and stenosis or dilation of the arterial lumen. Dissociation of vessel wall layers, particularly in the leptomeningeal small arteries, referred to as double barreling, could be produced as an artifact during tissue processing due to the different physical properties of tissue components (Figure 2.9A,B) [22–25].

The Aβ depositions lining capillary walls are referred to as capillary CAA (capCAA). The surrounding neuropil frequently shows Aβ depositions (Figure 2.10). Capillary CAA may show additional Aβ depositions in noncapillary blood vessels, whereas in large vessel CAA Aβ depositions are restricted to the cortical and leptomeningeal arteries, arterioles, and rarely veins, with the exception of capillaries [24]. Richard et al. [28] suggested that capCAA is pathologically and possibly pathogenetically distinct from larger vessel CAA.

A grading system for CAA proposed by Vonsattel et al. [29] is widely used in routine pathology. Mild indicates amyloid deposition in the tunica media without significant SMC disruption; moderate means replacement of the tunica media by amyloid causing thickening of media, with no evidence of blood leakage; and severe means extensive amyloid deposition with focal wall fragmentation and evidence of blood leakage.

Intracerebral hemorrhages associated with CAA are characterized by lobar hemorrhage. Incidence rises among the elderly, and intracerebral hemorrhages are not necessarily associated with hypertension. Therefore, a specific term, spontaneous intracerebral hemorrhage, is applied to this. Primary subarachnoid hemorrhage due to CAA is rare in spite of involvement of the superficial lobar vessels. Cerebellar hemorrhages also occur. Recurrence of lobar hemorrhages at multiple locations is common. Lobar hemorrhage is assumed to occur secondary to rupture of weakened blood vessel walls laden with Aβ or to microaneurysms (Figures 2.11–2.13) [22]. Vonsattel et al. [29] noted that a severe degree of CAA and the presence of fibrinoid necrosis, with or without microaneurysms, are consistently related to intracerebral hemorrhage. A serial section study by Wakai et al. [10] found ruptured microaneurysms associated with CAA. There is evidence that CAA is the risk factor for intracerebral hemorrhage associated

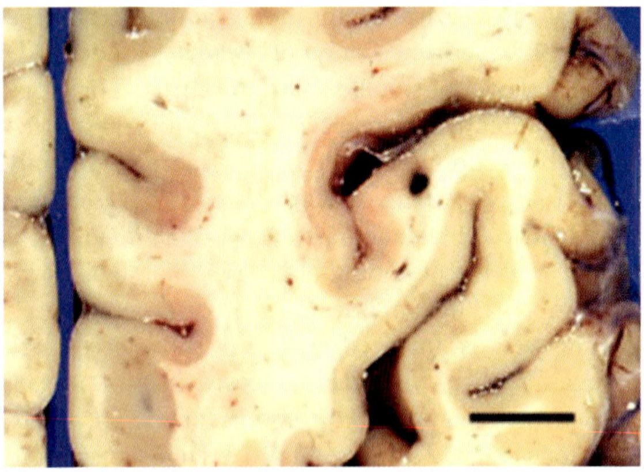

Figure 2.11 A horizontal section of the brain with a dark spot in the corticomedullary junction of the parietal lobe. This was a histologically aneurysmal enlargement of a β-amyloid laden artery occluded by a thrombus. Bar = 10 μm.

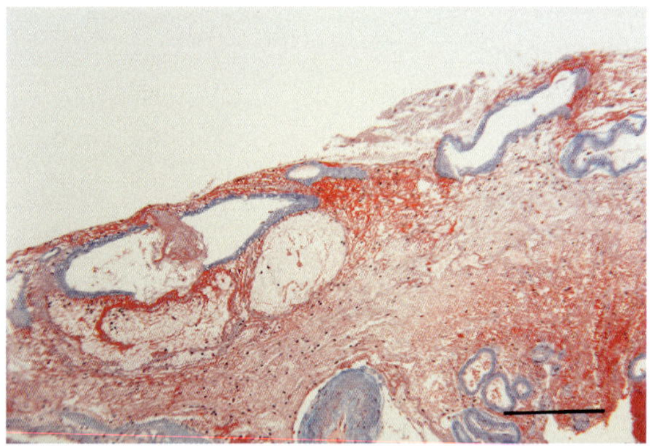

Figure 2.13 Small arteries in a surgically evacuated clot from a patient suffering from a parietal lobar hemorrhage. Arterial walls were heavily laden with β-amyloid in the immunostaining. Cracks in the arterial walls are seen. Masson trichrome (MT). Bar = 200 μm.

(A) (B)

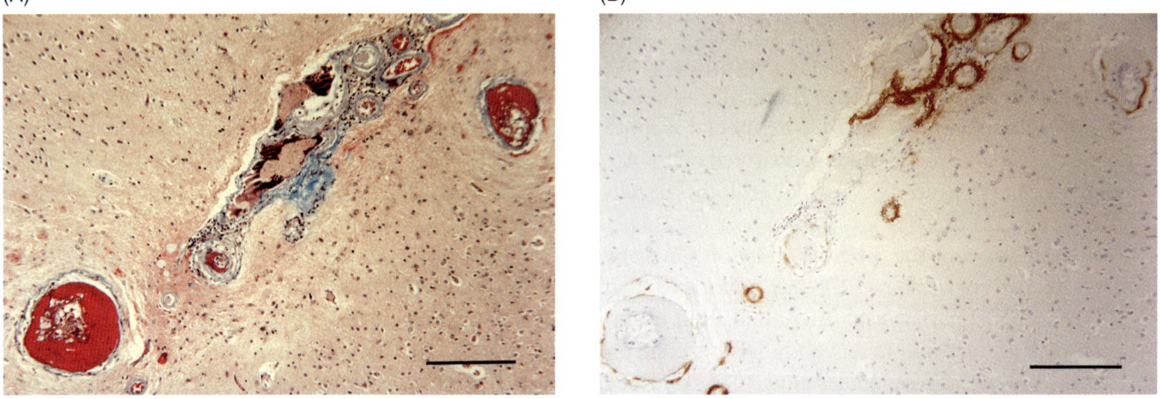

Figure 2.12 β-Amyloid depositions in intracortical and leptomeningeal vessels and microaneurysms in the parietal lobe. Microaneurysms are occluded with thrombi. (A) Masson trichrome (MT); (B) immunostain. Bar = 200 μm.

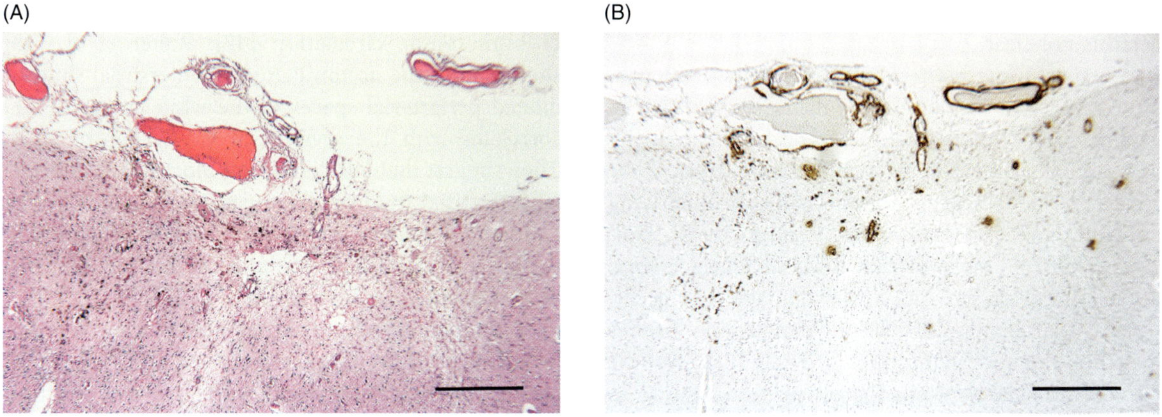

Figure 2.14 A microinfarct and hemosiderin-laden macrophages in the cortex and leptomeningeal space. β-Amyloid depositions in the vessels and double-barrel formation of the leptomeningeal vessels. (A) Hematoxylin and eosin (H&E); (B) immunostain. Bar = 0.5 mm.

with thrombolysis [30] and the use of warfarin [31] and antiplatelet agents [32].

Cerebral microbleeds (CMBs) are small areas of signal void on gradient echo T2*-weighted magnetic resonance images (MRIs). The punctuate signal voids have been observed in a number of diseases, the most common being hypertension and CAA. CMBs associated with hypertensive vasculopathy tend to be localized to the deep central gray matter, brainstem, and cerebellum, whereas those associated with CAA show lobar localization [33, 34]. Lobar CMBs have been proven to be a strong predictor of recurrent intracerebral hemorrhage in patients with CAA [35]. Meanwhile, a systematic review of studies on intracerebral hemorrhage among non-CAA antithrombotic drug users by Lovelock et al. [36] showed that the presence of CMBs is a potential risk factor for intracerebral hemorrhage and suggested that CMBs increase the risk of warfarin-associated intracerebral hemorrhage.

Fazekas et al. [37] performed MR imaging and correlative histologic examination in formalin-fixed brain slices to provide histologic support for the assumption that these represent remnants of previous microbleeds. Histopathologic examination showed focal accumulation of hemosiderin-laden macrophages in many areas of MR signal loss. All specimens from patients with hypertension had fibrohyalinosis, while CAA was present in some brains.

Schrag et al. [38] conducted a systemic correlation of high resolution, three-dimensional gradient echo T2*- and susceptibility-weighted imaging-identified hypodensities to tissue pathology in the slices of postmortem AD brains with varying degrees of CAA. The hypodensity spots were examined under a dissecting microscope before processing for serial sections. The common lesions were acute microhemorrhages, hemosiderin residua of old hemorrhages, small infarcts ringed by hemosiderin, and microaneurysms in the cerebral cortex, in areas just beneath the gray–white junction, deep white matter, and deep gray matter. Aβ was present in the lobar vessel wall.

Superficial hemosiderosis is hemosiderin deposition at the surface of the CNS. Feldman et al. [39] and Linn et al. [40] reported hemosiderin-laden macrophages in the subarachnoid space and superficial neocortex in AD patients with CAA. Gradient echo T2*-weighted MRIs showed a linear gyriform hypointense signal. There were lobar CMBs in close vicinity to the superficial siderosis. They suspected origin of the focal bleeding to be either spread from superficial neocortical hemorrhage or leak through leptomeningeal vessels into the subarachnoid space, or both. Vernooij et al. [41] supported the presumed link between superficial siderosis and CAA in elderly subjects without dementia in the Rotterdam Scan Study.

Microinfarcts are defined as regions of tissue necrosis not visible to the naked eye that are detectable on histologic sections (Figure 2.14A,B) [42, 43]. There are studies suggesting the location and number of microinfarcts contributes to the likelihood of dementia [43]. The microinfarcts are associated with advanced SVD including arteriosclerosis and CAA [43]. While occlusive vascular disease, embolism, hypoperfusion, blood–brain barrier impairment, and inflammation may be potential causes of microinfarcts, the pathogenesis of the development in detail is not clear.

Cerebral white matter damage appears to be promoted by CAA. Zhu et al. [44] demonstrated that in patients with CAA, white matter T2-hyperintensities preferentially appear in the occipital lobe, areas of the greatest CAA pathology. The mechanisms underlying the white matter damage are not entirely clear. Holland et al. [45] showed that lowered local cerebral perfusion can cause white matter damage. The occlusive vascular changes of the long penetrating arteries irrigating the underlying cerebral white matter at the intracortical and leptomeningeal portion appear to play a significant role [46]. The vessels involved with

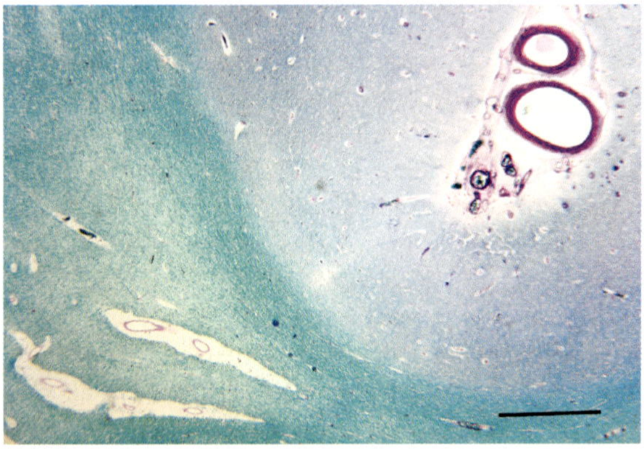

Figure 2.15 Dilatation of periarterial spaces in the occipital white matter. The leptomeningeal and cortical vessels were heavily deposited with β-amyloid, while the medullary arteries themselves were free from amyloid deposition. The white matter beneath the arcuate fiber zone shows myelin rarefaction. Luxol fast blue–periodic acid–Schiff (PAS). Bar = 1 mm.

Aβ deposition would also impair regulatory function of brain tissue circulation [47]. Roher et al. [48] showed that the accumulation of interstitial fluid in dilated periarterial spaces of the white mater in AD correlates with the severity of CAA (Figure 2.15). They suggest that Aβ deposition blocks the periarterial interstitial fluid drainage pathways at the cortical and leptomeningeal arteries, resulting in dilatation of the perivascular spaces in the white matter. This can be visualized on in vivo MRIs.

Inflammatory change of the vessels may be found in advanced CAA (Figure 2.16A,B) [22]. Eng et al. [49] reported inflammation with giant-cell reaction surrounding amyloid-laden vessels in cases showing subacute cognitive decline or seizure with radiographic white matter abnormalities. Some of the patients demonstrated clinical and radiographic improvement after immunosuppressive treatment. Eng et al. [49] suggest inflammation against Aβ, as a potential toxic response, can cause vascular dysfunction. Scolding et al. [50] made a clinicopathologic study of autopsy cases of Aβ-related angiitis and compared its features with those of primary angiitis of the CNS. Affected vessels revealed angiodestructive inflammation, often granulomatous, with meningeal lymphocytosis. Aβ was consistently present in abundance in affected vessels. They concluded that their findings help to dissect one separate clinicopathologic entity from the primary angiitis of the CNS, have important therapeutic implications for patients with amyloid-related vasculopathy, and may provide valuable insights into the development of amyloid-associated inflammation, related not only to

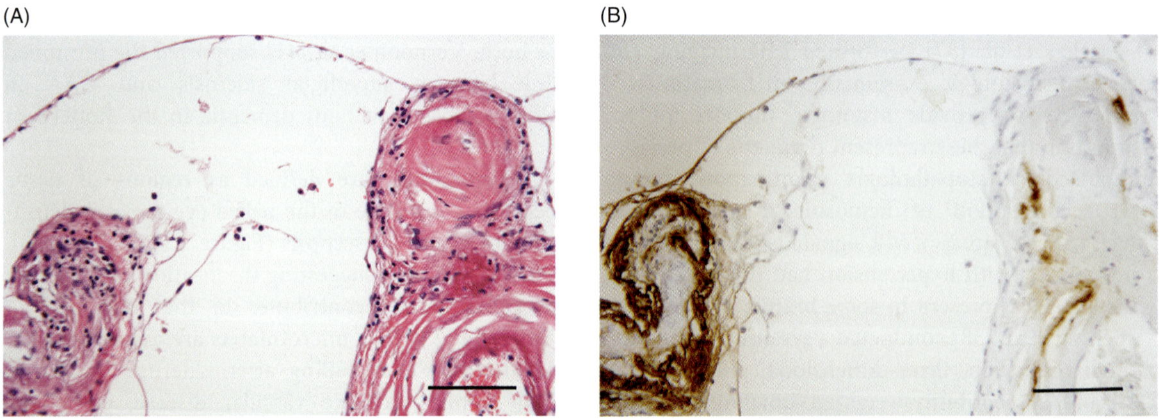

Figure 2.16 Intramural and perivascular cell infiltration of the leptomeningeal vessels in association with β-amyloid deposition in the occipital lobe of an 83-year-old patient with Alzheimer's disease. (A) Hematoxylin and eosin (H&E); (B) immunostain. Bar = 100 μm.

Table 2.1 Predominant pathologic findings of two major small vessel diseases: hypertensive vasculopathy and cerebral amyloid angiopathy

	Hypertensive vasculopathy	Cerebral amyloid angiopathy
Blood vessel pathology	Fibrinoid necrosis, arteriosclerosis, atherosclerosis	β-Amyloid deposition/associated vasculopathy in lobar cortical/leptomeningeal vessels
	Preference for basal ganglia, thalamus, pons, cerebellum	Preference for posterior lobe
Cerebral microbleeds	Basal ganglia, thalamus, pons, cerebellum, lobar	Lobar
Intracerebral gross hemorrhage	Basal ganglia, thalamus, pons, cerebellum, lobar	Lobar; coexistence of fresh/old lesions in multiple locations
Superficial siderosis	Rare	Subarachnoid/superficial cortical siderosis
Microinfarct	Basal ganglia, thalamus	Lobar
Subcortical white matter degeneration	Medullary vessel pathology	Cortical/leptomeningeal vessel pathology Dilated perivascular spaces
Lacunar infarct	Basal ganglia, thalamus, pons	None

Aβ-related angiitis but also Aβ-immunization-related meningoencephalitis and to AD.

Discussion

Table 2.1 compares the predominant pathologic findings of the two major SVDs, hypertensive vasculopathy and CAA. Hypertensive vasculopathy occurs in the basal central gray matter, pons, and cerebellum, whereas CAA and the associated vasculopathy appear in the lobar intracortical and leptomeningeal vessels. The development of the vascular changes is influenced by vascular risk factors and genetic predisposition, and they become manifest separately or in various combinations.

White matter degeneration in cases with hypertensive vasculopathy is associated with changes in the penetrating arteries within the cerebral white matter. In contrast, in cases with CAA, occlusive changes in the lobar vessels, periarterial space block-associated Aβ deposition to the lobar vessels, inflammation of the vessels, and toxic effects of amyloid may contribute to the development.

The importance of in vivo MRI examination of the CNS has been increasingly appreciated in determining the mechanisms of development of vascular and parenchymal lesions in SVD. The MR imaging studies on CMBs, enlarged perivascular spaces in the subcortical white matter, and superficial siderosis, among others, have led the advance in the understanding of SVD. MR imaging examination of postmortem brain slices before the neuropathologic analysis with microscopic tissue blocks of regular size has been performed to obtain the histologic counterpart of CMBs [37, 38]. This method appears very useful in analyzing histopathologic changes of the brain, including those of other etiologies.

Many points remain to be explained. Further studies are needed to elucidate the unsolved problems in longitudinal follow-up in a general population using neuroimaging techniques with postmortem brain examination.

Conclusion

Two major SVDs, hypertensive vasculopathy and CAA, are common and appear separately, or in combination. Recent developments in SVD research, especially those based on MR imaging, have permitted differentiation of the mechanisms involved in the development of these two different pathologies to a remarkable degree.

Acknowledgements

We express our particular appreciation to Ms. Y. Watanabe for her contribution in preparing the figures.

References

1. Ogata J, Yutani C, Otsubo R, et al. Heart and vessel pathology underlying brain infarction in 142 stroke patients. *Ann Neurol* 2008;63:770–781.
2. Ogata J, Yamanishi H, Ishibashi-Ueda H. Review: role of cerebral vessels in ischaemic injury of the brain. *Neuropathol Appl Neurobiol* 2011;37:40–55.
3. Ogata J, Fijishima M, Tamaki K, et al. Stroke-prone spontaneously hypertensive rats as an experimental model of malignant hypertension. I. A light- and electron-microscopic study of the brain. *Acta Neuropathol* 1980;51:179–184.
4. Amano S. Vascular changes in the brain of spontaneously hypertensive rats: hyaline and fibrinoid degeneration. *J Pathol* 1977;121:119–128.
5. Rosenblum WI. Fibrinoid necrosis of small brain arteries and arterioles and miliary aneurysms as causes of hypertensive hemorrhage: a critical reappraisal. *Acta Neuropathol* 2008;116:361–369.
6. Fisher CM. Cerebral miliary aneurysms in hypertension. *Am J Pathol* 1971;66:313–330.
7. Fisher CM. Pathological observations in hypertensive cerebral hemorrhage. *J Neuropathol Exper Neurol* 1971;30:536–550.
8. Takebayashi S, Kaneko M. Electron microscopic studies of ruptured arteries in hypertensive intracerebral hemorrhage. *Stroke* 1983;14:28–36.
9. Wakai S, Nagai M. Histological verification of microaneurysms as a cause of cerebral haemorrhage in surgical specimens. *J Neurol Neurosurg Psychiatry* 1989;52:595–599.
10. Wakai S, Kumakura N, Nagai M. Lobar intracerebral hemorrhage. A clinical, radiological, and pathological study of 29 consecutive operated cases with negative angiography. *J Neurosurg* 1992;76:231–238.
11. Naghavi M, Libby P, Falk E, et al. From vulnerable plaque to vulnerable patient. A call for new definitions and risk assessment strategies: part I. *Circulation* 2003;108:1664–1672.
12. Fisher CM. Capsular infarcts. The underlying vascular lesions. *Arch Neurol* 1979;36:65–73.
13. Caplan LR. Intracranial branch atheromatous disease: a neglected, understudied, and underused concept. *Neurology* 1989;39:1246–1250.
14. Fisher CM, Caplan LR. Basilar artery branch occlusion: a cause of pontine infarction. *Neurology* 1971;21:900–905.
15. Fisher CM. Lacunes: small, deep cerebral infarcts. *Neurology* 1964;15:774–784.
16. Fisher CM. The arterial lesions underlying lacunes. *Acta Neuropathol* 1969;12:1–15.
17. Akima M, Nonaka H, Kagesawa M, Tanaka K. A Study on the microvasculature of the cerebral cortex. Fundamental architecture and its senile change in the frontal cortex. *Lab Invest* 1986;55:482–489.
18. Thore CR, Anstrom JA, Moody DM, et al. Morphometric analysis of arteriolar tortuosity in human cerebral white matter of preterm, young, and aged subjects. *J Neuropathol Exper Neurol* 2007;66:337–345.
19. Challa VR, Bell MA, Moody DM. A combined hematoxylin–eosin, alkaline phosphatase and high-resolution microradiographic study of lacunes. *Clin Neuropathol* 1990;9:196–204.
20. Tanoi Y, Okeda R, Budka H. Binswanger's encephalopathy: serial sections and morphometry of the cerebral arteries. *Acta Neuropathol* 2000;100:347–355.
21. Pollock H, Hutchings M, Weller RO, Zhang E-T. Perivascular spaces in the basal ganglia of the human brain: their relation to lacunes. *J Anat* 1997;191:337–346.
22. Vinters HV. Cerebral amyloid angiopathy. A critical review. *Stroke* 1987;18:311–324.
23. Revesz T, Holton JL, Lashley T, et al. Genetics and molecular pathogenesis of sporadic and hereditary cerebral amyloid angiopathies. *Acta Neuropathol* 2009;118:115–30.
24. Attems J, Jellinger K, Thal DR, Van Nostrand W. Review: sporadic cerebral amyloid angiopathy. *Neuropathol Appl Neurobiol* 2011;37:75–93.
25. Biffi A, Greenberg SM. Cerebral amyloid angiopathy: a systematic review. *J Clin Neurol* 2011;7:1–9.
26. Vinters HV, Gilbert JJ. Cerebral amyloid angiopathy: incidence and complications in the aging brain. II. The distribution of amyloid vascular changes. *Stroke* 1983;14:924–928.
27. Weller RO, Massey A, Tracey A, et al. Cerebral amyloid angiopathy. Amyloid β accumulates in putative interstitial fluid drainage pathways in Alzheimer's disease. *Am J Pathol* 1998;153:725–733.
28. Richard E, Carrano A, Hoozemans JJ, et al. Characteristics of dyshoric capillary cerebral amyloid angiopathy. *J Neuropathol Exp Neurol* 2010;69:1158–1167.
29. Vonsattel JPG, Myers RH, Hedley-Whyte ET, et al. Cerebral amyloid angiopathy without and with cerebral hemorrhages: a comparative histological study. *Ann Neurol* 1991;30:637–649.
30. Ly JV, Rowe CC, Villemagne VL, et al. Cerebral β-amyloid detected by Pittsburgh compound B positron emission topography predisposes to recombinant tissue plasminogen activator-related

hemorrhage. *Ann Neurol* 2010;68:959–962.

31. Rosand J, Hylek EM, O'Donnell HC, Greenberg SM. Warfarin-associated hemorrhage and cerebral amyloid angiopathy: a genetic and pathologic study. *Neurology* 2000;55:947–951.
32. Biffi A, Halpin A, Towfighi A, et al. Aspirin and recurrent intracerebral hemorrhage in cerebral amyloid angiopathy. *Neurology* 2010;75:693–698.
33. Vernooij MW, van der Lugt A, Ikram MA, et al. Prevalence and risk factors of cerebral microbleeds. The Rotterdam Scan Study. *Neurology* 2008;70:1208–1214.
34. Greenberg SM, Vernooij MW, Cordonnier C, et al. Cerebral microbleeds: a field guide to their detection and interpretation. *Lancet Neurol* 2009;8:165–174.
35. Greenberg SM, Eng JA, Ning M, Smith EE, Rosand J. Hemorrhage burden predicts recurrent intracerebral hemorrhage after lobar hemorrhage. *Stroke* 2004;35:1415–1420.
36. Lovelock CE, Cordonnier C, Naka H, et al. Antithrombotic drug use, cerebral microbleeds, and intracerebral hemorrhage: a systematic review of published and unpublished studies. *Stroke* 2010;41:1222–1228.
37. Fazekas F, Kleinert R, Roob G, et al. Histopathologic analysis of foci of signal loss on gradient-echo T2*-weighted MR images in patients with spontaneous intracerebral hemorrhage: evidence of microangiopathy-related microbleeds. *AJNR Am J Neuroradiol* 1999;20;637–642.
38. Schrag M, McAuley G, Pomakian J, et al. Correlation of hypointensities in susceptibility-weighted images to tissue histology in dementia patients with cerebral amyloid angiopathy: a postmortem MRI study. *Acta Neuropathol* 2010;119:291–302.
39. Feldman HH, Maia LF, Mackenzie IRA, et al. Superficial siderosis. A potential diagnostic marker of cerebral amyloid angiopathy in Alzheimer disease. *Stroke* 2008;39:2894–2897.
40. Linn J, Herms J, Dichgans M, et al. Subarachnoid hemosiderosis and superficial cortical hemosiderosis in cerebral amyloid angiopathy. *AJNR Am J Neuroradiol* 2008;29:184–186.
41. Vernooij MW, Ikram MA, Hofman A, Krestin GP, Breteler MMB. Superficial siderosis in the general population. *Neurology* 2009;73:202–205.
42. Hachinski V, Iadecola C, Petersen RC, et al. National Institute of Neurological Disorders and Stroke–Canadian Stroke Network vascular cognitive impairment harmonization standards. *Stroke* 2006;37:2220–2241.
43. Smith EE, Schneider JA, Wardlaw JM, Greenberg SM. Cerebral microinfarcts: the invisible lesions. *Lancet Neurol* 2012;11:272–282.
44. Zhu YC, Chabriat H, Godin O, et al. Distribution of white matter hyperintensity in cerebral hemorrhage and healthy aging. *J Neurol* 2012;259: 530–536.
45. Holland CM, Smith EE, Csapo I, et al. Spatial distribution of white-matter hyperintensities in Alzheimer disease, cerebral amyloid angiopathy, and healthy aging. *Stroke* 2008;39:1127–1133.
46. Thal DR, Ghebremedhin E, Orantes M, Wiestler OD. Vascular pathology in Alzheimer disease: correlation of cerebral amyloid angiopathy and arteriosclerosis/lipohyalinosis with cognitive decline. *J Neuropathol Exp Neurol* 2003;62:1287–1301.
47. Dumas A, Dierksen GA, Gurol ME, et al. Functional magnetic resonance imaging detection of vascular reactivity in cerebral amyloid angiopathy. *Ann Neurol* 2012;72:76–81.
48. Roher AE, Kuo YM, Esh C, et al. Cortical and leptomeningeal cerebrovascular amyloid and white matter pathology in Alzheimer's disease. *Mol Med* 2003;9:112–122.
49. Eng JA, Frosch MP, Choi K, Rebeck GW, Greenberg SM. Clinical manifestations of cerebral amyloid angiopathy-related inflammation. *Ann Neurol* 2004;55:250–256.
50. Scolding NJ, Joseph F, Kirby PA, et al. Aβ-related angiitis: primary angiitis of the central nervous system associated with cerebral amyloid angiopathy. *Brain* 2005;128:500–515.

Chapter 3

Pathologic aspects of the ischemic consequences of small vessel disease on brain parenchyma

Margaret Esiri and Elisabet Englund

Introduction

Cerebrovascular disease has long been recognized as a contributor to dementia. but the manner in which it makes its contribution is still not fully understood. More than 100 years ago, Alzheimer and Binswanger described subcortical vascular pathology of demented individuals who had what they termed "arteriosclerotic dementia" or "arteriosclerosis senilis" [1]. In today's terminology these cases would fall into the category of small vessel disease (SVD). The later work of Tomlinson and colleagues in 1970 [2] attributed vascular dementia (VaD) to macroscopic infarction with a volume greater than 50–100 ml. Attempts to cover the entire spectrum of vascular ischemic brain changes pertinent to cognitive decline and dementia have been made many times. During some periods these attempts have been somewhat hampered by a reduced interest in the vascular ischemic field among researchers, such as the "Alzheimer-dominated" period of the 1980s. The successfully introduced concept of multi-infarct dementia (MID) [3] was brought into wide use in clinics as well as research, and increased awareness of VaD as a whole. In the light of MID conditions corresponding to earlier descriptions of arteriosclerotic dementia, and to the later-named SVD, MID was not prominent in the spectrum of disorders linked to cognitive impairment. However, from the 1990s onwards, we moved closer to a terminology that is inclined towards pathophysiology rather than eponyms, and hence attempts to link morphologic descriptions with clinical symptoms. In this way, vascular cognitive impairment, or VaD, appeared in conjunction with SVD. The work of Tatemichi [4], Brun [5], and Knopman et al. [6] further clarified some of the clinicopathologic correlations.

However, not only does nosology change over time, but to some extent so does the real disease spectrum. For instance, it appears that brain infarct volume greater than 50 ml is not commonly encountered nowadays in people thought clinically to be suffering from vascular cognitive impairment (VCI). Hence, new consensus criteria for attributing cognitive impairment to cerebrovascular disease are required.

Our understanding of the important contributors to VCI is unfortunately limited, a situation that needs to be addressed if we are to be able to intervene effectively to prevent or treat it. There are a number of factors responsible for this state of affairs, which have been frequently reviewed [7–9]. Briefly, heterogeneous forms of vascular disease occur at widely differing regions of the brain; often more than one form occurs together with another and it can be difficult to assign loss of function to one of these in any individual case. Furthermore, vascular disease often occurs with Alzheimer's disease (AD) of varying degrees of severity, and in this situation the vascular contribution can be difficult to evaluate. Also, until recently, cognitive assessment protocols relied heavily on testing functions that are impaired in AD but have less sensitivity to functional impairments that are characteristic of VCI. Finally, cerebrovascular disease, particularly SVD, is very common in elderly subjects with seemingly well-preserved cognition, casting doubt on its significance [10].

To combat these pitfalls requires careful neuropathologic analysis of large numbers of cases of elderly subjects with and without cognitive impairment. Different research centers need to employ common methods of assessment, both of cognition and pathology, if progress is to be made. In this chapter we describe the nature of the damage inflicted on the brain by SVD, which is thought likely to play an

Cerebral Small Vessel Disease, ed. Leonardo Pantoni and Philip B. Gorelick. Published by Cambridge University Press.

important part in VCI. At some sites the result is microinfarcts, which are found in the cerebral cortex, white matter, and deep gray matter of the basal ganglia, in the thalamus and pons, or lacunes, found in subcortical sites. However, some significant damage falls short of complete infarction and results in more diffuse damage, particularly in cerebral white matter.

For a comprehensive investigation of the vascular–ischemic burden of pathology in a brain, some form of whole brain examination is required. For certain purposes, a set of small sections from multiple locations may be sufficient – it allows for an easily correlated immunohistochemical antibody stain assessment in regions that are identical with the basal morphology staining hematoxylin and eosin. In certain situations, such as when neuropathologic correlations with imaging investigations prior to death are required, there may be an advantage to map the changes in large hemispheric or whole brain coronal sections, where all types of pathology may be identified and in detail related to specific cortical and lobar regions.

Such sections are generally also a prerequisite for the assessment of white matter pathology – due to the risk of deformation of small, cut-out, white matter samples and the irregular loosening of the fiber density around the edges of each sample. This is an effect of the histotechnical process, resulting in the shape of the cut white matter sample being much less well preserved than any gray matter sample. Consequently, any evaluation of white matter disease (WMD) on small samples must be done with great caution, with the experience of false positive pathology in mind.

Furthermore, if white matter samples are taken from one, or at most a limited number of locations, this will preclude the evaluation of most white matter pathology provided from large sections, hence preventing the assessment of subventricular, subcortical, and central white matter together.

Pathology

Focal lesions: subcortical lacunes

Cerebral lacunes are foci of ischemic necrosis visible to the naked eye in brain slices and in magnetic resonance images (MRIs), usually measuring less than 1.5 cm in diameter [1] (Figure 3.1). They can occur in the basal ganglia, thalamus, or white matter (Figure 3.2) and are

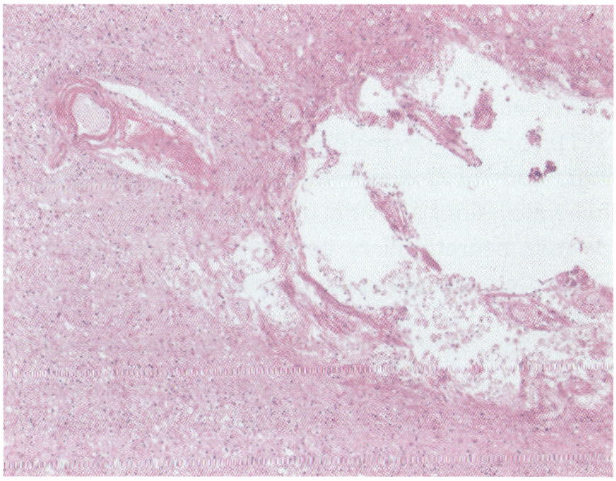

Figure 3.1 A cerebral white matter lacune, 2 × 3 mm. Hematoxylin and eosin (H&E) staining.

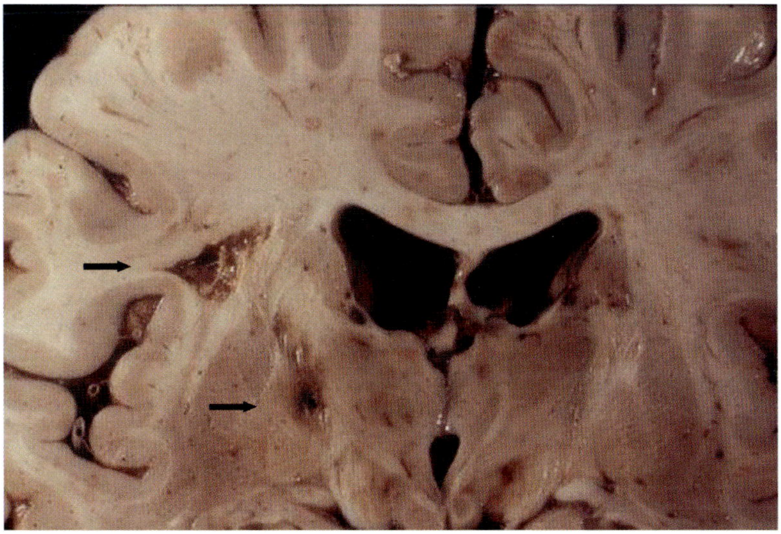

Figure 3.2 Fixed brain slice from an elderly subject showing a white matter lacune in left frontal lobe (top arrow) and a smaller lacune in the left globus pallidus, abutting on the left internal capsule (bottom arrow).

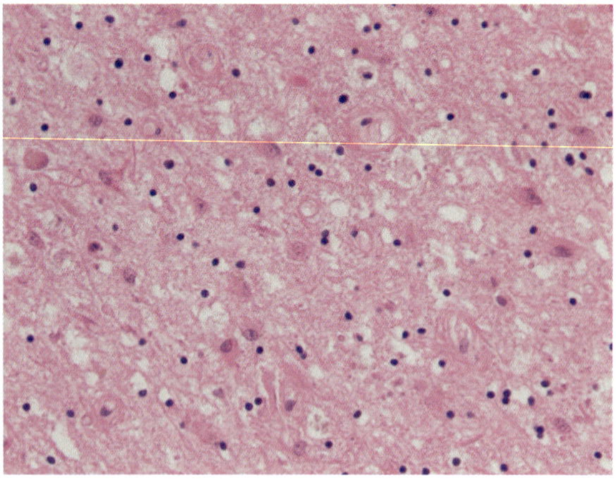

Figure 3.3 Reactive astrocytes and edema in the vicinity of a fresh white matter infarct.

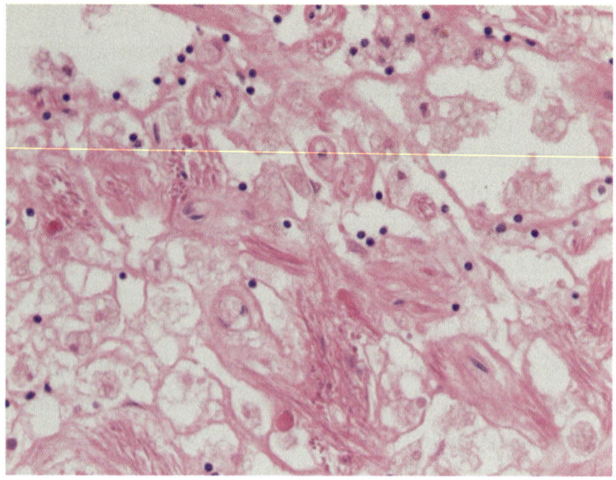

Figure 3.4 Macrophages within a lacunar infarct still undergoing cavity formation (part of the lacune in Figure 3.1).

generally the result of vascular occlusion (small vessel occlusion within the brain). They are strongly associated with the existence of other manifestations of SVD. They may be single or multiple. In a clinicopathologic study of 72 elderly subjects with no macroscopic ischemic lesions and only insignificant Alzheimer tau-positive neurofibrillary pathology of Braak grade II [11] or less, lacunes in the thalamus and basal ganglia, but not deep white matter, were associated with cognitive impairment [12]. In the community-based study by Strozyk et al. [13], lacunes were not associated with dementia, in contrast to diffuse white matter manifestations of SVD. However, lacunes were an element contributing to an overall vascular lesion score, which was related to risk of dementia.

The morphology of lacunes is determined by a number of factors, namely type of pathogenesis, age of the lesion, duration of ischemic event, and specific localization within the brain.

Lacunes, by definition, represent the pathology of a previous ischemic incident, having occurred weeks prior to their appearance. In the situation of an embolic vessel occlusion, there is generally a hemorrhagic component, which may range from a macroscopically visible perivascular bleed to minimal extravasation of erythrocytes. A "pale" lesion void of bleeding is typical of a thrombotic occlusion, but also appears in the nonocclusive stroke, i.e., the stroke emanating from hypoperfusion. Acute systemic hypotension, judged to have caused manifest stroke in a considerable proportion of fatal strokes in the elderly [14], is recognized as deserving more attention for its pathogenic importance in cerebrovascular disease and for cognitive impairment [15]. However, the hypotensive stroke may be difficult to discern among other plausible forms and has mostly been demonstrated in reports on cases with assumed etiology [16] or in single case reports [17, 18]. Acute or subacute lesions of a similar nature are within the first few days not yet lacunar and are hence less readily seen with brain imaging. These lesions comprise devitalized neuroglial tissue with pale and blurry cell contours and a variable edema that spreads diffusely and yet also forms a peripheral border of microvacuoles around the necrotic center. The appearance of such lesions depends on their localization in the white matter or in subcortical nuclei; lesions in the latter exhibiting more clearly delineated borders, due to relatively higher vascular density of the gray matter.

Lacunes are frequently accompanied by macrophages, reactive microglia, and astrocytes, and by coarse, angular astrocytic processes around their margins (Figure 3.3). Within the first few days, a variable amount of reactive blood cells and glia assembles, and macrophage activation occurs in a fashion seemingly proportional to the degree of regional reperfusion (Figure 3.4). During the post-ischemic period, the macrophage reaction gradually fades and leaves the empty lacune.

The type of SVD defines, to some extent, the type of tissue pathology occurring subsequent to the ischemic event. The most typical lacunar infarct seen in the situation of hypertensive angiopathy is accompanied by the remains of blood–brain barrier leakage, hence displaying hemosiderin-laden macrophages within the lacunar cavity and in the adventitial fibrosis of

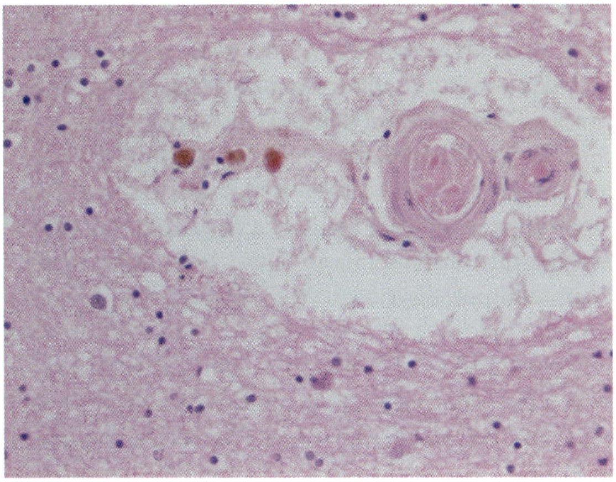

Figure 3.5 A widened perivascular space around a hypertension-degenerated and sclerotic arteriole, with adventitial fibrosis and hemosiderin-laden macrophages as signs of blood–brain barrier leakage.

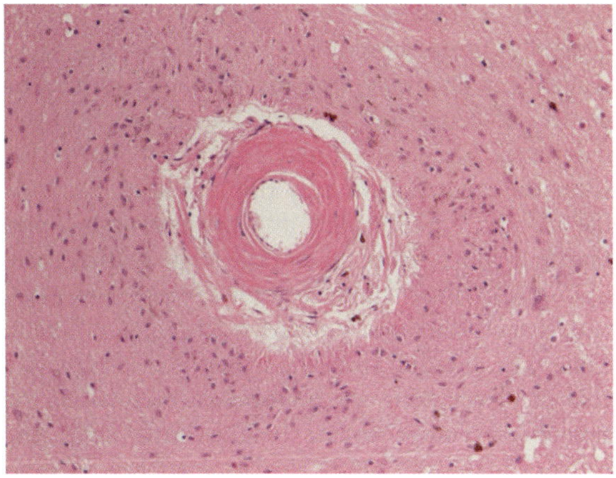

Figure 3.6 A vessel typical of hypertensive angiopathy in small vessel disease, exhibiting vessel wall degeneration, palissading glial cells, and hemosiderin deposits.

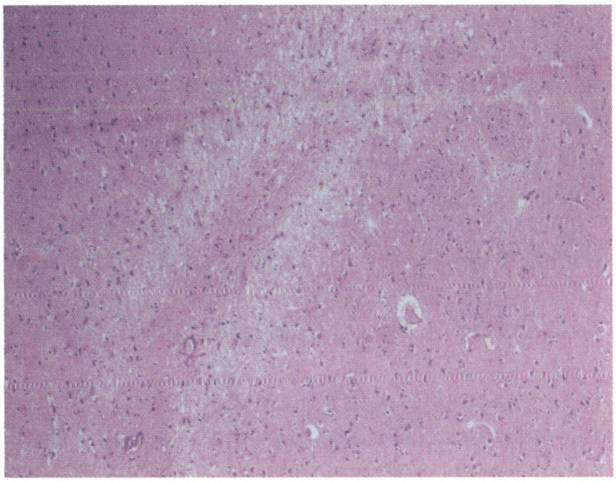

Figure 3.7 A cortical microinfarct forming a scar of 1.0 × 0.3 mm.

an adjacent arteriole (Figure 3.5). At some point, a glial cell reaction with formation of a cell palisade may also be seen, illustrating the brain's reaction to a recurrently opened blood–brain barrier (Figure 3.6). The leaking of plasma proteins through a degenerated vessel wall may be visualized, for example, by immunostaining with an antialbumin or antifibrinogen antibody, but in general this does not need to be demonstrated other than for evaluation in comparison with MR imaging (MRI)/diffusion tensor imaging (DTI) changes. A hemorrhagic component in the tissue is more prominent if there was previous rupture of a vascular microaneurysm or in the (non-hypertensive) situation of an embolic arteriolar occlusion. Another cause for small hemorrhages is the rarer situation of a vasculitis. This typically causes microscopic bleeding around vessels, the accumulation of leukocytes within and around the arteriolar walls, and sometimes fibrinoid necrosis in the vessel wall. Characteristic, and different from the hypertensive and/or embolic situation, is that the parenchymal changes with vasculitis are much more widespread and not unifocal.

Cognitive impairment attributable to lacunes is likely due to ischemic damage to neurons, myelin, and axons. It is possible that residual function relates to the volume of surviving tissue subserving the same function as the elements that have been destroyed, rather as in "cerebral reserve," a concept that is invoked when attempting to account for cases with neurodegenerative pathology but preserved cognition in some elderly subjects [19]. However, this aspect of the elderly brain, as applied to vascular disease, has not as yet been systematically studied.

Focal lesions: cortical microinfarcts

The cerebral cortex does not exhibit lacunes, but rather scarring with slightly elongated streaks of tissue condensation accompanied by reactive astrocytes and microglia. The cortical microinfarct (Figure 3.7) is often the result of a small vessel occlusion, although in a smaller arteriole than that in the embolic type of damage causing lacunes. It is seen both with hypertensive vascular pathology and with amyloid angiopathy [20–23], hence illustrating a more progressive decrement of vascular service over time. These lesions may be numerous and can be found in many hundreds within one whole coronal section. They are generally considerably smaller than the average lacunar infarct and may measure 1.0 × 0.3 mm. The density of vessels in the cortex, being much higher than in the white matter, may provide conditions that allow the formation of only tiny damaged areas. As the relative proportion of oligodendrocytes and myelin is much lower than in the white matter, there is much less tissue volume (on a microlevel) to be lost, and, hence, the macrophage reaction is different. Time (i.e., duration from the ischemic insult) plays a role in determining the appearance here, as in the subcortical compartment. In the acute state, the neurons may swell before shrinking as they undergo cell death, the type of which probably depends on the character, hence speed, of ischemic insult. A composite photograph (Figure 3.8) illustrates several aspects of micromorphology of SVD.

Nonfocal lesions

Nonfocal pathology of the vascular–ischemic type is typically seen in the white matter, and here it may be the predominating pathology, occurring in association with, as well as without, nearby lacunar infarcts. If a lacune is present, the diffuse white matter pathology, or incomplete infarction, generally represents a vast gradient area around a central clear-cut infarct (Figure 3.9), a perifocal lesion that may comprise well over 200 times the volume of the central lacune [24]. In the absence of lacunes, the diffuse white matter pathology may be the sole morphological alteration in a large region or even in the entire white matter compartment. There is a subtotal loss of axons, myelin, and oligodendroglia, and the presence of a moderate increase of reactive astrocytes (Figure 3.10), in some areas approaching the number of oligodendroglial cells, but not being nearly as predominant as the astrocyte reaction in an early phase of a lacunar infarct. The mild associated macrophage reaction marks the slow regressive tissue process. Nonfocal white matter pathology is accompanied by a stenosing arteriolosclerosis (Figure 3.11), exhibiting concentric hyaline fibrosis with collagen deposition, which replaces the degenerated smooth muscle layer of the vessel [25]. Even if the underlying cause for this type of lesion is ischemia per se, the particular pathogenesis may involve small vessel pathology and recurrent hypoperfusion, leading to recurrent subtotal oxygenation of the tissue, though not complete ischemia. Macroscopically, ischemic white matter pathology may go undetected, or in advanced cases exhibit a gray discoloration and a rough, pitted surface on cut brain slices. Microscopically, the myelin and the number of oligodendrocytes are reduced. The axons are similarly fewer and those that are left show, e.g., when silver stains are applied, a fiber thinning as well as fragmentation along with seemingly spared, normal-appearing fibers. Macrophages are generally present but to a limited extent, indicating a mild regressive process dissimilar to that of a frank infarct. When the nonfocal white matter lesions are mild, they may be too subtle for conventional microscopical grading of severity. In this situation, the counting of oligodendrocytes and astrocytes expressed as oligo/astro-cell ratios [26], or measuring myelin loss as change in optical density and level of degraded myelin basic protein [27], may help to delineate the damaged areas.

In the context of a marked vascular–ischemic brain disease, the nonfocal lesions are prominent and frequent components of the brain pathology, and they may be anticipated on the basis of clinical history, clinical symptoms, and imaging signs. Also, in primary neurodegenerative disease, vascular pathology appears and may pave the way for a secondary vascular–ischemic pathology. Such is the scenario in AD, in which nonfocal WMD of this type is found in a considerable proportion of cases [28]. The WMD occurs in addition to other region-specific white matter alterations, relating to neuronal–axonal degeneration in the adjacent cortex, which is particularly evident in the basal temporal lobes. Cerebral vascular amyloid, not generally appearing in the white matter, nevertheless seems to play a detrimental role for perfusion in the deep brain regions – as indicated from quantitation of leptomeningeal amyloid angiopathy correlating with degree of WMD in AD [21, 29].

A dilatation of perivascular spaces may be seen in many brains of mentally well-preserved elderly individuals; this may be perceived also with neuroradiology, especially as MRI findings [30]. The term cribriform state, or *état criblé* [1] (Figure 3.12), describes numerous widened perivascular spaces around more or less sclerotic arterioles (Figures 3.5 and 3.8). While this picture is not a pathologic condition that corresponds to defined clinical symptoms of cognitive decline, it is particularly prominent along with other manifestations of vascular disease in individuals with documented VCI.

(A)

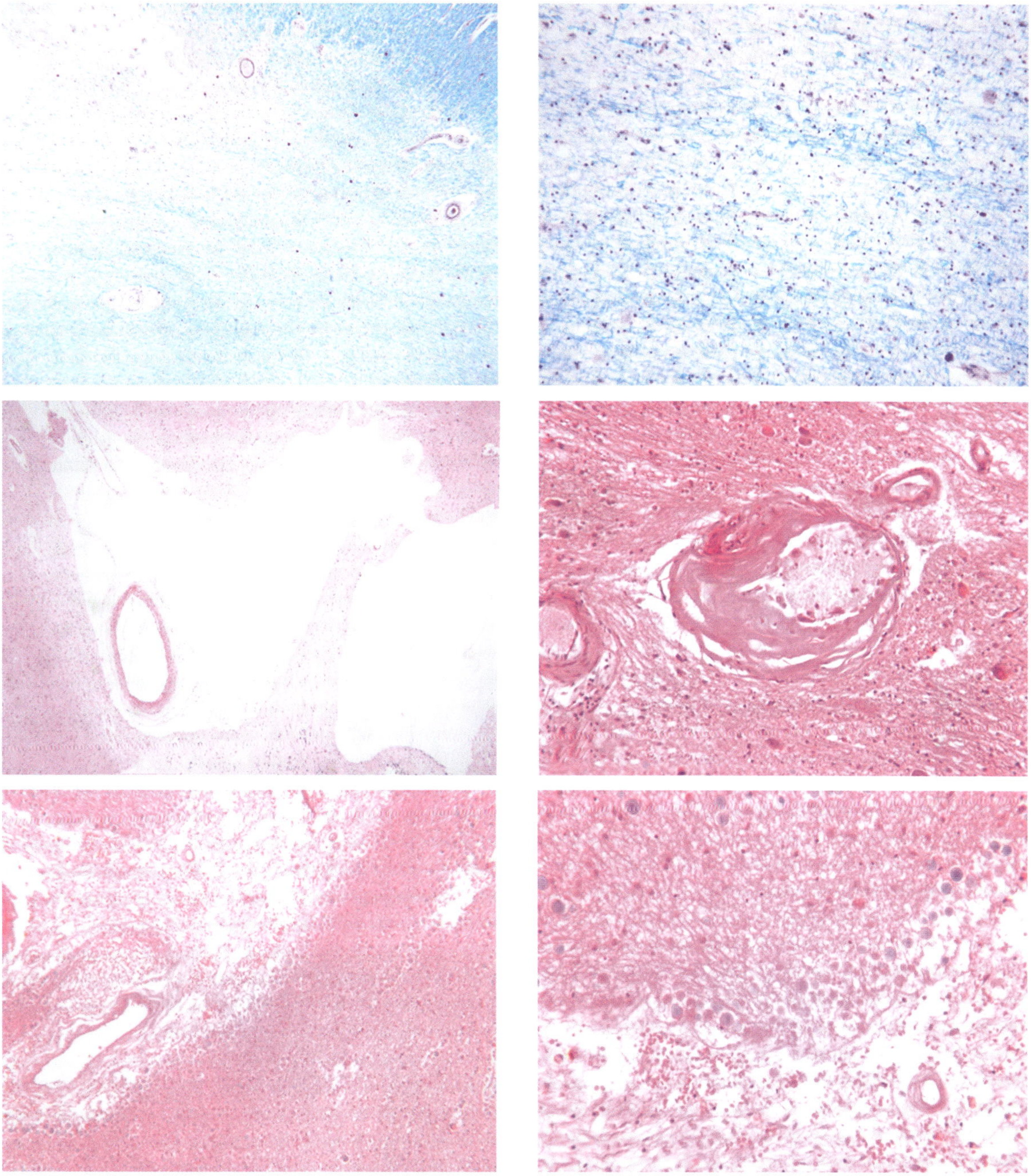

Figure 3.8 Examples of severe pathological features in small vessel disease. (A, top) Luxol fast blue-stained sections of white matter showing a region of severe white matter attenuation adjacent to a small lacune, visible in the left-hand panel with extensive macrophage infiltration evident in right-hand panel. (A, middle) Below this are hematoxylin and eosin (H&E)-stained sections showing widened perivascular spaces in the left-hand panel and a severely fibrotic small arterial wall in the right-hand panel. (A bottom) The panels below these show severe ischemic damage to deep gray matter at low power (left panel) and medium power (right panel). (B) (overleaf) These bottom two panels show examples of severely fibrotic and narrowed arterioles.

(B)

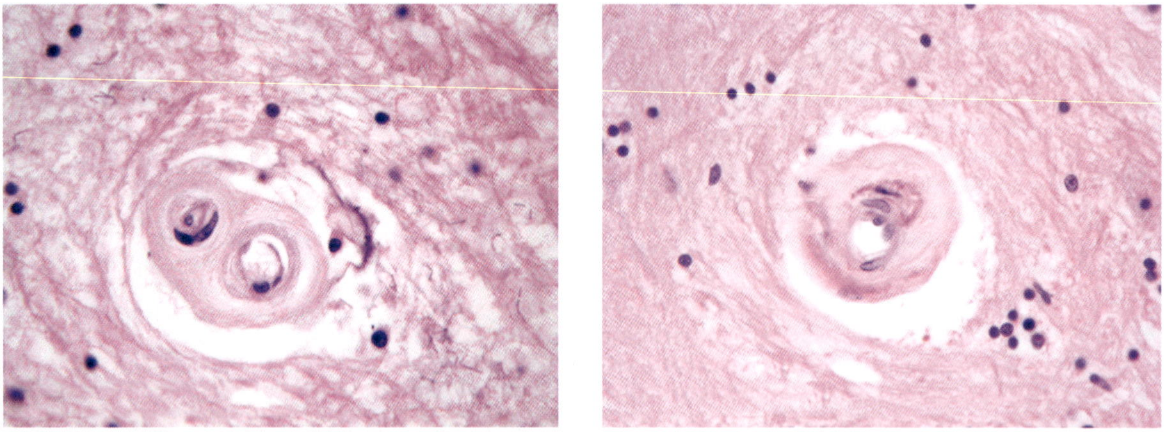

Figure 3.8 *(cont.)*

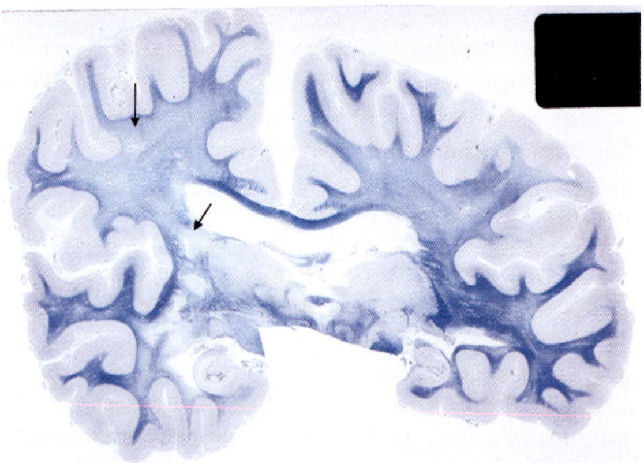

Figure 3.9 Coronal whole brain section of a hypoperfusive stroke, with multiple small foci of complete white matter infarct (circumscribed pale foci in the blue-colored white matter), surrounded by vast areas of diffuse, incomplete ischemic damage. Luxol fast blue myelin staining.

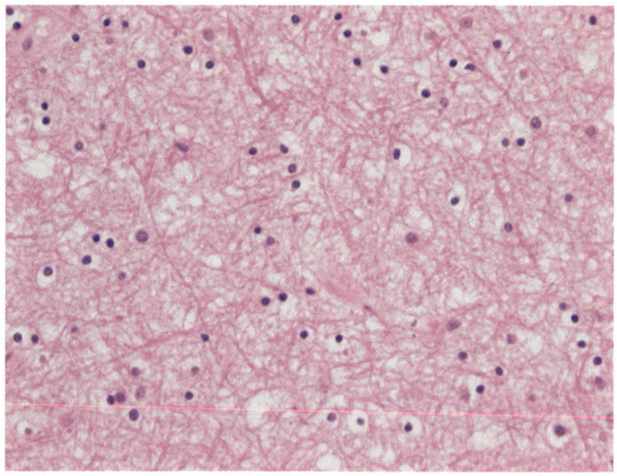

Figure 3.10 Nonfocal white matter lesion with subtotal loss of axons, myelin, and oligodendroglia as well as presence of enlarged reactive astrocytes.

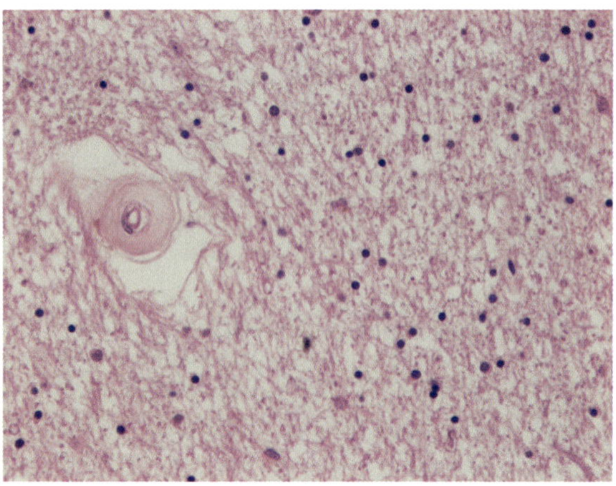

Figure 3.11 Nonfocal white matter pathology in small vessel disease exhibiting tissue attenuation and a fibrohyaline arteriolosclerosis.

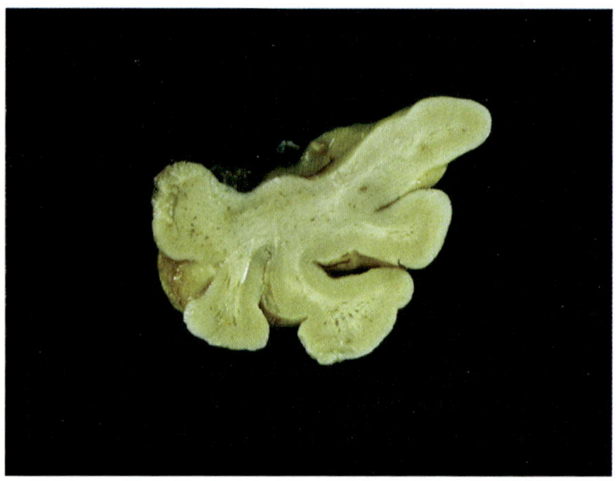

Figure 3.12 Macro-photograph of the temporal pole in an elderly individual with prominent cribriform state (*état criblé*) due to numerous widened perivascular spaces around sclerotic arterioles.

Focal lesions caused by global brain ischemia

When temporary global brain ischemia occurs, several forms of focal brain damage may appear. In contrast to occlusive vascular disease and repeated strokes, cerebral hypoperfusion is often the result of circulatory failure, which in turn may be caused by congestive heart failure, orthostatic hypotension, bradyarrhythmia, or from hypotension induced during cardiac surgery; for example, bypass grafting [31]. In these circumstances, the organization of the vascular tree, supplying both separate and shared regions, is the prerequisite for focal damage resulting from global perfusion impairment. Hence, in the situation of cardiac arrest or other severe cause of hypoperfusion, border-zone infarcts may be seen in the fronto-parietal territories supplied by both the anterior and middle cerebral arteries and in the arterial "triple boundary zone" of the posterior parieto-occipital lobes. Another major cause for focal damage stems from selective vulnerability in certain regions and neuronal populations [32]. The hippocampus is particularly prone to developing damage during cardiac arrest, and the hippocampal pathology may often be sharply delineated, seen as marked macroscopic, often bilateral atrophy, due to pyramidal neuronal loss in the cornu ammonis accompanied by focal gliosis and subsequent axonal degeneration with demyelination in the most proximal regions. Cardiac arrest may also result in selective neuronal death in specific regions, the extent of which depends on, e.g., the time of the arrest situation, hyperglycemia, and the level of regional pH [33, 32]. Areas particularly vulnerable to such lesions that target neurons only include the hippocampus, the cerebellar cortex, and the thalamus [32–34].

Small vessel pathology due to hypertension and/or diabetes is a highly prevalent component in individuals with this type of lesion, and is thought to contribute to its development. Due to selective vulnerability, neuronal death in brain areas pertinent to VCI is observed in the hippocampus and in the thalamus, whereas other areas known to be susceptible to such damage, such as the cerebellum, are less involved in cognitive functions. Global ischemia resulting in cognitive impairment is noted in some situations following severe circulatory impairment, such as a myocardial infarction with profound hypoperfusion, or subsequent to an abrupt onset of systemic hypotension due to another cause. This pathogenic situation has been described under names such as "cardiogenic dementia" [35] or "hypotensive stroke" [14]. It has been given relatively little attention, compared to the conditions related to hypertension and disorders due to different forms of vascular occlusion. Also here, SVD, namely a fibrohyaline arteriolosclerosis (Figures 3.8 and 3.11), is generally found in the white matter – whereas the neocortex and also central gray matter nuclei may exhibit ordinary vasculature. Hypertensive vascular pathology may, however, often also be found (Figures 3.6) in vast areas.

Brain pathology of a particular type of hypoperfusive–hypoxic pathogenesis is seen with cardiac arrest encephalopathy [33]. In cardiac arrest, the brain cells are exposed to noncirculating blood, and hence to the detrimental compounds normally cleared from the region, such as lactic acid. The result is generally that of selective eosinophilic neuronal death, targeting not only the hippocampus and the cerebellum but also specifically the thalamus and basal ganglia, which are regions otherwise relatively spared in ischemic situations. The manifestations of cardiac arrest encephalopathy may presumably add and contribute to the damage of selective vulnerability following a myocardial infarct. The propensity for not only hippocampal but also thalamic damage may result in the undercutting of corticothalamic pathways, i.e., frontothalamic circuits. This, in turn, may permit and be the structural counterpart of certain patterns of cognitive deficit.

Assessment of SVD and its contribution to motor and cognitive dysfunction in the elderly

There is a shortage of studies that attempt to optimize the assessment of SVD at the pathologic level. This is in contrast to the pathology in AD, and Parkinson's disease, which has been the subject of repeated attempts to refine categories of pathologic diagnosis. The key questions that need to be answered are: What types of pathology and what extent of pathology best correlate with clinical deficits attributable solely to SVD (and not to other pathology that may also be present)? And can these features be reliably recognized and quantified by different observers? Answering these questions requires large studies in which subjects have been carefully assessed for

Table 3.1 Clinicopathologic studies listed in chronological order correlating CVD with cognition

Clinical assessment	No. of autopsies	Assessment of CVD pathology	Clinicopathologic correlation	Ref.
Annual cognitive tests	102	Macroinfarcts and lacunes; also AD path	In cases with AD presence of additional infarcts or lacunes significantly reduced cognition	Snowdon et al. (1997) [38]
Prospective study with regular cognitive tests	103	Macroinfarcts and microinfarcts, subcortical lacunes, and diffuse subcortical SVD; also AD path	Presence of CVD lesions only significantly reduced cognition, compared to cases with AD pathology alone in Braak tau stages I/II	Esiri et al. (1999) [39]
Prospective AD center with yearly cognitive tests	237	Cortical and subcortical infarcts up to 10 cm^3 volume; also AD path	No significant difference (though trend was evident) for cases with AD pathology and infarct(s) to show greater cognitive impairment compared with those with AD path only	Lee et al. (2000) [40]
Community-based elderly subjects assessed for cognition at outset	209	Macroinfarcts, lacunes, and diffuse white matter damage; also AD path	Multiple forms of vascular pathology significantly more common in demented than nondemented group	Neuropathology Group (2001) [41]
Annual cognitive tests on elderly clergy (ROS)	153	Bilateral chronic infarcts; also AD path	Presence of macroinfarcts increased odds of dementia 2.8-fold	Schneider et al. (2004) [42]
Annual cognitive tests in ROS	180	Chronic cerebral macroinfarcts and lacunes; also AD and Lewy body path	Intermediate numbers of infarcts (as well as extent of AD path) in those with MCI compared with normal controls and those with dementia	Bennett et al. (2005) [43]
Prospective study of elderly with cognitive tests within 4 years of death	333	Cortical and subcortical macroinfarcts (nonagonal); also AD path	Risk of dementia increased in those with cerebrovascular lesions, especially in those with few neuritic plaques	Petrovitch et al. (2005) [44]
Prospectively assessed elderly subjects without significant AD path or macrovascular lesions	72	Bilateral microvascular pathology and lacunes; also AD path	Basal ganglia and thalamic lacunes (but not white matter lacunes) and cortical microinfarcts influenced cognition	Gold et al. (2005) [12]
Cases of clinical AD and VaD	79	Used a novel cerebrovascular parenchymal path score; also AD path and hippocampal sclerosis	Overall, only Braak tau stage was related to global neuropsychological measure of cognitive impairment	Chui et al. (2006) [45]

Table 3.1 *(cont.)*

Clinical assessment	No. of autopsies	Assessment of CVD pathology	Clinicopathologic correlation	Ref.
Prospective study of elderly with 2-yearly cognitive assessment	221	Cystic microinfarcts, lacunes and microinfarcts; also AD path	High Braak tau stage and high microinfarct score were main determinants of cognitive impairment	Sonnen et al. (2007) [46]
Prospective study of elderly with yearly cognitive tests	148	Bilateral, cortical, and subcortical microinfarcts and macroinfarcts; also AD path	Presence of cerebral cortical or subcortical infarcts increased odds of dementia by 5.06 and 3.93, respectively	Schneider et al. (2007) [47]
Prospective study of elderly with cognitive assessments every 12–18 months	190	Mainly unilateral cortical and subcortical macroinfarcts, diffuse white matter damage, microinfarcts and cribriform change; also AD path	Higher overall lesion score was correlated with dementia. Severity of white matter damage was particularly strongly correlated with dementia	Strozyk et al. (2010) [13]
Prospective study of cases with only mild AD path; all cognitively assessed within 2 years of death	70	Novel semiquantitative assessment of SVD; also AD path	Significant correlation between severity of subcortical SVD and cognitive score	Smallwood et al. (2012) [48]

AD, Alzheimer's disease; CVD, cerebrovascular disease; MCI, mild cognitive impairment; ROS, Religious Orders Study; SVD, small vessel disease; VaD, vascular dementia.

clinical features attributable to SVD in life and then the pathologic features that best correlate with these clinical features have been assessed in those subjects that are shown not to have any other pathology than SVD, or have such pathology statistically taken into account. In the few studies of this type that exist the clinical assessments that have been carried out have usually been restricted to cognitive testing. The cognitive testing itself has often been based on features more characteristic of AD, and has, therefore, risked underestimating the cognitive problems experienced by those with vascular impairment. Because many studies that encompass prospective follow-up of subjects with brain donation for research are based in memory clinics, the studies are likely to lead to an overemphasis on the importance of Alzheimer-type pathology and an underestimation of the importance of vascular pathology as a source of cognitive impairment. Other clinical features such as impaired gait, falls, depression, and incontinence have usually been only cursorily sought, if at all. Furthermore, there has been no widely accepted and validated way to assess the pathology so, in the studies that have been carried out, the methods used by pathologists have been variable [7, 8].

While all these deficiencies in clinicopathologic studies have become better recognized in recent years, the imaging of SVD has progressed apace [36, 37] and to such an extent that some investigators seem to regard actual pathology as redundant. This is not a helpful attitude as we shall only understand better the cellular and molecular underpinnings of SVD if tissue is studied at the microscopic level. In this section lessons that have been learnt from pathologic studies of SVD that incorporate both clinical and pathologic aspects will be summarized (Table 3.1 [12, 13, 38–48]).

Most elderly subjects have some SVD as well as some AD-type pathology. The presence of both types of pathology can summate, particularly at mild levels of AD pathology [39, 44], but there is no good evidence that one promotes the other. In a series of 70 cases that included elderly subjects with no more than Braak stage III tau pathology, and no other dementing pathology, and in which a semiquantitative score was given for the severity of SVD, the vascular pathology needed to be relatively severe to be associated with dementia (above the median score of 5/12) [48]. The score for dementia severity using the Mini Mental State Examination (MMSE) or the Cambridge Cognitive Examination (CAMCOG) was only mild to moderate in these cases. However, these cognitive tests are not as sensitive as others, such as the Montreal Cognitive Assessment (MoCA) [49], for capturing cognitive deficiencies due to SVD, and so this study may underestimate the contribution of SVD to dementia or cognitive impairment. Imaging studies have also suggested that the imaging correlates of SVD need to be relatively severe to give rise to dementia [50–52].

Conclusion

The pathologic consequences of SVD, as summarized here, have been recognized for many decades. It will, however, require well-designed future clinicopathologic and clinicoimaging studies to enable us to correctly recognize the features of SVD that bear particularly on difficulties experienced in later life in cognitive, affective, and motor functions. Recognition of a disease condition with regard to both clinical and structural features is a first essential step on the way to ameliorating or preventing its negative consequences.

References

1. Roman GC. On the history of lacunes, *ètat criblé* and the white matter lesions of vascular dementia. *Cerebrovasc Dis* 2002;13 (Suppl 2):1–6.
2. Tomlinson BE, Blessed G, Roth M. Observations on the brains of demented old people. *J Neurol Sci* 1970;11:205–242.
3. Hachinski VC, Lassen NA, Marschall J. Multi-infarct dementia. A cause of mental deterioration in the elderly. *J Amer Geriatr Soc* 1974;2:207–210.
4. Tatemichi TK. How acute brain failure becomes chronic. A view of the mechanisms and syndromes of dementia related to stroke. *Neurology* 1990;40:1652–1659.
5. Brun A. Pathology and pathophysiology of cerebrovascular dementia: pure subgroups of obstructive and hypoperfusive etiology. *Dementia* 1994;5:145–147.
6. Knopman DS, Parisi JE, Boeve BF, et al. Vascular dementia in a population-based autopsy study. *Arch Neurol* 2003;60:569–575.
7. Alafuzoff I, Gelpi E, Al-Sarraj S, et al. The need to unify neuropathological assessments of vascular alterations in the ageing brain: multicentre survey by the BrainNet Europe consortium. *Exp Gerontol* 2012;47:825–833.
8. Pantoni L, Sarti C, Alafuzoff I, et al. Postmortem examination of vascular lesions in cognitive impairment: a survey among neuropathological services. *Stroke* 2006;37:1005–1009.
9. Pantoni L, Poggesi A, Inzitari D. Cognitive decline and dementia related to cerebrovascular diseases: some evidence and concepts. *Cerebrovasc Dis* 2009;27 (Suppl 1):191–196.
10. Schneider JA, Bennett DA. Where vascular meets neurodegenerative disease. *Stroke* 2010;41(Suppl): S144–S146.
11. Braak H, Alafuzoff I, Arzberger T, Kretzschmar H, Del Tredici K. Staging of Alzheimer disease-associated neurofibrillary pathology using paraffin sections and immunohistochemistry. *Acta Neuropathol* 2006;112:389–404.
12. Gold G, Kövari E, Herrmann FR, et al. Cognitive consequences of thalamic, basal ganglia and deep white matter lacunes in brain aging and dementia. *Stroke* 2005;36:1184–1188.
13. Strozyk D, Dickson DW, Lipton RB, et al. Contribution of vascular pathology to the clinical expression of dementia. *Neurobiol Aging* 2010;31:1710–1720.
14. Mitchinson MJ. The hypotensive stroke. *Lancet* 1980;1(8162): 244–246.
15. Zuccalà G, Onder G, Pedone C, et al. Hypotension and cognitive impairment. Selective association in patients with heart failure. *Neurology* 2001;57:1986–1992.
16. Duggal N, Lach B. Selective vulnerability of the lumbosacral spinal cord after cardiac arrest and hypotension. *Stroke* 2001;33: 116–121.
17. Verbrugge SJ, Klinek M, Klein J. A cerebral watershed infarction after general anaesthesia in a patient with increased anti-cardiolipin antibody level. *Anesthesist* 2004;53:341–346.
18. Wang CJ, Cheng KI, Soo LY, Tang CS. Intraoperative stroke under epidural anesthesia for bipolar hemiarthroplasty in a patient with multiple myeloma: a case report. *Kaohsiung J Med Sci* 2001; 17:55–59.
19. Esiri MM, Chance SA. Cognitive reserve, cortical plasticity and resistance to Alzheimer's disease. *Alzheimers Res Ther* 2012;4:7.
20. Cadavid D, Mena H, Koeller K, Frommelt RA. Cerebral β amyloid angiopathy is a risk factor for cerebral ischemic infarction. A case control study in human brain biopsies. *J Neuropathol Exp Neurol* 2000;59:768–773.
21. Greenberg SM. Cerebral amyloid angiopathy and vessel dysfunction. *Cerebrovasc Dis* 2002;13 (Suppl 2):42–47.

22. Haglund M, Passant U, Sjöbeck M, Ghebremedin E, Englund E. Cerebral amyloid angiopathy and cortical microinfarcts as putative substrates of vascular dementia. *Int J Geriatr Psychiatry* 2006;21:681–687.

23. Kövari E, Hermann FR, Hof PR, Bouras C. The relationship between cerebral amyloid angiopathy and cortical microinfarcts in brain ageing and Alzheimer's disease. *Neuropathol Appl Neurobiol* 2013;39:498–509.

24. Englund E. Neuropathology of white matter lesions in vascular cognitive impairment. *Cerebrovasc Dis* 2002;13(Suppl) :11–15.

25. Olsson Y, Brun A, Englund E. Fundamental pathological lesions in vascular dementia. *Acta Neurol Scand* 1996;168(Suppl):31–38.

26. Sjöbeck M, Englund E. Glial levels determine severity of white matter changes in Alzheimer's disease: a neuropathological study of glial changes. *Neuropathol Appl Neurobiol* 2003;29:159–169.

27. Ihara M, Polvikoski TM, Hall R, et al. Quantification of myelin loss in frontal lobe white matter in vascular dementia, Alzheimer's disease and dementia with Lewy bodies. *Acta Neuropathol* 2010;119:579–589.

28. Sjöbeck M, Haglund M, Englund E. White matter mapping in Alzheimer's disease. A neuropathological study. *Neurobiol Aging* 2006;27:673–680.

29. Haglund M, Englund E. Cerebral amyloid angiopathy, white matter lesions and Alzheimer encephalopathy – a histopathological assessment. *Dement Geriatr Cogn Disord* 2002;14:161–166.

30. Schmidt R, Schmidt H, Haybeaeck J, et al. Heterogeneity in age-related white matter changes. *Acta Neuropathol* 2011;122:171–185.

31. Roman GC. Vascular dementia may be the most common form of dementia in the elderly. *J Neurol Sci* 2002;203:7–10.

32. Pulsinelli WA, Brierley JB, Plum F. Temporal profile of neuronal damage in a model of transient forebrain ischemia. *Ann Neurol* 1982;11:491–498.

33. Petito CK, Feldmann E, Pulsinelli WA, Plum F. Delayed hippocampal damage in humans following cardiorespiratory arrest. *Neurology* 1987;37:1281–1286.

34. Björklund E, Lindberg E, Rundgren M, et al. Ischemic brain damage after cardiac arrest and therapeutic hypothermia – a systematic description of selective neuronal death. *Resuscitation* 2013, Dec 6 [Epub ahead of print].

35. Rosenberg GA, Haaland RY. Cardiogenic dementia. *Lancet* 1981;318:368–372.

36. O'Sullivan M. Imaging small vessel disease: lesion topography, networks and cognitive deficits investigated with MRI. *Stroke* 2010;41(Suppl):S154–158.

37. Pantoni L. Cerebral small vessel disease: from pathogenesis and clinical characteristics to therapeutic challenges. *Lancet Neurol* 2010;9:689–701.

38. Snowdon DA, Greiner LH, Mortimer JA, et al. Brain infarction and the clinical expression of Alzheimer disease. The Nun Study. *JAMA* 1997;277: 813–817.

39. Esiri MM, Nagy Z, Smith MZ, Barnetson L, Smith AD. Cerebrovascular disease and threshold for dementia in the early stages of Alzheimer's disease. *Lancet* 1999;354 (9182):919–920.

40. Lee JH, Olichney JM, Hansen LA, Hofstetter CR, Thal LJ. Small concomitant vascular lesions do not influence rates of cognitive decline in patients with Alzheimer's disease. *Arch Neurol* 2000;57:1474–1479.

41. Neuropathology Group. Medical Research Council Cognitive Function and Aging Study. Pathological correlates of late-onset dementia in a multicentre, community-based population in England and Wales. *Lancet* 2001;357:169–175.

42. Schneider JA, Wilson RS, Bienias JL, Evans DA, Bennett DA. Cerebral infarctions and the likelihood of dementia from Alzheimer disease pathology. *Neurology* 2004;62:1148–1455.

43. Bennett DA, Schneider JA, Bienias JL, Evans DA, Wilson RS. Mild cognitive impairment is related to Alzheimer disease pathology and cerebral infarctions. *Neurology* 2005;64:834–841.

44. Petrovitch H, Ross GW, Steinhorn SC, et al. AD lesions and infarcts in demented and non-demented Japanese-American men. *Ann Neurol* 2005;57:98–103.

45. Chui HC, Zarow C, Mack WJ, et al. Cognitive impact of subcortical vascular and Alzheimer's disease pathology. *Ann Neurol* 2006;60:677–687.

46. Sonnen JA, Larson EB, Crane PK, et al. Pathological correlates of dementia in a longitudinal, population-based sample of aging. *Ann Neurol* 2007; 62:406–413.

47. Schneider JA, Arvanitakis Z, Bang W, Bennett DA. Mixed brain pathologies account for most dementia cases in community-dwelling older persons. *Neurology* 2007;69:2197–2204.

48. Smallwood A, Oulhaj A, Joachim C, et al. Cerebral subcortical vessel disease and its relation to cognition in elderly subjects: a pathological study in the Oxford Project to Investigate Memory and Ageing (OPTIMA) cohort. *Neuropathol Appl Neurobiol* 2012;38:337–343.

49. Nasreddine ZS, Phillips NA, Bédirian V, et al. The Montreal Cognitive Assessment, MoCA: a brief screening tool for mild cognitive impairment. *J Am Geriatr Soc* 2005; 53:695–699.

50. Erkinjuntti T. Subcortical vascular dementia. *Cerebrovasc Dis* 2002;13 (Suppl 2):58–60.

51. Frisoni GB. Dementia: important advances in research in 2006. *Lancet Neurol* 2007;6:4–5.

52. Lee AY. Vascular dementia. *Chonnam Med J* 2011;47:66–71.

Chapter 4

Pathologic aspects of the hemorrhagic consequences of small vessel disease on the brain

Johannes Attems and Kurt A. Jellinger

Introduction

Cerebrovascular disease (CVD) encompasses both large vessel disease, which may cause cortical ischemic and hemorrhagic infarcts, and subcortical small vessel disease (SVD). CVD may be present in demented and nondemented individuals. However, SVD is increasingly recognized as a predictor of cognitive impairment and dementia [1].

Intracranial hemorrhages, including large lobar hemorrhages, deep bleeds in the basal ganglia, microscopic brain hemorrhages or cerebral microbleeds (CMBs), and subarachnoid hemorrhages (SAHs) may all be caused by SVD. Small vessel disease may also cause white matter hyperintensities (WMHs), lacunes, and ischemic as well as hemorrhagic infarcts. While the latter two lesions are usually complications of cerebral large vessel disease, all the others may occur in association with various types of SVD, the pathology of which has been summarized in Chapter 2. The prevalence and incidence of SVD increases with age, and SVD is most frequently diagnosed in subjects aged over 60 years. However, the prevalence of the various pathologic lesions that may be caused by SVD varies in the oldest-old: macroscopic ICHs are comparatively rare in the very elderly, while microscopic brain hemorrhages and CMBs, that are often associated with severe cerebral amyloid angiopathy (CAA) [2], are frequent and of considerable clinical importance. In nondemented elderly subjects, lacunes, CMBs, and WMHs have been associated with cognitive decline, including reduced mental speed, and impaired executive functions [3], as well as with other neuropsychiatric symptoms. SVD is even more common in subjects with Alzheimer's disease (AD), and might interact with the neurodegenerative changes in AD as either independent of each other [4] or due to additive or synergistic effects on cognitive decline [5]. A better understanding of the underlying pathologic mechanisms that link SVD and its associated consequences is of paramount importance as some of these consequences could potentially be treated and/or prevented. The present chapter will present an update of the morphological aspects and pathogenesis of the hemorrhagic consequences of SVD, with a focus on different types of CAA-related cerebral hemorrhages.

Intracerebral hemorrhage

Neuropathology of intracerebral hemorrhage

The pathologic features of intracerebral hemorrhage (ICH) include accumulations of fresh blood dissecting through the tissue planes (Figure 4.1A) and along tracts, deformation of the brain, perihematomal necrosis, edema formation, and blood–brain barrier (BBB) disruption; after 2–3 days, accumulation of hematogenous inflammatory cells (Figure 4.1B), including neutrophils (initially) and macrophages (later), and phagocytosis of the erythrocytes by phagocyting cells occur. These events are followed by hematoma reabsorption and finally formation of a scar or cavity. Hemosiderin-laden or so called "foamy" macrophages and hematoidin remain visible for months or years within the lesion or in gliotic walls of the cavity (Figure 4.1C–G).

ICHs variably account for 6.5–30.0% of first-time strokes, are most frequently caused by hypertension, and are hence associated with hypertension-related risk factors [6]. While saccular arterial aneurysms and arteriovenous malformations are often seen in ICHs caused by large vessel disease, ICHs caused by

Cerebral Small Vessel Disease, ed. Leonardo Pantoni and Philip B. Gorelick. Published by Cambridge University Press.

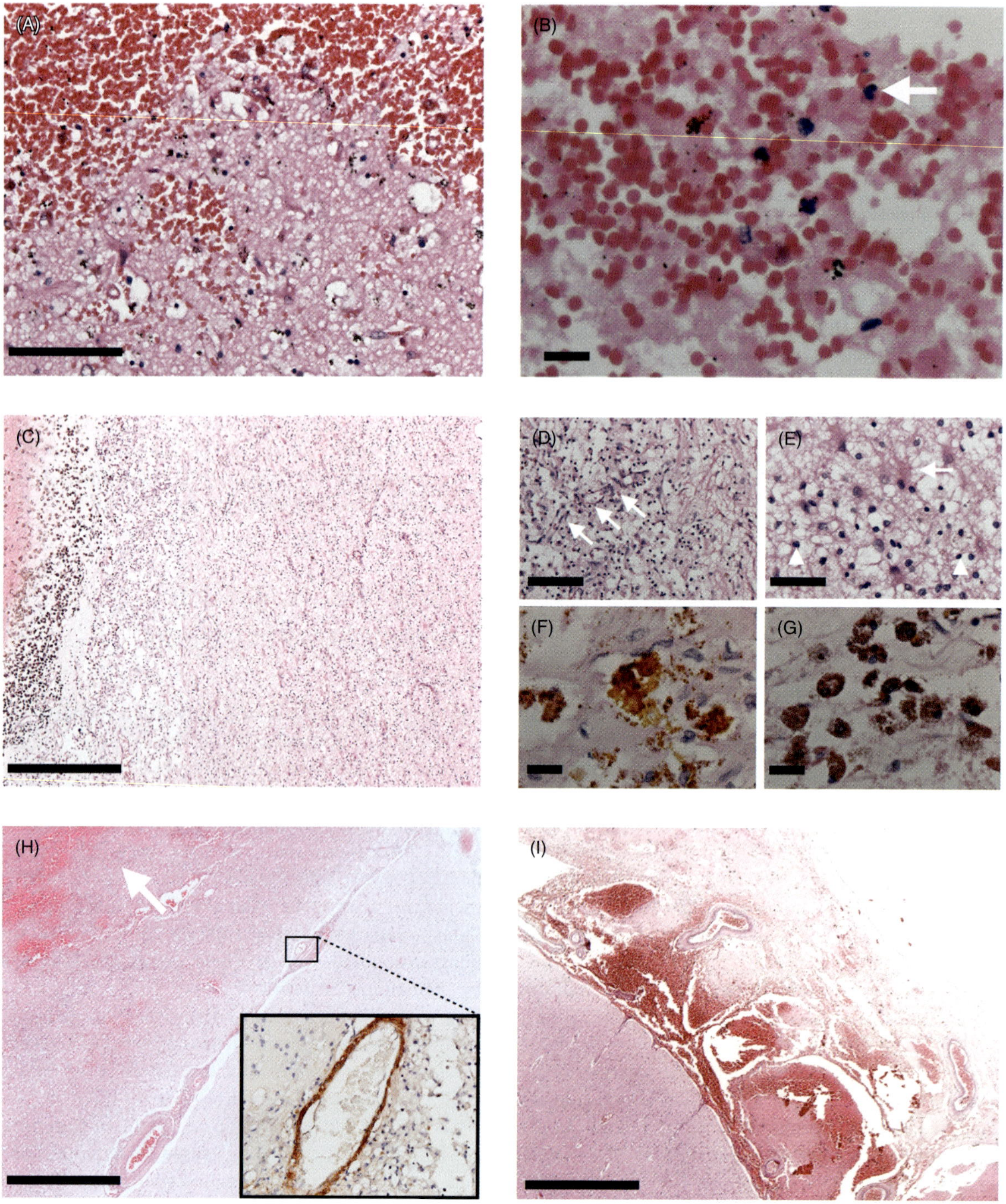

Figure 4.1 (A,B) Fresh intracerebral hemorrhage (ICH) invading brain tissue with accumulation of neutrophilic granulocytes (arrow in B). (C) Gliotic wall of a cavity resulting from an ICH; directly adjacent to the cavity is a brownish rim consisting of accumulations of hemosiderin/hemosiderin-laden macrophages (left in C and high magnification in G). The gliotic scar shows prominent capillaries (arrows in D) and proliferation of glial cells including astrocytes (arrow in E) and microglia (arrowheads in E). (F) Hematoidin depositions. (H) Cerebral amyloid angiopathy (CAA) and ICH; a meningeal vessel in close vicinity to an ICH (arrow) shows β-amyloid (Aβ) deposition (inset in H) indicating an association between CAA and ICH in this case. (I) Subarachnoid hemorrhage.

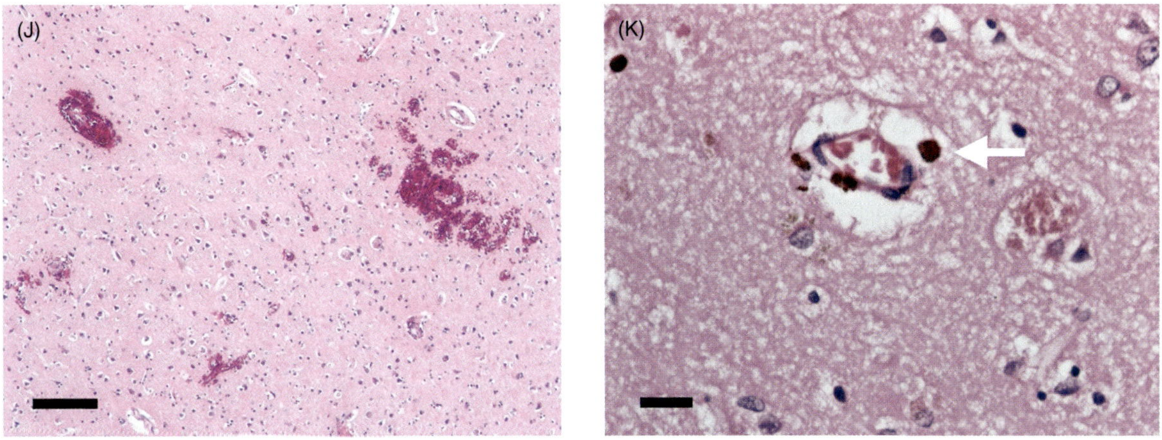

Figure 4.1 *(cont.)* (J) Fresh cerebral microbleeds and (K) small perivascular hemosiderin depositions (arrow in K) that are assumed to represent old cerebral microbleeds and appear as small signal voids on T2*-weighted magnetic resonance imaging (MRI). Slides stained with hematoxylin and eosin (H&E), except inset in (H), Aβ antibody 4G8. Original magnifications: 20×, H and I; 100×, J and C; 200×, A and D; 400×, B, E, and K; 600, F and G. Scale bars: 20 μm, B, F, G, and K; 50 μm, E; 100 μm, A, D, and J; 500 μm, C; 1000 μm, H and I. Figure J was kindly provided by Dr. Tuomo Polvikoski.

rupture of a small vessel frequently occurs in the presence of hypertension, CAA (Figure 4.1H), or anticoagulation. The majority of ICHs (>75%) in the elderly are classified as spontaneous (sometimes also termed primary or nontraumatic), resulting from rupture of small arteries affected by either of two main pathologic lesions: hypertensive arteriopathy or CAA.

Hypertensive arteriopathy, CAA, and ICH

Hypertensive arteriopathy is characterized by fibrinoid necrosis and lipohyalinosis of small lenticulostriate arterial perforators, and is considered to be an important cause of spontaneous ICH in deep- or infra-tentorial locations (basal ganglia, thalamus, and pons) [7]. By contrast, CAA-related ICHs preferentially affect cortical–subcortical (lobar) regions, in particular the occipital and temporal lobes [8], while the cerebellum and deep or brainstem structures are rarely involved. The predilection sites for CAA-associated ICH reflect the distribution of the underlying microangiopathy [9]. The frequent involvement of the occipital lobe in CAA is not well understood, but it has been hypothesized that greater tortuosity of occipital small arteries impairs perivascular drainage [10].

It is generally accepted that CAA is an important risk factor for spontaneous nontraumatic ICHs in the elderly. Clinicopathologic correlative studies suggest that CAA-related ICH account for 5–20% of all spontaneous ICH [9, 11]. In the Vantaa 85+ study, only 2.3% of the oldest-old subjects (mean age at death 92.4 ± 3.7 years) had macroscopic ICH; three (1%) each had basal ganglia hemorrhage and lobar hemorrhage, while one had SAH. Interestingly, of those with basal ganglia hemorrhages none had been hypertensive [2]. The prevalence of macroscopic ICH (of any type) in this oldest-old cohort was low (2.3%) when compared with a previous population-based study (demented 6%, nondemented 3%) [12], and a retrospective consecutive study of 2060 elderly patients showing 5.6% macroscopically detected ICHs excluding CMBs [13]. Among the oldest-old, the apolipoprotein E (*APOE*) ε4 allele was common in patients with lobar hemorrhages, similar to a previous study [14], and, in contrast to other studies [15], there was no over-representation of the *APOE* ε2 allele [2]. However, several studies retrospectively compared CAA-positive with CAA-negative cohorts and did not find significant differences regarding the prevalence of ICH, while significant differences were seen when the comparison was made between groups with no or low-grade versus moderate- to high-grade CAA, respectively [11, 13, 16–18], suggesting that mild CCA is not an important risk factor for ICH. On the other hand, CAA was more severe in the brains with ICH than in those without, and microaneurysms and fibrinoid necrosis, which both indicate severe CAA, were seen exclusively in brains with ICH [11]. Moreover, CAA-associated ICHs were restricted to lobar regions, while ICHs in both lobar and deep cerebral regions were seen in CAA-positive cases in which no direct topographic co-localization between vessels that were affected with CAA and the site of hemorrhage were identified. Studies investigating the progression of white matter lesions (or WMHs) in subjects with CAA indicated their association with incident lobar hemorrhages reflecting the progressive nature of this microangiopathy [19]. Like other markers of CVD, cerebral microinfarcts are associated with both advanced SVD and ICH, and silent ischemic infarcts are associated with hemorrhage burden in CAA [20].

In contrast to hypertensive microangiopathy, the risk of CAA is not influenced by conventional cardiovascular risk factors other than age [9]. Hypertension is not considered a risk factor for developing CAA, but may increase the risk of CAA-related ICH. Therefore, the important question must be asked as to whether hypertension in association with CAA confers a greater risk for ICH compared to CAA alone? Some studies of autopsy-proven CAA found the prevalence of hypertension to be around 32% [9], while another pathologic study reported that CAA patients with ICH were more frequently hypertensive (50%) than those without ICH (23%), suggesting that hypertension may contribute to CAA-related ICH [11]. In a recent multicenter cohort of patients with spontaneous ICH, the prevalence of hypertension in CAA-related ICH was significantly lower (62%) than in non-CAA-related ICHs (85%) [21]. Evidence from the Perindopril Protection aGainst REcurrent Stroke Study (PROGRESS) trial of blood pressure lowering after stroke showed that a mean blood pressure of 120 (systolic)/70 (diastolic) mmHg reduced the risk of subsequent CAA-related ICH by about 77%, supporting the important causal role of hypertension in CAA-related hemorrhage [22].

In a postmortem study of 394 patients with detailed clinical information, CAA-associated ICH was present in 15.8% of cases with severe CAA compared with 12.2% with no or moderate CAA. Of the cases with CAA-associated ICH, only four showed no signs of hypertension [17]. This indicates that in only four of 54 cases CAA might have been the only cause of ICH, confirming previous statements that the high frequency of CAA in many patients without hemorrhage suggests that in many instances the presence of CAA alone is not sufficient to explain the occurrence of hemorrhages [11].

Since many elderly individuals have subclinical CAA without hemorrhage, mild CAA may not be sufficient to be regarded as the single cause for lobar ICH, but may contribute to ICH via interaction with other factors for ICH, such as hypertension or the use of anticoagulant drugs [11, 13, 16, 18, 23]. Besides arterial hypertension, several other factors might facilitate ICH in CAA. *APOE* ε4 in both postmortem and clinical series has been shown to increase the risk of sporadic CAA related to lobar ICH [14, 24, 25]. The *APOE* ε2 genotype was associated with severe pathomorphological changes in CAA, such as "double barreling," fibrinoid necrosis, and evidence of perivascular bleeding [26, 27], as well as with increased risk of CAA-related spontaneous lobar ICH [26–29]. Both of these risk alleles are also associated with a younger age of first ICH [30], and a higher risk of recurrence [29]. The ε2 and ε4 alleles might promote CAA-related hemorrhage through distinct mechanisms: ε4 by promoting β-amyloid (Aβ) deposition and ε2 by inducing structural changes in amyloid-laden vessels, making them prone to rupture [26, 27, 31, 32]. Other, as yet unidentified, genetic polymorphisms relating to amyloid metabolic pathways may also play a role in sporadic CAA (for a review see [33]).

Furthermore, the influence of Aβ on matrix metalloproteinases (MMPs), a family of zinc-dependent endopeptidases, may also play a role in the association between ICH and CAA. MMPs are responsible for degradation and remodeling of extracellular matrices and are involved in the regulation of vascular integrity [34]. Aβ peptides induce MMP-2 and MMP-9 activation and that of MMP-2 coincided with the appearance of Aβ degradation fragments and reduced fibril formation, while silencing MMP-2 expression resulted in reduced Aβ degradation and enhanced apoptosis in cell cultures [35]. However, MMP-2 also cleaves components of vascular basement membranes such as collagen IV and V, laminin, and proteoglycan [36]. MMP-9 immunostaining of CAA vessels that showed evidence of microhemorrhage was demonstrated in APPsw transgenic mice, suggesting that spontaneous hemorrhage in CAA might be, at least in part, caused by Aβ-induced MMP activation [37]. The presence of the Kunitz protease inhibitor (KPI) domain in certain isoforms of Aβ precursor protein (AβPP) could also contribute to bleeding in CAA, as it inactivates several proteins involved in blood clotting [38, 39]. This could explain why many patients with even severe CAA do not suffer from ICHs, as it may be more related to the levels of KPI-containing AβPP rather than Aβ. However, further studies are warranted to test this possibility in human postmortem brains.

Anticoagulation-related ICH

CAA may represent an important risk factor or cause for ICH related to oral anticoagulatant use. Over the past decade there has been a fivefold increase in the incidence of anticoagulation-related ICHs, which now account for about 15% of all ICHs [40]. This trend is probably due to an increasing use of warfarin to prevent cardioembolic stroke in elderly persons with atrial fibrillation. The excess of CMBs in warfarin users with ICH compared to other groups suggests that CMBs increase the risk of warfarin-associated ICHs [41]. Anticoagulant use per se should not cause ICH if cerebral vessels are intact, but the presence of CAA, or other microarteriopathies that render vessel walls fragile, is a plausible aggravating factor for such hemorrhages. An otherwise harmless, minor, and self-limiting vessel leak could give raise to a dangerous hematoma if the leaking occurs in a vessel that is damaged by advanced CAA. Evidence supporting a link between CAA and anticoagulation linked ICH includes the following: (1) most such ICHs occur within the therapeutic range of anticoagulant drug levels [42] suggesting that an intrinsic disorder of small cerebral vessels (e.g., SVD) could be important; and (2) the *APOE* ε2 allele is more common in patients with warfarin-related ICH than in patients treated with warfarin but lacking ICH. Given that *APOE* ε2 is associated with CAA-related ICH, this finding supports the role of CAA in ICH related to anticoagulation therapy [42]. However, although retrospective data point towards the possibility that CAA might indeed represent a major underlying pathology, prospective studies that benefit from reliable *intra vitam* diagnosis of CAA (e.g., by MRI evidence of CMBs) in cohorts treated with anticoagulants are needed to further elucidate the role of CAA in the co-occurrence of ICH and anticoagulation therapy.

CAA may also be a risk factor for ICH after thrombolysis, as ICH after thrombolysis shares some characteristics with CAA-associated ICH; both types show a predilection for lobar regions, multiplicity of hemorrhages, age-dependency, and an association with dementia and white matter lesions [43]. In a small study, two of five cases of ICH after thrombolysis for acute myocardial infarction had severe CAA [44]. ICHs are not common in cerebral autosomal dominant arteriopathy with subcortical infarcts and leukoencephalopathy (CADASIL) without additional risk factors for ICH, as they occur most often in patients treated with anticoagulants or antiaggregants, or who have been subjected to arteriography [45], while others reported ICHs in 25% of symptomatic CADASIL patients, closely related to the number of CMBs [46].

SAH and superficial siderosis

Isolated, nontraumatic cortical subarachnoid hemorrhage (cSAH) is a localized bleed (Figure 4.1I), usually in up to several adjacent sulci, frequently involving the central sulcus, without other subarachnoid bleeding at the base of the brain in the pattern typically associated with saccular aneurysm rupture [47, 48]. cSAH alone is rare but more frequently seen in CAA, where it often results from lobar ICH extending to the cortical surface [49, 50]. The literature contains some cases of pathologically proven CAA-associated acute SAH [49, 51, 52]. The largest cohort of patients with isolated cSAH ($N = 29$) found that CAA is a frequent apparent cause in patients over age 60 [47] [53] and acute SAH was observed in 50% of CAA patients [54]. A retrospective analysis of consecutive patients admitted to a tertiary stroke unit with cSAH suggested that CAA could be a common cause for cSAH in the elderly [48]. This assumption is supported by another recent study of a cohort of patients presenting with cSAH [55].

Superficial siderosis presents as hemosiderin deposits in the superficial layers of the cerebral cortex, spinal cord, and nerves [56], and may follow repeated episodes of bleeding in the subarachnoid space, for example cSAH [49]. Compared with the well-described syndrome of central nervous system superficial siderosis, which typically affects the brainstem and posterior fossa, CAA-related superficial siderosis has a predilection for the cerebral convexity [57]. On T2-weighted gradient-recalled echo (GRE) magnetic resonance imaging (MRI) sequences, cortical superficial siderosis is defined as a linear gyriform pattern of hypointense signal [58, 59]. Among 270 cases of superficial siderosis, 3% were considered to be caused by CAA [60]. However, recently, cortical superficial siderosis was detected in 60.5% of patients with a clinical diagnosis of CAA (mean age 70 years), while it was absent in all controls (mean age 54 years), suggesting that it may be helpful for the clinical diagnosis of CAA, enhancing the sensitivity of the Boston criteria for CAA without loss of specificity [54].

Cerebral microbleeds

The term CMBs refers to small signal voids detected by MRI; these signal voids indicate perivascular accumulation of hemosiderin/hemosiderin-laden macrophages assumed to represent past hemorrhages.

Epidemiology of CMBs

The increasing use of T2*-weighted MRI sequences and of susceptibility-weighted MRI has led to increasing detection of CMBs. CMBs are small, well-demarcated, hypointense, rounded lesions that cannot be detected on conventional MRI [61–65]. MRI has a higher sensitivity for CMBs than for cerebral microinfarcts, thereby allowing for the distinction between those two lesions [20]. In particular 7-Tesla MRI may have a significant impact on CMB early detection [66, 67] mainly in cortical–subcortical regions [68]. Long-term follow-up MRI studies show dynamic temporal change of most CMBs [69].

Prevalence rates of CMBs in elderly people are strongly influenced by the choice of MRI method and range from 3.1 [70] to 35% [71], or from 4.7 to 24.4% of community-based subjects [72]. Pooling data from various studies revealed a prevalence of CMBs of 5% in healthy adults. This value is raised to 20% in the elderly (>60 years) [73], to 34% in people with ischemic stroke, and to 60–80% in subjects with nontraumatic ICHs (52% with first ICH and 83% with recurrent ICH) [74]. CMBs are associated with hypertension (odds ratio [OR] 3.0) and diabetes mellitus (OR 2.2) in otherwise healthy adults [75]. The prevalence rates of CMBs reported in patients suffering from various types of ischemic strokes and ICHs vary between 19.4 and 68.5% [72], and between 16 and 32% in AD, respectively [75], while they are rare in transient ischemic attacks. The prevalence of CMBs in Binswanger's disease is 77%, and in patients with multiple lacunar strokes the prevalence is between 51 and 68%.

CMBs have been observed in 31% of symptomatic CADASIL patients, predominantly located in the thalamus, with significant increase in prevalence with age, probably indicating an increased risk for ICH, but were not reported in preclinical or early CADASIL [76]. Corresponding to prevalence rates of CMBs indicated by *intra vitam* imaging studies, perivascular deposits of hemosiderin-containing macrophages were histologically detected in 86% of CADASIL brains [77]. Supratentorial CMBs in hereditary cerebral hemorrhage with amyloidosis, Dutch type, occur independently of the presence of hypertension, whereas infratentorial CMBs correlate with hypertension [78].

In the Vantaa 85+ study, microscopic ICHs were frequent and not associated with any of the clinical, genetic, or neuropathologic variables investigated, while in contrast, the frequency of microscopic brain hemorrhages (a subgroup of microscopic hemorrhages defined as deposits with >5 siderophages) was low (5.3%) even when compared with the frequency of CMBs in population-based MRI studies of younger patients (15.3 and 11.1%) [79, 80]. Infratentorial CMBs are associated with loss in cognitive functioning [81] and their presence is associated with increased mortality [82, 83].

Neuropathologic correlates of neuroimaging

Despite the relatively high prevalence rates of CMBs in MRI studies, the histologic correlates of CMBs have not been frequently examined in postmortem brains, and only a few studies have correlated postmortem MRI with the respective histologic findings to establish the morphological correlates of MRI hypointensities [84, 85]. A recent study that systematically correlated susceptibility-weighted imaging on advanced T2*-MRI sequence with tissue pathology of hypointensities in AD patients found that most lesions appeared indeed to be CMBs, while a minority corresponded to small lacunes, dissections of a vessel wall, or to microaneurysms. CMBs potentially could also correspond to focal accumulations of hemosiderin-containing macrophages in the perivascular space that are unrelated to previous bleeds; there is evidence of heme degradation activity within a surrounding inflammatory reaction with activated microglial cells, late complement activations, and apoptosis [86].

Histologically CMBs are defined as blood extravasations into the perivascular and/or Virchow–Robin space usually without disruption of the surrounding tissue and/or very small ICH usually measuring less than 5 mm in diameter (Figure 4.1J). Hemosiderin-laden macrophages and hemosiderin depositions within the perivascular space (Figure 4.1K) are generally considered to indicate prior CMBs [87]. CMBs were found to be occasionally surrounded by gliosis and incomplete ischemic changes. The walls of ruptured arterioles may show CAA-related vascular damage, with thickened acellular morphology, lack of the muscular layer, and Aβ deposition. In addition, ruptured microvessels affected by hypertensive angiopathy or atherosclerosis have been found to be associated with CMBs [64, 80, 88]. A systemic review of five studies on the histopathologic correlation between CMBs and neuroimaging findings (N total = 18) [89] found that hemosiderin deposition was reported in 49% to correlate with CMBs as diagnosed by MRI, while 19% corresponded to old hematomas which stained for iron, 15% had no associated specific pathology, 13% contained intact erythrocytes, and 1% each was due to vascular pseudocalcification, microaneurysm, or distended dissected vessel. Here, lipofibrohyalinosis was the most frequent associated vascular pathology.

Pathogenesis of CMBs

Lobar CMBs in CAA are likely to be caused by vessel wall fragility and rupture due to the deposition of amyloid within the media and adventia of small- or medium-sized cerebral arteries, and have been studied extensively in CAA [30, 90]. In elderly patients presenting with lobar ICH, the frequency of CMBs is more than double the respective frequency seen in other types of macrohemorrhages [90].

The topographic distributions of CMBs follow those that are typical for the associated vascular disease as MRI histology correlation studies have shown that hypertensive vasculopathy is associated with CMBs in deep brain regions (basal ganglia, thalamus, brainstem, and cerebellum), whereas in CAA CMBs are characterized by a lobar distribution [61, 86, 91, 92] showing a predilection for parietal and occipital lobes [8]. Additionally, lesions tended to cluster in the same lobe in subjects with multiple lesions [8]. Moreover, the *APOE* ε4 genotype, which is closely related to CAA-type 1 [93], has been associated with lobar CMBs [94] but not with deep hemispheric or infratentorial CMBs that have been associated with systolic blood pressure, hypertension, and lacunar infarcts [64, 80]. In the Vantaa 85+ study, the subjects with microscopic brain hemorrhages overexpressed the *APOE* ε4 alleles [2], as has been previously shown in subjects with CMBs [64, 79, 95]. In the Framingham study, no relationship between CMBs and cardiovascular risk factors, ApoE status, brain volume, or WMHs was found [96].

Besides age, hypertension, diabetes mellitus, and low serum cholesterol have so far been identified as risk factors for CMBs, and the presence of an *APOE* ε4 allele is the only genetic factor that was consistently shown to increase the risk for CMB development (see [72]). In AD brains, CMBs are not related to common hemorrhagic risk factors, but their significant relation with white matter pathology suggested that CMBs in AD may be associated with CAA but not with hypertension or other cerebrovascular diseases [97]. New CMBs develop rapidly after acute ischemic stroke. Baseline CMBs and severe SVD are predictors for the development of new CMBs. The relevance of CMBs for cognitive impairment remains uncertain [98].

Examination of the densities and size of Aβ deposits and heme-rich deposits, and their relationship to blood vessels in the aging human brain showed marked variation between cases, particularly between demented and nondemented subjects. The frequency of heme deposits showed a correlation with the frequency of Aβ deposits; both formed adjacent to or encircling small vessels, often at branch points, and a spatial proximity analysis confirmed that both were found close to or co-localizing with microvessels. Since heme is an established marker of cerebral bleeding, and Aβ a marker of senile plaques, these data suggest that senile plaques are the sites of microhemorrhages and raise the question as to whether microhemorrhages are early events in plaque formation [99].

Presence of multiple CMBs, especially in a strict lobar location, is associated with worse cognitive function. In stroke patients, CMBs are consistently associated with executive impairment and may have prognostic relevance for long-term cognitive impairment whereas absence of CMBs predicts reversible cognitive impairment [100].

It has been suggested that there is a topographic association between the radiologically detected CMBs and CAA [101], especially in AD subjects [97], similar to respective findings that have been reported for ICHs [90]. In some studies the prevalence of CMB and CAA was highest in the parietal lobes [2, 95].

Indeed, the high frequency of CMBs in the parietal lobe may be due to CAA that is frequent in the parietal lobe. According to a recent postmortem study on the prevalence of CMBs in neurodegenerative dementias, CMBs are most frequent in AD brains and often associated with CAA. CMBs were also frequent in dementia with Lewy bodies (DLB), possibly due to the high frequency of AD pathology (e.g., CAA) as a comorbid condition in DLB. However, occasionally CMBs were observed in up to 60% of elderly controls.

The topographic distribution of CAA-affected vessels differs from that of CMBs associated with CAA; while severe CAA is usually associated with the presence of CAA-affected vessels in all lobes, CMBs are more localized. Moreover, within a given brain that shows both severe CAA and CMBs, not all vessels affected by severe CAA show surrounding CMBs. Therefore, it is likely that other additional factors promote CMBs in a given vessel affected by severe CAA.

A recent study in clinically probable CAA, using noninvasive amyloid imaging with Pittsburgh Compound B (PiB), found that CMBs correspond to areas with high concentration of amyloid [101]. They correlate with the risk of lobar ICH recurrence [90], suggesting their important role in prognosis in CAA [98]. CMBs located in the lobar regions in CAA have been shown to be related to disease progression, recurrent ICH, and CAA-related cognitive impairment [90]. Large numbers of CMBs and *APOE* ε2 or ε4 genotype were the only predictors of new CMBs, and both the number of hemorrhages at baseline and the number of CMBs at follow-up increased the risk of recurrent hemorrhage (3-year cumulative risk of 14–51% in subjects with one and more than six baseline hemorrhages, respectively). The distribution of new CMBs at follow-up has been correlated with the distribution of baseline CMBs [8].

CMBs, which are regionally strongly associated with the presence and development of ICHs [102], are not only a predictor of future ICH [33, 103], but are also independently associated with cognitive decline [104–106].

The precise relationship between CMBs and macrohemorrhages in CAA is currently being investigated. A recent study suggested that CAA subjects with very high (over 50) CMB counts have increased vessel wall thickness compared to those with relatively few CMBs [61]. This suggests that increasing wall thickness may predispose vessels to CMBs when they rupture. In support of this hypothesis, severe wall thickening occurs in Iowa-type hereditary CAA, which is characterized by multiple microbleeds without symptomatic hemorrhage [107]. Although increased vessel wall thickness and luminal narrowing in CAA is a well-described phenomenon [108, 109], little is known about the factors that determine degree of vessel thickness and its clinical impact [5]. These and other questions about CAA in the elderly were reviewed recently [110].

Relationship between ICH and CMBs

CMBs are a strong predictor of impending ICH in patients with infective endocarditis, representing related vascular vulnerability [111]. Moreover, they are more frequent in patients receiving platelet inhibitors [112], in which only aspirin administration has been associated with strictly CAA-related lobar CMBs, while carbasalate calcium therapy was not [113]. Asymptomatic CMBs may be a risk factor for aspirin-associated CHs [114]. CMBs are an increased risk factor for ICH following thrombolysis for acute ischemic stroke especially in patients with multiple lobar CMBs suggestive of CAA, but further studies are warranted [115, 116]. Although CMBs are significantly more frequent in warfarin-treated stroke patients with ICH, there is not enough evidence to consider them as a contraindication for antithrombotic agents in stroke prevention [72]. Previous studies suggested that CMBs are not more frequent in patients receiving anticoagulant therapy [113], but a new prospective observational inception cohort study (Clinical Relevance of Microbleeds in Stroke; CROMIS-2, unpublished, but see [103]) is intended to assess the value of MRI markers in SVD (including CMBs) and genetic factors for the risk of oral anticoagulation-associated ICHs [33, 103]. The role of CMBs in immunization therapy for AD is unclear, although patients with advanced CAA and CMBs might be less eligible for Aβ immunization therapy, and their role in the development of vasogenic edema after bapineuzumab therapy is also unclear [117]. Despite a strong increase of publications on CMBs, their diagnostic and prognostic values remain to be explored, and new definitions and diagnostic criteria for vascular cognitive impairment are warranted and should take into account both microinfarcts and CMBs.

References

1. Smallwood A, Oulhaj A, Joachim C, et al. Cerebral subcortical small vessel disease and its relation to cognition in elderly subjects: a pathological study in the Oxford Project to Investigate Memory and Ageing (OPTIMA) cohort. *Neuropathol Appl Neurobiol* 2012;38:337–343.
2. Tanskanen M, Makela M, Myllykangas L, et al. Intracerebral hemorrhage in the oldest old: a population-based study (Vantaa 85+). *Front Neurol* 2012;3:103.
3. Seo SW, Hwa Lee B, et al. Clinical significance of microbleeds in subcortical vascular dementia. *Stroke* 2007;38:1949–1951.
4. Esiri MM, Joachim C, Sloan C, et al. Cerebral subcortical small vessel disease in subjects with pathologically confirmed Alzheimer's disease: a clinicopathological study in the Oxford Project to Investigate Memory and Ageing (OPTIMA). *Alzheimer Dis Assoc Disord* 2013, Jul 8 [Epub ahead of print].
5. Zekry D, Duyckaerts C, Belmin J, et al. Cerebral amyloid angiopathy in the elderly: vessel wall changes and relationship with dementia. *Acta Neuropathol* 2003;106: 367–373.
6. Ferrer I, Kaste M, Kalimo H. Vascular diseases. In Love S, Louis DN, Ellison DW, eds. *Greenfield's Neuropathology*, 8th edn. London: Hodder Arnold; 2008: pp. 121–240.
7. Pantoni L. Cerebral small vessel disease: from pathogenesis and clinical characteristics to therapeutic challenges. *Lancet Neurol* 2010;9:689–701.
8. Rosand J, Muzikansky A, Kumar A, et al. Spatial clustering of hemorrhages in probable cerebral amyloid angiopathy. *Ann Neurol* 2005;58:459–462.
9. Vinters HV. Cerebral amyloid angiopathy. A critical review. *Stroke* 1987;18:311–324.
10. Attems J, Jellinger K, Thal DR, Van Nostrand W. Review: sporadic cerebral amyloid angiopathy. *Neuropathol Appl Neurobiol* 2011;37:75–93.
11. Vonsattel JP, Myers RH, Hedley-Whyte ET, et al. Cerebral amyloid angiopathy without and with cerebral hemorrhages: a comparative histological study. *Ann Neurol* 1991;30:637–649.
12. Neuropathology Group. Medical Research Council Cognitive Function and Ageing Study. Pathological correlates of late-onset dementia in a multicentre, community-based population in England and Wales. *Lancet* 2001;357:169–175.
13. Attems J, Lauda F, Jellinger KA. Unexpectedly low prevalence of intracerebral hemorrhages in sporadic cerebral amyloid angiopathy: an autopsy study. *J Neurol* 2008;255:70–76.
14. Biffi A, Sonni A, Anderson CD, et al. Variants at ApoE influence risk of deep and lobar intracerebral hemorrhage. *Ann Neurol* 2010;68:934–943.
15. McCarron MO, Nicoll JA. High frequency of apolipoprotein E ε2 allele is specific for patients with cerebral amyloid angiopathy-related haemorrhage. *Neurosci Lett* 1998;247:45–48.
16. Olichney JM, Hansen LA, Hofstetter CR, et al. Association between severe cerebral amyloid angiopathy and cerebrovascular lesions in Alzheimer disease is not a spurious one attributable to apolipoprotein E ε4. *Arch Neurol* 2000;57:869–874.
17. Jellinger KA, Lauda F, Attems J. Sporadic cerebral amyloid angiopathy – no frequent cause of spontaneous brain haemorrhage. *Neuropathol App Neurobiol* 2008;34:S1–14.
18. Jellinger KA, Lauda F, Attems J. Sporadic cerebral amyloid angiopathy is not a frequent cause of spontaneous brain hemorrhage. *Eur J Neurol* 2007;14:923–928.
19. Chen YW, Gurol ME, Rosand J, et al. Progression of white matter lesions and hemorrhages in cerebral amyloid angiopathy. *Neurology* 2006;67:83–87.
20. Smith EE, Schneider JA, Wardlaw JM, Greenberg SM. Cerebral microinfarcts: the invisible lesions. *Lancet Neurol* 2012;11:272–282.
21. Gregoire SM, Charidimou A, Gadapa N, et al. Acute ischaemic brain lesions in intracerebral haemorrhage: multicentre cross-sectional magnetic resonance imaging study. *Brain* 2011;134:2376–2386.
22. Arima H, Tzourio C, Anderson C, et al. Effects of perindopril-based lowering of blood pressure on intracerebral hemorrhage related to amyloid angiopathy: the PROGRESS trial. *Stroke* 2010;41:394–396.
23. Revesz T, Holton JL, Lashley T, et al. Genetics and molecular pathogenesis of sporadic and hereditary cerebral amyloid angiopathies. *Acta Neuropathol* 2009;118:115–130.
24. Verghese PB, Castellano JM, Holtzman DM. Apolipoprotein E in Alzheimer's disease and other neurological disorders. *Lancet Neurol* 2011;10:241–252.
25. Greenberg SM, Rebeck GW, Vonsattel JP, Gomez-Isla T, Hyman BT. Apolipoprotein E ε4 and cerebral hemorrhage associated with amyloid angiopathy. *Ann Neurol* 1995;38:254–259.
26. Greenberg SM, Vonsattel JP, Segal AZ, et al. Association of apolipoprotein E ε2 and vasculopathy in cerebral amyloid angiopathy. *Neurology* 1998;50:961–965.
27. McCarron MO, Nicoll JA, Stewart J, et al. The apolipoprotein E ε2 allele and the pathological features

in cerebral amyloid angiopathy-related hemorrhage. *J Neuropathol Exp Neurol* 1999;58:711–718.

28. Nicoll JA, Burnett C, Love S, et al. High frequency of apolipoprotein E ε2 allele in hemorrhage due to cerebral amyloid angiopathy. *Ann Neurol* 1997;41:716–721.
29. O'Donnell HC, Rosand J, Knudsen KA, et al. Apolipoprotein E genotype and the risk of recurrent lobar intracerebral hemorrhage. *N Engl J Med* 2000;342:240–245.
30. Greenberg SM, Briggs ME, Hyman BT, et al. Apolipoprotein E ε4 is associated with the presence and earlier onset of hemorrhage in cerebral amyloid angiopathy. *Stroke* 1996;27:1333–1337.
31. Biffi A, Anderson CD, Jagiella JM, et al. *APOE* genotype and extent of bleeding and outcome in lobar intracerebral haemorrhage: a genetic association study. *Lancet Neurol* 2011;10:702–709.
32. Montaner J. Genetics of intracerebral haemorrhage: a tsunami effect of *APOE* ε2 genotype on brain bleeding size? *Lancet Neurol* 2011;10:673–675.
33. Charidimou A, Gang Q, Werring DJ. Sporadic cerebral amyloid angiopathy revisited: recent insights into pathophysiology and clinical spectrum. *J Neurol Neurosurg Psychiatry* 2012;83:124–137.
34. Sumii T, Lo EH. Involvement of matrix metalloproteinase in thrombolysis-associated hemorrhagic transformation after embolic focal ischemia in rats. *Stroke* 2002;33:831–836.
35. Hernandez-Guillamon M, Mawhirt S, Fossati S, et al. Matrix metalloproteinase 2 (MMP-2) degrades soluble vasculotropic amyloid-β e22q and l34v mutants, delaying their toxicity for human brain microvascular endothelial cells. *J Biol Chem* 2010;285:27144–27158.
36. Rosenberg GA. Matrix metalloproteinases and their multiple roles in neurodegenerative diseases. *Lancet Neurol* 2009;8:205–216.
37. Lee JM, Yin KJ, Hsin I, et al. Matrix metalloproteinase-9 and spontaneous hemorrhage in an animal model of cerebral amyloid angiopathy. *Ann Neurol* 2003;54:379–382.
38. Del Zoppo GJ. Bleeding in the brain: amyloid-β may keep clots away. *Nat Med* 2009;15:1132–1133.
39. Xu F, Previti ML, Nieman MT, et al. Aβ APP/APLP2 family of Kunitz serine proteinase inhibitors regulate cerebral thrombosis. *J Neurosci* 2009;29:5666–5670.
40. Flaherty ML, Kissela B, Woo D, et al. The increasing incidence of anticoagulant-associated intracerebral hemorrhage. *Neurology* 2007;68:116–121.
41. Lovelock CE, Cordonnier C, Naka H, et al. Antithrombotic drug use, cerebral microbleeds, and intracerebral hemorrhage: a systematic review of published and unpublished studies. *Stroke* 2010;41:1222–1228.
42. Rosand J, Hylek EM, O'Donnell HC, Greenberg SM. Warfarin-associated hemorrhage and cerebral amyloid angiopathy: a genetic and pathologic study. *Neurology* 2000;55:947–951.
43. McCarron MO, Nicoll JA. Cerebral amyloid angiopathy and thrombolysis-related intracerebral haemorrhage. *Lancet Neurol* 2004;3:484–492.
44. Sloan MA, Price TR, Petito CK, et al. Clinical features and pathogenesis of intracerebral hemorrhage after RT-PA and heparin therapy for acute myocardial infarction: the Thrombolysis In Myocardial Infarction (TIMI) (ii) pilot and randomized clinical trial combined experience. *Neurology* 1995;45:649–658.
45. Kalimo H, Miao Q, Tikka S, et al. CADASIL: the most common hereditary subcortical vascular dementia. *Future Neurol* 2008;3:683–704.
46. Choi JC, Kang SY, Kang JH, Park JK. Intracerebral hemorrhages in CADASIL. *Neurology* 2006;67:2042–2044.
47. Kumar S, Goddeau RP, Jr., Selim MH, et al. Atraumatic convexal subarachnoid hemorrhage: clinical presentation, imaging patterns, and etiologies. *Neurology* 2010;74:893–899.
48. Raposo N, Viguier A, Cuvinciuc V, et al. Cortical subarachnoid haemorrhage in the elderly: a recurrent event probably related to cerebral amyloid angiopathy. *Eur J Neurol* 2011;18:597–603.
49. Linn J, Herms J, Dichgans M, et al. Subarachnoid hemosiderosis and superficial cortical hemosiderosis in cerebral amyloid angiopathy. *AJNR Am J Neuroradiol* 2008;29:184–186.
50. Cuvinciuc V, Viguier A, Calviere L, et al. Isolated acute nontraumatic cortical subarachnoid hemorrhage. *AJNR Am J Neuroradiol* 2010;31:1355–1362.
51. Katoh M, Yoshino M, Asaoka K, et al. A restricted subarachnoid hemorrhage in the cortical sulcus in cerebral amyloid angiopathy: could it be a warning sign? *Surg Neurol* 2007;68:457–460.
52. Karabatsou K, Lecky BR, Rainov NG, Broome JC, White RP. Cerebral amyloid angiopathy with symptomatic or occult subarachnoid haemorrhage. *Eur Neurol* 2007;57:103–105.
53. Kase CS, Nguyen TN. The clinical conundrum of convexal subarachnoid hemorrhage. *Neurology* 2010;74:874–875.
54. Linn J, Halpin A, Demaerel P, et al. Prevalence of superficial siderosis in patients with cerebral

amyloid angiopathy. *Neurology* 2010;74:1346–1350.

55. Beitzke M, Gattringer T, Enzinger C, et al. Clinical presentation, etiology, and long-term prognosis in patients with nontraumatic convexal subarachnoid hemorrhage. *Stroke* 2011;42:3055–3060.
56. Fearnley JM, Stevens JM, Rudge P. Superficial siderosis of the central nervous system. *Brain* 1995;118 (Pt 4):1051–1066.
57. Kumar N, Cohen-Gadol AA, Wright RA, et al. Superficial siderosis. *Neurology* 2006;66:1144–1152.
58. Feldman HH, Maia LF, Mackenzie IR, et al. Superficial siderosis: a potential diagnostic marker of cerebral amyloid angiopathy in Alzheimer disease. *Stroke* 2008;39:2894–2897.
59. Vernooij MW, Ikram MA, Hofman A, et al. Superficial siderosis in the general population. *Neurology* 2009;73:202–205.
60. Levy M, Turtzo C, Llinas RH. Superficial siderosis: a case report and review of the literature. *Nat Clin Pract Neurol* 2007;3:54–58; quiz 59.
61. Greenberg SM, Vernooij MW, Cordonnier C, et al. Cerebral microbleeds: a guide to detection and interpretation. *Lancet Neurol* 2009;8:165–174.
62. Haacke EM, DelProposto ZS, Chaturvedi S, et al. Imaging cerebral amyloid angiopathy with susceptibility-weighted imaging. *AJNR Am J Neuroradiol* 2007;28:316–317.
63. Kellner CP, Connolly ES, Jr. Neuroprotective strategies for intracerebral hemorrhage: trials and translation. *Stroke* 2010;41: S99–S102.
64. Vernooij MW, van der Lugt A, Ikram MA, et al. Prevalence and risk factors of cerebral microbleeds: the Rotterdam Scan Study. *Neurology* 2008;70:1208–1214.
65. Nandigam RN, Viswanathan A, Delgado P, et al. MR imaging detection of cerebral microbleeds: effect of susceptibility-weighted imaging, section thickness, and field strength. *AJNR Am J Neuroradiol* 2009;30:338–343.
66. Theysohn JM, Kraff O, Maderwald S, et al. Seven Tesla MRI of microbleeds and white matter lesions as seen in vascular dementia. *J Magn Reson Imaging* 2011;33:782–791.
67. Conijn MM, Geerlings MI, Luijten PR, et al. Visualization of cerebral microbleeds with dual-echo T2*-weighted magnetic resonance imaging at 7.0 T. *J Magn Reson Imaging* 2010;32:52–59.
68. De Reuck J, Auger F, Cordonnier C, et al. Comparison of 7.0-T T(2)*-magnetic resonance imaging of cerebral bleeds in postmortem brain sections of Alzheimer patients with their neuropathological correlates. *Cerebrovasc Dis* 2011;31:511–517.
69. Lee SH, Lee ST, Kim BJ, et al. Dynamic temporal change of cerebral microbleeds: long-term follow-up MRI study. *PLoS One* 2011;6:e25930.
70. Tsushima Y, Tanizaki Y, Aoki J, Endo K. MR detection of microhemorrhages in neurologically healthy adults. *Neuroradiology* 2002;44:31–36.
71. Cordonnier C. Brain microbleeds: more evidence, but still a clinical dilemma. *Curr Opin Neurol* 2011;24:69–74.
72. Loitfelder M, Seiler S, Schwingenschuh P, Schmidt R. Cerebral microbleeds: a review. *Panminerva Med* 2012;54:149–160.
73. Hofman A, Breteler MM, van Duijn CM, et al. The Rotterdam Study: 2010 objectives and design update. *Eur J Epidemiol* 2009;24:553–572.
74. Koennecke HC. Cerebral microbleeds on MRI: prevalence, associations, and potential clinical implications. *Neurology* 2006;66:165–171.
75. Cordonnier C, Al-Shahi Salman R, Wardlaw J. Spontaneous brain microbleeds: systematic review, subgroup analyses and standards for study design and reporting. *Brain* 2007;130:1988–2003.
76. Chabriat H, Joutel A, Dichgans M, Tournier-Lasserve E, Bousser MG. CADASIL. *Lancet Neurol* 2009;8:643–653.
77. Dichgans M, Holtmannspotter M, Herzog J, et al. Cerebral microbleeds in CADASIL: a gradient-echo magnetic resonance imaging and autopsy study. *Stroke* 2002;33:67–71.
78. Van den Boom R, Bornebroek M, Behloul F, et al. Microbleeds in hereditary cerebral hemorrhage with amyloidosis-Dutch type. *Neurology* 2005;64:1288–1289.
79. Sveinbjornsdottir S, Sigurdsson S, Aspelund T, et al. Cerebral microbleeds in the population based ages – Reykjavik study: prevalence and location. *J Neurol Neurosurg Psychiatry* 2008;79:1002–1006.
80. Poels MM, Vernooij MW, Ikram MA, et al. Prevalence and risk factors of cerebral microbleeds: an update of the Rotterdam Scan Study. *Stroke* 2010;41:S103–106.
81. Van Es AC, van der Grond J, de Craen AJ, et al. Cerebral microbleeds and cognitive functioning in the PROSPER study. *Neurology* 2011;77:1446–1452.
82. Henneman WJ, Sluimer JD, Cordonnier C, et al. MRI biomarkers of vascular damage and atrophy predicting mortality in a memory clinic population. *Stroke* 2009;40:492–498.
83. Altmann-Schneider I, Trompet S, de Craen AJ, et al. Cerebral microbleeds are predictive of

mortality in the elderly. *Stroke* 2011;42:638–644.

84. Fazekas F, Kleinert R, Roob G, et al. Histopathologic analysis of foci of signal loss on gradient-echo T2*-weighted MR images in patients with spontaneous intracerebral hemorrhage: evidence of microangiopathy-related microbleeds. *AJNR Am J Neuroradiol* 1999; 20:637–642.
85. Tanaka A, Ueno Y, Nakayama Y, Takano K, Takebayashi S. Small chronic hemorrhages and ischemic lesions in association with spontaneous intracerebral hematomas. *Stroke* 1999;30:1637–1642.
86. Schrag M, McAuley G, Pomakian J, et al. Correlation of hypointensities in susceptibility-weighted images to tissue histology in dementia patients with cerebral amyloid angiopathy: a postmortem MRI study. *Acta Neuropathol* 2010;119:291–302.
87. Grinberg LT, Thal DR. Vascular pathology in the aged human brain. *Acta Neuropathol* 2010;119:277–290.
88. Hommet C, Mondon K, Constans T, et al. Review of cerebral microangiopathy and Alzheimer's disease: relation between white matter hyperintensities and microbleeds. *Dement Geriatr Cogn Disord* 2011;32:367–378.
89. Shoamanesh A, Kwok CS, Benavente O. Cerebral microbleeds: histopathological correlation of neuroimaging. *Cerebrovasc Dis* 2011;32:528–534.
90. Greenberg SM, Eng JA, Ning M, Smith EE, Rosand J. Hemorrhage burden predicts recurrent intracerebral hemorrhage after lobar hemorrhage. *Stroke* 2004;35:1415–1420.
91. Knudsen KA, Rosand J, Karluk D, Greenberg SM. Clinical diagnosis of cerebral amyloid angiopathy: validation of the Boston criteria. *Neurology* 2001;56:537–539.
92. Roob G, Lechner A, Schmidt R, et al. Frequency and location of microbleeds in patients with primary intracerebral hemorrhage. *Stroke* 2000; 31:2665–2669.
93. Thal DR, Ghebremedhin E, Rub U, et al. Two types of sporadic cerebral amyloid angiopathy. *J Neuropathol Exp Neurol* 2002;61:282–293.
94. Maxwell SS, Jackson CA, Paternoster L, et al. Genetic associations with brain microbleeds: systematic review and meta-analyses. *Neurology* 2011;77:158–167.
95. Poels MM, Ikram MA, van der Lugt A, et al. Incidence of cerebral microbleeds in the general population: the Rotterdam Scan Study. *Stroke* 2011; 42:656–661.
96. Jeerakathil T, Wolf PA, Beiser A, et al. Cerebral microbleeds: prevalence and associations with cardiovascular risk factors in the Framingham Study. *Stroke* 2004;35:1831–1835.
97. Nakata-Kudo Y, Mizuno T, Yamada K, et al. Microbleeds in Alzheimer disease are more related to cerebral amyloid angiopathy than cerebrovascular disease. *Dement Geriatr Cogn Disord* 2006;22:8–14.
98. Charidimou A, Werring DJ. Cerebral microbleeds: detection, mechanisms and clinical challenges. *Future Neurol* 2011;6:587–611.
99. Cullen KM, Kocsi Z, Stone J. Microvascular pathology in the aging human brain: evidence that senile plaques are sites of microhaemorrhages. *Neurobiol Aging* 2006; 27:1786–1796.
100. Tang WK, Chen YK, Lu JY, et al. Absence of cerebral microbleeds predicts reversion of vascular "cognitive impairment no dementia" in stroke. *Int J Stroke* 2011;6:498–505.
101. Dierksen GA, Skehan ME, Khan MA, et al. Spatial relation between microbleeds and amyloid deposits in amyloid angiopathy. *Ann Neurol* 2010;68:545–548.
102. Lee SH, Bae HJ, Kwon SJ, et al. Cerebral microbleeds are regionally associated with intracerebral hemorrhage. *Neurology* 2004;62:72–76.
103. Charidimou A, Shakeshaft C, Werring DJ. Cerebral microbleeds on magnetic resonance imaging and anticoagulant-associated intracerebral hemorrhage risk. *Front Neurol* 2012;3:133.
104. Charidimou A, Werring DJ. Cerebral microbleeds and cognition in cerebrovascular disease: an update. *J Neurol Sci* 2012.
105. Gold G, Kovari E, Herrmann FR, et al. Cognitive consequences of thalamic, basal ganglia, and deep white matter lacunes in brain aging and dementia. *Stroke* 2005;36:1184–1188.
106. Werring DJ. Cerebral microbleeds: clinical and pathophysiological significance. *J Neuroimaging* 2007;17:193–203.
107. Grabowski TJ, Cho HS, Vonsattel JP, Rebeck GW, Greenberg SM. Novel amyloid precursor protein mutation in an Iowa family with dementia and severe cerebral amyloid angiopathy. *Ann Neurol* 2001;49:697–705.
108. Mandybur TI. Cerebral amyloid angiopathy: the vascular pathology and complications. *J Neuropathol Exp Neurol* 1986;45:79–90.
109. Okoye MI, Watanabe I. Ultrastructural features of cerebral amyloid angiopathy. *Hum Pathol* 1982;13:1127–1132.
110. Viswanathan A, Greenberg SM. Cerebral amyloid angiopathy in the elderly. *Ann Neurol* 2011;70:871–880.
111. Okazaki S, Sakaguchi M, Hyun B, et al. Cerebral microbleeds predict

impending intracranial hemorrhage in infective endocarditis. *Cerebrovasc Dis* 2011;32:483–488.

112. Gregoire SM, Jager HR, Yousry TA, et al. Brain microbleeds as a potential risk factor for antiplatelet-related intracerebral haemorrhage: hospital-based, case-control study. *J Neurol Neurosurg Psychiatry* 2010;81:679–684.

113. Vernooij MW, Haag MD, van der Lugt A, et al. Use of antithrombotic drugs and the presence of cerebral microbleeds: the Rotterdam Scan Study. *Arch Neurol* 2009;66:714–720.

114. Wong KS, Chan YL, Liu JY, Gao S, Lam WW. Asymptomatic microbleeds as a risk factor for aspirin-associated intracerebral hemorrhages. *Neurology* 2003;60:511–513.

115. Charidimou A, Kakar P, Fox Z, Werring DJ. Cerebral microbleeds and the risk of intracerebral haemorrhage after thrombolysis for acute ischaemic stroke: systematic review and meta-analysis. *J Neurol Neurosurg Psychiatry* 2013;84:277–280.

116. Shoamanesh A, Kwok CS, Lim PA, Benavente OR. Postthrombolysis intracranial hemorrhage risk of cerebral microbleeds in acute stroke patients: a systematic review and meta-analysis. *Int J Stroke* 2013;8:348–356.

117. Cordonnier C, van der Flier WM. Brain microbleeds and Alzheimer's disease: innocent observation or key player? *Brain* 2011;134:335–344.

Chapter 5

Experimental animal models of cerebral small vessel disease

Atticus H. Hainsworth and Hugh S. Markus

Introduction

An important factor underlying the lack of specific treatments in small vessel disease (SVD) is the lack of good animal models in which to test potential therapies [1]. Animal models have been widely used to study acute cerebral ischemia, but such models tend to produce large areas of predominantly gray matter infarction and are not representative of SVD for a number of reasons [1]. Firstly, SVD pathology is primarily in the white matter and deep gray matter nuclei, where ischemic mechanisms may differ from those in cortical gray matter [2, 3]. Secondly, chronic ischemic damage, seen on neuroimaging as leukoaraiosis, is an important component of SVD and this is not seen in standard models of acute ischemia. Thirdly, lacunar infarcts in SVD are, relative to brain size, much smaller than those in most acute infarct models such as the middle cerebral artery occlusion model. Fourthly, chronic arterial pathology occurs in SVD while almost all acute ischemic models involve acute ischemia in previously normal vessels. A useful model in SVD must describe at least some of the characteristic pathologic features of clinical disease, either the arterial changes, or white matter changes and lacunar infarcts seen in the brain, or both.

The different pathologic mechanisms underlying SVD/lacunar stroke [4] suggest that one animal model is unlikely to describe all disease features. Neuropathologic, neuroimaging, and epidemiologic data suggest that there may be at least two major categories of SVD with different clinical prognoses [4–7]. Firstly, microatheroma in the larger intracerebral arteries at the origins of the perforating vessels or within the proximal perforating arteries has been associated with one or a few larger lacunar infarcts in the absence of leukoaraiosis. Secondly, a diffuse arteriopathy affecting the smaller perforating arteries has been associated with multiple smaller lacunar infarcts [6] and leukoaraiosis [5]. In this second subtype, cerebral blood flow (CBF) and cerebral reactivity/autoregulation are reduced [8, 9] and endothelial dysfunction has been implicated [10, 11]. It has been suggested that this could result in pathology by hypoperfusion [8] and/or blood–brain barrier permeability [12]. Histopathology and transcranial Doppler data suggest that thromboembolism is not a common cause of SVD lesions [6, 13, 14].

We and others have carried out systematic reviews on animal models relevant to SVD [1], lacunar stroke [15, 16], and vascular cognitive impairment (VCI) [17]. We previously identified 15 animal models relevant to some aspect of SVD [1]. We categorized these based on four types of injury stimuli: "embolic," "hypoperfusion," "hypertensive," or "vessel damage." Here we summarize these classes, highlighting areas of progress since our previous review [1].

Embolic models

With a rationale of small artery occlusion to induce a lacune-like ischemic lesion, there is a large literature on acute embolization. Cerebral embolic lesions have been induced by intravascular injections of cholesterol, agarose, plastic microspheres, or autologous blood clot emboli, in rats, rabbits, and primates [1, 17, 18]. These resulted in scattered small infarcts or a more extensive territorial infarct. However, lesions include both cortical and subcortical infarcts and such embolic models do not represent a specific model of SVD.

Cerebral Small Vessel Disease, ed. Leonardo Pantoni and Philip B. Gorelick. Published by Cambridge University Press.

Hypoperfusion-based models

These include lesions induced by either a brief period of severe global hypoperfusion, or less severe hypoperfusion applied over a much longer timescale (weeks to months), or a focal ischemic insult. Global hypoperfusion produces white matter lesions in many animal models, reflecting the low regional CBF in white matter internal border-zone regions.

Acute global ischemic challenge

Brief global ischemia has been produced by transient occlusion of both common carotid arteries (CCA; duration 5–30 min) in gerbils and in mice of the C57BL6 strain, which have a poorly developed posterior communicating artery [19–21]. Animals show impaired learning on standard tests [17] accompanied by neuropathologic lesions in hippocampi and white matter areas [20, 21]. Oligodendrocyte death and depletion of myelin basic protein (MBP) were seen in corpus callosum and caudate white matter bundles from 3 to 7 days [19].

Chronic hypoperfusion

Bilateral surgical occlusion of both common carotid arteries (BCCAo) in adult rats produces a chronic hypoperfusion state, leading to a post-acute evolution of brain lesions and cognitive change, over a period of weeks [17]. The animals develop white matter lesions, and cognitive impairment though ischemic damage to hippocampal neurons and optic tracts is likely to contribute to the observed cognitive changes. Unsurprisingly these surgically induced models do not develop SVD-like vasculopathy, though thickening and fibrosis of capillary walls has been reported >12 months after occlusion [22].

Variants have been developed that produce less severe hypoperfusion and thus minimize hippocampal damage [23, 24]. A recent modification is "two-vessel gradual occlusion" (2-VGO), in which ameroid constrictor cuffs are placed around each CCA. The cuffs gradually swell to produce complete occlusion of the arteries at 2–3 days [25]. Following 2-VGO rats developed white matter lesions and working memory impairment over a 28-day period. They had reduced inflammatory responses, and less hippocampal and optic tract damage, relative to standard BCCAo rats [25].

Chronic carotid stenosis

Chronic carotid stenosis using surgical microcoils has been characterized in mice [26, 27]. After 30 days of chronic hypoperfusion, animals showed impaired performance on a working memory task, while maintaining normal neurologic function in a battery of behavioral tests [26, 28]. Microglial and astrocyte proliferation was seen as early as three days, with white matter vacuolation in the corpus callosum from around 14 days, but no gray matter lesions [27, 28]. In white matter areas there were some apoptotic cells and loss of MBP, with minimal damage to the optic tract and hippocampus. Chronically, some hippocampal hypometabolism was seen on positron emission tomography (PET) imaging, and hippocampal atrophy seen histologically after eight months [26, 29]. In mice with more severe stenosis, locomotor damage was observed [26, 27, 29].

Mouse unilateral common carotid occlusion

Modest cerebral hypoperfusion was achieved by surgical occlusion of only the right common carotid artery (mouse unilateral common carotid occlusion [UCCAo]) in C57BL6 mice [30]. Shortly after surgery these mice showed reduced CBF (to 50–70%) in the ipsilateral hemisphere without change in the contralateral hemisphere, recovering to approximately 80% by four weeks [30, 31]. At four weeks, novel object recognition was substantially impaired (relative to sham-operated mice), though T-maze learning and motor activity were normal [30]. No hippocampal cellular damage was seen at seven days [31]. Immunohistochemical labeling showed reduced neurofilament density, suggesting loss of axons, and elevation of microglia, in the corpus callosum but not in caudate white matter [30].

Focal hypoperfusion models

Intracerebral injections of the vasoconstrictor endothelin-1 in rats produce a transient local ischemia (1–2 h) and a focal infarct [32, 33]. Animals with a unilateral striatal injection showed the expected neurologic deficits, with forelimb asymmetry and impaired motor performance at 14 days [33]. Similar strategic infarcts have been produced in the internal capsule [32].

Hypertensive models

Hypertensive primates

Nonhuman primates have large gyrencephalic brains, abundant white matter, and complex behaviors that resemble aspects of human cognition [34–37]. Macaque monkeys with surgical narrowing of the thoracic aorta developed chronic hypertension and, from approximately 12 months post-operatively, a decline in cognitive function [37]. As well as short-term memory deficit, monkeys showed impairment in attention and executive function. Impairment in cognitive function correlated with increased systolic and diastolic blood pressure [37]. Neuropathologically the most prominent lesions were microinfarcts (<500 μm diameter) of irregular shape, associated with local gliosis, scattered through gray and white matter in cerebral cortex, brainstem, and cerebellum, particularly in forebrain white matter [34, 37]. Apart from some local microglial activation, no blood vessel pathology was seen [34].

Stroke-prone spontaneously hypertensive rats

Spontaneously hypertensive stroke-prone rats (SHRSP) were derived from the Wistar–Kyoto strain by selective breeding for high arterial blood pressure and incidence of stroke lesions in adulthood. They develop progressive hypertension from the approximate age of eight weeks, reaching severe hypertension from approximately 12 weeks, and are suggested to resemble a variety of vascular disease states [1, 15–17]. The molecular cause of their phenotype is still unknown. Lesions occur in diverse brain areas and have a range of size and severity, a substantial fraction being hemorrhagic. Lesion occurrence is unpredictable and a modified diet (elevated sodium, low potassium) is often used to precipitate stroke events. Probably due to their chronically hypertensive state, SHRSP develop arterial wall thickening, particularly in their large leptomeningeal arteries. There are few investigations of white matter changes in SHRSP, prior to stroke events [1]. Magnetic resonance imaging (MRI) studies suggest that leukoaraiosis-like white matter changes are not a feature of stroke-free SHRSP [38–40]. In a longitudinal MRI study, focal leakage of intravascular contrast agent (indicative of local blood–brain barrier breakdown) was seen up to 14 days prior to a stroke lesion in the affected brain area [41].

Vessel damage-based models

Hyperhomocysteinemic rodents

Mild to moderate hyperhomocysteinemia can be induced by elevated dietary homocysteine or its precursor methionine. Mice exposed to high methionine diet (for 10 weeks) developed learning and memory impairment [42]. Histopathologic changes included hippocampal endothelial damage and reduced numbers of microglia, but no detectable neurodegeneration [42, 43].

Hyperhomocysteinemia is also observed in transgenic mice deficient in methylenetetrahydrofolate reductase (MTHFR) or cystathionine-β-synthase (CBS), both enzymes involved in homocysteine metabolism [44–46]. Homozygous null mice have severe phenotype and substantial elevation of total plasma homocysteine (30 μM in MTHFR$^{-/-}$ and up to 200 μM in CBS$^{-/-}$ animals, relative to ~3 μM in wild type mice) [47]. Heterozygotes, however, have only mild hyperhomocysteinemia (5–10 μM) [47]. Wall thickening in cerebral arteries with some modest increase in blood–brain permeability was seen in CBS$^{+/-}$ mice [45, 46].

CADASIL *NOTCH3* transgenic mice

Cerebral autosomal dominant arteriopathy with subcortical infarcts and leukoencephalopathy (CADASIL) is a rare, monogenic form of SVD caused by mutations in *NOTCH3*, a large transmembrane receptor found in vascular myocytes of adult arteries [48]. CADASIL has many similarities to hypertension-related SVD with lacunar infarcts and leukoaraiosis, in terms of neuroimaging, clinical profile, and neuropathology, but is earlier in onset and less hypertension dependent [48].

Recently two groups have reported transgenic mice with phenotype relevant to CADASIL [49, 50]. One strain carries an artificial chromosome to express the rat homolog of *NOTCH3* with the CADASIL-causing R169C-point mutation (Notch3^{R169C}) [49, 51]. The other carries the equivalent mutation in the murine *Notch3* gene (referred to as Notch3^{Arg170Cys}) [50]. Both strains developed granular osmiophilic (GOM) deposits (a hallmark of CADASIL) in vessel myocytes, and had normal lifespan [49, 50]. In Notch3^{R169C} mice, vascular pathology including GOM deposits was seen from five months, and astrogliosis from 12 months. Aged Notch3^{R169C} mice (18–20 months) showed extensive white matter lesions in the corpus callosum, striatum, internal capsule, and hippocampus. There was no change in blood–brain barrier permeability and no stroke lesions were observed [49]. Abnormal myogenic and autoregulatory responses were noted from age six months, and reduced resting CBF was present at 12 months. Cerebrovascular response to the hypercapnic carbon dioxide challenge was also impaired [49].

The Notch3^{Arg170Cys} strain exhibited GOM deposits at nine months and, later, some evidence of stroke-like lesions. Motor impairments (limb paresis, staggering gait) were seen from age 13 months in some individuals (~12%, 9 in a cohort of 73) [50]. In aged animals (20–22 months) brain parenchymal lesions were present in a substantial proportion (17/73, 23%) including microhemorrhages, microinfarction, and small cystic cavities [50]. As the authors point out, the presence of brain lesions in only a subgroup (<30% of individuals) suggests that modifying factors additional to genotype determine disease incidence [50].

These are interesting transgenic models, displaying vasculopathy prior to white matter lesions and – in the case of Notch3^{Arg170Cys} – prior to stroke symptoms. Although the molecular basis likely differs from sporadic SVD, the mechanisms by which cerebral small vessel arteriopathy causes white matter lesions may well be similar. Both strains may be useful for testing therapeutic interventions.

M5R$^{-/-}$ transgenic mice

Muscarinic acetylcholine receptor M5-null mice exhibit constitutive vasoconstriction of the cerebral arteries, with globally attenuated CBF [52, 53]. Relative to wild type littermates, M5R$^{-/-}$ mice showed impaired performance in cognitive tests [52, 53]. Electrophysiologic measures of synaptic strengthening (long-term potentiation, paired pulse facilitation) were also impaired [52]. Histopathologically, M5R$^{-/-}$ mice had reduced dendritic branching in cortical neurons, and swelling of astrocytes in the cortex and hippocampus [52, 53].

Comorbidities

Advanced age

Aged animals can display cognitive and neuropathologic changes resembling those in aged humans. These are seen in rats and mice from age approximately 12 months [54, 55]. In aged dogs a "canine cognitive dysfunction syndrome" is recognized, encompassing decreased attention and activity, sleep disruption, spatial disorientation, and incontinence [56, 57]. Relative to young controls, aged dogs (8–18 years) exhibited worse scores on learning tasks [56, 58]. These were accompanied by vascular lesions, including vessel wall fibrosis with focal thickening in both venous and arterial vessels, cerebral amyloid angiopathy (CAA), parenchymal β-amyloid (Aβ) deposits, widened cerebral ventricles and sulci, and reduced CBF in gray matter and white matter [56–58].

Aged squirrel monkeys (>13 years) develop a striking pattern of cortical gray matter CAA, and a lesser degree of parenchymal Aβ plaques [59]. CAA was particularly evident in capillaries. Microhemorrhages, fibrinoid exudation, and white matter lesions were rare, even in aged animals with severe CAA [59]. In cynomologus macaques no cognitive differences were seen between "middle-aged" (10–12 years) and "aged" animals (15–17 years) [36]. Aged animals showed improved cognitive performance relative to age-matched sedentary controls, following a five-month regime of daily physical exercise, accompanied by a modest increase in vascularity of the motor cortex [36].

Amyloid disease

Cerebral amyloid disorders, including CAA, are reproduced in a range of transgenic mouse strains. CAA is also evident in aged dogs and primates (see above). There are authoritative recent reviews of animal models of Alzheimer's disease [60] and of the vascular effects of amyloidopathy in animals [61].

Diabetes mellitus

Chronic experimental diabetes mellitus (DM) is observed in rodents following a single intraperitoneal injection of streptazocin (a model of type 1 DM) or in transgenic murine strains, such as KK-A^{y} or ob/ob (type 2 DM) [62, 63]. Double transgenic mice were obtained by crossing APP23 Alzheimer mice with two diabetic strains (leptin-deficient ob/ob, or polygenic NSY) [63]. As early as eight weeks of age, learning deficits were seen in double transgenic mice (but not in APP23 or ob/ob single transgenics) that were independent of visual dysfunction or obesity [63]. In APP23-ob/ob mice histopathologic changes included depletion of hippocampal cholinergic axons and marked astrogliosis, vascular inflammation, and amyloid angiopathy. No amyloid plaques were seen in these animals. Expression of receptor for advanced glycation end-products (RAGE) was evident in cerebral vessels from age three months, with CAA evident from age six months, and severe brain atrophy at age 12 months [63].

The effects of diabetic disease combined with hypertension have also been explored [64]. Over a five-month timescale, rats with type 1 DM exhibited reduced oligodendrocyte density while hypertensive rats (SHR strain) showed no such reduction. The combination of DM and hypertension gave more pronounced oligodendrocyte loss than DM alone. The potentiating effects of hypertension were similar in both type 1 and type 2 DM models [64]. The effects of DM, and the interaction with hypertension, appeared to be independent of changes in CBF or tissue ischemia.

Intervention studies

Recent years have seen increased awareness of the need for standardization in preclinical testing of drugs and other interventions [65, 66]. While there is no clear predictive model of SVD, recent studies have addressed some aspects of SVD. Rats subjected to chronic hypoperfusion (BCCAo) developed white matter lesions and cognition deficits that were ameliorated by treatment with cholinergic agents [54, 67], or by the phosphodiesterase (PDE3) inhibitor cilostazol [68]. In a well-conducted study, adult rats were randomized to vehicle or cilostazol (provided orally in chow, equivalent to 50 mg/kg per day) for 28 days following BCCAo surgery [68]. Drug-treated animals exhibited improved performance on the Morris water maze and, on histologic examination of white matter areas, reduced apoptotic cell numbers and elevated density of oligodendroglia [68]. Another study found white matter preservation in SHRSP following 20 weeks of cilostazol treatment [69]. These white matter-sparing effects appear to be independent of changes in arterial blood pressure [68, 69].

In another recent example, effects of combination therapy in severe hypertension were explored [70]. SHRSP fed a high sodium diet for 28 days were treated with either amlodipine (a calcium channel antagonist) or valsartan (an angiotensin receptor blocker), or both drugs. In vehicle-treated animals mortality was greater than 80% and incidence of neurologic impairment greater than 90% by the end of the 28-day study period. Either drug reduced both mortality and morbidity, while the combination of drugs reduced both mortality and morbidity to nil [70]. The additive effect of the two drugs was evident in terms of improved endothelial function and reduced arterial thickening, white matter astrocytosis, and microgliosis (Figures 5.1 and 5.2 [70]). While these beneficial effects were clearly mediated in part by antihypertensive action, there were also effects on brain parenchymal cells (such as reduced AT1R expression on astrocytes and microglia) that may contribute to the observed treatment effects.

Perspective

As concluded by previous systematic reviews [1, 15, 71], no animal model reproduces all features of human SVD. This is likely to result from the differences between animals and humans in lifespan, brain size, cerebral development, white : gray matter volume ratio, and vessel dimensions. While capillaries are similar in scale across species, a "deep penetrating artery" in mouse caudate–putamen bears little resemblance to the human deep penetrating arteries that manifest SVD [4, 13, 72].

The utility of experimental animal models lies in three areas. Firstly, animals allow us to explore SVD-related pathologic processes at the cell/molecular level in vivo. Examples are fibrotic thickening of artery walls [49, 63, 70], or ischemic white matter damage [25, 39, 49, 73, 74]. There is a clear caveat that such models do not necessarily equate to the chronology and causality of human SVD pathogenesis, though similar chronic pathologic pathways may apply in aged humans and aged primates [34–37], and in other large mammals [56–58]. Secondly, animal models have potential benefit for testing the effects of drugs and other interventions on specific pathologic processes. Well-defined preclinical studies in validated in vivo models will improve subsequent clinical trial design [65, 66]. Recent examples are given above [54, 62, 67–70]. Thirdly, experimental models allow us to examine the interactions of different pathologic pathways. The interactions of SVD with comorbidities such as Alzheimer's disease, DM, and obesity, as well as normal aging, are likely to be clinically relevant. Prospective animal studies offer a testing ground in which to tease apart the risk factors

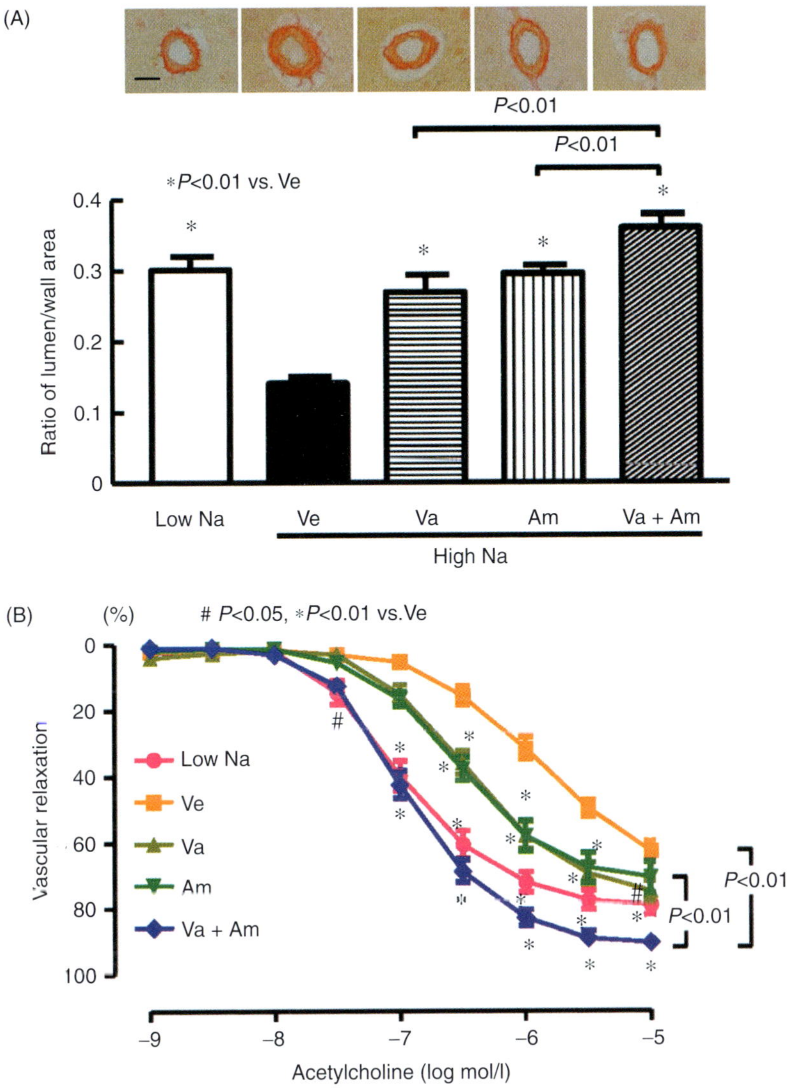

Figure 5.1 Effects of valsartan, amplodipine, or the combination of both drugs in spontaneously hypertensive stroke-prone rats (SHRSP). Cerebral vascular remodeling in cerebral cortical arterioles (A) and acetylcholine-induced, endothelium-dependent relaxation of isolated carotid arteries (B) were studied in adult male SHRSP. (A) Top panel shows representative small arteries stained with Sirius red. Animals on high salt diet (High Na) exhibited vessel wall thickening, reflected in lumen : wall area ratio, relative to SHRSP on normal diet (Low Na). Treatment with valsartan (Va) or amplodipine (Am) reduced vessel thickening, relative to vehicle-treated (Ve) animals. Drugs were administered orally (both 2 mg/kg per day) for four weeks. The combination of both drugs (Va + Am) was more effective than either agent alone ($P < 0.01$, one-way analysis of variance [ANOVA]). (B) Bottom panel shows potency of acetylcholine (as a measure of endothelium-dependent vessel relaxation) and exhibited a similar pattern. Symbols show mean ± standard error of mean [SEM] (N = 5–8). From reference [70], reproduced with permission.

involved, with a degree of control that would not be feasible in the multifactorial clinical setting. Recent examples explored the interaction of diabetic and obesity-related disease with amyloidopathy [63], or with hypertension [64]. Others combined surgically induced hypoperfusion with genetic hypertension (SHRSP) to produce specific and predictable white matter lesions [39].

In conclusion, no one model describes all the features of human SVD – different models offer the potential to model different aspects of the human disease [1]. The choice of model will depend on the research question being asked. For example, interventions designed to reduce arterial damage may require different models from those required by interventions designed to prevent white matter damage. SHRSP and Notch3 transgenic mice (discussed above) reproduce some aspects of the arteriopathy of human SVD. To study leukoaraiosis-like white matter damage, there are a number of potentially useful models based on hypoperfusion. Although differing in underlying molecular pathology from sporadic SVD, the CADASIL transgenic model may represent a useful model to determine how small vessel arteriopathy results in ischemic damage, and to test the effect of therapeutic interventions.

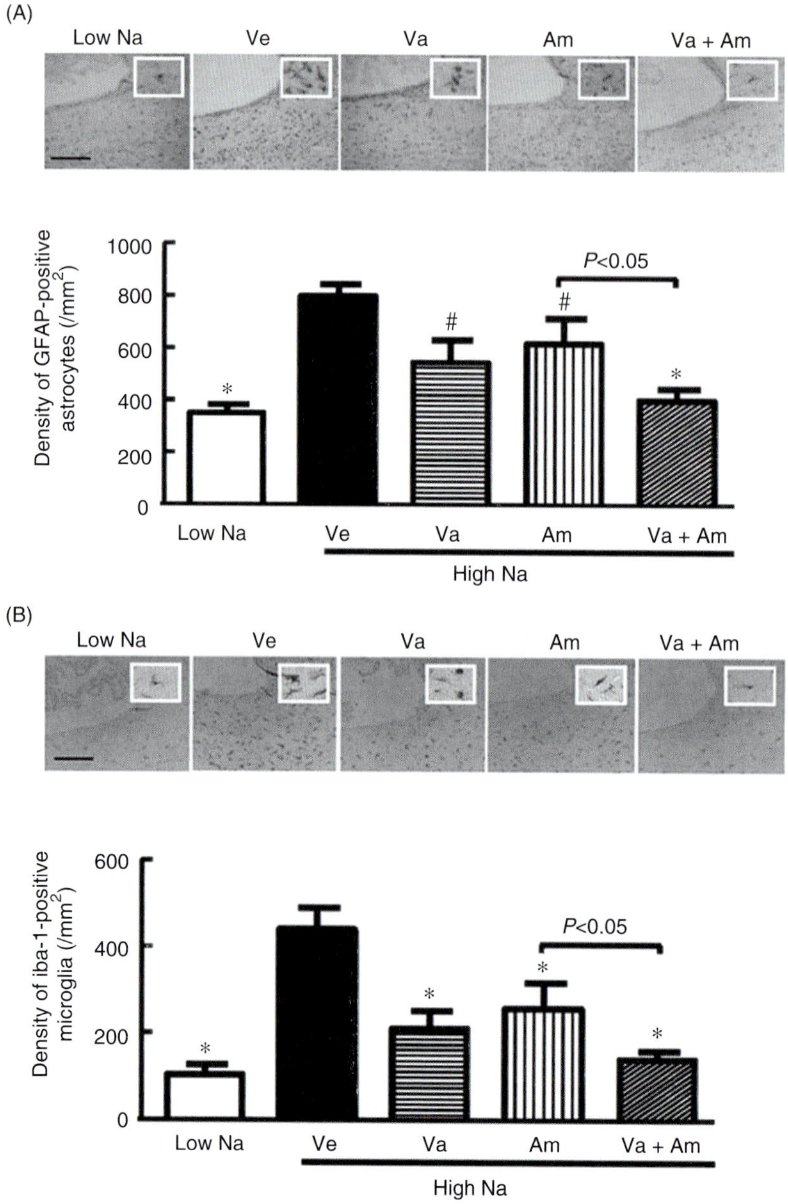

Figure 5.2 Astrocyte and microglial density in white matter of spontaneously hypertensive stroke-prone rats (SHRSP): effects of valsartan, amplodipine, or the combination of both drugs. Density of astrocytes (A, labeled with glial fibrillary acidic protein [GFAP]) or microglia (B, labeled with Iba-1) were studied in adult male SHRSP. Upper panels show representative micrographs, scale bars: 200 µm. Inset panels show enlarged images. Animals on high salt diet (High Na) exhibited increased astrocyte density (A) and microglial density (B) relative to SHRSP on normal diet (Low Na). Treatment with valsartan (Va) or amplodipine (Am), or both drugs (Va + Am) reduced cell density, relative to vehicle-treated animals (Ve). Drugs were administered orally (both 2 mg/kg per day) for four weeks. Bars show mean + standard error of mean [SEM] (N = 6–9). #*P* <0.05, **P* <0.01 relative to Ve (one-way analysis of variance [ANOVA]). From reference [70], reproduced with permission.

References

1. Hainsworth AH, Markus HS. Do in vivo experimental models reflect human cerebral small vessel disease? A systematic review. *J Cereb Blood Flow Metab* 2008;28:1877–1891.
2. Imai H, Masayasu H, Dewar D, et al. Ebselen protects both gray and white matter in a rodent model of focal cerebral ischemia. *Stroke* 2001;32:2149–2154.
3. Sarti C, Pantoni L. Experimental models of vascular dementia: a focus on white matter disease and incomplete infarction. In Bowler JV, Hachinski V, eds. *Vascular Cognitive Impairment: Preventable Dementia*. Oxford: Oxford University Press; 2003: pp. 76–92.
4. Pantoni L. Cerebral small vessel disease: from pathogenesis and clinical characteristics to therapeutic challenges. *Lancet Neurol* 2010;9:689–701.
5. Boiten J, Lodder J, Kessels F. Two clinically distinct lacunar infarct

entities? A hypothesis. *Stroke* 1993;24:652–656.

6. Fisher CM. The arterial lesions underlying lacunes. *Acta Neuropathol* 1968;12:1–15.
7. Khan U, Porteous L, Hassan A, Markus HS. Risk factor profile of cerebral small vessel disease and its subtypes. *J Neurol Neurosurg Psychiatry* 2007;78:702–706.
8. O'Sullivan M, Lythgoe DJ, Pereira AC, et al. Patterns of cerebral blood flow reduction in patients with ischemic leukoaraiosis. *Neurology* 2002;59:321–326.
9. Terborg C, Gora F, Weiller C, Rother J. Reduced vasomotor reactivity in cerebral microangiopathy: a study with near-infrared spectroscopy and transcranial Doppler sonography. *Stroke* 2000;31:924–929.
10. Fernando MS, Simpson JE, Matthews F, et al. White matter lesions in an unselected cohort of the elderly: molecular pathology suggests origin from chronic hypoperfusion injury. *Stroke* 2006;37:1391–1398.
11. Hassan A, Hunt BJ, O'Sullivan M, et al. Markers of endothelial dysfunction in lacunar infarction and ischaemic leukoaraiosis. *Brain* 2003;126:424–432.
12. Wardlaw JM, Sandercock PA, Dennis MS, Starr J. Is breakdown of the blood–brain barrier responsible for lacunar stroke, leukoaraiosis, and dementia? *Stroke* 2003;34:806–812.
13. Giwa MO, Williams J, Elderfield K, et al. Neuropathologic evidence of endothelial changes in cerebral small vessel disease. *Neurology* 2012;78:167–174.
14. Kaposzta Z, Young E, Bath PM, Markus HS. Clinical application of asymptomatic embolic signal detection in acute stroke: a prospective study. *Stroke* 1999;30:1814–1818.
15. Bailey EL, McCulloch J, Sudlow C, Wardlaw JM. Potential animal models of lacunar stroke: a systematic review. *Stroke* 2009;40: e451–e458.
16. Bailey EL, Wardlaw JM, Graham D, et al. Cerebral small vessel endothelial structural changes predate hypertension in stroke-prone spontaneously hypertensive rats: a blinded, controlled immunohistochemical study of 5- to 21-week-old rats. *Neuropathol Appl Neurobiol* 2011;37:711–726.
17. Jiwa NS, Garrard P, Hainsworth AH. Experimental models of vascular dementia and vascular cognitive impairment. A systematic review. *J Neurochem* 2010;115:814–828.
18. Sato Y, Chin Y, Kato T, et al. White matter activated glial cells produce BDNF in a stroke model of monkeys. *Neurosci Res* 2009;65:71–78.
19. Walker EJ, Rosenberg GA. Divergent role for MMP-2 in myelin breakdown and oligodendrocyte death following transient global ischemia. *J Neurosci Res* 2010;88:764–773.
20. Yamamoto Y, Shioda N, Han F, et al. Nobiletin improves brain ischemia-induced learning and memory deficits through stimulation of CaMKII and CREB phosphorylation. *Brain Res* 2009;1295:218–229.
21. Lai M, Horsburgh K, Bae SE, et al. Forebrain mineralocorticoid receptor overexpression enhances memory, reduces anxiety and attenuates neuronal loss in cerebral ischaemia. *Eur J Neurosci* 2007;25:1832–1842.
22. Farkas E, Luiten PG, Bari F. Permanent, bilateral common carotid artery occlusion in the rat: a model for chronic cerebral hypoperfusion-related neurodegenerative diseases. *Brain Res Rev* 2007;54:162–180.
23. Ohta H, Nishikawa H, Kimura H, Anayama H, Miyamoto M. Chronic cerebral hypoperfusion by permanent internal carotid ligation produces learning impairment without brain damage in rats. *Neuroscience* 1997;79:1039–1050.
24. Sarti C, Pantoni L, Bartolini L, Inzitari D. Persistent impairment of gait performances and working memory after bilateral common carotid artery occlusion in the adult Wistar rat. *Behav Brain Res* 2002;136:13–20.
25. Kitamura A, Fujita Y, Oishi N, et al. Selective white matter abnormalities in a novel rat model of vascular dementia. *Neurobiol Aging* 2012;33:1012–1035.
26. Nishio K, Ihara M, Yamasaki N, et al. A mouse model characterizing features of vascular dementia with hippocampal atrophy. *Stroke* 2010;41:1278–1284.
27. Shibata M, Ohtani R, Ihara M, Tomimoto H. White matter lesions and glial activation in a novel mouse model of chronic cerebral hypoperfusion. *Stroke* 2004;35:2598–2603.
28. Shibata M, Yamasaki N, Miyakawa T, et al. Selective impairment of working memory in a mouse model of chronic cerebral hypoperfusion. *Stroke* 2007;38:2826–2832.
29. Miki K, Ishibashi S, Sun L, et al. Intensity of chronic cerebral hypoperfusion determines white/gray matter injury and cognitive/motor dysfunction in mice. *J Neurosci Res* 2009;87:1270–1281.
30. Yoshizaki K, Adachi K, Kataoka S, et al. Chronic cerebral hypoperfusion induced by right unilateral common carotid artery occlusion causes delayed white matter lesions and cognitive impairment in adult mice. *Exp Neurol* 2008;210:585–591.
31. Kitagawa K, Yagita Y, Sasaki T, et al. Chronic mild reduction of cerebral perfusion pressure induces ischemic tolerance in focal cerebral ischemia. *Stroke* 2005;36:2270–2274.

32. Lecrux C, McCabe C, Weir CJ, et al. Effects of magnesium treatment in a model of internal capsule lesion in spontaneously hypertensive rats. *Stroke* 2008;39:448–454.

33. Whitehead SN, Hachinski VC, Cechetto DF. Interaction between a rat model of cerebral ischemia and β-amyloid toxicity: inflammatory responses. *Stroke* 2005;36:107–112.

34. Kemper TL, Blatt GJ, Killiany RJ, Moss MB. Neuropathology of progressive cognitive decline in chronically hypertensive rhesus monkeys. *Acta Neuropathol (Berl)* 2001;101:145–153.

35. Ndung'u M, Hartig W, Wegner F, et al. Cerebral Aβ42 deposits and microvascular pathology in ageing baboons. *Neuropathol Appl Neurobiol* 2012;38:487–499.

36. Rhyu IJ, Bytheway JA, Kohler SJ, et al. Effects of aerobic exercise training on cognitive function and cortical vascularity in monkeys. *Neuroscience* 2010;167: 1239–1248.

37. Moss MB, Jonak E. Cerebrovascular disease and dementia: a primate model of hypertension and cognition. *Alzheimers Dement* 2007;3: S6–S15.

38. Henning EC, Warach S, Spatz M. Hypertension-induced vascular remodeling contributes to reduced cerebral perfusion and the development of spontaneous stroke in aged SHRSP rats. *J Cereb Blood Flow Metab* 2010;30:827–836.

39. Jalal FY, Yang Y, Thompson J, Lopez AC, Rosenberg GA. Myelin loss associated with neuroinflammation in hypertensive rats. *Stroke* 2012;43:1115–1122.

40. Schreiber S, Bueche CZ, Garz C, et al. The pathologic cascade of cerebrovascular lesions in SHRSP: is erythrocyte accumulation an early phase? *J Cereb Blood Flow Metab* 2012;32:278–290.

41. Lee JM, Zhai G, Liu Q, et al. Vascular permeability precedes spontaneous intracerebral hemorrhage in stroke-prone spontaneously hypertensive rats. *Stroke* 2007;38:3289–3291.

42. Troen AM, Shea-Budgell M, Shukitt-Hale B, et al. B-vitamin deficiency causes hyperhomocysteinemia and vascular cognitive impairment in mice. *Proc Natl Acad Sci USA* 2008;105:12474–12479.

43. Lee H, Kim JM, Kim HJ, Lee I, Chang N. Folic acid supplementation can reduce the endothelial damage in rat brain microvasculature due to hyperhomocysteinemia. *J Nutr* 2005;135:544–548.

44. Mikael LG, Wang XL, Wu Q, et al. Hyperhomocysteinemia is associated with hypertriglyceridemia in mice with methylenetetrahydrofolate reductase deficiency. *Mol Genet Metab* 2009;98:187–194.

45. Baumbach GL, Sigmund CD, Bottiglieri T, Lentz SR. Structure of cerebral arterioles in cystathionine β-synthase-deficient mice. *Circ Res* 2002;91:931–937.

46. Kamath AF, Chauhan AK, Kisucka J, et al. Elevated levels of homocysteine compromise blood–brain barrier integrity in mice. *Blood* 2006;107:591–593.

47. Troen AM. The central nervous system in animal models of hyperhomocysteinemia. *Prog Neuropsychopharmacol Biol Psychiatry* 2005;29:1140–1151.

48. Chabriat H, Joutel A, Dichgans M, Tournier-Lasserve E, Bousser MG. CADASIL. *Lancet Neurol* 2009;8:643–653.

49. Joutel A, Monet-Lepretre M, Gosele C, et al. Cerebrovascular dysfunction and microcirculation rarefaction precede white matter lesions in a mouse genetic model of cerebral ischemic small vessel disease. *J Clin Invest* 2010;120:433–445.

50. Wallays G, Nuyens D, Silasi-Mansat R, et al. Notch3 Arg170Cys knock-in mice display pathologic and clinical features of the neurovascular disorder cerebral autosomal dominant arteriopathy with subcortical infarcts and leukoencephalopathy. *Arterioscler Thromb Vasc Biol* 2011;31:2881–2888.

51. Ayata C. CADASIL: experimental insights from animal models. *Stroke* 2010;41:S129–S134.

52. Araya R, Noguchi T, Yuhki M, et al. Loss of M5 muscarinic acetylcholine receptors leads to cerebrovascular and neuronal abnormalities and cognitive deficits in mice. *Neurobiol Dis* 2006;24:334–344.

53. Kitamura N, Araya R, Kudoh M, et al. Beneficial effects of estrogen in a mouse model of cerebrovascular insufficiency. *PLoS One* 2009;4:e51–e59.

54. Storozheva ZI, Proshin AT, Sherstnev VV, et al. Dicholine salt of succinic acid, a neuronal insulin sensitizer, ameliorates cognitive deficits in rodent models of normal aging, chronic cerebral hypoperfusion, and β-amyloid peptide-(25–35) β-induced amnesia. *BMC Pharmacol* 2008;8:1.

55. Park L, Anrather J, Girouard H, Zhou P, Iadecola C. Nox2-derived reactive oxygen species mediate neurovascular dysregulation in the aging mouse brain. *J Cereb Blood Flow Metab* 2007;27:1908–1918.

56. Cummings BJ, Head E, Ruehl W, Milgram NW, Cotman CW. The canine as an animal model of human aging and dementia. *Neurobiol Aging* 1996;17:259–268.

57. Borras D, Ferrer I, Pumarola M. Age-related changes in the brain of the dog. *Vet Pathol* 1999;36:202–211.

58. Head E, Mehta R, Hartley J, et al. Spatial learning and memory as a function of age in the dog. *Behav Neurosci* 1995;109:851–858.
59. Elfenbein HA, Rosen RF, Stephens SL, et al. Cerebral β-amyloid angiopathy in aged squirrel monkeys. *Histol Histopathol* 2007;22:155–167.
60. LaFerla FM, Green KN. Animal models of Alzheimer disease. *Cold Spring Harb Perspect Med* 2012;2: a006320.
61. Hamel E, Nicolakakis N, Aboulkassim T, Ongali B, Tong XK. Oxidative stress and cerebrovascular dysfunction in mouse models of Alzheimer's disease. *Exp Physiol* 2008;93:116–120.
62. Tsukuda K, Mogi M, Li JM, et al. Amelioration of cognitive impairment in the type-2 diabetic mouse by the angiotensin II type-1 receptor blocker candesartan. *Hypertension* 2007;50:1099–1105.
63. Takeda S, Sato N, Uchio-Yamada K, et al. Diabetes-accelerated memory dysfunction via cerebrovascular inflammation and Aβ deposition in an Alzheimer mouse model with diabetes. *Proc Natl Acad Sci USA* 2010;107:7036–7041.
64. Yang C, Devisser A, Martínez JA, et al. Differential impact of diabetes and hypertension in the brain: adverse effects in white matter. *Neurobiol Dis* 2011;42:446–458.
65. Landis SC, Amara SG, Asadullah K, et al. A call for transparent reporting to optimize the predictive value of preclinical research. *Nature* 2012;490: 187–191.
66. Kilkenny C, Browne WJ, Cuthill IC, Emerson M, Altman DG. Improving bioscience research reporting: the ARRIVE guidelines for reporting animal research. *PLoS Biol* 2010;8: e1000412.
67. Wang J, Zhang HY, Tang XC. Huperzine a improves chronic inflammation and cognitive decline in rats with cerebral hypoperfusion. *J Neurosci Res* 2010;88:807–815.
68. Miyamoto N, Tanaka R, Shimura H, et al. Phosphodiesterase III inhibition promotes differentiation and survival of oligodendrocyte progenitors and enhances regeneration of ischemic white matter lesions in the adult mammalian brain. *J Cereb Blood Flow Metab* 2010; 30:299–310.
69. Fujita Y, Lin JX, Takahashi R, Tomimoto H. Cilostazol alleviates cerebral small-vessel pathology and white-matter lesions in stroke-prone spontaneously hypertensive rats. *Brain Res* 2008;1203:170–176.
70. Dong YF, Kataoka K, Tokutomi Y, et al. Beneficial effects of combination of valsartan and amlodipine on salt-induced brain injury in hypertensive rats. *J Pharmacol Exp Ther* 2011;339:358–366.
71. Bailey EL, Smith C, Sudlow CL, Wardlaw JM. Is the spontaneously hypertensive stroke prone rat a pertinent model of subcortical ischemic stroke? A systematic review. *Int J Stroke* 2011;6:434–444.
72. Lammie GA. Hypertensive cerebral small vessel disease and stroke. *Brain Pathol* 2002;12:358–370.
73. Holland PR, Bastin ME, Jansen MA, et al. MRI is a sensitive marker of subtle white matter pathology in hypoperfused mice. *Neurobiol Aging* 2011;32:2325–2326.
74. Brittain JF, McCabe C, Khatun H, et al. An MRI-histological study of white matter in stroke-free SHRSP. *J Cereb Blood Flow Metab* 2013;33:760–763.

Chapter 6

Sporadic small vessel disease: pathogenic aspects

Joanna M. Wardlaw and Leonardo Pantoni

Introduction

As detailed in the first chapter of this book, the term small vessel disease (SVD) refers to many different types of parenchyma lesions. According to the most recent position paper [1], six types of SVD lesions are described: (1) recent small subcortical infarcts; (2) lacunes of presumed vascular origin; (3) white matter hyperintensities (WMHs) of presumed vascular origin; (4) perivascular spaces; (5) cerebral microbleeds; and (6) brain atrophy. These lesions have rather different pathologic aspects and possibly different pathogenic mechanisms – as is the case for lesions of putative ischemic origin (lacunar infarcts) and of those with a hemorrhagic nature such as microbleeds. Moreover, some lesions, such as perivascular spaces, have been known for many years, but only recently have they become encompassed under the "umbrella" term SVD, and their pathogenesis has not been investigated in such a detailed way as have other SVD lesions so far. The handling of the pathogenesis of each single lesion seems difficult, may be very theoretical, and in addition some mechanisms may be common to different lesion types. Therefore, in this chapter we will restrict this review to those mechanisms for which more evidence exists and data are available to review.

In a previous review paper, one of us provided a general overview of the pathogenic aspects of SVD [2]. This scheme foresees, at the basic level, an interaction between genetic and risk factors (including, in a broad sense, also aging) to determine the typical pathologic changes of the small vessels of the brain. The main concepts based on pathologic observations that are essential to understand the possible pathogenesis of sporadic SVD are:

1. There are striking changes in small arteries and arterioles, summarized by in the loss of smooth muscle cells and the replacement of wall constituents by other materials (e.g., collagen, not otherwise defined hyaline material, or amyloid).
2. The vessel lumen is restricted or dilated – the general architecture of the vascular tree is disrupted with increased vessel tortuosity and elongation, and formation of aneurysmal sacs.

The subsequent mechanisms leading to the brain parenchyma damage are:

1. There is a reduced or dysregulated blood flow that can be focal and severe in some areas leading to small infarcts.
2. Some areas suffer from a state of more chronic ischemia that is not severe enough to determine tissue pan-necrosis but causes selective damage to some cell populations (such as neurons or oligodendrocytes).
3. The wall of some vessels ruptures and parenchymal hemorrhage occurs.
4. The changes in small vessels lead to damage to the blood–brain barrier and this leads, secondarily, to extravasation of fluids and different molecules into the brain parenchyma.

In the following paragraphs we will review some of these mechanisms. We will not touch upon the mechanisms of hemorrhage since this topic is dealt with in other chapters of this book.

Ischemia and SVD

The hypothesis that ischemia plays an important role in SVD originates from two main groups of observations: (1) the original work of C. Miller Fisher in relation to lacunar infarcts [3, 4]; and (2) the theory about the vascular pathogenesis of white matter lesions (leukoaraiosis) [2, 5, 6]. Concerning the first one, the word "infarct" directs us to the presence of an ischemic insult; the presence of pathologic alterations of small arterial vessel as described by Fisher, and mainly characterized by marked lumen restriction, reinforced and integrated such a view. Of note, the precise mechanisms leading from the vessel wall damage to the supposedly ischemic insult of the parenchyma remain at present unknown, as local thrombosis has not been documented and other possible mechanisms such as local vasospasm or lumen occlusion without thrombosis are difficult to prove. It is interesting to remember, however, that systemic thrombolysis is effective also in lacunar infarcts [7, 8], and this could indirectly support the thrombotic hypothesis. It is possible that thrombosis is a late secondary phenomenon triggered by the disrupted arteriolar endothelium.

Data supporting an ischemic origin of white matter lesions (leukoaraiosis) are various. Many of them have been described in detail in two previous papers [5, 6]. Here we provide a brief itemized summary:

1. White matter lesions are localized in a border-zone blood supply area that is, therefore, at higher risk of reductions in blood flow [9].
2. In epidemiologic studies, leukoaraiosis is almost invariably associated with vascular risk factors, at both the cross-sectional and longitudinal level, and with a history and incidence of cerebrovascular events, the most common of which are lacunar and hemorrhagic strokes [10, 11], and, in addition, patients with leukoaraiosis have an increased risk of vascular death [12].
3. At the pathologic level, many studies have found, in association with the typical histologic correlates of leukoaraiosis, alterations of the small vessel. More recently, histologic markers have been described that support a hypoxic environment within white matter lesions [13].
4. A high susceptibility of the main white matter components (oligodendrocytes and myelin sheaths) to ischemia has been documented [14, 15].
5. There are a few observations based on positron emission tomography (PET) studies showing an ischemic status of areas of leukoaraiosis [16, 17].
6. Perfusion magnetic resonance imaging (MRI) data point to an oligemic status in white matter areas of patients with leukoaraiosis [18].

The type of ischemia possibly responsible for white matter changes is not entirely known. In the white matter, two types of histologic alterations can be found:

1. Areas of true cavitation; this is not conceptually different from the ischemic hypothesis of lacunar infarct in the gray matter structures.
2. Areas of pallor in which the myelin appears rarefied.

The first type of lesion is assumed to result from focal ischemic insults of severe grade that cause necrosis of all the cellular elements (pan-necrosis); the second type is reputed to be a form of incomplete ischemia, i.e., an ischemic insult that is able to produce only selective necrosis of some elements, particularly of oligodendrocytes. The temporal and spatial dissemination of these insults would lead to the typical diffuse pale appearance of white matter in areas corresponding to leukoaraiosis. This mechanism has been called "incomplete infarct of the white matter" [19–21].

According to this view, SVD would result, in the first instance, in the acute occlusion of the vessels; the more selective and diffuse damage would be caused by the progressive stenosis of the vessels and by a subliminal ischemic state. In addition, SVD can lead to incapacity of the vessels to dilate and constrict following changes in systemic blood pressure and, therefore, to a loss of autoregulation. The parenchyma would, thus, suffer from blood flow fluctuations in response to changes of systemic blood pressure. This damage would be increased because of the terminal type vascularization in the white matter with scarce anastomoses among perforating blood vessels [22, 23]. The presence of disturbed autoregulation in patients with vascular white matter hyperintensities, as shown by altered acetazolamide challenge, is documented [24].

Blood–brain barrier and SVD

Normal blood–brain barrier

The blood–brain barrier (BBB) is a very important structure; its importance perhaps indicated by the presence of a BBB in many different species from *Drosophila* to human [25]. It is represented by the endothelial lining of the cerebral capillaries and the junctions between endothelial cells, the underlying supporting basement membranes, pericytes, and astrocytic end-feet [26]. The endothelial lining the capillaries is continuous with the endothelium lining the perforating arterioles and venules. The endothelium varies in structure along the cerebral vascular tree, which may partly explain why some features of SVD (such as small subcortical infarcts) due to disease in the perforating arterioles develop earlier, while other features (such as WMHs) develop later and in the territory of the terminal arterioles and capillaries [27].

The endothelium has important barrier functions underpinned by active and passive transport mechanisms [28]. Normal function of the BBB is essential to maintain the optimal milieu for neurons, glia, astrocytes, and other cells within the brain to function properly. Plasma components that cross the normal BBB into the cerebral extracellular compartment leave the extracellular space either by crossing back across the BBB into the venules or via the perivascular spaces into the cerebrospinal fluid (CSF) [28]. The full cellular and molecular components are still not fully understood [29]. However, the important components in terms of structures that fail, which we have some understanding of, and that provide targets for intervention, are listed above. This section will take an overview of current knowledge about the BBB from a clinical perspective, and how its dysfunction may lead to SVD. Data come from several sources.

The human BBB does not maintain a constant integrity across the life course but changes during normal aging [30]. Generally, nonspecific BBB integrity can be assessed by comparing the amount of albumin in the CSF with the amount in the plasma. Normally, albumin is not (as far as is known) manufactured in the brain and is at very low levels in the CSF. Albumin is a medium-sized protein that crosses the BBB passively and so increasing amounts of albumin in the CSF indicate a general loss of BBB integrity. Amongst 10 studies of 700 cognitively normal subjects with no major medical disorder, increasing age was associated with increasing permeability of the BBB, as demonstrated by the increasing CSF : plasma albumin ratio (standardized mean difference [SMD], across all ages 1.2; 95% confidence interval [CI], 0.6–1.8; $P < 0.01$) (Figure 6.1) [31].

The increased BBB permeability accelerated with advancing age, there being a nearly twofold difference between the "younger old" and the "older old" (SMD, 1.91; 95% CI, 0.55–3.28). Therefore, the older the subject, the greater the vulnerability to additional insults that affect BBB integrity and the more likely it is that plasma components can cross the BBB to the perivascular spaces and interstitial tissues.

Experimental models in SVD

There are few valid experimental models of SVD, one reason being the lack of clarity concerning mechanisms of SVD [32, 33]. However, acknowledging all that we know from human SVD pathologically and epidemiologically, the animal model that most closely matches the features seen in humans is the spontaneous strokes experienced by the spontaneously hypertensive stroke-prone rat (SHRSP) [34]. Elderly dogs [35] and primates [36] have also provided some insights into SVD mechanisms.

The SHRSP was selectively inbred to develop spontaneous hypertension and to develop spontaneous stroke, but is also vulnerable to developing large territorial infarcts when used in middle cerebral artery occlusion models. The brain histopathology is very similar to human SVD. So it is as close to a "natural" (i.e., noninduced, nontransgenic) model as we have. It becomes hypertensive from seven to eight weeks of age, has established hypertension from 12 weeks, and starts to develop stroke-like lesions and symptoms from 20 weeks. Increased dietary salt accelerates the development of all features. The brain damage has largely been attributed to the hypertension, although many brain vascular abnormalities are present prior to any measureable rise in blood pressure (see below) [34, 37]. There are also spontaneously hypertensive stroke-resistant rats (SHRSR), indicating that the hypertension alone is not the sole cause of the vascular disease or stroke.

In the SHRSP, an early feature in the development of perforating arteriolar, capillary, and related brain disease, demonstrated on contrast enhanced MRI or with Evans blue dye and histology, is increased BBB permeability (Figure 6.2 [38]).

This is seen prior to the development of overt small vessel pathology or stroke, and is exacerbated by salt administration [38]. A further prominent feature is inflammatory cell infiltration into the vessel walls and perivascular tissues associated with abnormal plasma inflammatory proteins, again exacerbated by salt loading [38, 39]. A hypothesis-driven analysis

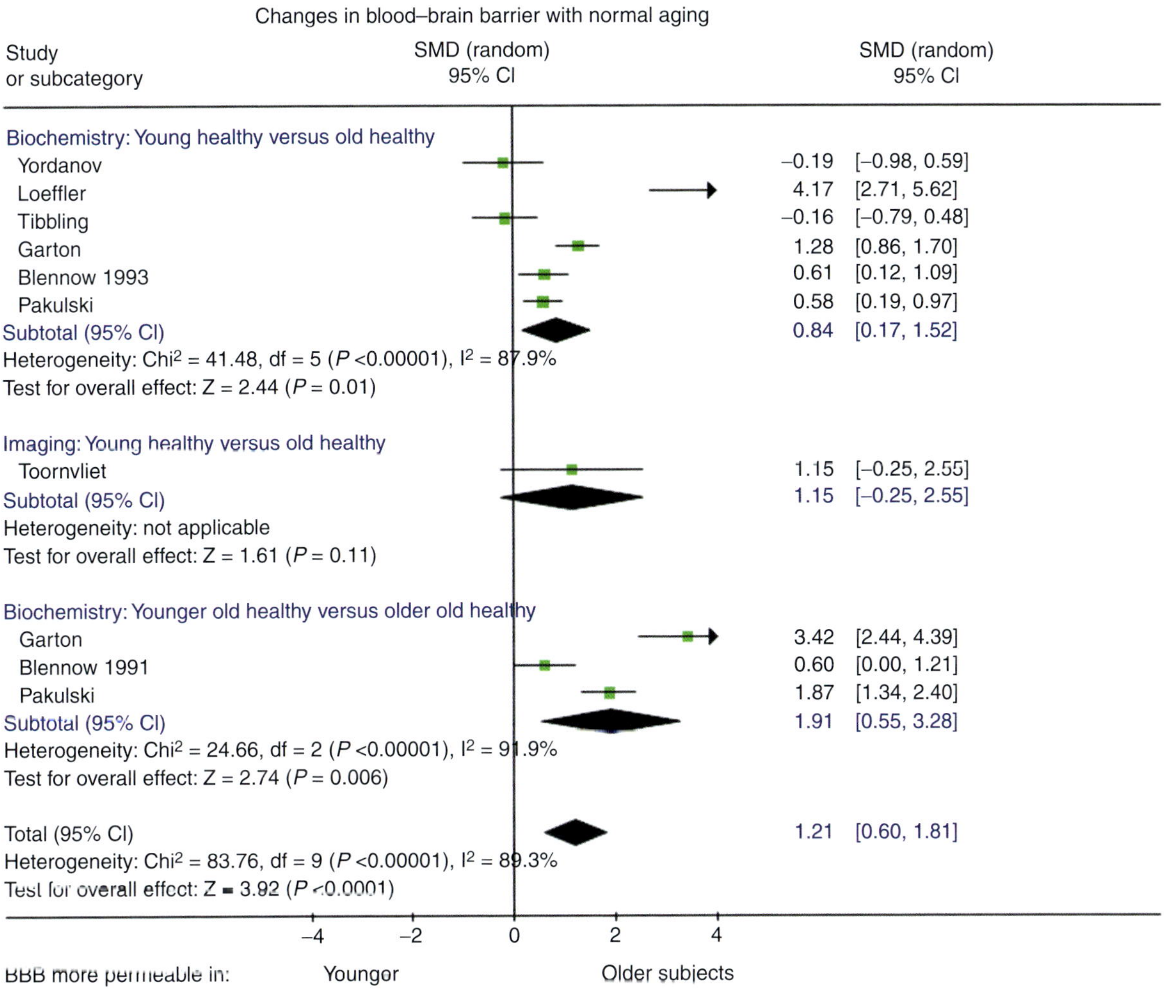

Figure 6.1 Changes in the human blood–brain barrier (BBB) with normal aging. Systematic review of studies comparing older with younger healthy subjects using the cerebrospinal fluid : plasma albumin ratio to assess BBB permeability. Adapted from Farrall and Wardlaw [31].

of immunohistochemistry [37] and messenger ribonucleic acid (mRNA) expression [40] targeted at components of the neurovascular unit, demonstrated that the SHRSP had multiple abnormalities at multiple sites across the neurovascular unit that would increase its vulnerability to SVD. These abnormalities are detectable at five weeks of age, well before the onset of hypertension, and suggest an inherent vulnerability. Compared with the parent control strain from which it was bred (Wistar Kyoto rat), the SHRSP has abnormal endothelial tight junction proteins (claudins), activated microglia and acute phase response gene activation, impaired myelination, abnormal matrix metalloproteinases, overactive glial fibrosis, lack of bioavailability of nitric oxide, and reduced albumin, all present at five weeks of age – well before the development of hypertension [37, 40].

How do each of these features increase vulnerability to SVD? The abnormal tight junctions would be less able to sustain the BBB integrity; the microglial activation is in keeping with the inflammatory cell infiltrate seen pathologically and consistently for over a century on human pathology (see below), and may indicate a chronically overactive immune system that promotes damage [41]; the impaired myelination indicates less ability to withstand white matter damage; the increased glial scarring indicates a tendency to tissue damage; the reduced nitric oxide availability may be secondary to increased nitric oxide destruction through inflammation (as there

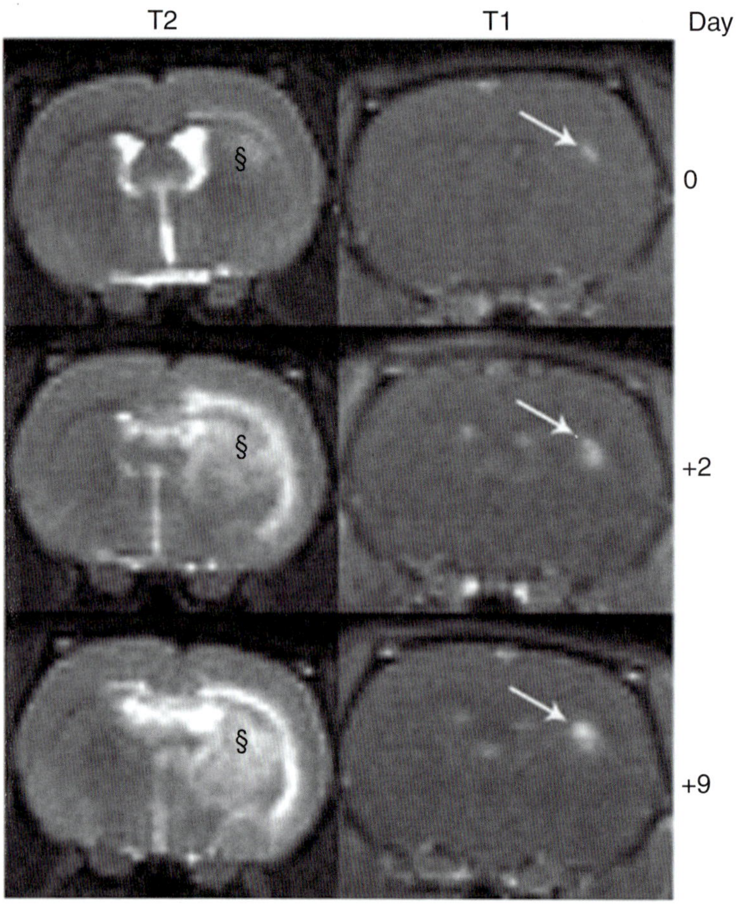

Figure 6.2 Coronal brain section of a spontaneously hypertensive stroke prone rat (SHRSP) sampled at the first detection of brain abnormalities (day 0) and two and nine days later. T2-weighted magnetic resonance imaging (MRI) shows vasogenic edema (left column; §), and T1-weighted MRI after gadolinium injection shows leakage through the blood–brain barrier (BBB) (right column; arrows). From Sironi et al. [38], reproduced with permission.

was no evidence of reduced production), but the net result is impaired ability to vasodilate or autoregulate when necessary, increasing the risk of secondary ischemic damage; and the reduced albumin suggests reduced plasma oncotic pressure increasing the tendency for fluid to leak into the interstitial space. An abnormality in any one of these elements alone might not cause too much trouble, but, in combination, it is not difficult to see how even two or three of these abnormalities together could increase vulnerability to brain damage just through general wear and tear without any additional stressors such as hypertension. Specific vascular risk factors like hypertension would then accelerate the damage. Interestingly, although SVD is thought of as a "vascular" disease, a gene pathway analysis showed that the most differentially expressed genes were in *neurologic* (including BBB) and *inflammatory* (including complement activation) pathways, not in vascular disease or hypertension pathways [40].

Human data: pathology

Pathologic descriptions of small vessel lesions date back to the mid-1800s. The commonest abnormality described pathologically [41] over this time is a diffuse, intrinsic disease of the smaller (40–200 μm diameter) arterioles, referred to by Fisher as "arteriolosclerosis," "lipohyalinosis," or "fibrinoid necrosis" depending on its severity. The original term used by Fisher was "segmental" [4], which well describes the areas of vessel narrowing due to the thickened wall and also of luminal dilatation; loss of normal architecture in the smooth muscle and external layers; and extravasation of red cells, proteins [42], and other blood components into the perivascular space. The vessel wall changes include transudation and exudation of plasma components [43], including inflammatory cells, perivascular edema [44], and vessel wall and brain tissue damage [41, 45]. Many of these features were recognized over 100 years ago, including the inflammatory cell component [41].

When described in the 1950s and 1960s, these changes were thought largely to result from hypertension, partly as hypertension was perhaps more extreme when present and there were fewer effective antihypertensive agents than there are today. Many consider the individual components of SVD still to be almost entirely a consequence of hypertension, which leads to arteriolar stiffening and, through chronic vasospasm, creates fixed defects like fibrinoid necrosis. However, epidemiology indicates that patients with lacunar stroke are equally likely to be hypertensive as are patients with nonlacunar ischemic stroke [46–48], any apparent increased association between lacunar stroke and hypertension being an artifact of the use of risk factor-based stroke classifications such as TOAST (Trial of Org 10172 in Acute Stoke Treatment) [49]. Lacunar stroke remains equally prevalent as an ischemic stroke subtype (25%), and stroke rates have generally not declined particularly, despite much improved control of blood pressure in the last half century (at least as far as the stroke epidemiology data allow us to say). Furthermore, there are many people with lacunar stroke and/or WMHs who are not hypertensive, even allowing for underdiagnosis. Of a consecutive autopsy series of patients with histologic evidence of SVD, 31% had no indication of hypertension in life on stringent criteria; 9% had been nonelderly, nondiabetic, and normotensive; and five of six cases lacking classic risk factors had systemic conditions known to increase BBB permeability [50].

The intrinsic SVD has also been variously attributed to "microatheroma," i.e., diffuse deposition of lipid in arteriolar walls, hence "lipohyalinosis," or discrete lipid deposits in microplaques near the arteriolar origin. There is little direct evidence that lipohyalinosis is due to lipid deposition. Hypercholesterolemia is not a particular feature of lacunar stroke or WMHs. Additionally, there is little direct association between known atheroma such as carotid stenosis and either ipsilateral lacunar stroke [51] or WMHs [52], any apparent association being due to shared co-association with common vascular risk factors. Small atheromatous plaques at the lenticulostriate artery origin are seen pathologically [53, 54] and on imaging, particularly with increasing use of 7-Tesla MR scanners [55], but it is unclear what proportion of lacunar infarcts are caused by either middle cerebral artery or lenticulostriate atheroma. In one trial of stroke prevention in patients with intracranial stenosis, only 38 patients out of 347 (11%) had a lacunar stroke, the rest being cortical territorial, and all recurrent strokes in these were nonlacunar [56]. Intracranial stenosis would also not account for most lacunar infarcts or WMHs in ethnic groups where the prevalence of intracranial atheroma is low, for example white northern Europeans.

The alternative possibility, that of vascular endothelial and BBB loss of integrity, such that the small arteriolar and capillary walls become permeable to substances which would normally remain within the blood and outside the brain, is more recent but provides a plausible explanation for much of the data [57]. The substances – proteins, inflammatory cells, other plasma components, and red cells – result both in damage to the small vessel wall and in perivascular edema [44]. The perivascular edema, which is toxic to neurons, glia, astrocytes, and, in fact, all "brain" cells [44, 58], would lead to insidious perivascular cumulative tissue damage resulting eventually in demyelination seen in WMHs pathologically, and on imaging [59]. The endothelial disruption and luminal distortion could lead to late secondary perforating arteriolar thrombosis and traditional "infarction." Thickened, stiffened arterioles may have impaired autoregulatory ability and contribute further to brain damage through reduced ability to vasodilate when required, as described in the opening paragraphs of this chapter. Both of these late-stage consequences [60] could be superimposed on the background initiating process of endothelial failure. This constellation of events could explain the pathologic and imaging features of the abnormal small arteriolar walls, lacunar infarcts [61], WMHs, prominent perivascular spaces [62, 63], and microhemorrhages [64].

Human clinical data

Lack of recognition of the potential role of BBB and endothelial failure in the genesis of SVD means that direct evidence for a causative role is limited, although there is reasonable evidence for a strong association [57, 64].

First, in a systematic review where BBB permeability was assessed by a variety of methods, mostly the CSF : plasma albumin ratio, having any dementia (26 studies, 1060 patients, Alzheimer's disease, vascular or mixed) was associated with increased BBB permeability compared with normal age-matched controls (SMD 0.8, 95% CI 0.4–1.3, $P < 0.01$) [31]. Having vascular dementia as opposed to Alzheimer's disease

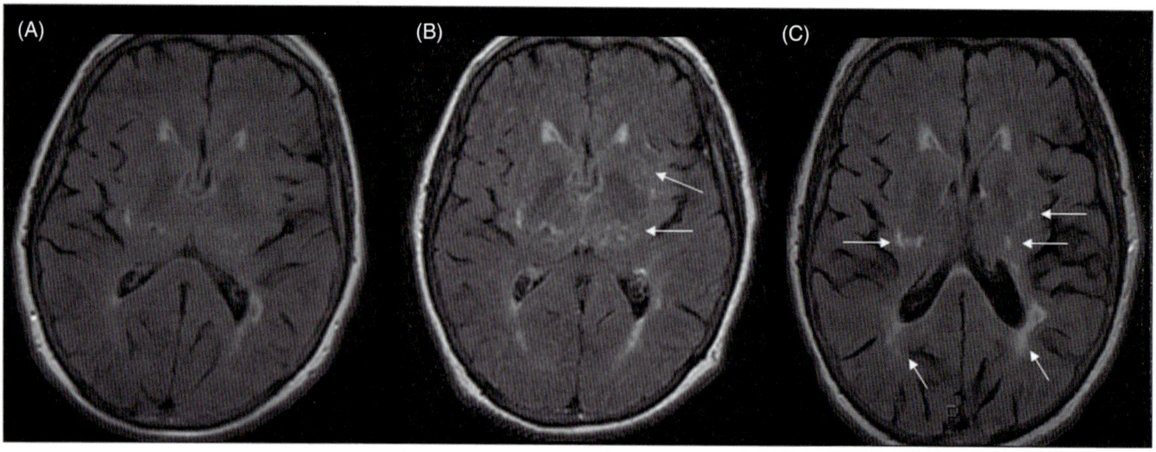

Figure 6.3 Blood–brain barrier (BBB) imaging in a patient with a lacunar stroke. (A) Fluid-attenuated inversion recovery (FLAIR) imaging at presentation shows some hyperintensities in the basal ganglia region. (B) FLAIR imaging two months later at 35 minutes after intravenous gadolinium contrast injection shows contrast in the perivascular spaces (arrows) in the lentiform nucleus and thalamus, indicating BBB leak. (C) Two years later, FLAIR imaging shows an increase in the number of hyperintensities in the basal ganglia.

(10 studies, 460 patients) was associated with further increases in BBB permeability (SMD 0.7, 95% CI 0.1–1.3, $P < 0.01$) [31]. Finally, having more WMHs on imaging (five studies, 200 patients) was also associated with increasing BBB permeability (SMD 0.6, 95% CI 0.3–0.9, $P < 0.01$), although there were few studies up to the first decade of the twenty-first century that had examined BBB and WMHs [31].

BBB permeability imaging with MR (or computed tomography [CT]) is a developing technique. Several studies in the systematic review [31], and since [65–67], used MRI following an injection of intravenous gadolinium to assess BBB permeability. There are several gadolinium contrast agents in current use, but they are all relatively nonspecific markers of general BBB failure that are widely used clinically. These recent studies await more widespread replication, but suggest that there is increased contrast leakage diffusing into the white matter in 97 patients with lacunar stroke (versus nonlacunar stroke controls [65]) in 60 patients with vascular dementia (vs. age-matched normal controls [67]), and in the normal-appearing white matter of SVD patients with more WMHs (versus fewer WMHs) [66]. Increased contrast leak was also detected in older maturity-onset diabetics versus controls [68] and in patients with early Alzheimer's disease compared with age-matched normal controls [69], though not in one other small study in patients with dementia (though this used a less sensitive method) [70]. The increased BBB permeability seen on MRI correlated with increased CSF albumin levels, one of the first direct confirmations that the MR BBB imaging technique is valid [67]. The BBB permeability increased with age and with increased numbers of perivascular spaces in the patients with lacunar stroke (Figure 6.3) [65], consistent with known associations between BBB change and age [30, 31], and interstitial fluid drainage [28, 71].

The MRI post-contrast method is relatively insensitive to the very low-level changes that represent BBB failure in SVD, and several groups are currently working on improved methods of image acquisition and of extracting reliable signal changes [72, 73]. Agents that increase sensitivity to subtle BBB nonspecific leak, as well as to failure of specific processes such as inflammation/microglial activation, would be very valuable and are the subject of intensive research at present.

In the absence of more specific data, other evidence is supportive. Two studies assessed the association between BBB permeability at entry to the study and disease progression long term. Skoog et al. [74] found that higher CSF : plasma albumin ratios in subjects who were normal at presentation were associated with increased risk of progression to cognitive impairment and dementia over three years of follow-up. We found that patients with stroke who had higher basal ganglia BBB permeability on MRI at entry to the study were more likely to be dependent at three years (Figure 6.3) [75].

Currently, several studies are assessing BBB permeability and SVD using imaging and their findings will be reported over the next few years. Wider use of imaging methods in population studies will also help provide more information on brain water content as an indirect measure of BBB leak. The foregoing provides some evidence in support of the concept that vulnerability to cerebral vascular endothelial and BBB damage, with increased permeability, leads to the arteriolar and brain tissue pathologies that we recognize as lacunar infarction, lacunes, WMHs, and perivascular spaces. The hypothesis that a variety of conditions enhancing small vessel permeability may contribute to pathogenesis of SVD merits consideration [50]. Secondary pathologies superimposed on this initiating step – particularly thrombosis secondary to the abnormal damaged endothelium, leading to luminal thrombosis and arteriolar occlusion, and impaired vascular responsiveness, leading to secondary tissue ischemia through failure to vasodilate in response to increased neuronal activity – may precipitate symptoms and worsen disease. Similarly exposure to vascular risk factors, particularly hypertension, will probably accelerate the damage. Other as yet unknown factors may also contribute: in experimental models several endogenous agents may increase endothelial permeability, including pain [76] and inflammation [77–78], both common nonspecific stimuli present in older people with joint problems and the altered immunity that accompanies aging. Whether the inflammation is a consequence of systemic nonspecific inflammatory processes, or brain specific [27, 78] is unknown.

If BBB failure is the initiating factor, then prevention of progression of SVD features, notably WMHs and recurrent lacunar stroke, will require alternative approaches to those currently used for prevention of cardioembolic and atheromatous stroke. Avoidance of dual antiplatelet agents may be important, as this appears to be hazardous in patients with lacunar stroke due to intrinsic SVD [79]. Optimal management of blood pressure, of other vascular risk factors, such as diabetes, lipids, and smoking cessation, is important as these actions are likely to reduce vascular disease risk in general, although direct evidence of their benefit in SVD would be valuable. Other approaches, such as methods to increase vasoreactivity, e.g., through drugs that increase the bioavailability of nitric oxide, or reduction in dietary salt, or improved exercise tolerance, should be evaluated in randomized clinical trials. Anti-inflammatory agents may also need to be evaluated. Indeed, several drugs currently used in stroke prevention (some statins, dipyridamole) have pleiotropic effects that include anti-inflammatory and vasoactive properties, which may be beneficial and should be evaluated specifically in SVD.

Other possible pathogenic mechanisms in cerebral SVD

Besides ischemia and blood–brain barrier dysfunction, other mechanisms have been proposed that might link the pathologic changes of the small vessels to brain parenchyma damage. A list of some of these possible mechanisms is reported in Table 6.1.

Venous pathology and dysfunction

A disturbance of venous efflux rather than of arterial blood flow has been hypothesized as a possible cause of white matter alterations. The first observation in this context was a pathologic one. Moody et al. [80] found noninflammatory collagenous thickening of venous walls resulting in severe periventricular venous stenosis in 13 out of 20 patients older than 60 years. Advanced leukoaraiosis was found in 10 of these 13 patients and was associated with more severe venous disease.

The finding of similar changes in the blood flow and fluid pulsatility in leukoaraiosis and normal pressure hydrocephalus (NPH) has led Bateman [81] to hypothesize that pulse-wave encephalopathy, resulting from alteration of intracranial pulse pressure, may have a causal role in the development of white matter changes also in patients without NPH.

Table 6.1 Possible pathogenic mechanisms for small vessel disease-related parenchyma damage (with particular reference to nonhemorrhagic lesions)

- Diffuse subnecrotic ischemia (incomplete infarct of the white matter)
- Selective neuronal necrosis (incomplete infarct of the gray matter)
- Blood–brain barrier damage
- Impairment of venous return flow and venous stagnation (jugular venous reflux; venous collagenosis)
- Pulse wave encephalopathy
- Increased arterial pulsatility
- Apoptosis

He found that leukoaraiosis and NPH share increased arterial and sinus pulsatility. According to this hypothesis, in leukoaraiosis, cortical vein compliance is initially increased but in severe leukoaraiosis and NPH it is reduced [81]. This hypothesis has been tested in other MRI studies [82].

Recently, Chung et al. [83] found that subjects with severe jugular venous reflux exhibit more severe age-related white matter changes in comparison with those with mild to moderate reflux. The background of this study was the observation of the occurrence of white matter changes and cognitive decline in patients with parenchyma venous engorgement caused by dural arteriovenous fistulas.

Increased arterial pulsatility

Arterial stiffening produced by aging and vascular risk factors may reduce damping of the arterial waveform and increase pulsatility of cerebral blood flow (CBF). This may expose the small vessels in the brain to abnormal flow pulsations and may contribute to the pathogenesis of cerebral SVD. Some older studies suggested a relationship between increased middle cerebral artery pulsatility and leukoaraiosis or lacunar infarction in patients with hypertension [84] and diabetes [85].

This topic has been recently revisited with new observations. Webb et al. [86] found that, in 100 patients, middle cerebral artery pulsatility as measured with transcranial ultrasound was significantly greater in patients with leukoaraiosis than in patients without leukoaraiosis. Moreover, the severity of leukoaraiosis was associated with middle cerebral artery pulsatility and aortic pulse wave velocity for periventricular and deep white matter lesions independent of aortic systolic blood pressure, diastolic blood pressure, pulse pressure, and middle cerebral artery transit time. Middle cerebral artery pulsatility was the strongest physiologic correlate of leukoaraiosis, independent of age, and was dependent on aortic diastolic blood pressure, pulse pressure, and aortic and middle cerebral artery stiffness, supporting the hypothesis that large artery stiffening results in increased arterial pulsatility with transmission to the cerebral small vessels resulting in leukoaraiosis [86].

In their large population-based cohort, Poels et al. [87] studied aortic pulse wave velocity and correlated these data with brain MRI. They found that increased arterial stiffness was associated with a larger volume of white matter lesions [87]. No similar association was instead found with lacunar infarcts or microbleeds. Similar results were found in another study, performed in China [88].

Apoptosis

The occurrence of apoptosis in brains from two patients with leukoaraiosis on MRI was investigated by Brown et al. [89]. Their study, based on the TUNEL assay and other methods for detecting DNA fragmentation, revealed that apoptotic cells were more numerous in areas corresponding to leukoaraiosis than in nearby unaffected white matter. However, the authors also found apoptotic cells in the cortex and in the walls of blood vessels, so the specificity of this finding to explain WMHs remains to be proven [89]. However, the fact that some oligodendrocytes die by apoptosis would nicely explain the absence of complete necrosis and the possibility of having progressive loss of myelin sheaths.

Conclusions

The pathogenic mechanisms linking the pathologic changes seen in patients with cerebral SVD and the consequent parenchyma changes is likely very complex. In this chapter, we have tried to outline some of the main mechanisms that have, in various ways and with different evidence levels, been proposed and tested (Table 6.1). It is possible that these mechanisms are not mutually exclusive and that rather they contemporaneously act in the determination of the pathologic picture. A better comprehension of these mechanisms is important as it might yield therapeutic implications for the future [2].

References

1. Wardlaw JM, Smith EE, Biessels GJ, et al. STandards for ReportIng Vascular changes on nEuroimaging (STRIVE v1). Neuroimaging standards for research into small vessel disease and its contribution to ageing and neurodegeneration. *Lancet Neurol* 2013;12:822–838.
2. Pantoni L. Cerebral small vessel disease: from pathogenesis and clinical characteristics to therapeutic challenges. *Lancet Neurol* 2010;9:689–701.
3. Fisher CM. Lacunes: small, deep cerebral infarcts. *Neurology* 1965;15:774–84.

4. Fisher CM. Lacunar strokes and infarcts: a review. *Neurology* 1982;32:871–876.

5. Pantoni L, Garcia JH. Pathogenesis of leukoaraiosis: a review. *Stroke* 1997;28:652–659.

6. Pantoni L. Pathophysiology of age-related cerebral white matter changes. *Cerebrovasc Dis* 2002;13 (Suppl. 2):7–10.

7. Pantoni L, Fierini F, Poggesi A. Thrombolysis in acute stroke patients with cerebral small vessel disease. *Cerebrovasc Dis* 2014;37:5–13.

8. IST-3 Collaborative Group. The benefits and harms of intravenous thrombolysis with recombinant tissue plasminogen activator within 6 h of acute ischaemic stroke (the Third International Stroke Trial [IST-3]): a randomised controlled trial. *Lancet* 2012;379:2352–2363.

9. De Reuck J. The human periventricular arterial blood supply and the anatomy of cerebral infarctions. *Eur Neurol* 1971;5:321–334.

10. Basile AM, Pantoni L, Pracucci G, et al. Age, hypertension, and lacunar stroke are the major determinants of the severity of age-related white matter changes. The LADIS (Leukoaraiosis And DISability in the elderly) study. *Cerebrovasc Dis* 2006;21:315–22.

11. Folsom AR, Yatsuya H, Mosley TH Jr, Psaty BM, Longstreth WT Jr. Risk of intraparenchymal hemorrhage with magnetic resonance imaging-defined leukoaraiosis and brain infarcts. *Ann Neurol* 2012;71:552–559.

12. Inzitari D, Cadelo M, Marranci ML, Pracucci G, Pantoni L. Vascular deaths in elderly neurological patients with leukoaraiosis. *J Neurol Neurosurg Psychiatry* 1997;62:177–181.

13. Fernando MS, Simpson JE, Matthews F, et al.; MRC Cognitive Function and Ageing Neuropathology Study Group. White matter lesions in an unselected cohort of the elderly: molecular pathology suggests origin from chronic hypoperfusion injury. *Stroke* 2006;37:1391–1398.

14. Pantoni L, Garcia JH, Gutierrez JA. Cerebral white matter is highly vulnerable to ischemia. *Stroke* 1996;27:1641–1646.

15. Petito CK, Olarte JP, Roberts B, Nowak TS, Jr., Pulsinelli WA. Selective glial vulnerability following transient global ischemia in rat brain. *J Neuropathol Exp Neurol* 1998;57:231–238.

16. Yao H, Sadoshima S, Ibayashi S, et al. Leukoaraiosis and dementia in hypertensive patients. *Stroke* 1992;23:1673–1677.

17. Nezu T, Yokota C, Uehara T, et al. Preserved acetazolamide reactivity in lacunar patients with severe white-matter lesions: ^{15}O-labeled gas and H_2O positron emission tomography studies. *J Cereb Blood Flow Metab* 2012;32:844–850.

18. O'Sullivan M, Lythgoe DJ, Pereira AC, et al. Patterns of cerebral blood flow reduction in patients with ischemic leukoaraiosis. *Neurology* 2002;59:321–326.

19. Brun A, Englund E. A white matter disorder in dementia of the Alzheimer type: a pathoanatomical study. *Ann Neurol* 1986;19:253–262.

20. Lammie GA, Brannan F, Wardlaw JM. Incomplete lacunar infarction (Type Ib lacunes). *Acta Neuropathol* 1998;96:163–171.

21. Ma K-C, Olsson Y. Structural and vascular permeability abnormalities associated with lacunes of the human brain. *Acta Neurol Scand* 1993;88:100–107.

22. Rowbotham GF, Little E. Circulation of the cerebral hemispheres. *Brit J Surg* 1965;52:8–21.

23. Van den Bergh R, van der Eecken H. Anatomy and embryology of cerebral circulation. *Progr Brain Res* 1968;30:1–26.

24. Tomura N, Sasaki K, Kidani H, et al. Reduced perfusion reserve in leukoaraiosis demonstrated using acetazolamide challenge ^{123}I-IMP SPECT. *J Comput Assist Tomogr* 2007;31:884–887.

25. Mayer F, Mayer N, Chinn L, et al. Evolutionary conservation of vertebrate blood–brain barrier chemoprotective mechanisms in *Drosophila. J Neurosci* 2009;29:3538–3550.

26. Neuwelt E, Abbott NJ, Abrey L, et al. Strategies to advance translational research into brain barriers. *Lancet Neurol* 2008;7: 84–96.

27. Bechmann I, Galea I, Perry VH. What is the blood–brain barrier (not)? *Trends Immunol* 2007;29:5–11.

28. Abbott NJ. Evidence for bulk flow of brain interstitial fluid: significance for physiology and pathology. *Neurochem Int* 2004;45:545–552.

29. Iadecola C. Neurovascular regulation in the normal brain and in Alzheimer disease. *Nat Rev Neurosci* 2004;5:347–360.

30. Mooradian AD. Effect of aging on the blood–brain barrier. *Neurobiol Aging* 1988;9:31–39.

31. Farrall AJ, Wardlaw JM. Blood brain barrier: ageing and microvascular disease – systemic review and meta-analysis. *Neurobiol Aging* 2007;30:337–352.

32. Bailey EL, McCulloch J, Sudlow C, Wardlaw JM. Potential animal models of lacunar stroke: a systematic review. *Stroke* 2009;40: e451–e458.

33. Hainsworth AH, Markus HS. Do in vivo experimental models reflect human cerebral small vessel disease? A systematic review. *J Cereb Blood Flow Metab* 2008;28:1877–1891.

34. Bailey EL, Smith C, Sudlow CLM, Wardlaw JM. Is the spontaneously

hypertensive stroke prone rat a pertinent model of subcortical ischaemic stroke? A systematic review. *Int J Stroke* 2011; 6:434–444.

35. Su MY, Head E, Brooks WM, et al. Magnetic resonance imaging of anatomic and vascular characteristics in a canine model of human aging. *Neurobiol Aging* 1998;19:479–485.

36. Kemper TL, Blatt GJ, Killiany RJ, Moss MB. Neuropathology of progressive cognitive decline in chronically hypertensive rhesus monkeys. *Acta Neuropathol* 2001;101:145–153.

37. Bailey E, Wardlaw J, Graham D, et al. Cerebral small vessel endothelial structural changes predate hypertension in stroke prone spontaneously hypertensive rats: a blinded, controlled immunohistochemical study of 5- to 21-week old rats. *Neuropathol Appl Neurobiol* 2011;37:711–726.

38. Sironi L, Guerrini U, Tremoli E, et al. Analysis of pathological events at the onset of brain damage in stroke-prone rats: a proteomics and magnetic resonance imaging approach. *J Neurosci Res* 2004; 78:115–122.

39. Sironi L, Tremoli E, Miller I, et al. Acute-phase proteins before cerebral ischemia in stroke-prone rats: identification by proteomics. *Stroke* 2001;32:753–760.

40. Bailey EL, McBride MW, Crawford W, et al. Differential gene expression in multiple neurological, inflammatory and connective tissue pathways explains vulnerability to cerebral small vessel disease in a spontaneous model of human disease. *Neuropathol Appl Neurobiol*, in press.

41. Bailey EL, Smith C, Sudlow CLM, Wardlaw JM. Pathology of lacunar ischaemic stroke in humans – a systematic review. *Brain Pathol* 2012;22:583–591.

42. Tomimoto H, Akiguchi I, Suenaga T, et al. Alterations of the blood–brain barrier and glial cells in white matter lesions in cerebrovascular and Alzheimer's disease patients. *Stroke* 1996;27:2069–2074.

43. Young VG, Halliday GM, Kril JJ. Neuropathologic correlates of white matter hyperintensities. *Neurology* 2008;71:804–811.

44. Lammie GA, Brannan F, Wardlaw JM. Incomplete lacunar infarction (type 1b lacunes). *Acta Neuropathol* 1998;96:163–171.

45. Gouw AA, Seewann A, van der Flier WM, et al. Heterogeneity of small vessel disease: a systematic review of MRI and histopathology correlations. *J Neurol Neurosurg Psychiatry* 2011;82:126–135.

46. Jackson CA, Sudlow CLM. Are lacunar strokes really different? A systematic review of differences in risk factor profiles between lacunar and non-lacunar infarcts. *Stroke* 2005;36:891–904.

47. Jackson CA, Hutchison A, Dennis MS, et al. Differences between ischemic stroke subtypes in vascular outcomes support a distinct lacunar ischemic stroke arteriopathy. A prospective, hospital-based study. *Stroke* 2009;40:3679–3684.

48. Jackson CA, Hutchison A, Dennis MS, et al. Differing risk factor profiles of ischemic stroke subtypes: evidence for a distinct lacunar arteriopathy? *Stroke* 2010;41:624–629.

49. Landau WM, Nassief A. Editorial comment – time to burn the TOAST. *Stroke* 2005;36:902–904.

50. Lammie GA, Brannan F, Slattery J, Warlow C. Nonhypertensive cerebral small-vessel disease. An autopsy study. *Stroke* 1997;28:2222–2229.

51. Mead GE, Lewis SC, Wardlaw JM, Dennis MS, Warlow CP. Severe ipsilateral carotid stenosis and middle cerebral artery disease in lacunar ischaemic stroke: innocent bystanders? *J Neurol* 2002;249:266–271.

52. Potter GM, Doubal FN, Jackson CA, et al. Lack of association of white matter lesions with ipsilateral carotid artery stenosis. *Cerebrovasc Dis* 2012;33:378–384.

53. Fisher CM. Capsular infarcts: the underlying vascular lesions. *Arch Neurol* 1979;36:65–73.

54. Lammie GA, Wardlaw JM. Small centrum ovale infarcts – a pathological study. *Cerebrovasc Dis* 1999;9:82–90.

55. Kang CK, Park CA, Park CW, et al. Lenticulostriate arteries in chronic stroke patients visualised by 7 T magnetic resonance angiography. *Int J Stroke* 2010;5:374–380.

56. Khan A, Kasner SE, Lynn MJ, Chimowitz MI. Risk factors and outcome of patients with symptomatic intracranial stenosis presenting with lacunar stroke. *Stroke* 2012;43:1230–1233.

57. Wardlaw JM, Sandercock PA, Dennis MS, Starr J. Is breakdown of the blood–brain barrier responsible for lacunar stroke, leukoaraiosis, and dementia? *Stroke* 2003;34:806–812.

58. Silberberg DH, Manning MC, Schreiber AD. Tissue culture demyelination by normal human serum. *Ann Neurol* 1984; 15:575–580.

59. Fazekas F, Ropele S, Enzinger C, et al. MRI of white matter hyperintensities. *Brain* 2005;128:2926–2932.

60. Simpson JE, Wharton SB, Cooper J, et al. Alterations of the blood–brain barrier in cerebral white matter lesions in the ageing brain. *Neurosci Lett* 2010;486:246–251.

61. Wardlaw JM, Dennis MS, Warlow CP, Sandercock PA. Imaging appearance of the symptomatic perforating artery in patients with lacunar infarction: occlusion or other vascular pathology? *Ann Neurol* 2001;50:208–215.

62. Doubal FN, MacLullich AM, Ferguson KJ, Dennis MS, Wardlaw JM. Enlarged perivascular spaces on MRI are a feature of cerebral small vessel disease. *Stroke* 2010;41:450–454.

63. Potter GM, Doubal FN, Jackson CA, et al. Enlarged perivascular spaces and cerebral small vessel disease. *Int J Stroke* 2013, May 22 [Epub ahead of print].

64. Wardlaw JM, Smith C, Dichgans M. Mechanisms of sporadic cerebral small vessel disease: insights from neuroimaging. *Lancet Neurol* 2013;12:483–497.

65. Wardlaw JM, Doubal F, Armitage P, et al. Lacunar stroke is associated with diffuse blood–brain barrier dysfunction. *Ann Neurol* 2009;65:194–202.

66. Topakian R, Barrick TR, Howe FA, Markus HS. Blood–brain barrier permeability is increased in normal-appearing white matter in patients with lacunar stroke and leucoaraiosis. *J Neurol Neurosurg Psychiatry* 2010;81:192–197.

67. Taheri S, Gasparovic C, Huisa BN, et al. Blood–brain barrier permeability abnormalities in vascular cognitive impairment. *Stroke* 2011;42:2158–2163.

68. Starr JM, Wardlaw J, Ferguson K, et al. Increased blood–brain barrier permeability in type II diabetes demonstrated by gadolinium magnetic resonance imaging. *J Neurol Neurosurg Psychiatry* 2003;74:70–76.

69. Starr JM, Farrall AJ, Armitage P, McGurn B, Wardlaw J. Blood–brain barrier permeability in Alzheimer's disease: a case-control MRI study. *Psychiatry Res* 2009;171:232–241.

70. Wahlund LO, Bronge L. Contrast-enhanced MRI of white matter lesions in patients with blood–brain barrier dysfunction. *Ann N Y Acad Sci* 2000;903:477–481.

71. Weller RO, Djuanda E, Yow HY, Carare RO. Lymphatic drainage of the brain and the pathophysiology of neurological disease. *Acta Neuropathol* 2009;117:1–14.

72. Taheri S, Gasparovic C, Shah NJ, Rosenberg GA. Quantitative measurement of blood–brain barrier permeability in human using dynamic contrast-enhanced MRI with fast T1 mapping. *Magn Reson Med* 2011;65:1036–1042.

73. Armitage PA, Farrall AJ, Carpenter TK, Doubal FN, Wardlaw JM. Use of dynamic contrast-enhanced MRI to measure subtle blood–brain barrier abnormalities. *Magn Reson Imaging* 2011;29:305–314.

74. Skoog I, Wallin A, Fredman P, et al. A population study on blood–brain barrier function in 85-year-olds: relation to Alzheimer's disease and vascular dementia. *Neurology* 1998;50: 966–971.

75. Wardlaw JM, Doubal FN, Valdes-Hernandez MC, et al. Blood–brain barrier permeability and long term clinical and imaging outcomes in cerebral small vessel disease. *Stroke* 2013;44:525–527.

76. Hawkins BT, Davis TP. The blood–brain barrier/ neurovascular unit in health and disease. *Pharmacol Rev* 2005;57:173–185.

77. Abbott NJ. Inflammatory mediators and modulation of blood–brain barrier permeability. *Cell Mol Neurobiol* 2000; 20:131–147.

78. Huber JD, Witt KA, Hom S, et al. Inflammatory pain alters blood–brain barrier permeability and tight junctional protein expression. *Am J Physiol Heart Circ Physiol* 2001;280:H1241–H1248.

79. The SPS3 Investigators. Effects of clopidogrel added to aspirin in patients with recent lacunar stroke. *N Engl J Med* 2012;367:817–825.

80. Moody DM, Brown WR, Challa VR, Anderson RL. Periventricular venous collagenosis: association with leukoaraiosis. *Radiology* 1995;194:469–476.

81. Bateman GA. Pulse-wave encephalopathy: a comparative study of the hydrodynamics of leukoaraiosis and normal-pressure hydrocephalus. *Neuroradiology* 2002;44:740–748.

82. Henry Feugeas MC, De Marco G, Peretti II, et al. Age-related cerebral white matter changes and pulse-wave encephalopathy: observations with three-dimensional MRI. *Magn Reson Imaging* 2005;23:929–937.

83. Chung CP, Wang PN, Wu YH, et al. More severe white matter changes in the elderly with jugular venous reflux. *Ann Neurol* 2011;69:553–559.

84. Sierra C, de la Sierra A, Chamorro A, et al. Cerebral hemodynamics and silent cerebral white matter lesions in middle-aged essential hypertensive patients. *Blood Press* 2004;13:304–309.

85. Lee KY, Sohn YH, Baik JS, Kim GW, Kim JS. Arterial pulsatility as an index of cerebral microangiopathy in diabetes. *Stroke* 2000;31:1111–1115.

86. Webb AJ, Simoni M, Mazzucco S, et al. Increased cerebral arterial pulsatility in patients with leukoaraiosis: arterial stiffness enhances transmission of aortic pulsatility. *Stroke* 2012; 43:2631–2636.

87. Poels MM, Zaccai K, Verwoert GC, et al. Arterial stiffness and cerebral small vessel disease: the Rotterdam Scan Study. *Stroke* 2012;43:2637–2642.

88. Mok V, Ding D, Fu J, et al. Transcranial Doppler ultrasound for screening cerebral small vessel disease: a community study. *Stroke* 2012;43:2791–2793.

89. Brown WR, Moody DM, Challa VR, Thore CR, Anstrom JA. Apoptosis in leukoaraiosis lesions. *J Neurol Sci* 2002;203:169–171.

Chapter 7

Pathogenic aspects of hereditary small vessel disease of the brain

Anne Joutel

Introduction

Cerebral small vessel disease (SVD) of the brain is currently recognized as a major burden of diseases responsible for cognitive impairment and motor disability in the adult. Despite its importance, there are currently no specific treatments, and therapeutic options for secondary prevention are particularly limited compared to other common causes of stroke. One obstacle to developing therapies is the diversity of diseases and pathologic processes under the umbrella of cerebral SVD. Another major obstacle is a limited understanding of the key molecular events that provoke vascular and brain lesions. Although the majority of SVD is sporadic, specific genetic defects have been identified in rare familial cases. The discovery of genes responsible for these rare but highly penetrant causes of SVD is particularly exciting because it can provide unique insights into pathogenesis. Particularly, it allows the generation of animal models with definite significance to specific forms of the human diseases. Importantly, these genes and the processes that they regulate are potential therapeutic targets that can be assessed in these models.

This chapter focuses on hereditary forms of SVD with an adult onset, whose causative gene has been identified. After briefly discussing their cliniconeuropathologic characteristics, current concepts of their etiology and pathogenesis are reviewed.

Hereditary SVD predominantly predisposing to ischemic strokes

Cerebral autosomal dominant arteriopathy with subcortical infarcts and leukoencephalopathy

Clinical, neuroimaging, and pathologic aspects

Cerebral autosomal dominant arteriopathy with subcortical infarcts and leukoencephalopathy (CADASIL) is an archetypal ischemic SVD. The four cardinal manifestations are: (1) migraine with aura, present in 20–40% of patients and often the first clinical manifestation around 30 years; (2) recurrent ischemic strokes in 60–85% of patients with an onset around 50 years; (3) mood disturbance in 20% of patients; and (4) cognitive decline in nearly all patients after 50 years. Patients become unable to walk around age 60, and die around 65–70 years. White matter hyperintensities, lacunar lesions, microhemorrhages, brain atrophy, and tissue microstructural changes are detected on brain magnetic resonance imaging (MRI). Leukoaraiosis is the earliest change, preceding the onset of symptoms by 10–15 years and is always present after the age of 35, whereas lacunar infarcts and other lesions occur later in life [1]. Studies in a large cohort of patients have shown that the volume of lacunar lesions, whole brain mean apparent-diffusion coefficient, and brain parenchymal fraction, each have an independent influence on global cognitive function

Cerebral Small Vessel Disease, ed. Leonardo Pantoni and Philip B. Gorelick. Published by Cambridge University Press.

and disability, with brain atrophy being the strongest contributor to clinical impairment [2]. Importantly, there are multiple lines of evidence that cortical lesions may be related to subcortical lacunar and tissue microstructural lesions [3].

The arteriopathy involves primarily the leptomeningeal and small penetrating arteries, and is characterized by progressive loss of vascular smooth muscle cells (vSMCs), prominent thickening of the vessel wall by various types of collagens, and extracellular accumulation of the so-called granular osmiophilic material (GOM). Remarkably, GOM deposits are observed all along the vascular tree, including the peripheral arteries [4].

Molecular genetics

The disease is caused by dominant mutations in the *NOTCH3* gene and emerges as the most common causative diagnosis of hereditary ischemic SVD [1, 5]. *NOTCH3* encodes a 2321-amino-acid-long protein belonging to the evolutionarily conserved NOTCH receptor family. The NOTCH3 receptor comprises a large extracellular domain containing 34 epidermal growth factor-like repeats (EGFR), a single transmembrane domain, and an intracellular domain containing seven ankyrin repeats flanked by two nuclear localization signals [5]. *NOTCH3* has 33 exons but all CADASIL mutations occur in the exons 2–24 that encode the EGFR, with strong clustering, in some populations, in exons 3–4 encoding EGFR2–5. The vast majority of mutations are missense mutations; others are splice site mutations or small inframe deletions. Virtually all mutations hitherto reported result in an odd number of cysteine residues within a given EGFR [5, 6]. There have been a few reports of mutations which do not affect cysteine residues; however, there is neither genetic nor experimental evidence that these sequence variants are pathogenic.

NOTCH3 synthesis, expression, and functions

NOTCH3 is initially synthesized as a ~280-kDa precursor, which then undergoes proteolytic processing, resulting in the formation of a mature heterodimeric transmembrane receptor, consisting of a 210-kDa extracellular domain ($\text{Notch3}^{\text{ECD}}$) noncovalently attached to the 97-kDa transmembrane intracellular domain ($\text{Notch3}^{\text{TMIC}}$) [7].

NOTCH3 is predominantly expressed in vSMCs of small arteries in the adult. There are four NOTCH receptors (NOTCH1–4) in mammals, but multiple lines of evidence indicate that NOTCH3 is the predominant NOTCH receptor in SMCs of distal arteries, particularly in the brain arteries. Experimental studies have demonstrated that NOTCH3 is critically required for arterial differentiation and postnatal maturation of SMCs in these vessels [8]. NOTCH3 is also required for the proper function of small arteries. Distal arteries and arterioles constrict or dilate when intravascular pressure increases or decreases, respectively. This phenomenon, known as myogenic reactivity, is in the brain a major contributor to the maintenance of cerebral blood flow (CBF) (autoregulation) in face of variations in systemic blood pressure. In mice completely lacking NOTCH3, myogenic tone of distal arteries including brain arteries is strongly reduced, autoregulation of CBF is altered, and susceptibility to ischemic stroke upon challenge is increased [8–10].

Signal activation of NOTCH receptors is initiated by the binding of NOTCH to transmembrane ligands, Delta or Jagged. Upon activation, NOTCH undergoes a series of proteolytic cleavages resulting in the release of its intracellular domain (NICD) from the plasma membrane. After translocation to the nucleus, NICD binds to the transcription factor RBPJ and coactivator Mastermind to activate transcription of genes [11]. In cerebral arteries, NOTCH3 controls expression of genes important for the regulation of myogenic tone [12].

Mechanisms of disease

Pathogenicity of *NOTCH3* mutations

Mechanisms linking *NOTCH3* mutations to the arteriopathy are incompletely understood. Contrasting with the highly stereotyped nature of CADASIL-associated mutations, cell-based and in-vivo studies have shown that mutations differently affect NOTCH3/RBPJ activity. Where functional analysis has been performed, NOTCH3 receptors bearing a mutation in the mutational hotspot (EGFR2–5) have preserved function and are able to activate RBP-Jκ transcription at wild type levels, while mutations located in the two EGFR (10 and 11) required for ligand binding (present in ~4% of CADASIL families) result in a loss of NOTCH3 receptor function [13–15]. However, mice lacking NOTCH3 do not develop brain lesions as typically seen in the recently generated CADASIL mouse model [8]. Additionally, genotype–phenotype correlation analyses unexpectedly suggest that loss-of-function mutations are associated with an attenuated clinical phenotype [14]. Thus, the dominant view is that an impaired NOTCH3 activity is unlikely to contribute to the disease phenotype, although this is still a matter of debate [16].

On the other hand, mutant NOTCH3 spontaneously forms higher order multimers in vitro [17]. Patients and mice carrying the so-called cysteine mutations invariably harbor extracellular deposition of $NOTCH3^{ECD}$ in small blood vessels. $NOTCH3^{ECD}$ accumulates as microscopic extracellular aggregates around vSMCs and brain pericytes, and $NOTCH3^{ECD}$ has been recently recognized as a component of GOM [7, 18, 19]. Vascular deposition of $NOTCH3^{ECD}$ aggregates is regarded as one of the earliest events in the disease process, suggesting that it might be the proximate cause of cellular pathology [19]. There is a body of literature indicating that protein aggregates may promote aberrant interactions with proteins having essential cellular function, resulting in their sequestration and functional impairment. Hence, sequestration of proteins into $NOTCH3^{ECD}$-containing deposits may be critical in CADASIL pathogenesis. As such, clearance of $NOTCH3^{ECD}$ aggregates may represent a valuable therapeutic approach.

Modeling CADASIL in the mouse

Animal models that recapitulate aspects of the corresponding human disease are instrumental in studying disease mechanisms. Attempts at modeling CADASIL in the mouse have used knock-in and transgenesis approaches. What these mice develop well are $Notch3^{ECD}$ aggregates or GOM deposits [20]. Moreover, enhanced cortical spreading depression, the electrophysiologic substrate of migraine aura, has been demonstrated in one of these mouse models [21]. Importantly, only transgenic mice (PAC-Notch3R169C) overexpressing a mutant NOTCH3 protein, approximately fourfold over NOTCH3 endogenous levels with an endogenous-like expression pattern, further develop fully penetrant brain lesions. Specifically, PAC-Notch3R169C transgenic mice exhibit $Notch3^{ECD}$ accumulation and GOM deposits by one and five months of age respectively, and white matter lesions after 12 months of age. Prior to the appearance of brain lesions, mutant mice exhibit moderate and widespread reduction (10–20%) of the resting CBF [19].

Mechanisms of brain lesions

Studies in patients had suggested that chronic hypoperfusion might be important in the pathogenesis of white matter lesions; however, the causal relationship, i.e., chronic subcortical ischemia as the primary cause of white matter changes, had not been demonstrated. Furthermore, it had been put forward, from neuropathologic and functional neuroimaging studies in CADASIL patients, that subcortical ischemia was related to narrowing of the vascular lumen and impaired arteriolar dilation because of vessel wall fibrosis, particularly in arterioles of the white matter, and smooth muscle cell loss. We learned from the PAC-Notch3R169C transgenic mouse model that white matter lesions and cerebral hypoperfusion occur in the absence of overt SMC degeneration and fibrosis of cerebral arteries, as well as in the absence of blood–brain barrier breakdown [19]. However, this is not to say that, once present, they may not aggravate cerebrovascular dysfunction and exacerbate brain lesions already in progress. On the other hand, it was found in these mutant mice that cerebrovascular autoregulation and functional hyperemia (i.e., the increase in local CBF which accompanies increased cellular activity to satisfy enhanced glucose and oxygen demand) were compromised, prior to the occurrence of white matter damages. Further experiments showed that myogenic responses and mechanical properties of brain arteries were altered early in mutant mice. Finally, progressive rarefaction of brain capillaries in the white matter was likewise an early manifestation. Altogether these studies provide compelling evidence for cerebrovascular dysfunction and microcirculatory failure as the earliest consequences of pathogenic mutant NOTCH3, culminating in progressive hypoperfusion and white matter damage [19] (Figure 7.1).

Cerebral autosomal recessive arteriopathy with subcortical infarcts and leukoencephalopathy

Clinical, neuroimaging, and pathologic aspects

Cerebral autosomal recessive arteriopathy with subcortical infarcts and leukoencephalopathy (CARASIL) is a very rare autosomal recessive SVD predominantly reported in Japanese families, with a phenotype more complex and more severe than CADASIL. Clinical landmarks are cognitive deficit, motor dysfunction, and subcortical stroke, in association with diffuse alopecia and attacks of severe low back pain due to spondylosis deformans and/or disk degeneration. Alopecia frequently occurs as early as adolescence and most

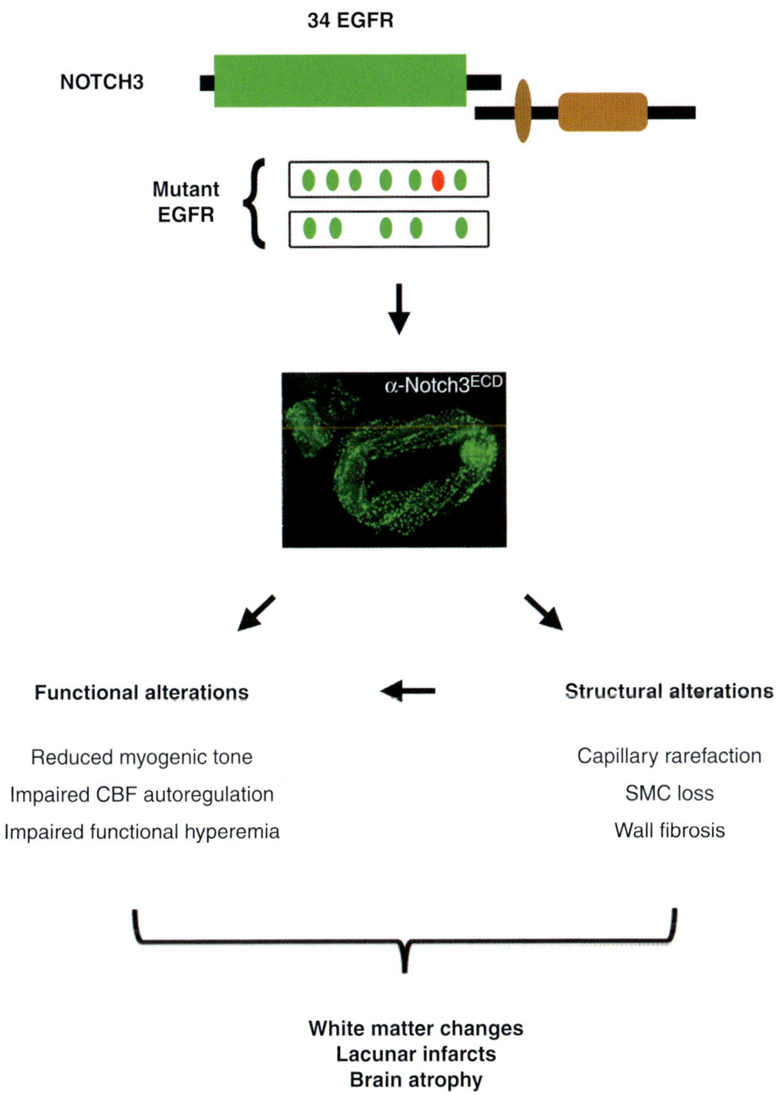

Figure 7.1 Hypothetical effect of CADASIL-associated *NOTCH3* mutations on cerebral vessels. Cysteine mutations in the epidermal growth factor-like repeat (EGFR) of NOTCH3 cause deposition of NOTCH3^{ECD} aggregates around smooth muscle cells, inducing structural and function alterations of cerebral blood vessels, which ultimately result in white matter degeneration, lacunar infarcts, and brain atrophy. CBF, cerebral blood flow; SMC, smooth muscle cell.

patients become demented and bedridden in the fourth decade [22]. The cerebral arteriopathy is mostly predominant in the white matter and basal ganglia. It is characterized by strong thinning of the adventitia and the media, with extensive loss of smooth muscle cells, fibrous intimal proliferation, splitting of the internal elastica lamina, and frequent double barreling of the wall (configuration of concentric vessel within a vessel) [23].

Molecular genetics

CARASIL is caused by recessive mutations in HTRA1, a member of a unique family of oligomeric serine proteases that are conserved from bacteria to humans. *HTRA1* consists of nine exons encoding a 480-amino-acid-long secreted serine protease, which comprises, from the N- to the C-terminus, a signal peptide that is required to permit secretion from the cell, an N-terminal domain of unknown function, a serine protease domain (aa 204–342), and one PDZ domain (aa 381–473). Yet, very few mutations have been reported; they include homozygous nonsense mutations as well as homozygous missense mutations in the serine protease domain. Nonsense mutations result in the loss of HTRA1 protein by nonsense mediated decay of messenger RNA and missense mutations strongly compromise HTRA1 protease activity. Hence, CARASIL likely arises from a reduced activity of HTRA1 [24].

HTRA1 functions

HTRA1 is ubiquitously expressed in adult mammalian tissues. A variety of potential substrates have been identified, including extracellular matrix proteins such as aggregan [25] or fibronectin [26], as well as fibroblast growth factor or transforming growth factor-β (TGF-β) family members [27, 28]. Crystal structure revealed an autoactivation mechanism of HTRA1, by showing that substrate binding to the protease domain is sufficient to stimulate proteolytic activity [29]. As yet, physiologic functions of HTRA1 in vivo remain largely unknown. In vitro studies suggest that HTRA1 inhibits matrix calcification [30]; however, these data have been recently challenged by a study showing opposite effects of HTRA1 [31]. Other studies suggest that HTRA1 may repress signaling by TGF-β family members through binding to the pro-region (latency-associated peptide [LAP]) of the TGF-β1 precursor and its cleavage [28, 32].

Mechanisms of disease

Much work remains to be done to further our understanding of how *HTRA1* mutations contribute to the disease phenotype. At present, there is no reported mouse model mimicking the human disease. The only documented phenotype of mice carrying a constitutive inactivation of the *HtrA1* gene is a reduced capillary density in the retina [33]. At the molecular level, immunohistochemical analysis of cerebral arteries from CARASIL patients as well as in vitro studies are consistent with an abnormally elevated TGF-β signaling activity via reduced cleavage of proTGF-β1 [24, 28]. However, this must be further substantiated and, more importantly, it is unknown whether an abnormally increased TGF-β signaling activity can drive the CARASIL-associated arteriopathy.

Retinal vasculopathy with cerebral leukodystrophy

Clinical, neuroimaging, and pathologic aspects

Cerebroretinal vasculopathy (CRV), hereditary endotheliopathy, retinopathy and nephropathy, and stroke (HERNS), and hereditary vascular retinopathy (HVR) are also extremely rare diseases identified as allelic disorders and, now, designated as autosomal dominant retinal vasculopathy with cerebral leukodystrophy (RVCL) (OMIM 192315) [34]. Clinical symptoms begin in middle age with progressive visual impairment, followed by stroke-like episodes, migraine-like headache, and cognitive decline. Death usually occurs 5–10 years later. Fluorescein angiograms show characteristic capillary obliteration, avascular areas in the retinal periphery, microaneuryms, and telangiectatic capillaries. Brain MRI displays white matter hyperintensities and may show contrast enhancing mass lesions, also called pseudotumors, within the deep white matter. Neuropathology of these pseudotumors demonstrates areas of coagulative necrosis, often centered on small blood vessels occluded by fibrin thrombi, surrounded by edematous white matter with minimal inflammatory infiltrates but prominent reactive astrogliosis, that are highly reminiscent of delayed radiation necrosis. Small vessels exhibit marked abnormalities with fibrinoid necrosis, thickened and fibrotic walls. On ultrastructural analysis, the capillary basement membranes exhibit a multilayered appearance. A subset of affected patients has systemic vasculopathy as evidenced by biologic or histologic abnormalities of the skin, kidney, liver, or intestine, although not as clinically prominent as in the brain [35–37]. Of note, patients with HVR exhibit distinctive features with highly prevalent Raynaud's phenomenon, absence of brain pseudotumors, and apparently normal life expectancy [38].

Molecular genetics

RVCL is caused by heterozygous mutations in the *TREX1* gene, which encodes a 3′ DNA exonuclease (former DNAse III) [34]. TREX1 is a 314-amino-acid-long protein containing three conserved exonuclease motifs (Exo I, II, and III), which form the active site of the enzyme, and a prolin-rich motif involved in protein–protein interactions. Remarkably, all RVCL-associated TREX1 mutations hitherto reported are frameshift mutations in the C-terminus. Since TREX1 is encoded by a single exon, frameshift mutations are predicted to escape the nonsense-mediated mRNA decay pathway [39], and thus to result in the expression of truncated proteins lacking the C-terminal region [34].

TREX1 expression and functions

TREX1 is the most abundant DNA exonuclease in mammalian cell. It is an autonomous exonuclease that can hydrolyze its target sequence independently. TREX1 functions as a homodimer with a preference for single-stranded DNA (ssDNA) to which it binds avidly. Unexpectedly for a DNA exonuclease, TREX1 is mainly cytosolic and localized to the endoplasmic reticulum (ER) [40, 41]. It was initially suspected that TREX1 was an integral transmembrane protein based on the presence of a predicted transmembrane helix at its C-terminus. Biochemical experiments suggest instead that TREX1 interacts with membranes of the ER or another resident protein of the ER, through its C-terminus [41].

It was initially thought that TREX1 might serve a DNA-editing role in DNA replication or gap filling during DNA repair [42]. However, the observation that genetic ablation of Trex1 in the mouse does not cause an increased frequency of spontaneous mutations or cancers does not support this possibility [43]. Nonetheless, genetic studies linking TREX1 mutations in humans with a spectrum of autoimmune diseases and further analysis of TREX1 null mice and TREX1-deficient cells have unraveled significant mechanistic insights on its functional role. In the human, homozygous and heterozygous loss-of-function mutations within the TREX1 active site cause Aicardi–Goutières syndrome and familial chilblain lupus, respectively. Aicardi–Goutières syndrome is a rare recessive early-onset progressive encephalopathy, mimicking congenital viral infection without evidence of an infectious agent. Familial chilblain lupus is a dominant form of cutaneous lupus erythematosus beginning in early childhood that shares significant phenotypic overlap with Aicardi–Goutières syndrome, including increased levels of interferon-α and circulating antinuclear antibodies [44–46]. In the mouse, loss of TREX1 causes an autoimmune myocarditis responsible for strongly reduced postnatal survival [43]. Importantly, experimental studies provided compelling evidence that TREX1 was an essential negative regulator of the interferon-α stimulatory DNA response. Specifically, in the absence of TREX1, single-stranded endogenous DNA polynucleotides, which should have been processed in the presence of TREX1, abnormally accumulate in the cytoplasm, leading to the activation of the innate immune system, which in turn triggers a lethal autoinflammatory response [41].

Several other potential functions of TREX1 have been identified. For example, TREX1 has been reported to be a member of the ER-associated SET complex, involved in granzyme A-mediated cell death, a caspase-independent pathway [47]. Also, Yang et al. [40] reported that cells deficient for Trex1 have cell-cycle abnormalities, being defective in G1/S transition as a result of chronic activation of the ATM-mediated DNA-damage checkpoint signaling. It is likely that additional functions of TREX1 will be discovered in the coming years.

Mechanisms of disease

The prediction is that RCVL-associated *TREX1* mutations result in the expression of TREX1 proteins truncated of their C-terminus, a region critically important for the normal localization of TREX1 in the endoplasmic reticulum (ER). Where functional analysis has been performed, RCVL-associated TREX1 mutations cause cellular mislocalization rather than a loss of enzymatic activity. Actually, mutant TREX1 forms lacking their carboxy termini are no longer localized to the ER but, instead, appear to be disseminated throughout the cell [34]. However, there are several caveats in these experiments to definitely rule out a loss-of-function mechanism. For example, expression of truncated TREX1 protein in patients with RCVL has not been demonstrated. Moreover, enzymatic activity of the mutant protein has been analyzed in a cell-free system, which did not take into account the defective cellular localization. Hence, the mutations could just result in insufficient quantities of TREX1 in the correct place to execute its function. An alternative mechanism could be a detrimental gain-of-function mutation acquired by truncated TREX1 proteins. Hence, although there have been remarkable discoveries during the last five years on the role of TREX1, the mechanisms linking TREX1 mutations to the RCVL disease phenotype are yet unclear. Further investigation of patients with RCVL, as well as generation and analysis of cellular and animal models of RCVL-associated *TREX1* mutations, are needed.

Hereditary SVD predominantly predisposing to hemorrhagic strokes

Hereditary cerebral amyloid angiopathies

Pathology

Cerebral amyloid angiopathy (CAA) is defined by the finding on neuropathologic examination of amyloid fibrils in the walls of cerebral small blood vessels. CAA affects predominantly the small- and medium-sized arteries and arterioles of the leptomeninges, cerebrum, and cerebellar cortex. Amyloid deposition, which is typically patchy and segmental, begins in the adventitia and around SMCs in its abluminal portion, and then gradually infiltrates the whole vessel wall replacing SMCs. In severe CAA, the vessel wall is strongly disrupted with prominent SMC loss, fragmentation, and even double-barreling, microaneurysm formation, fibrinoid necrosis, and leakage of blood through the wall. Perivascular inflammation with activated microglia, astrocytes, and activation of the complement cascade can be seen around amyloid-laden vessels. CAA occurs mostly as a sporadic disease fairly common in the elderly, with or without morphological evidence of additional Alzheimer's disease. It is responsible for spontaneous large lobar intracerebral hemorrhages (ICHs) (macrohemorrhages) as well as small microhemorrhages, cortical microinfarctions, and subcortical white matter lesions, which likely contribute to cognitive impairment. In sporadic CAA, amyloid is composed of 39–43-amino-acid β-amyloid (Aβ) peptides, which are proteolytic products of the amyloid precursor protein (APP) [48].

Clinical aspects and molecular genetics

Beside the common sporadic forms, very rare familial forms of CAAs have been identified. Hereditary CAAs include genetically and biochemically diverse conditions that can be classified as Aβ-CAA and non-Aβ-CAA, depending on the identity of the main component of amyloid deposits. Hereditary cerebral hemorrhage with amyloidosis–Dutch type (HCHWA-D) is an archetype of familial Aβ-CAA. It is caused by a point mutation at codon 693 of APP resulting in a glutamine for glutamic acid substitution (E693Q) at position 22 of Aβ. Mutations within residues 21–23 and 34 of the Aβ peptide are similarly associated with prominent CAA and cerebral hemorrhages. Other mutations in the APP gene flanking the Aβ coding region or duplication of the APP locus, as well as mutations in the catalytic subunit of the γ-secretase protein complex (presenilin-1 or presenilin-2 encoded by *PSEN1* and *PSEN2* genes, respectively) that generates Aβ can also cause severe CAA; however, early-onset Alzheimer's disease rather than cerebral hemorrhages may dominate the clinical phenotype [49]. Non-Aβ cerebral amyloidosis includes very rare autosomal dominant conditions. Familial British dementia (FBD) and familial Danish dementia (FDD), with deposition of 34 amino-acid-long C-terminal proteolytic fragments of the mutated BRI proteins (ABri and ADan in FBD and FDD, respectively), arise from a point mutation of the normal stop codon and a 10-nt duplication one codon before the normal stop codon of the *BRI2* gene respectively. Both mutations result in larger-than-normal BRI proteins containing 277 amino acids instead of 266 amino acids [50]. hereditary cerebral hemorrhage with amyloidosis–Icelandic type (HCHWA-I), with deposition of N-terminal degradation products of the mutated Cystatin-C protein, is caused by a founder mutation (L68Q) in the Cystatin-C gene [51]. Familial transthyretin (TTR)-related amyloidosis with accumulation of variants of transthyretin is due to mutations in the *TTR* gene [52]. Familial amyloidosis–Finnish type (FAF) is caused by missense mutations at residue 187 of Gelsolin; amyloidogenic fragments (5 and 8 kDa) in this form derive from aberrant processing, first in the Golgi and later outside the cell of the secreted form of Gelsolin [53]. Prion-related cerebral amyloidosis, with deposition of a N- and C-terminally truncated 70 amino-acid-long PrP peptide, has been identified in two families carrying a nonsense mutation at codon 145 and 163 respectively [54].

Overall, hereditary CAAs have an autosomal dominant mode of inheritance, occur at an earlier age of onset, and have a more severe clinical course than sporadic CAAs. Common features include lobar hemorrhages, frequently recurrent, cognitive decline, extensive white matter lesions, cortical infarcts, and microhemorrhages. Hereditary non-Aβ-CAAs exhibit distinguishing features. Particularly, cognitive decline rather than lobar ICH can dominate the clinical picture, with the exception of HCHWA-I, and amyloid deposits are usually found also in peripheral tissues. Pathogenesis of hereditary Aβ-CAA, only, will be further discussed herein. We refer the reader to several excellent textbooks and other reviews for hereditary non-Aβ-CAA.

Aβ peptide synthesis and clearance

APP is a single-pass transmembrane protein expressed by almost all cell types in the brain, of still unclear physiologic function. In the major pathway, APP is sequentially cleaved by the α-secretase and then the γ-secretase, liberating fragments that may convey the normal function of APP. In the so-called amyloidogenic pathway, APP is cleaved by the β-secretase instead of the α-secretase, and then by the γ-secretase, liberating the Aβ peptide(s). The γ-secretase protein complex can cleave APP at different positions, producing Aβ peptides of distinct lengths and C-termini, with Aβ40 and Aβ42 ending at residue Val-40 and Ala-42, respectively, being the two major species. Aβ peptides are soluble components present naturally in the brain interstitial fluid, cerebrospinal fluid, and the blood [55]. They are maintained in the brain at nonamyloidogenic levels by at least three mechanisms: (1) drainage with interstitial fluid along perivascular spaces to cervical lymph nodes [56]; (2) active transport across the blood–brain barrier to the blood, essentially mediated by the low density lipoprotein receptor-related protein 1 [57]; and (3) degradation by several proteases including neprilysin, endothelin-converting enzyme, insulin-degrading enzyme, plasmin, and cathepsin B [55].

Mechanisms of disease

Aβ peptide aggregation

Recent experimental evidence suggests that amyloid fibrils form by a "nucleated conformational conversion" mechanism whereby Aβ peptides rapidly aggregate into spherical oligomers that slowly convert into amyloid fibrils [58]. Importantly, Aβ species have different aggregation propensity; in particular Aβ42 aggregates more readily while Aβ40 is more soluble and less fibrillogenic [59]. Data suggest that APP and PSEN mutations differentially promote Aβ aggregation. Aβ peptides mutated in the center, like the archetypal Dutch mutant Aβ, exhibit a higher aggregation propensity than wild type Aβ, a slower clearance across the blood–brain barrier and perivascular drainage, and are more resistant to proteolytic degradation [60]. APP mutations near the β-secretase cleavage site or duplication of the APP locus increase the production of Aβ peptides, which also favors its aggregation, while APP mutations near the γ-secretase cleavage site or PSEN mutations increase the relative amount of Aβ42 versus Aβ40 [61–63].

Aβ vascular deposition

Multiple transgenic mouse models overexpressing various mutant human APP or PSEN have been generated. The majority of these models develop age-dependent parenchymal amyloid plaques and varying degrees of Aβ-CAA, which usually occur at an advanced age. Among these, the APPDutch transgenic mice, which overexpress (~5-fold) APP with the E693Q mutation, are interesting because mutant mice, like patients harboring this mutation, exhibit significant CAA, microhemorrhages, and neuroinflammation, with virtually no parenchymal amyloid plaques [64]. The other mouse model, which shows significant vascular amyloid deposits, is the APP23 mouse model, which overexpresses (~7-fold) APP with a double mutation near the β-secretase site, also called the "Swedish" double mutation. These mice develop parenchymal amyloid plaques by the age of six months and first lesions of CAA are detectable by eight months of age [65]. Despite a number of limitations, these models have proven invaluable to decipher some key mechanisms of vascular amyloid deposition (Figure 7.2). Particularly, it was uncertain whether vascular amyloid had a neuronal, vessel wall, or blood origin. The use of a variety of transgenic mice, overexpressing mutant APP under various promoters, provided experimental proof that neuronal source of Aβ peptides is sufficient to cause CAA [64]. Secondly, these models pinpointed the critical importance of the Aβ40 : Aβ42 ratio in determining the preferential site (parenchyma vs. vessel) of Aβ deposition. Aβ40 is the predominant species of vascular amyloid, while Aβ42 is the major molecular species deposited in brain parenchyma [66]. Moreover, brains from human HCHWA-D and APPDutch mice exhibit a high Aβ40 : Aβ42 ratio as compared to those of Alzheimer's disease patients and APPwt mice respectively. To establish that a high Aβ40 : Aβ42 ratio favors the formation of CAA over parenchymal plaque pathology, the Jucker laboratory conducted the following elegant experiment. They crossed the APPDutch mice with transgenic mice producing a mutant Presenilin-1 known to increase Aβ42 production, to artificially shift the AβDutch40 : AβDutch42 ratio toward AβDutch42 in the APPDutch mice. Remarkably, it was found that decreasing the Aβ40 : Aβ42 ratio in APPDutch mice resulted in the redistribution of the amyloid pathology from the vasculature to the parenchyma [64]. Further experimental studies revealed that Aβ40 may not be sufficient for amyloid deposition since mice overexpressing high levels of Aβ1–40, in the absence of APP overexpression, did not develop overt amyloid pathology. On the other hand, Aβ42 has been shown to be essential for amyloid deposition in both the parenchyma and vessels of mice and the data suggest that Aβ42 may act as a seed for amyloid deposition [67]. Also, studies have provided direct evidence that apolipoprotein E (ApoE), a key lipoprotein regulating

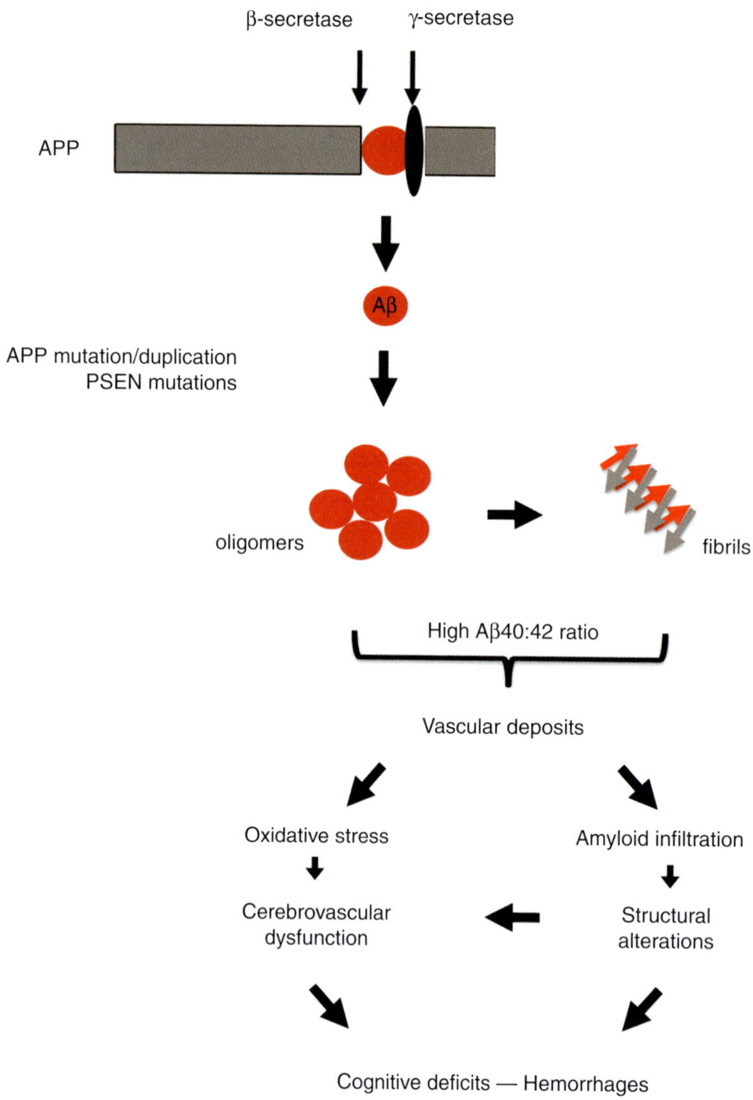

Figure 7.2 Putative mechanisms of clinical manifestations in hereditary β-amyloid (Aβ) cerebral amyloid angiopathy. Amyloid precursor protein (APP) produced in neurons is cleaved by β- and γ-secretases to produce soluble Aβ peptides. *APP* mutations, duplication of the *APP* locus, or Presenilin (*PSEN*) mutations increase the propensity of Aβ peptides to form Aβ oligomers and amyloid fibrils. A high Aβ40 : Aβ42 ratio favors vascular deposition of Aβ amyloid, inducing structural alterations of cerebral arteries, which may ultimately cause blood vessel leakage and lobar hemorrhage. Vascular deposition of Aβ peptides or amyloid also induces cerebrovascular dysfunction, because of increased oxidative stress, which may ultimately cause white matter degeneration and lacunar infarcts, and contribute to cognitive deficits.

the metabolism of lipids, plays a prominent role in vascular amyloid deposition, in an isoform-specific fashion. Studies in humans have established that the ε2 and ε4 isoforms of ApoE are associated with sporadic CAA risk and risk for brain hemorrhage [68]. ApoE interacts with soluble and aggregated Aβ in vitro and in vivo. Invalidation of the *ApoE* gene in two different transgenic mouse models with Aβ deposition strongly reduces vascular amyloid, despite significant parenchymal plaque deposition [69]. Notably, replacement of the *ApoE* murine gene with the human ApoE4 isoform results in a redistribution of Aβ deposition from the brain parenchyma to the cerebral vasculature [70]. It is worthy of note that a series of biochemical and in vivo studies have revealed that amyloidogenic peptides involved in non-Aβ CAA can bind Aβ and modulate Aβ deposition [71–73].

Mechanisms of brain lesions

Intuitively, amyloid deposition in the vessel wall and further SMC loss can weaken vessel walls, causing rupture and leading to micro- and macrohemorrhages. Actually, Aβ-CAA animal models have established that vascular amyloid deposition is sufficient to cause hemorrhages [64]. In particular, these studies have shown a positive temporal and spatial correlation between hemorrhages and vascular amyloid deposition. Beside these structural alterations, there is a significant body of evidence suggesting that vascular amyloid also causes cerebrovascular dysfunction that could be the mechanism by which CAA is associated with microinfarcts, white matter lesions, and cognitive decline. Specifically, mouse models of Aβ deposition have an attenuation of endothelium-dependent cerebrovascular vasodilation [74]. Moreover, functional hyperemia and CBF autoregulation are strongly compromised in these mice. Importantly, topical superfusion of Aβ40, but not of Aβ42, on the neocortex of normal mice can recapitulate vascular dysfunction observed in mouse models of Aβ deposition. Pharmacologic and genetic approaches further suggest that the deleterious effects of Aβ involve oxidative stress which is mediated, for the most part, by reactive oxygen species produced by an abnormal activation of the NADPH oxidase [75]. Vascular dysfunction manifests long before the development of vascular amyloid deposition, suggesting that elevated Aβ levels may be sufficient to disrupt vascular function; however, this point remains controversial [76]. Remarkably, functional transcranial Doppler and functional MRI analysis are consistent with an impaired vascular reactivity in patients with advanced CAA [77]. Functional and structural alterations of blood vessels may act to reduce the compensatory capacity of the cerebral circulation and increase the susceptibility of the brain to vascular insufficiency. It has been noticed that periventricular white matter, which is located at the boundary between the territory of penetrating arteries and basal ganglia arteries, is most susceptible to ischemic damage.

Anti-Aβ immunotherapy

Anti-Aβ immunotherapy has emerged as a promising therapeutic option for Alzheimer's disease since the pioneer study, from Schenk et al. in 1999 [78], showed that active peripheral immunization with the Aβ42 peptide in a transgenic mouse model of Alzheimer's disease resulted in both prevention of plaque formation and removal of existing plaques. However, it rapidly turned out that immunotherapy could have an impact on vascular amyloid. Although controversial, a rise in CAA severity accompanying the fall in plaque load has been documented in several reports, a finding consistent with the translocation of solubilized plaque Aβ42 to the vasculature according to the perivascular drainage hypothesis. Furthermore, the occurrence of microhemorrhages upon vaccination was repeatedly reported, both in mice and humans [79, 80]. Yet, the mechanism of microhemorrhage remains unclear since pathologic analysis did not reveal overt structural changes of the vessels and the severity of CAA does not appear to be correlated with the number of microhemorrhages. Hence, although there have been tremendous advances in our understanding of the pathogenesis of hereditary CAA, this field has yet to translate these insights into treatments.

SVD associated with *COL4A1* or *COL4A2* mutations

Basement membrane, also called basal lamina, forms the limiting boundaries of many organs such as the nervous system, underlies epithelium and vascular endothelium, and surrounds individual cells such as smooth or skeletal muscle cells or functional units in many tissues. Basement membrane is assembled as enmeshed polymers of laminins and type IV collagens that are tethered to nidogens and heparan sulfate proteoglycans (agrin and perlecan). Type IV collagen is one of the major components of basement membrane. It comprises up to six genetically distinct alpha chains designated alpha 1 (IV) to alpha 6 (IV), which interact and assemble with a remarkable specificity to form only three distinct heterotrimers: [α1α1α2], [α3α4α5], and [α5α5α6]. The alpha-1 and alpha-2 chains are present in the basement membrane of all tissues, whereas the other four chains have restricted tissue distribution during development [81].

Clinical, neuroimaging, and pathologic aspects

Phenotypic manifestations associated with mutations in the gene encoding the alpha-1 (IV) chain were initially described in mutant mice and subsequently recognized in patients. A first report documented *COL4A1* mutations in families with porencephaly, a rare neurologic disease characterized by fluid-filled cysts or cavities in the cerebral parenchyma that typically manifests in infants with hemiplegia and intellectual disability [82]. The same laboratory reported the following year a dominant *COL4A1* mutation segregating in a family with clinical and neuroimaging features of cerebral SVD in the adult, in association with ocular manifestations [83]. Since then, a broader range of phenotypes involving the brain and eyes most commonly, but also the kidney and skeletal muscle, presenting from the fetal period until late adulthood, has been associated with inherited or de novo mutations in *COL4A1* or, more recently, in the gene encoding the alpha-2 chain of collagen IV (*COL4A2*). Common neurologic features include porencephaly, schizencephaly, prenatal and perinatal ICHs, macro- and microhemorrhages in young and old patients, patchy to diffuse leukoaraiosis, dilated periventricular spaces, and, less frequently, small deep infarcts. Ocular manifestations include retinal arteriolar tortuosity, most commonly, anterior segment dysgenesis including Axenfeld–Rieger anomaly, congenital cataract, and juvenile-onset glaucoma. Kidney abnormalities range from albuminuria, hematuria, to renal cysts and agenesis of the kidney [84–87]. The hereditary angiopathy with nephropathy, aneurysms, and cramps (HANAC) syndrome has been coined to describe preferential phenotypic association, including the presence of arterial aneurysms, a high prevalence of eye, kidney, and skeletal manifestations, and Raynaud's phenomenon [88, 89]. It appears that the expressivity of *COL4A1* and *COL4A2* mutations is extremely variable, even between members of the same family. Furthermore, several case reports have documented the existence of clinically asymptomatic mutation carriers with or without brain MRI abnormalities.

As yet, there is no neuropathologic study of patients with *COL4A1* or *COL4A2* mutations. However, electron microscopy analysis of skin or kidney biopsies has repeatedly shown focal areas of fragmentation, duplication, and even herniation of the basement membrane [88–90].

Molecular genetics

Human *COL4A1* and *COL4A2* genes are composed of 52 and 48 exons respectively; the two genes sit head to head on chromosome 13, sharing a bi-directional promoter. The alpha-1 and alpha-2 chains are composed of three structurally distinct domains: (1) an N-terminal domain (7S) rich in cysteine and lysine residues; (2) a ~1400 residue long collagenous domain made of Gly–Xaa–Yaa triple repeats where Xaa is variable amino acid and Yaa is often a proline or a lysine residue; followed by (3) ~230 residue long C-terminal globular domain (NC1). A characteristic feature of collagen IV is the presence, in the collagenous domain, of natural short (1–24 residue) noncollagenous interruptions, which confer flexibility and may also serve as binding sites with partners and interchain crosslinking.

A recent survey of *COL4A1* and *COL4A2* mutations in patients indicates that a large proportion of these mutations are missense mutations resulting in substitution for one of the invariant glycine residues within the Gly-Xaa-Yaa repeats in the collagenous domain [84, 87]. On the other hand, significance of several missense mutations in the collagenous domain that do not affect glycine residues is more questionable and awaits additional studies. Although the still limited number of reported mutations precludes serious genotype–phenotype correlation analysis, it is remarkable that HANAC syndrome-associated *COL4A1* mutations are clustered within 30 amino-acid residues in the N-terminus of the collagenous domain, a binding site for VHL and other proteins (integrins, heparin, VWF) involved in angiogenesis [91].

Collagen type IV synthesis, structure, and functions

The triple-helical molecule of collagen type IV assembles intracellularly from the NC1 domain, which is important for correct assembly of two alpha-1 chains with one alpha-2 chain. The assembled trimer then folds from the C- to the N-terminus. Glycine residues play a crucial role in helix formation and stabilization. During chain synthesis and helix formation, proline and lysine residues undergo post-translational modifications, which are also critical for triple helix stabilization. Particularly, many proline at the Y position undergo hydroxylation to produce hydroxyproline. Once secreted into the extracellular matrix, molecules self-assemble into a highly covalently crosslinked network. NC1 domains of two triple-helical molecules form end to end interactions and 7S domains of four triple-helical molecules form antiparallel interactions; supramolecular twisting, and lateral associations of collagenous domains further enhance the network. This provides a molecular scaffold on which other components of the basement membrane can interact [81].

Collagen IV has both structural and nonstructural roles. In contrast with laminin proteins, collagen IV is dispensable for deposition and initial assembly of components of the basement membranes during early development. Indeed, targeted inactivation of *Col4a1/2* in the mouse does not impair early embryonic development and organogenesis. However, *Col4a1/2* knockout mice die at mid-gestation with strong alterations of the basement membrane structures, indicating that collagen IV is fundamental later on, for the maintenance of basement membrane integrity [92]. In addition to its structural role, collagen IV participates in cell–cell and cell–matrix interactions, through integrin and nonintegrin receptors, such as cell surface heparin sulfate proteoglycan, mannose receptors, and discoidin domain receptors. Cell–matrix interaction is critically important for cell adhesion, migration, proliferation, and differentiation [81].

Mouse models

A variety of mouse lines carrying mutations in the *Col4a1* or *Col4a2* genes, arising from chemical mutagenesis, has been identified. It is noticeable that mutations include, like in patients, a majority of glycine substitutions in the collagenous domain. Remarkably, heterozygous mutant mice develop pleiotropic phenotypes that closely resemble the human disease [82, 83, 93–96]. Among these, the Col4a1$^{+/\Delta ex41}$ mice (formerly named Col4a$^{1+/\Delta ex40}$) have been the most extensively characterized. These mice express a mutant *Col4a1* transcript, in which exon 40 is directly spliced to exon 42, because of a mutation in the splice acceptor site of exon 41 (formerly named exon 40). The resulting mutant collagen alpha-1 (IV) chain contains an inframe deletion (p.G1169_K1185del) of 17 amino-acid residues in the triple helix. At birth, all heterozygous Col4a1$^{+/\Delta ex41}$ mutant pups have cerebral hemorrhage and about half of them die within a day. A small proportion of young adult mice have porencephalic cavities. Adult mice also develop spontaneous multifocal recurrent ICHs, predominantly in the basal ganglia, that can be symptomatic or clinically silent. Col4a1$^{+/\Delta ex41}$ mice also have focal and variable cerebral cortex lamination defects with focal breaches of the pial basement membranes, particularly in vicinity to ectopias. Like humans with *COL4A1* mutations, mutant mice also exhibit eye (retinal arterial tortuosity, ocular anterior segment dysgenesis, optic nerve hypoplasia), kidney (microalbuminuria, hematuria), and muscle abnormalities. Electron microscopy analysis demonstrated basement membrane defects in the cerebral vessels as well as in other tissues of the mutant mice. Specifically, basement membranes showed uneven edges, variable density and thickness, and also focal disruption, splitting, and even herniations (Figure 7.3) [82, 83, 93, 94].

Mechanisms of disease

Pathogenicity of *COL4A1/2* mutations

At the cellular level, putative mechanisms of *COL4A1/2* mutation pathogenicity encompass the protein defect, the collagen alteration, and dysfunction at the cellular, matrix, and tissue level. The alpha-chain's stoichiometry predicts that *COL4A1* and *COL4A2* heterozygous mutations result in the production of 75% and 50% abnormal collagen IV molecules, respectively. There is in-vitro and in-vivo experimental evidence that *Col4a1* mutations can cause extracellular deficiency of both alpha-1 and alpha-2 chains of collagen type IV, and thus that the pathogenicity may arise from a quantitative defect of collagen IV. In vitro, the ratio of secreted : intracellular collagen alpha 1 and alpha 2 (IV) is reduced in cells stably expressing mutant COL4A1 [97]. Notably, mutation of alpha-1 (IV) chain has been shown to impair secretion of alpha-2 (IV) chain and vice versa. In vivo, deposition of collagen alpha 1 and alpha 2 (IV) is almost absent in the Reichert's membrane, a basement membrane of embryonic origin, in embryos homozygous for the Col4a1$^{\Delta ex41}$ mutation [82]. From this experiment, it is speculated, but not proven, that deposition may be half-reduced in mice carrying the mutation at the heterozygous state. These findings are consistent with previous studies showing that substitution of a glycine residue within the triple helix of collagen type I delays the folding and results in overmodified collagen, which may compromise its secretion [98]. Furthermore, a recent report has documented an apparent lack of expression of mutated *COL4A1* transcript in the fibroblasts of affected patients from two families carrying a frameshift and a splice site *COL4A1* mutation, respectively, because of nonsense-mediated mRNA decay [99]. However, the lack of overt phenotype in mice heterozygous for null alleles of *Col4a1* and *Col4a2*, although mice have not been analyzed in detail, suggests that haploinsufficiency (i.e., quantitative defect) may not solely account for the disease phenotype [92]. One possibility is that mutant molecules also exert a deleterious effect responsible for qualitative defects. Several studies have documented an intracellular retention of the alpha-1 and alpha-2 chains in cells stably expressing mutant COL4A1 or COL4A2 and in tissues of mutant mice, which in some cases led to reticulum endoplasmic stress [93]. Alternatively, some mutant molecules may reach the extracellular space and exert dominant negative effect over the various partners of collagen IV, which may compromise the matrix structure and promote abnormal cell–matrix and cell–cell interactions. Improving our knowledge in this field may be an interesting entry point for therapeutic interventions.

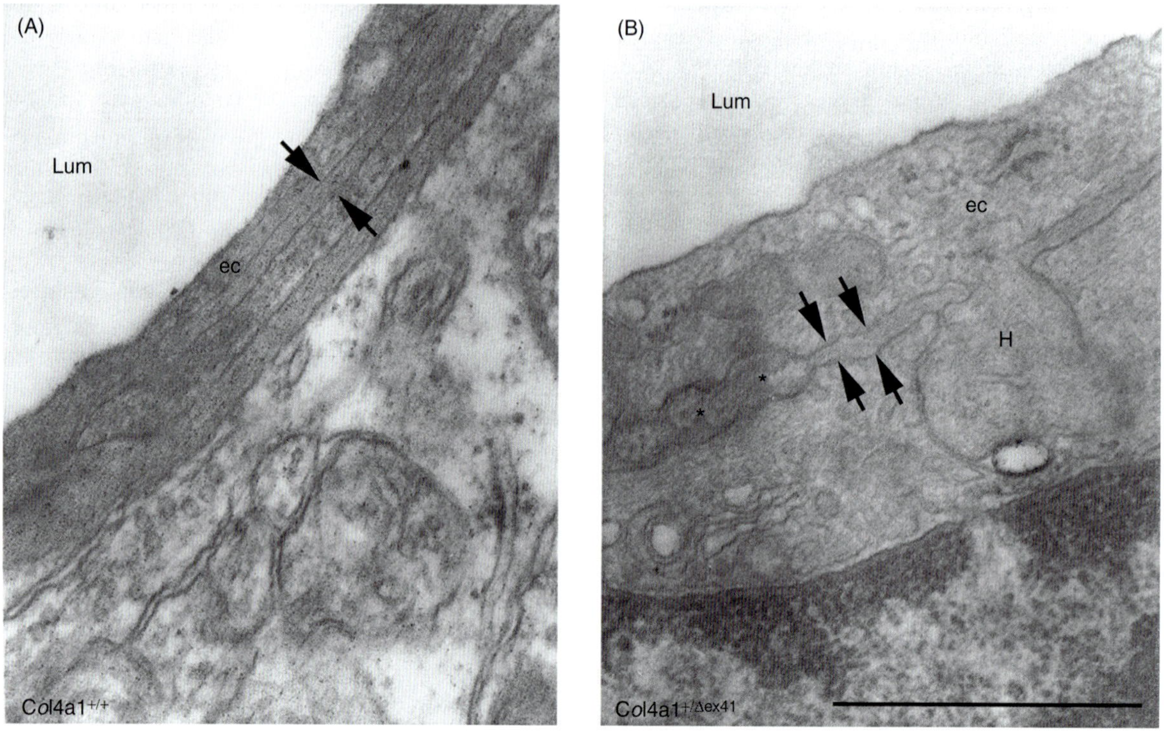

Figure 7.3 (A,B) *Col4a1* mutation in the mouse induces basement membrane defects in the cerebral vasculature. Vascular basement membrane in the Col4a1$^{+/\Delta ex41}$ mutant mouse exhibits variable thickness, inconsistent density, and uneven edges (B, between arrows), focal disruptions (asterisks), and herniation (H) as compared to the control Col4a1$^{+/+}$ mouse (A). (Lum, lumen; ec, endothelial cell; scale bar, 0.5 μm). Adapted from Gould et al. [82].

Environmental and genetic modifiers of the disease phenotype

In addition to playing a key role in the discovery of *COL4A1/2* mutations in patients with SVD, *Col4a1/2* mouse models proved valuable in elucidating important aspects of the disease. Head trauma, particularly during delivery, was clearly demonstrated to be a predisposing factor for cerebral hemorrhages. Gould et al. [83] nicely showed that surgical delivery of *Col4a1* mutant mice strongly reduced severe perinatal cerebral hemorrhages. Moreover, mouse studies have pinpointed genetic modifiers as likely contributors to variable expressivity of the disease. Gould et al. [83] demonstrated that the phenotype resulting from the *Col4a1* mutation varied greatly among mice depending on genetic background. For example, retinal arteriolar tortuosity and ocular anterior segment dysgenesis were highly penetrant in mice with the C57BL/6J genetic background and almost absent in mice with the mixed CAST-BL/6 background. Further genetic analyses identified a locus on mouse chromosome 1, which likely contains the modifier gene(s) [83, 93]. However, mechanisms of porencephalic cavities and cerebral hemorrhages in *Col4a1/2* mutants remain incompletely understood. Porencephalic cavities are thought to arise as a consequence of ante or perinatal ICHs, but the exact mechanisms are unclear. Also it is yet unknown whether hemorrhages arise from veins, arteries, or capillaries and from structural versus nonstructural alterations of vascular basement membranes. Moreover, it is unknown why the brain is the most severely affected organ while collagen alpha-1 and alpha-2 (IV) chains are ubiquitously expressed.

Summary

One breakthrough in the field of SVD has been the discovery of causative genes of rare Mendelian SVD, opening new research avenues and providing new concepts in the etiology and pathogenesis of these diseases. One critical step when studying the pathogenesis of a disease is the generation of animal models recapitulating the human form of the disease. However, the expectation that introducing the same genetic alteration in the mouse would be sufficient to achieve this has not been realized. With the exception of *Col4a1* mutant mice, existing genetically engineered mouse models only partially recapitulate the complex features of the human diseases. This is something that is not unusual in the mouse and that is also encountered in many neurodegenerative diseases with an adult age-of-onset. It is well known that the mouse has a smaller brain, a lower amount of white matter, a shorter lifespan, and many other distinctive features from humans. Nevertheless, incomplete mouse models, of, e.g., CADASIL and hereditary Aβ-CAA, proved useful to decipher some key mechanisms initiating the disease process and will certainly constitute invaluable tools for assessing therapeutic strategies.

Study of these rare Mendelian SVD must be encouraged, because they may be a powerful platform from which to gain insights into the sporadic diseases. There is a close resemblance between some sporadic and hereditary forms of SVD; for example, between hereditary and sporadic CAA, and between CADASIL and ischemic sporadic SVD. This suggests that monogenic and common non-Mendelian forms of SVD may have some of the same molecular and pathophysiologic underpinnings. Hence, research in this field may change the gloomy picture of SVD.

References

1. Chabriat H, Joutel A, Dichgans M, Tournier-Lasserve E, Bousser MG. CADASIL. *Lancet Neurol* 2009;8:643–653.
2. Viswanathan A, Godin O, Jouvent E, et al. Impact of MRI markers in subcortical vascular dementia: a multi-modal analysis in CADASIL. *Neurobiol Aging* 2010;31:1629–1636.
3. Duering M, Righart R, Csanadi E, et al. Incident subcortical infarcts induce focal thinning in connected cortical regions. *Neurology* 2012;79:2025–2028.
4. Ruchoux MM, Guerouaou D, Vandenhaute B, et al. Systemic vascular smooth muscle cell impairment in cerebral autosomal dominant arteriopathy with subcortical infarcts and leukoencephalopathy. *Acta Neuropathol (Berl)* 1995; 89:500–512.
5. Joutel A, Vahedi K, Corpechot C, et al. Strong clustering and stereotyped nature of Notch3 mutations in CADASIL patients. *Lancet* 1997;350:1511–1515.
6. Peters N, Opherk C, Bergmann T, et al. Spectrum of mutations in biopsy-proven CADASIL: implications for diagnostic strategies. *Arch Neurol* 2005;62:1091–1094.
7. Joutel A, Andreux F, Gaulis S, et al. The ectodomain of the NOTCH3 receptor accumulates within the cerebrovasculature of CADASIL patients. *J Clin Invest* 2000;105:597–605.
8. Domenga V, Fardoux P, Lacombe P, et al. NOTCH3 is required for arterial identity and maturation of vascular smooth muscle cells. *Genes Dev* 2004;18:2730–2735.
9. Belin de Chantemele EJ, Retailleau K, Pinaud F, et al. NOTCH3 is a major regulator of vascular tone in cerebral and tail resistance arteries. *Arterioscler Thromb Vasc Biol* 2008;28:2216–2224.
10. Arboleda-Velasquez JF, Zhou Z, Shin HK, et al. Linking NOTCH signaling to ischemic stroke. *Proc Natl Acad Sci USA* 2008; 105:4856–4861.
11. Kopan R, Ilagan MX. The canonical NOTCH signaling pathway: unfolding the activation mechanism. *Cell* 2009; 137:216–233.
12. Fouillade C, Baron-Menguy C, Domenga-Denier V, et al. Transcriptome analysis for NOTCH3 target genes identifies GRIP2 as a novel regulator of myogenic response in the cerebrovasculature. *Arterioscler Thromb Vasc Biol* 2013;33:76–86.
13. Monet M, Domenga V, Lemaire B, et al. The archetypal R90C CADASIL-NOTCH3 mutation retains NOTCH3 function in vivo. *Hum Mol Genet* 2007;16:982–992.
14. Monet-Lepretre M, Bardot B, Lemaire B, et al. Distinct phenotypic and functional features of CADASIL mutations in the NOTCH3 ligand binding domain. *Brain* 2009; 132:1601–1612.
15. Peters N, Opherk C, Zacherle S, et al. CADASIL-associated NOTCH3 mutations have differential effects both on ligand binding and ligand-induced NOTCH3 receptor signaling through RBP-J. *Exp Cell Res* 2004;299:454–464.
16. Arboleda-Velasquez JF, Manent J, Lee JH, et al. Hypomorphic NOTCH 3 alleles link notch signaling to ischemic cerebral small-vessel disease. *Proc Natl Acad Sci U S A* 2011;108:E128–135.
17. Duering M, Karpinska A, Rosner S, et al. Co-aggregate formation of CADASIL-mutant NOTCH3: a single-particle analysis. *Hum Mol Genet* 2011;20:3256–3265.
18. Ishiko A, Shimizu A, Nagata E, et al. NOTCH3 ectodomain is a major component of granular osmiophilic material (GOM) in CADASIL. *Acta Neuropathol* 2006;112:333–339.
19. Joutel A, Monet-Lepretre M, Gosele C, et al. Cerebrovascular

dysfunction and microcirculation rarefaction precede white matter lesions in a mouse genetic model of cerebral ischemic small vessel disease. *J Clin Invest* 2010;120:433–445.

20. Joutel A. Pathogenesis of CADASIL: transgenic and knock-out mice to probe function and dysfunction of the mutated gene, *NOTCH3*, in the cerebrovasculature. *Bioessays* 2011;33:73–80.
21. Eikermann-Haerter K, Yuzawa I, Dilekoz E, et al. Cerebral autosomal dominant arteriopathy with subcortical infarcts and leukoencephalopathy syndrome mutations increase susceptibility to spreading depression. *Ann Neurol* 2011;69:413–418.
22. Fukutake T. Cerebral autosomal recessive arteriopathy with subcortical infarcts and leukoencephalopathy (CARASIL): from discovery to gene identification. *J Stroke Cerebrovasc Dis* 2011;20:85–93.
23. Oide T, Nakayama H, Yanagawa S, et al. Extensive loss of arterial medial smooth muscle cells and mural extracellular matrix in cerebral autosomal recessive arteriopathy with subcortical infarcts and leukoencephalopathy (CARASIL). *Neuropathology* 2008;28:132–142.
24. Hara K, Shiga A, Fukutake T, et al. Association of HTRA1 mutations and familial ischemic cerebral small-vessel disease. *N Engl J Med* 2009;360:1729–1739.
25. Chamberland A, Wang E, Jones AR, et al. Identification of a novel HtrA1-susceptible cleavage site in human aggrecan: evidence for the involvement of HtrA1 in aggrecan proteolysis in vivo. *J Biol Chem* 2009;284:27352–27359.
26. Grau S, Richards PJ, Kerr B, et al. The role of human HtrA1 in arthritic disease. *J Biol Chem* 2006;281:6124–6129.
27. Kim GY, Kim HY, Kim HT, et al. HtrA1 is a novel antagonist controlling fibroblast growth factor (FGF) signaling via cleavage of FGF8. *Mol Cell Biol* 2012;32:4482–4492.
28. Shiga A, Nozaki H, Yokoseki A, et al. Cerebral small-vessel disease protein HTRA1 controls the amount of TGF-β1 via cleavage of proTGF-β1. *Hum Mol Genet* 2011;20:1800–1810.
29. Truebestein L, Tennstaedt A, Monig T, et al. Substrate-induced remodeling of the active site regulates human HTRA1 activity. *Nat Struct Mol Biol* 2011; 18:386–388.
30. Hadfield KD, Rock CF, Inkson CA, et al. HtrA1 inhibits mineral deposition by osteoblasts: requirement for the protease and PDZ domains. *J Biol Chem* 2008;283:5928–5938.
31. Tiaden AN, Breiden M, Mirsaidi A, et al. Human serine protease HTRA1 positively regulates osteogenesis of human bone marrow-derived mesenchymal stem cells and mineralization of differentiating bone-forming cells through the modulation of extracellular matrix protein. *Stem Cells* 2012;30:2271–2282.
32. Oka C, Tsujimoto R, Kajikawa M, et al. HtrA1 serine protease inhibits signaling mediated by TGFβ family proteins. *Development* 2004;131: 1041–1053.
33. Zhang L, Lim SL, Du H, et al. High temperature requirement factor A1 (*HTRA1*) gene regulates angiogenesis through transforming growth factor-β family member growth differentiation factor 6. *J Biol Chem* 2012;287:1520–1526.
34. Richards A, van den Maagdenberg AM, Jen JC, et al. C-terminal truncations in human 3′-5′ DNA exonuclease TREX1 cause autosomal dominant retinal vasculopathy with cerebral leukodystrophy. *Nat Genet* 2007;39:1068–1070.
35. Weil S, Reifenberger G, Dudel C, et al. Cerebroretinal vasculopathy mimicking a brain tumor: a case of a rare hereditary syndrome. *Neurology* 1999;53:629–631.
36. Grand MG, Kaine J, Fulling K, et al. Cerebroretinal vasculopathy. A new hereditary syndrome. *Ophthalmology* 1988;95:649–659.
37. Jen J, Cohen AH, Yue Q, et al. Hereditary endotheliopathy with retinopathy, nephropathy, and stroke (HERNS). *Neurology* 1997;49:1322–1330.
38. Terwindt GM, Haan J, Ophoff RA, et al. Clinical and genetic analysis of a large Dutch family with autosomal dominant vascular retinopathy, migraine and Raynaud's phenomenon. *Brain* 1998;121(Pt 2):303–316.
39. Khajavi M, Inoue K, Lupski JR. Nonsense-mediated mRNA decay modulates clinical outcome of genetic disease. *Eur J Hum Genet* 2006;14:1074–1081.
40. Yang YG, Lindahl T, Barnes DE. TREX1 exonuclease degrades ssDNA to prevent chronic checkpoint activation and autoimmune disease. *Cell* 2007;131:873–886.
41. Stetson DB, Ko JS, Heidmann T, Medzhitov R. TREX1 prevents cell-intrinsic initiation of autoimmunity. *Cell* 2008;134:587–598.
42. Hoss M, Robins P, Naven TJ, et al. A human DNA editing enzyme homologous to the *Escherichia coli* DnaQ/MutD protein. *EMBO J* 1999;18:3868–3875.
43. Morita M, Stamp G, Robins P, et al. Gene-targeted mice lacking the TREX1 (DNase III) 3′->5′ DNA exonuclease develop inflammatory myocarditis. *Mol Cell Biol* 2004;24:6719–6727.
44. Crow YJ, Hayward BE, Parmar R, et al. Mutations in the gene encoding the 3′-5′ DNA

exonuclease TREX1 cause Aicardi–Goutières syndrome at the AGS1 locus. *Nat Genet* 2006;38:917–920.

45. Rice G, Patrick T, Parmar R, et al. Clinical and molecular phenotype of Aicardi–Goutières syndrome. *Am J Hum Genet* 2007; 81:713–725.

46. Rice G, Newman WG, Dean J, et al. Heterozygous mutations in TREX1 cause familial chilblain lupus and dominant Aicardi–Goutières syndrome. *Am J Hum Genet* 2007;80:811–815.

47. Chowdhury D, Beresford PJ, Zhu P, et al. The exonuclease TREX1 is in the SET complex and acts in concert with NM23-H1 to degrade DNA during Granzyme A-mediated cell death. *Mol Cell* 2006;23:133–142.

48. Viswanathan A, Greenberg SM. Cerebral amyloid angiopathy in the elderly. *Ann Neurol* 2011;70:871–880.

49. Revesz T, Holton JL, Lashley T, et al. Genetics and molecular pathogenesis of sporadic and hereditary cerebral amyloid angiopathies. *Acta Neuropathol* 2009;118:115–130.

50. Garringer HJ, Murrell J, D'Adamio L, Ghetti B, Vidal R. Modeling familial British and Danish dementia. *Brain Struct Funct* 2010;214:235–244.

51. Levy E, Lopez-Otin C, Ghiso J, Geltner D, Frangione B. Stroke in Icelandic patients with hereditary amyloid angiopathy is related to a mutation in the cystatin C gene, an inhibitor of cysteine proteases. *J Exp Med* 1989;169:1771–1778.

52. Plante-Bordeneuve V, Said G. Familial amyloid polyneuropathy. *Lancet Neurol* 2011;10:1086–1097.

53. Solomon JP, Page LJ, Balch WE, Kelly JW. Gelsolin amyloidosis: genetics, biochemistry, pathology and possible strategies for therapeutic intervention. *Crit Rev Biochem Mol Biol* 2012; 47:282–296.

54. Rostagno A, Holton JL, Lashley T, Revesz T, Ghiso J. Cerebral amyloidosis: amyloid subunits, mutants and phenotypes. *Cell Mol Life Sci* 2010;67:581–600.

55. De Strooper B. Proteases and proteolysis in Alzheimer disease: a multifactorial view on the disease process. *Physiol Rev* 2010; 90:465–494.

56. Iliff JJ, Wang M, Liao Y, et al. A paravascular pathway facilitates CSF flow through the brain parenchyma and the clearance of interstitial solutes, including amyloid β. *Sci Transl Med* 2012;4:147.

57. Deane R, Bell RD, Sagare A, Zlokovic BV. Clearance of amyloid-β peptide across the blood–brain barrier: implication for therapies in Alzheimer's disease. *CNS Neurol Disord Drug Targets* 2009;8:16–30.

58. Lee J, Culyba EK, Powers ET, Kelly JW. Amyloid-β forms fibrils by nucleated conformational conversion of oligomers. *Nat Chem Biol* 2011;7:602–609.

59. Kim J, Onstead L, Randle S, et al. Aβ40 inhibits amyloid deposition in vivo. *J Neurosci* 2007; 27:627–633.

60. Levy E, Prelli F, Frangione B. Studies on the first described Alzheimer's disease amyloid β mutant, the Dutch variant. *J Alzheimers Dis* 2006;9:329–339.

61. De Jonghe C, Esselens C, Kumar-Singh S, et al. Pathogenic APP mutations near the γ-secretase cleavage site differentially affect Aβ secretion and APP C-terminal fragment stability. *Hum Mol Genet* 2001;10:1665–1671.

62. Citron M, Oltersdorf T, Haass C, et al. Mutation of the β-amyloid precursor protein in familial Alzheimer's disease increases β-protein production. *Nature* 1992;360:672–674.

63. Chavez-Gutierrez L, Bammens L, Benilova I, et al. The mechanism of γ-secretase dysfunction in familial Alzheimer disease. *EMBO J* 2012;31:2261–2274.

64. Herzig MC, Winkler DT, Burgermeister P, et al. Aβ is targeted to the vasculature in a mouse model of hereditary cerebral hemorrhage with amyloidosis. *Nat Neurosci* 2004;7:954–960.

65. Calhoun ME, Burgermeister P, Phinney AL, et al. Neuronal overexpression of mutant amyloid precursor protein results in prominent deposition of cerebrovascular amyloid. *Proc Natl Acad Sci USA* 1999;96: 14088–14093.

66. Castano EM, Prelli F, Soto C, et al. The length of amyloid-β in hereditary cerebral hemorrhage with amyloidosis, Dutch type. Implications for the role of amyloid-β1–42 in Alzheimer's disease. *J Biol Chem* 1996;271:32185–32191.

67. McGowan E, Pickford F, Kim J, et al. Aβ42 is essential for parenchymal and vascular amyloid deposition in mice. *Neuron* 2005;47:191–199.

68. Verghese PB, Castellano JM, Holtzman DM. Apolipoprotein E in Alzheimer's disease and other neurological disorders. *Lancet Neurol* 2011;10:241–252.

69. Fryer JD, Taylor JW, DeMattos RB, et al. Apolipoprotein E markedly facilitates age-dependent cerebral amyloid angiopathy and spontaneous hemorrhage in amyloid precursor protein transgenic mice. *J Neurosci* 2003;23:7889–7896.

70. Fryer JD, Simmons K, Parsadanian M, et al. Human apolipoprotein E4 alters the amyloid-β 40 : 42 ratio and promotes the formation of cerebral amyloid angiopathy in an amyloid precursor protein transgenic model. *J Neurosci* 2005;25:2803–2810.

71. Choi SH, Leight SN, Lee VM, et al. Accelerated Aβ deposition in

APPswe/PS1deltaE9 mice with hemizygous deletions of TTR (transthyretin). *J Neurosci* 2007;27:7006–7010.

72. Kaeser SA, Herzig MC, Coomaraswamy J, et al. Cystatin C modulates cerebral β-amyloidosis. *Nat Genet* 2007;39:1437–1439.

73. Coomaraswamy J, Kilger E, Wolfing H, et al. Modeling familial Danish dementia in mice supports the concept of the amyloid hypothesis of Alzheimer's disease. *Proc Natl Acad Sci USA* 2010;107:7969–7974.

74. Iadecola C, Zhang F, Niwa K, et al. SOD1 rescues cerebral endothelial dysfunction in mice overexpressing amyloid precursor protein. *Nat Neurosci* 1999; 2:157–161.

75. Park L, Anrather J, Zhou P, et al. NADPH-oxidase-derived reactive oxygen species mediate the cerebrovascular dysfunction induced by the amyloid β peptide. *J Neurosci* 2005;25:1769–1777.

76. Shin HK, Jones PB, Garcia-Alloza M, et al. Age-dependent cerebrovascular dysfunction in a transgenic mouse model of cerebral amyloid angiopathy. *Brain* 2007;130:2310–2319.

77. Dumas A, Dierksen GA, Gurol ME, et al. Functional magnetic resonance imaging detection of vascular reactivity in cerebral amyloid angiopathy. *Ann Neurol* 2012;72:76–81.

78. Schenk D, Barbour R, Dunn W, et al. Immunization with amyloid-β attenuates Alzheimer-disease-like pathology in the PDAPP mouse. *Nature* 1999;400:173–177.

79. Pfeifer M, Boncristiano S, Bondolfi L, et al. Cerebral hemorrhage after passive anti-Aβ immunotherapy. *Science* 2002;298:1379.

80. Boche D, Zotova E, Weller RO, et al. Consequence of Aβ immunization on the vasculature of human Alzheimer's disease brain. *Brain* 2008;131:3299–3310.

81. Khoshnoodi J, Pedchenko V, Hudson BG. Mammalian collagen IV. *Microsc Res Tech* 2008; 71:357–370.

82. Gould DB, Phalan FC, Breedveld GJ, et al. Mutations in *Col4a1* cause perinatal cerebral hemorrhage and porencephaly. *Science* 2005;308:1167–1171.

83. Gould DB, Phalan FC, van Mil SE, et al. Role of *COL4A1* in small-vessel disease and hemorrhagic stroke. *N Engl J Med* 2006;354:1489–1496.

84. Kuo DS, Labelle-Dumais C, Gould DB. *COL4A1* and *COL4A2* mutations and disease: insights into pathogenic mechanisms and potential therapeutic targets. *Hum Mol Genet* 2012;21:R97–R110.

85. Meuwissen ME, de Vries LS, Verbeek HA, et al. Sporadic *COL4A1* mutations with extensive prenatal porencephaly resembling hydranencephaly. *Neurology* 2011;76:844–846.

86. Yoneda Y, Haginoya K, Arai H, et al. De novo and inherited mutations in *COL4A2*, encoding the type IV collagen alpha-2 chain cause porencephaly. *Am J Hum Genet* 2012;90:86–90.

87. Yoneda Y, Haginoya K, Kato M, et al. Phenotypic spectrum of *COL4A1* mutations: porencephaly to schizencephaly. *Ann Neurol* 2013;73:48–57.

88. Alamowitch S, Plaisier E, Favrole P, et al. Cerebrovascular disease related to *COL4A1* mutations in HANAC syndrome. *Neurology* 2009;73:1873–1882.

89. Plaisier E, Gribouval O, Alamowitch S, et al. *COL4A1* mutations and hereditary angiopathy, nephropathy, aneurysms, and muscle cramps. *N Engl J Med* 2007; 357:2687–2695.

90. Verbeek E, Meuwissen ME, Verheijen FW, et al. *COL4A2* mutation associated with familial porencephaly and small-vessel disease. *Eur J Hum Genet* 2012;20:844–851.

91. Parkin JD, San Antonio JD, Pedchenko V, et al. Mapping structural landmarks, ligand binding sites, and missense mutations to the collagen IV heterotrimers predicts major functional domains, novel interactions, and variation in phenotypes in inherited diseases affecting basement membranes. *Hum Mutat* 2011;32:127–143.

92. Poschl E, Schlotzer-Schrehardt U, Brachvogel B, et al. Collagen IV is essential for basement membrane stability but dispensable for initiation of its assembly during early development. *Development* 2004;131:1619–1628.

93. Gould DB, Marchant JK, Savinova OV, Smith RS, John SW. *Col4a1* mutation causes endoplasmic reticulum stress and genetically modifiable ocular dysgenesis. *Hum Mol Genet* 2007;16:798–807.

94. Labelle-Dumais C, Dilworth DJ, Harrington EP, et al. *COL4A1* mutations cause ocular dysgenesis, neuronal localization defects, and myopathy in mice and Walker–Warburg syndrome in humans. *PLoS Genet* 2011;7: e1002062.

95. Favor J, Gloeckner CJ, Janik D, et al. Type IV procollagen missense mutations associated with defects of the eye, vascular stability, the brain, kidney function and embryonic or postnatal viability in the mouse, *Mus musculus*: an extension of the *Col4a1* allelic series and the identification of the first two *Col4a2* mutant alleles. *Genetics* 2007;175:725–736.

96. Van Agtmael T, Schlotzer-Schrehardt U, McKie L, et al. Dominant mutations of *Col4a1* result in basement membrane defects which lead to anterior segment dysgenesis and

glomerulopathy. *Hum Mol Genet* 2005;14:3161–3168.

97. Weng YC, Sonni A, Labelle-Dumais C, et al. *COL4A1* mutations in patients with sporadic late-onset intracerebral hemorrhage. *Ann Neurol* 2012;71:470–477.

98. Forlino A, Cabral WA, Barnes AM, Marini JC. New perspectives on osteogenesis imperfecta. *Nat Rev Endocrinol* 2012;7:540–557.

99. Lemmens R, Maugeri A, Niessen HW, et al. Novel *COL4A1* mutations cause cerebral small vessel disease by haploinsufficiency. *Hum Mol Genet* 2013; 22:391–397.

Chapter 8

Hereditary cerebral small vessel disease and the role of genetic factors

Christian Opherk and Martin Dichgans

Introduction

Similar to ischemic stroke in general, genetic factors have been recognized to have a significant impact on cerebral small vessel disease (SVD). Heritability estimates for cerebral white matter lesions as a surrogate marker of cerebral SVD range from 50 to 80% [1]. Furthermore, several monogenic conditions are closely associated with cerebral SVD. Some of these do have important implications for patient counseling and treatment. This chapter will give an overview on the most common monogenic conditions associated with cerebral SVD and recent data from genetic studies on sporadic cerebral SVD.

Monogenic conditions associated with cerebral SVD

Monogenic disorders are caused by highly penetrant mutations in a *single* gene. The presence of cerebral SVD in young patients and individuals without classical vascular risk factors should raise the suspicion of a monogenic condition. In some of these disorders cerebral SVD is the main manifestation, in others SVD is part of a wider phenotypic spectrum (Table 8.1). In order to recognize monogenic forms of SVD, it is essential to perform a systematic family history and to search for associated neurologic and non-neurologic signs and symptoms in index cases and relatives. The diagnosis may have implications both for therapeutic decisions and genetic counseling. Detailed information about pathogenetic and clinical aspects as well as specific diagnostic strategies of hereditary SVD will be provided in Chapters 7, 16, and 23.

Cerebral autosomal dominant arteriopathy with subcortical infarcts and leukoencephalopathy

Cerebral autosomal dominant arteriopathy with subcortical infarcts and leukoencephalopathy (CADASIL) is an autosomal-dominantly inherited nonamyloid systemic angiopathy, caused by mutations in the *NOTCH3* gene [2]. The prevalence has been estimated to be $>4:100\,000$ [3]. CADASIL is the most common hereditary SVD and has been reported to account for roughly 2% of cases of lacunar stroke with leukoaraiosis in patients younger than 65 years and for 11% of cases in those younger than 50 years [4].

The main clinical symptoms are migraine with aura, recurrent transitory ischemic attacks (TIAs) and cerebral ischemia, progressive cognitive deficits, as well as psychiatric disturbance. Although the disease is of systemic nature, clinically relevant manifestations outside the brain have not been described.

Pathologically, CADASIL patients show multiple cerebral ischemic lesions and diffuse white matter changes. The mean age of onset for first stroke is 46 years, which may be preceded by migraine with aura in about 30–40% of the cases [5, 6]. Cerebral lesions lead to both physical disability and cognitive dysfunction. Over 70% of patients are demented in their sixth decade of life. Gender seems to influence the clinical phenotype: migraine with aura is more frequent in women and stroke is more frequent in men before the age of menopause [7]. The long-term prognosis for disability and death is worse for men compared to women [6].

Cerebral Small Vessel Disease, ed. Leonardo Pantoni and Philip B. Gorelick. Published by Cambridge University Press.

Table 8.1 Monogenic conditions associated with cerebral SVD

Condition	Gene (inheritance)	Protein	Age at onset	Clinical symptoms	Imaging findings
CADASIL	*NOTCH3* (autosomal dominant)	NOTCH3 receptor	30–50	Recurrent TIAs and strokes, migraine, mood disorders, progressive dementia	Leukoencephalopathy (prominent involvement of temporal poles, external capsule), microbleeds
CARASIL	*HTRA1* (autosomal recessive)	HTRA1 serine protease	20–30	Recurrents TIAs and strokes, mood disorders, progressive cognitive dysfunction, alopecia, orthopedic symptoms	Leukoencephalopathy
Fabry's disease	*GLA* (X-linked)	α-Galactosidase A	Childhood	Acroparesthesia, polyneuropathy, angiokeratoma, hypohidrosis with heat intolerance, corneal and lenticular opacities, proteinuria, cardiomyopathy, TIAs and strokes	Leukoencephalopathy, ectasia of large vessels, embolic infarcts
COL4A1-associated angiopathy	*COL4A1* (autosomal dominant)	Type IV collagen alpha-1 chain	All ages	Recurrent TIAs and strokes, brain hemorrhage, retinal arteriolar tortuosity, cataracts, Axenfeld–Rieger anomaly, muscle cramps, Raynaud's syndrome, kidney dysfunction	Intracerebral hemorrhage, leukoencephalopathy, in some cases porencephaly
RVCL	*TREX1* (autosomal dominant)	Exonuclease DNAse III	20–40	Recurrent TIAs and strokes, retinal vasculopathy, headaches, migraine, psychiatric disturbance, progressive cognitive dysfunction, kidney dysfunction	Leukoencephalopathy, contrast enhancing lesions with vasogenic edema ("pseudotumors")

CADASIL, cerebral autosomal dominant arteriopathy with subcortical infarcts and leukoencephalopathy; CARASIL, cerebral autosomal recessive arteriopathy with subcortical infarcts and leukoencephalopathy; RVCL, retinal vasculopathy with cerebral leukodystrophy; SVD, small vessel disease; TIA, transient ischemic attack.

Cerebral magnetic resonance imaging (MRI) in CADASIL patients shows all features of cerebral SVD, including lacunar lesions, white matter hyperintensities, and cerebral microbleeds. An early involvement of the anterior temporal poles and the external capsule is indicative of CADASIL [8]. There is considerable variability of both cerebral white matter lesion load and clinical symptoms [6, 9], even within families. This variability does not seem to be caused by different *NOTCH3* mutations. Since heritability for T2-lesion volumes in CADASIL has been estimated to be 74%, additional genetic modifiers seem to be relevant [9].

CADASIL is caused by mutations in the *NOTCH3* gene, which encodes a large type-I transmembrane receptor [2]. In the postnatal period, NOTCH3 (N3) seems to exert a critical role in the differentiation and maturation of the arterial vascular smooth muscle cells (vSMCs) [10]. In adulthood, N3 is mainly expressed by vSMCs and pericytes. The exact pathophysiologic mechanism of CADASIL is still uncertain. Virtually all CADASIL mutations described so far result in an odd number of cysteines within the extracellular domain of N3 [6, 11]. Therefore, it has been proposed that abnormal disulfide bridge formation might mediate receptor multimerization and/or interaction with other proteins. Indeed, the pathologic hallmark of the disease is (diagnostically relevant) N3-immunopositive deposits (granular osmiophilic material [GOM] on electron microscopy) at the cell surface of vSMCs. These cells degenerate over the course of the disease. In vitro studies in transfected cells and rescue experiments in transgenic mice suggest that CADASIL-associated mutations do not lead to a classic gain- or loss-of-function mechanism [12–14]. Instead, CADASIL-associated mutations may act through a neomorphic effect, i.e., a novel function of the mutated receptor. Consistent with this hypothesis, it has been shown that CADASIL-mutated N3 fragments are able to sequestrate other proteins into the aggregates [15].

Currently, no targeted treatment exists that would slow down progression of the primary disease process. Migraine in CADASIL rarely requires specific treatment as attack frequency is commonly low. If prophylactic treatment is warranted, the usual agents such as beta-blockers or antiepileptics can be used. For acute treatment, triptanes should be avoided due to their vasoconstrictive properties. With the lack of a well-documented prevention of ischemic attacks, standard stroke prevention therapy is currently administered using antiplatelet drugs, statins, and control of general vascular risk factors. In some cases, patients are placed on a B-vitamin complex and a low dose of a blood pressure lowering agent that is thought to protect the vessel wall (e.g., a calcium channel blocking agent), though none of these strategies has been proven to reduce the risk of stroke in CADASIL. Patients should be advised to ensure adequate fluid intake in order prevent dehydration.

The only randomized trial to be performed so far in CADASIL tested the efficacy of donepezil in CADASIL patients with cognitive impairment [16]. In this trial donepezil showed no effect on the primary endpoint (the Vascular Dementia Assessment Scale – cognitive subscale [VADAS-cog]). However, with donepezil treatment improvement of several subscales of executive function was noted. The clinical relevance of this finding is not clear.

Cerebral autosomal recessive arteriopathy with subcortical infarcts and leukoencephalopathy

Cerebral autosomal recessive arteriopathy with subcortical infarcts and leukoencephalopathy (CARASIL) is an autosomal *recessive* syndrome similar to CADASIL, with cerebral SVD in combination with orthopedic problems and alopecia, that has been described in families predominantly of Asian origin as the Maeda syndrome [17, 18]. This disorder is very rare. Only one white family has been described so far [19].

Similar to CADASIL patients, these patients develop recurrent strokes and cognitive decline, ultimately leading to vascular dementia. Orthopedic complications include intervertebral disk disease and miscellaneous manifestations of osseous structures, in particular kyphosis, degenerative arthropathy, ossification of intraspinal canal ligaments, and deformity of elbows. Brain imaging shows symmetrical T2-hyperintense white matter signal abnormalities and small lacunar lesions [17].

Pathologically, affected vessels show vSMC loss with fragmentation of the elastica interna with lumen narrowing, intimal thickening, as well as accumulation of collagen fibers and hyaline degeneration of the medial layers of small arteries [18]. In contrast to CADASIL, no GOM is detectable on electron microscopy.

CARASIL is caused by mutations in the *HTRA1* gene encoding a serine protease known to influence transforming growth factor-beta (TGF-β) signaling [20]. Most mutations described result in a stop codon and lead to decreased protease activity. Since TGF-β is one of the substrates of HTRA1, increased TGF-β activity had been proposed to be a central factor of the disease. Accordingly, TGF-β1 immunoreactivity is elevated in brain vessels from CARASIL patients [20]. There is no specific treatment so far.

Fabry's disease

Fabry's disease is an X-linked disorder resulting from mutations of the *GLA* gene leading to a very low specific activity of the lysosomal enzyme hydrolase α-galactosidase A (GLA) [21]. This leads to progressive accumulation of glycosphingolipids (primarily

Gb3) in various organs, predominantly in the vascular endothelial and smooth muscle cells, myocardium, renal epithelium, and the central nervous system. Dermal vessels undergo dilation and proliferation to form angiokeratoma. The incidence has been estimated to be 2.5 : 100 000. Despite X-linked inheritance, women can be affected, though usually with a milder phenotype.

Clinical symptoms of the disease usually start in adolescence with severe neuropathic pain in the extremities with acroparesthesia, anhidrosis, and skin and mucosal angiokeratoma. Ophthalmologic examination often reveals corneal opacities, retrolenticular cataracts, and tortuous retinal blood vessels. Morbidity is primarily determined by cardiac, renal, and cerebrovascular involvement, which tends to occur in the fourth decade [21]. Prior to the introduction of enzyme replacement therapy the median age at death was 55 years in males.

Cerebrovascular symptoms seem to be mediated by both large and small artery involvement with a preference for the posterior circulation [22]. Small artery involvement is characterized by progressive occlusion of blood vessels, secondary to deposition of Gb3 within the vascular wall. Prevalence of Fabry's disease in young male patients with cryptogenic stroke has been estimated to be as high as 5% [23]. Stroke may be the first obvious clinical manifestation of Fabry's disease. A dolichoectatic vertebrobasilar artery complex may be a manifestation of the disease.

Fabry's disease can be diagnosed by determination of GLA enzyme activity in blood (in women GLA activity is not a reliable marker due to inconstant X-chromosomal inactivation). Establishing the diagnosis has therapeutic implications: enzyme replacement therapy has been shown to be effective in terms of renal and cardiac outcomes [24], but a positive effect on cerebrovascular complications is still lacking. However, some guidelines recommend enzyme replacement therapy for the management of stroke in infants and children with this disorder [25].

COL4A1-associated angiopathy

Mutations in the *COL4A1* gene encoding the alpha-1 chain of type IV collagen have been recently described in the context of cerebral SVD [26]. The disease shows autosomal dominant inheritance and is rare with fewer than 20 families described.

Clinically, four major phenotypes of COL4A1-associated angiopathy have been described: (1) a condition exhibiting perinatal hemorrhage with porencephaly [27]; (2) SVD with hemorrhage and hemiparesis [28]; (3) SVD with Axenfeld–Rieger anomaly [29]; and (4) hereditary angiopathy with nephropathy, aneurysms, and muscle cramps (HANAC) syndrome [30]. Apart from brain hemorrhage, patients with *COL4A1* mutations typically show ophthalmologic manifestations with retinal artery tortuosity, cataracts, glaucoma, and anterior segment dysgenesis of the eye (e.g., Axenfeld–Rieger anomaly). HANAC-associated *COL4A1* mutations seem to lead to a broader clinical phenotype with involvement of large arteries with aneurysms, Raynaud's syndrome, kidney defects, and cardiac arrhythmia.

Brain hemorrhage is often the first manifestation of the disease. Brain MRI reveals typical cerebral SVD. Cases with porencephaly are characterized by large, fluid-filled cavities in the periventricular regions. There is no specific treatment thus far.

Retinal vasculopathy with cerebral leukodystrophy

Hereditary endotheliopathy with retinopathy, nephropathy, and stroke (HERNS) [31], cerebroretinal vasculopathy (CRV) [32], and hereditary vascular retinopathy (HVR) [33] were reported independently, but identification of the responsible gene has revealed that they are different phenotypic spectra of the same disease (retinal vasculopathy with cerebral leukodystrophy [RVCL]). A consistent feature of all three is SVD affecting the brain and the retina. RVCL is exceptionally rare.

Clinical symptoms usually commence in the fourth decade of life with visual disturbances ("blind spots"), migrainous headache, transient ischemic attacks, strokes, and behavioral abnormalities. Most affected individuals in later disease stages suffer from severe cognitive impairment. Neurologic complications of HERNS and CRV usually lead to death before the age of 55; patients with HVR live longer.

Apart from typical cerebral SVD, brain MRI often reveals contrast-enhancing lesions with surrounding vasogenic edema, most commonly in the frontoparietal region, which can be misinterpreted as brain tumors. Upon biopsy, brain pathologic changes are consistent with coagulative necrosis secondary to an obliterative vasculopathy but with negligible inflammatory infiltrates. Small intracerebral vessels exhibit multilayered capillary basal membranes, and amorphous thickening of their walls with adventitial fibrosis. Retinal abnormalities include telangiectatic capillaries and microaneurysms, which may be seen even in asymptomatic individuals on fluorescein angiography [33]. Advanced stages are characterized by occlusion of branches of large retinal arteries and avascular areas in the retinal periphery. In HERNS, renal insufficiency and proteinuria have been a consistent feature.

Linkage analyses demonstrated that HERNS, CRV, and HVR are allelic disorders mapped to the same locus on chromosome 3p21.1–p21.3. They are now described as autosomal dominant RVCL [34]. Pathogenic mutations affect the *TREX1* gene, which encodes an autonomous (nonprocessive) 3′–5′ DNA-specific exonuclease found in all mammalian cells. While heterozygous mutations result in RVCL, homozygous mutations are the cause of the recessive form of Aicardi–Goutières syndrome (AGS) [35]. AGS manifests as a progressive encephalopathy of early onset, brain atrophy, demyelination, basal ganglia calcifications, and chronic lymphocytic proliferation in the cerebrospinal fluid (CSF).

Hereditary forms of cerebral amyloid angiopathy

Several hereditary forms of cerebral amyloid angiopathy (CAA) have been described. They show autosomal dominant inheritance and may be differentiated based on clinicopathologic, biochemical, and genetic findings [36, 37]. The primary manifestation of these disorders is cerebral hemorrhage. Some of the most relevant forms show cerebral SVD and are summarized in Table 8.2.

Amyloid precursor protein (APP)-related CAA

Several point mutations within the amyloid precursor protein (*APP*) gene have been shown to be associated with enhanced deposition of β-amyloid (Aβ), a 39–43-amino-acid fragment of APP. Mutations associated with severe CAA are typically located within the Aβ region itself and are associated with a higher Aβ40 : Aβ42 ratio, while mutations associated primarily with senile plaques (Alzheimer's disease type pathology) flank the Aβ region. Typical CAA mutations affect three neighboring codons close to the α-cleavage site (Table 8.2).

The most thoroughly characterized form of familial CAA is the Dutch type (also called hereditary cerebral hemorrhage with amyloidosis–Dutch type, HCHWA-D). Affected individuals typically present with recurrent strokes with onset between the ages of 40 and 75 years (mean 50 years) [38]. With at least 80% of the cases, brain hemorrhage is the main clinical manifestation. Another prominent feature is dementia, which may develop in the absence of clinically overt stroke. Most patients show cerebral SVD on brain imaging with occipital predominance [38]. The exact mechanisms by which CAA may cause stroke and dementia are unknown. In an autopsy study, cognitive function was associated with the severity of CAA (CAA-load and vessel wall thickening) but was independent of plaques and neurofibrillary tangles, i.e., AD-like pathologic changes [39]. However, neither the number of focal infarcts nor the extent of white matter lesions were directly associated with cognitive decline [40]. Therefore, the dementia in HCHWA-D may be classified as vascular dementia, but likely involves other mechanisms than infarcts or white matter lesions. Other APP-related hereditary CAA forms associated with cerebral SVD are the Flemish, the Iowa, and the Piedmont types (Table 8.2).

Cystatin C-related CAA

Hereditary cerebral hemorrhage with amyloidosis–Icelandic type (HCHWA-I) has been described in several families from Iceland [37]. The disease is characterized by severe amyloid deposition within small arteries and arterioles of the leptomeninges, cerebral cortex, basal ganglia, brainstem, and cerebellum. The main clinical manifestation is recurrent intracerebral hemorrhage (ICH) starting between age 20 and 40 years. Cognitive deficits are frequent and typically slowly progressive. In some patients dementia may be the sole manifestation.

Pathologic and MRI examination of the brain shows single or multiple hemorrhages, diffuse white matter changes, and occasional ischemic infarctions. The main amyloid component in HCHWA-I is cystatin C, a type II cysteine protease inhibitor (Table 8.2) produced by many cell types including neurons. Affected individuals carry a missense mutation at position 68 of the *CST3* gene.

ABri precursor protein (ABriPP)-related CAA

Two specific mutations of the *BRI2* gene have been associated with familial British dementia (FBD) and familial Danish dementia (FDD). The wild-type

Table 8.2 Hereditary forms of CAA-associated with cerebral SVD

Type	Gene (chr.)	Precursor protein	Mutation(s)	Amyloid component	Cerebral hemorrhage	Ischemic white matter lesions (MRI)	Dementia	Brain parenchymal changes other than CAA
Amyloidois–Flemish	*APP* (21)	Amyloid precursor protein (APP)	A692G	Aβ (4 kDa)	+	+	++ (AD-like)	NP (++), NFT (++)
HCHWA–Dutch			E693Q		++	++	+ (VD-like)	Diffuse plaques rare: NP and NFT
Amyloidosis–Iowa			D694N		(+) Microhemorrhages	++ Posterior calcifications	++ Aphasic dementia	NP (+) NFT (++)
Amyloidosis–Piedmont			L705V		+	+	+	–
HCHWA–Icelandic	*CST3* (20)	Cystatin C (Cys C)	L68Q	Acys (20 kDA)	++	+	+	–
FBD	*BRI2* (13)	ABri precursor protein (ABriPP)	STOP267R	ABri (4 kDa)	Relatively rare (+)	++	++	Amyloid plaques, neuronal degeneration
FDD			Decamer duplication	ADan (4 kDa)				
FAF	*GEL* (9)	Gelsolin (Gel)	D187N	AGel (7 kDa)	–	++	Cognitive impairment	–

Aβ, β-amyloid; chr., chromosome; AD, Alzheimer's disease; FAF, familial amyloidosis–Finnish type; FBD, familial British dementia; FDD, familial Danish dementia; HCHWA, hereditary cerebral hemorrhage with amyloidosis; NFT, neurofibrillary tangles; NP, neuritic plaques; SVD, small vessel disease; VD, vascular dementia.

ABriPP precursor protein is a type-II, single-pass transmembrane protein. Disease-causing mutations in FBD or FDD lead to deposition of an ABriPP c-terminal fragment as amyloid in leptomeningeal vessels and in blood vessels of the cortex, white matter and spinal cord [41].

FBD has been described in a few pedigrees from Great Britain. Clinically, patients develop progressive memory loss or dementia (>95%), spastic tetraparesis (>90%), and cerebellar ataxia (75%) [42]. Additional manifestations include stroke-like episodes and headache, whereas intracerebral hemorrhages or epileptic seizures are rather uncommon. Mean age of onset is 48 years with a mean disease duration of nine years (mean age at death is 56 years).

FDD was originally described in a large family from Denmark. Affected patients typically present with cataracts and other ocular disorders including ocular hemorrhages in the third decade followed by severe hearing loss. Cerebellar ataxia usually develops around the age of 40. Psychiatric symptoms occur in the sixth decade and are followed by dementia in the majority of cases. Most patients die in their fifth to sixth decade [41].

Neuropathologically, FBD and FDD are characterized by a diffuse atrophy of the brain (including the cerebellum), cranial nerves, and spinal cord. Another prominent feature is the presence of ischemic white matter changes and lacunar infarcts [41, 42], whereas cerebral hemorrhages are relatively rare. Ischemic lesions are connected with extensive CAA [41, 43].

Histopathologic findings further include parenchymal plaques and neurofibrillary tangles. Thus, the pathology in FBD and FDD comprises both vascular (predominantly ischemic) and neurodegenerative alterations. Most likely, both components contribute to the development of dementia in ABriPP-related CAAs.

Susceptibility loci for the common forms of sporadic SVD

Heritability of white matter lesions

Previous studies have demonstrated that white matter lesions (WMLs) are highly heritable [44]. Heritability is a measure indicating the interindividual difference of a trait due to additive genetic factors. WML heritability estimates have been published for male twins [45], for a population-based sample of middle-aged elderly sibships [46], among hypertensive siblings [47, 48], and in siblings discordant for Alzheimer's disease [49]. In these studies heritability measures ranged between 50 and 80%. Comparable studies for lacunes have not been published, although a recent study that applied genome-wide complex trait analysis to genome-wide data from 3752 patients with ischemic strokes and 5972 controls found a low heritability of small-vessel-related stroke [50].

In light of the apparently high contribution of genetic factors in the pathogenesis of WML linkage studies have identified several loci which were significantly associated with WML volume: on chromosome 4 [51] in a population-based sample and at chromosome 1q24 in hypertensive sibships [48]. Additional suggestive loci were reported on chromosomes 11, 21, and 22.

Common variants associated with WMLs (results from candidate gene studies and genome-wide association studies)

Candidate gene studies

Until recently the most widely used method to identify genetic variants associated with WMLs was the candidate gene approach. Numerous studies have been published and were recently reviewed in a meta-analysis [52]. One of the most replicated findings is polymorphisms in the renin–angiotensin–aldosterone system. The angiotensin-converting enzyme (*ACE*) gene I/D polymorphism has been investigated in nine studies including 2396 individuals. The DD genotype was a significant predictor of WML volume. The M235T variant of the angiotensinogen (*AGT*) gene was assessed in six candidate gene studies including 2702 individuals and was shown not to be a predictor of WML load [52]. However, since its chromosomal location (1q42) was previously found in linkage studies and a recent genome-wide association study (GWAS) [53] has replicated the N235T variant as a predictor for WMLs, it is likely that a neighboring variant in linkage disequilibrium is causative. A longitudinal study reported that WML progression might be related to polymorphisms in the angiotensin receptor (*AGTR*) 1 and 2 genes [54], partly in combination with the N235T *AGT* variant [55]. Numerous other candidate genes have been evaluated in the past, yet most of these studies could not be replicated [52].

Recently, several variants in the *NOTCH3* gene, the gene responsible for CADASIL, were reported to be associated with WML load in a community-dwelling elderly cohort. Among the nine common single-nucleotide polymorphisms (SNPs), four were found to be associated with WML volume, although only in hypertensives [56]. The most robust SNP was replicated in the Cohorts for Heart and Aging Research in Genome Epidemiology (CHARGE) consortium on an independent sample of hypertensives. Among the 33 rare SNPs, nine were only found in subjects with severe WMLs, and six of these were predicted to be functional by protein modeling tools [56]. These results argue for a possible role of *NOTCH3* mutations also in sporadic cerberal SVD.

Genome-wide association studies

In contrast to the candidate analysis, genome-wide association studies (GWAS) take an unbiased approach to sequence variants. A recent GWAS on ischemic WMLs performed by the CHARGE consortium included 9361 individuals of European descent [53]. Genome-wide significance was found for six SNPs on chromosome 17q25. This locus was later confirmed in independent samples, including the Rotterdam Study [57]. The chromosomal region on 17q25 spans roughly 100 kb and harbors several genes: two tripartite motif-containing genes, *TRIM65* and *TRIM47*; the WW domain-binding protein 2 gene (*WBP2*); the mitochondrial ribosomal protein L38 gene (*MRPL38*); the Fas-binding factor 1 gene (*FBF1*); the acyl-coenzyme A oxidase 1 gene (*ACOX1*); and the *Caenorhabditis elegans* homolog *UNC13D* gene. Three additional SNPs with suggestive statistical significance were identified. These are located in genes coding for the polyamine-modulated factor 1 gene (*PMF1*), the collagen type XXV alpha gene (*COL25A1*), and the methylentetrahydrofolate dehydrogenase 1 gene (*MTHFD1*).

Conclusions

Recent studies have provided evidence of substantial progress toward the understanding of genetic factors in the pathogenesis of cerebral SVD. Monogenic variants can serve as important model conditions for sporadic cerebral SVD. They are diagnosed by careful assessment of the family history, different and sometimes specific clinical features, pathologic findings, and genetic testing. GWAS, in combination with next-generation sequencing tools, will provide further insights into the genetic architecture of cerebral SVD. This may then provide the basis for novel biomarkers and potential therapeutic targets.

References

1. Dichgans M. Genetics of ischaemic stroke. *Lancet Neurol* 2007;6:149–161.
2. Joutel A, Corpechot C, Ducros A, et al. Notch3 mutations in CADASIL, a hereditary adult-onset condition causing stroke and dementia. *Nature* 1996;383:707–710.
3. Narayan SK, Gorman G, Kalaria RN, Ford GA, Chinnery PF. The minimum prevalence of CADASIL in northeast England. *Neurology* 2012;78:1025–1027.
4. Dong Y, Hassan A, Zhang Z, et al. Yield of screening for CADASIL mutations in lacunar stroke and leukoaraiosis. *Stroke* 2003;34:203–205.
5. Chabriat H, Joutel A, Dichgans M, Tournier-Lasserve E, Bousser MG. CADASIL. *Lancet Neurol* 2009;8:643–653.
6. Opherk C, Peters N, Herzog J, Luedtke R, Dichgans M. Long-term prognosis and causes of death in CADASIL: a retrospective study in 411 patients. *Brain* 2004;127:2533–2539.
7. Gunda B, Herve D, Godin O, et al. Effects of gender on the phenotype of CADASIL. *Stroke* 2012;43:137–141.
8. Yamamoto Y, Ihara M, Tham C, et al. Neuropathological correlates of temporal pole white matter hyperintensities in CADASIL. *Stroke* 2009;40:2004–2011.
9. Opherk C, Peters N, Holtmannspotter M, et al. Heritability of MRI lesion volume in CADASIL: evidence for genetic modifiers. *Stroke* 2006;37:2684–2689.
10. Domenga V, Fardoux P, Lacombe P, et al. Notch3 is required for arterial identity and maturation of vascular smooth muscle cells. *Genes Dev* 2004;18:2730–2735.
11. Peters N, Opherk C, Bergmann T, et al. Spectrum of mutations in biopsy-proven CADASIL: implications for diagnostic strategies. *Arch Neurol* 2005;62:1091–1094.
12. Joutel A, Monet M, Domenga V, Riant F, Tournier-Lasserve E. Pathogenic mutations associated with cerebral autosomal dominant arteriopathy with subcortical infarcts and leukoencephalopathy differently affect Jagged1 binding and Notch3 activity via the RBP/JK signaling pathway. *Am J Hum Genet* 2004;74:338–347.
13. Monet M, Domenga V, Lemaire B, et al. The archetypal r90c CADASIL-notch3 mutation retains notch3 function in vivo. *Hum Mol Genet* 2007;16:982–992.
14. Peters N, Ebert A, Freilinger T, et al. Postoperative amnesic state with impairment of static visual perception. *Eur J Neurol* 2008;15: e44–45.
15. Duering M, Karpinska A, Rosner S, et al. Co-aggregate formation of CADASIL-mutant notch3: a single-particle analysis. *Hum Mol Genet* 2011;20:3256–3265.
16. Dichgans M, Markus HS, Salloway S, et al. Donepezil in patients with subcortical vascular cognitive impairment: a randomised double-blind trial in CADASIL. *Lancet Neurol* 2008;7:310–318.
17. Fukutake T. Cerebral autosomal recessive arteriopathy with subcortical infarcts and leukoencephalopathy (CARASIL): from discovery to gene identification. *J Stroke Cerebrovasc Dis* 2011;20:85–93.
18. Arima K, Yanagawa S, Ito N, Ikeda S. Cerebral arterial pathology of CADASIL and CARASIL (Maeda syndrome). *Neuropathology* 2003;23:327–334.
19. Mendioroz M, Fernandez-Cadenas I, Del Rio-Espinola A, et al. A missense *HTRA1* mutation expands CARASIL syndrome to the Caucasian population. *Neurology* 2010;75:2033–2035.
20. Hara K, Shiga A, Fukutake T, et al. Association of *HTRA1* mutations and familial ischemic cerebral small-vessel disease. *N Engl J Med* 2009;360:1729–1739.
21. Brady RO, Schiffmann R. Clinical features of and recent advances in therapy for Fabry disease. *JAMA* 2000;284:2771–2775.
22. Moore DF, Herscovitch P, Schiffmann R. Selective arterial distribution of cerebral hyperperfusion in Fabry disease. *J Neuroimaging* 2001;11:303–307.
23. Rolfs A, Bottcher T, Zschiesche M, et al. Prevalence of Fabry

disease in patients with cryptogenic stroke: a prospective study. *Lancet* 2005;366:1794–1796.

24. Parenti G. Treating lysosomal storage diseases with pharmacological chaperones: from concept to clinics. *EMBO Mol Med* 2009;1:268–279.
25. Roach ES, Golomb MR, Adams R, et al. Management of stroke in infants and children: Scientific Statement from a Special Writing Group of the American Heart Association Stroke Council and the Council on Cardiovascular Disease in the Young. *Stroke* 2008;39:2644–2691.
26. Yamamoto Y, Craggs L, Baumann M, Kalimo H, Kalaria RN. Review: molecular genetics and pathology of hereditary small vessel diseases of the brain. *Neuropath Applied Neurobiol* 2011;37:94–113.
27. Gould DB, Phalan FC, Breedveld GJ, et al. Mutations in COL4A1 cause perinatal cerebral hemorrhage and porencephaly. *Science* 2005;308:1167–1171.
28. Vahedi K, Kubis N, Boukobza M, et al. COL4A1 mutation in a patient with sporadic, recurrent intracerebral hemorrhage. *Stroke* 2007;38:1461–1464.
29. Sibon I, Coupry I, Menegon P, et al. COL4A1 mutation in Axenfeld–Rieger anomaly with leukoencephalopathy and stroke. *Ann Neurol* 2007;62:177–184.
30. Plaisier E, Gribouval O, Alamowitch S, et al. COL4A1 mutations and hereditary angiopathy, nephropathy, aneurysms, and muscle cramps. *N Engl J Med* 2007;357:2687–2695.
31. Jen J, Cohen AH, Yue Q, et al. Hereditary endotheliopathy with retinopathy, nephropathy, and stroke (HERNS). *Neurology* 1997;49:1322–1330.
32. Terwindt GM, Haan J, Ophoff RA, et al. Clinical and genetic analysis of a large Dutch family with autosomal dominant vascular retinopathy, migraine and Raynaud's phenomenon. *Brain* 1998;121(Pt 2):303–316.
33. Ophoff RA, DeYoung J, Service SK, et al. Hereditary vascular retinopathy, cerebroretinal vasculopathy, and hereditary endotheliopathy with retinopathy, nephropathy, and stroke map to a single locus on chromosome 3p21.1-p21.3. *Am J Hum Genet* 2001;69:447–453.
34. Richards A, van den Maagdenberg AM, Jen JC, et al. C-terminal truncations in human 3′-5′ DNA exonuclease TREX1 cause autosomal dominant retinal vasculopathy with cerebral leukodystrophy. *Nat Genet* 2007;39:1068–1070.
35. Crow YJ, Hayward BE, Parmar R, et al. Mutations in the gene encoding the 3′-5′ DNA exonuclease TREX1 cause Aicardi–Goutieres syndrome at the AGS1 locus. *Nat Genet* 2006;38:917–920.
36. Biffi A, Greenberg SM. Cerebral amyloid angiopathy: a systematic review. *J Clin Neurol* 2011;7:1–9.
37. Revesz T, Holton JL, Lashley T, et al. Genetics and molecular pathogenesis of sporadic and hereditary cerebral amyloid angiopathies. *Acta Neuropathol* 2009;118:115–130.
38. Maat-Schieman M, Roos R, van Duinen S. Hereditary cerebral hemorrhage with amyloidosis–Dutch type. *Neuropathology* 2005;25:288–297.
39. Natte R, Maat-Schieman ML, Haan J, et al. Dementia in hereditary cerebral hemorrhage with amyloidosis–Dutch type is associated with cerebral amyloid angiopathy but is independent of plaques and neurofibrillary tangles. *Ann Neurol* 2001;50:765–772.
40. Bornebroek M, Haan J, van Buchem MA, et al. White matter lesions and cognitive deterioration in presymptomatic carriers of the amyloid precursor protein gene codon 693 mutation. *Arch Neurol* 1996;53:43–48.
41. Holton JL, Lashley T, Ghiso J, et al. Familial Danish dementia: a novel form of cerebral amyloidosis associated with deposition of both amyloid-Dan and amyloid-β. *J Neuropathol Exp Neurol* 2002;61:254–267.
42. Mead S, James-Galton M, Revesz T, et al. Familial British dementia with amyloid angiopathy: early clinical, neuropsychological and imaging findings. *Brain* 2000;123 (Pt 5):975–991.
43. Revesz T, Holton JL, Lashley T, et al. Sporadic and familial cerebral amyloid angiopathies. *Brain Pathol* 2002;12:343–357.
44. Freudenberger P, Schmidt R, Schmidt H. Genetics of age-related white matter lesions from linkage to genome wide association studies. *J Neurol Sci* 2012;322:82–86.
45. Carmelli D, DeCarli C, Swan GE, et al. Evidence for genetic variance in white matter hyperintensity volume in normal elderly male twins. *Stroke* 1998;29:1177–1181.
46. Atwood LD, Wolf PA, Heard-Costa NL, et al. Genetic variation in white matter hyperintensity volume in the Framingham Study. *Stroke* 2004;35:1609–1613.
47. Turner ST, Jack CR, Fornage M, et al. Heritability of leukoaraiosis in hypertensive sibships. *Hypertension* 2004;43:483–487.
48. Turner ST, Fornage M, Jack CR, Jr., et al. Genomic susceptibility loci for brain atrophy, ventricular volume, and leukoaraiosis in hypertensive sibships. *Arch Neurol* 2009;66:847–857.
49. Cuenco KT, Green RC, Zhang J, et al. Magnetic resonance imaging traits in siblings discordant for Alzheimer disease. *J Neuroimaging* 2008;18:268–275.

50. Bevan S, Traylor M, Adib-Samii P, et al. Genetic heritability of ischemic stroke and the contribution of previously reported candidate gene and genomewide associations. *Stroke* 2012;43:3161–3167.

51. DeStefano AL, Atwood LD, Massaro JM, et al. Genome-wide scan for white matter hyperintensity: the Framingham Heart Study. *Stroke* 2006; 37:77–81.

52. Paternoster L, Chen W, Sudlow CL. Genetic determinants of white matter hyperintensities on brain scans: a systematic assessment of 19 candidate gene polymorphisms in 46 studies in 19 000 subjects. *Stroke* 2009;40:2020–2026.

53. Fornage M, Debette S, Bis JC, et al. Genome-wide association studies of cerebral white matter lesion burden: the charge consortium. *Ann Neurol* 2011;69:928–939.

54. Taylor WD, Steffens DC, Ashley-Koch A, et al. Angiotensin receptor gene polymorphisms and two-year change in hyperintense lesion volume in men. *Mol Psychiatry* 2010;15:816–822.

55. Van Rijn MJ, Bos MJ, Isaacs A, et al. Polymorphisms of the renin–angiotensin system are associated with blood pressure, atherosclerosis and cerebral white matter pathology. *J Neurol Neurosurg Psychiatry* 2007;78:1083–1087.

56. Schmidt H, Zeginigg M, Wiltgen M, et al. Genetic variants of the *NOTCH3* gene in the elderly and magnetic resonance imaging correlates of age-related cerebral small vessel disease. *Brain* 2011;134:3384–3397.

57. Verhaaren BF, de Boer R, Vernooij MW, et al. Replication study of chr17q25 with cerebral white matter lesion volume. *Stroke* 2011;42:3297–3299.

Chapter 9

The link between large artery aging and cerebral small vessel disease

Angelo Scuteri and Edward G. Lakatta

Heterogeneity of the arterial system

When we were students of medicine, we learned that the fundamental law of static fluid dynamics is a variant of Ohm's law:

$$\Delta P = -RQ$$

where the determinants of blood pressure (*P*) are peripheral resistance (*R*) and cardiac output (*Q*). For decades we have based our conceptualization of blood pressure therapy and prevention of cardiovascular (CV) events in terms of peripheral resistance and cardiac output [1]. According to Ohm's Law, arterial properties between the center (heart) and the periphery (tissue) are not taken into account. In other terms, central elastic arteries play only the passive role of conduit tubes, delivering the blood from the center to the periphery. The microcirculation, in contrast, i.e., the peripheral arterial district whose diameter is around 300 μm and characterized by high resistance, governs a steady blood flow [2].

This idea is consistent with the etymology of the word artery – from "air." At that time, knowledge in medicine was based mainly upon anatomic observation, and arteries were found empty at autopsy; thus it was surmised that these were to just transport air in the body. However, what transforms the pulsatile flow at the tissue level into a steady flow in the periphery is the large central arteries, the aorta, and its major branches.

Effectiveness of such a cushioning function depends on the viscoelastic properties of arterial walls and on the arterial geometry [2]. Large artery structure and function are not independent from one another [3]. The Moens–Korteweg equation directly correlates pulse wave velocity (PWV) with arterial wall thickness and arterial distensibility, and inversely with the arterial radius. Thus, changes in the composition of the wall and changes in geometry impact large artery structure and function. In population studies, we have previously described specific patterns of large artery structural and functional properties [4], and how these patterns independently predict subsequent CV events [5].

Moving from the heart to the periphery, changes occur in artery structure and function. Arteries become smaller, progressively less elastic (a decrease in the elastin to collagen fiber ratio), and richer in vascular smooth muscle. In the proximal aorta, elastin is the principal component of the extracellular matrix, whereas collagen predominates in the distal aorta. In the distal compartment, vascular smooth muscle cells predominate. The functional properties of arterial wall components also change along the arterial tree [6]. Arterial smooth muscle cells in the proximal and distal aorta likely have a different embryonic origin [7] and differing synthetic phenotypes in terms of elastin or collagen fiber production [8]. Endothelial function becomes impaired predominantly in the proximal, but not the distal, aorta with aging [9].

Thus, the arterial system is characterized by *heterogeneity* that significantly impacts the functional cross-talk between large arteries and the microcirculation, arbitrarily defined as vessels smaller than 300 μm in diameter. In fact, the homogeneous mismatch within the arterial system, particularly at dividing branches, becomes a source of reflection sites. When large arteries become stiffer, reflecting sites are located closer to the heart, and thus the reflected wave returns to the central aorta in early systole rather than at the end of diastole, thus augmenting central arterial pressure [10]. Of note, this increment to central pulse

Cerebral Small Vessel Disease, ed. Leonardo Pantoni and Philip B. Gorelick. Published by Cambridge University Press.

pressure is not evident from the change in peripheral pulse pressure assessed during routine blood pressure measurement. The progressive age-associated increase in large artery stiffness exposes the microcirculation to higher pulsatility, and progressive microcirculation rarefaction occurs [10, 11]. On converging, microcirculation damage and rarefaction may lead to proximalization of reflection of the incident pulse wave, and thus, there is an increase in arterial stiffness [11]. Therefore, increased arterial stiffness is a contemporaneous cause and a consequence of microcirculatory damage.

Evidence of a link between microvascular brain damage and large arteries aging

Although the brain is only 2% of body weight, it accounts for 20% of oxygen consumption and 25% of total glucose utilization. Given the lack of cerebral energy reserve, the brain is dependent on adequate cerebral blood flow (CBF) and perfusion. Cerebrovascular autoregulation maintains CBF relatively constant in the face of changes in arterial pressure within a certain range, protecting the brain from sudden changes in perfusion pressure [12]. Neurovascular coupling, the regulation of CBF, includes local neuronal activity and metabolism, and requires intact circulation in pial arteries [13].

With aging and resting hypertension, CBF decreases regionally and cerebrovascular reactivity is impaired, the cerebrovascular autoregulation curve is shifted to the right and becomes steeper [14]. As a result of large artery aging, high pulse pressure is transmitted into the small cerebral arteries. This greater pulsatility promotes an initial increase in the small artery myogenic tone, and later, an inward remodeling of small cerebral vessels [15]. The progressive encroachment of arterial lumen is aimed to protect the microcirculation from pulsatile stress [16]. However, cerebral small vessel inward remodeling increases minimal resistance and reduces vasodilator responses, and thus contributes also to an increased susceptibility to chronic hypoperfusion resulting in focal ischemia and in the genesis of white matter lesions (WMLs) [17, 18].

Therefore, even brief episodes of hypotension that are very common in older subjects [19] may trigger cerebral hypoperfusion and WML progression [20]. Indeed, WMLs, identified as areas of hypodensity on computed tomography (CT) or hyperintensity on T2-weighted magnetic resonance imaging (MRI) sequences, are recognized as one of the manifestations of microvascular brain disease [21].

Studies in humans show associations of large artery aging, WMLs, and hypotension with cognitive dysfunction. Specifically, arterial stiffness, measured as PWV, has emerged as a significant risk factor for cognitive decline, even after controlling for age, gender, education, and blood pressure level [22–26]. Blood pressure variability and hypotensive episodes occurring in the context of a stiffer arterial system have been associated with reduced cognitive function in older subjects [27, 28]. WMLs are associated with cognitive deterioration or dementia [11, 29].

The complexity of the cross-talk between aging large arteries, and microvascular brain damage becomes evident when considering the many clinical vascular and hemodynamic markers shown to be associated with cognitive dysfunction and that are inter-related. These factors are summarized in Figure 9.1. Arterial stiffness is linked to blood pressure level and profile over a 24-hour period [10, 30]. Both arterial stiffness and blood pressure variability are associated with increased left ventricular mass (LVM) [31]. Furthermore, LVM has been associated with a twofold higher likelihood of having dementia, independent of blood pressure level [32], and with the occurrence of WMLs [33, 34]

Of note, our studies indicate that not only were arterial stiffness, presence of WMLs at neuroimaging, and episodes of hypotension significantly associated with poorer cognitive function and progression to dementia after controlling for age, sex, education, depression, traditional cardiovascular risk factors, and medications, but also that there is a synergistic effect between these three parameters. In other words, the occurrence of any two of the trilogy of exaggerated arterial stiffening, presence of WMLs, or hypotension was associated with lower Mini Mental State Examination (MMSE) score, and in the presence of all three factors, there is a further significant decline in cognitive function [35].

Towards a “common soil” hypothesis

In 1995, Stern [36] used the expression “common soil” to suggest that both diabetes mellitus and atherosclerosis may have common genetic and

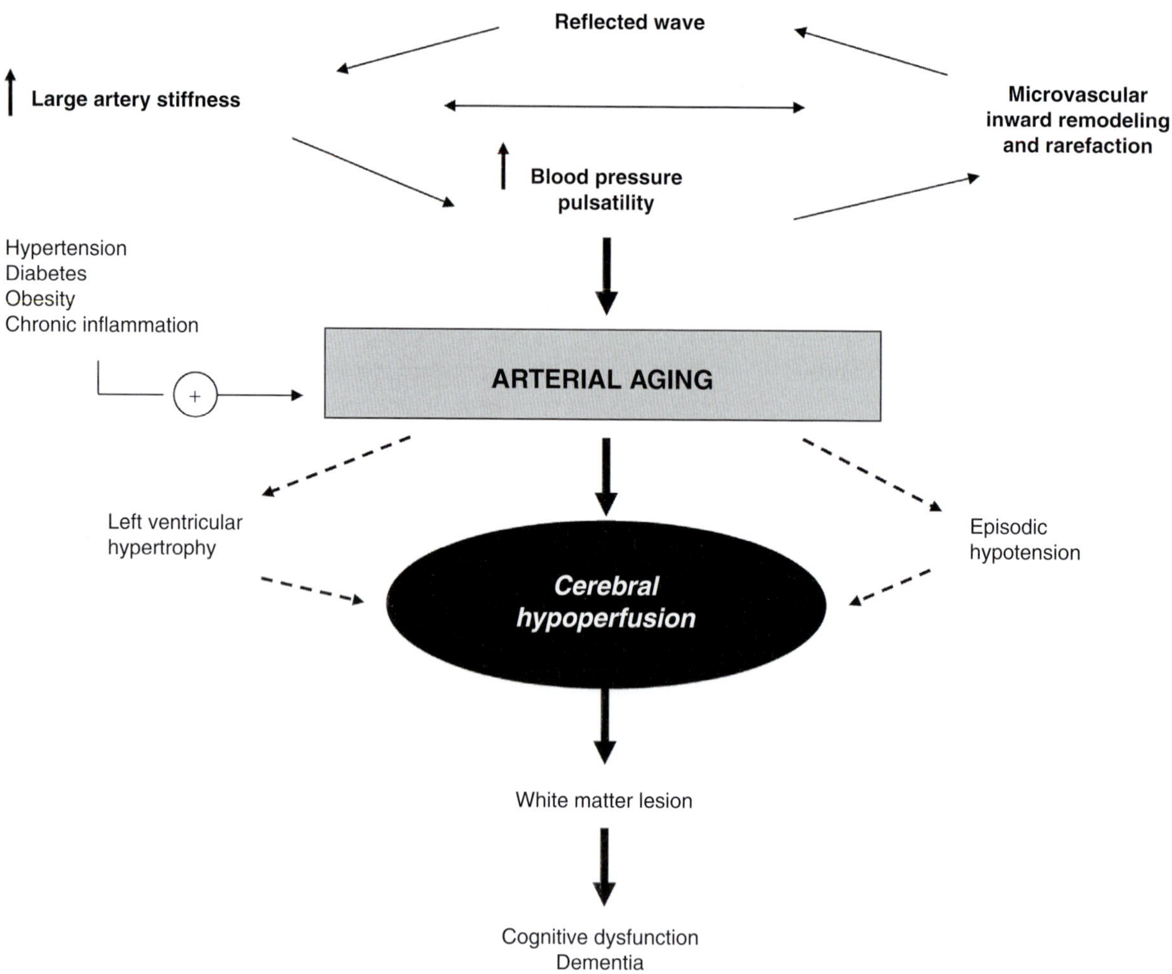

Figure 9.1 Inter-relationship of clinical vascular and hemodynamic markers known to be associated with cognitive dysfunction.

environmental antecedents, given that diabetes can precede the development of atherosclerosis, and vice versa.

It is also possible that alterations in common pathogenetic pathway(s) impact on the rate of large artery aging, microvascular brain damage, and cognitive decline. There are appealing candidates to mediate this relationship, whose roles in brief are presented below.

Genetic

Specific congenital small vessel disease, characterized by cognitive dysfunction, porencephaly, and leukoencephalopathy, is caused by mutations of the *COL4A1* (type IV collagen alpha-1 chain) gene [37]. Of note, variants of the same *COL4A1* gene have been associated with arterial stiffness in the general population [38].

Endothelial dysfunction

Endothelial dysfunction initiates and promotes atherosclerosis and premature arterial aging [39]. In some models, endothelial dysfunction occurs earlier or to a greater extent in the cerebral circulation than in blood vessels outside of the brain [40]. Additionally, in a mouse model of dementia [41], impairment of endothelium-dependent regulation of cortical microcirculation precedes β-amyloid neuronal accumulation.

Endothelial dysfunction may contribute to brain aging by impairing neurogenesis, altering neuronal transmission, inhibiting amyloidogenic processing of amyloid precursor protein, or affecting survival and growth of oligodendrocyte precursor cells [42, 43].

Angiotensin II

Angiotensin II (AngII) accelerated aging of the aorta in old monkeys and humans [44], and chronic pharmacologic inhibition of the renin–angiotensin system significantly retarded arterial aging [45]. Cerebral arteries show an exaggerated oxidative stress in response to AngII compared to extracranial vessels [46] with consequent loss of blood–brain barrier integrity, altered neurovascular coupling, and inward vascular remodeling that increases susceptibility to cerebral focal ischemia [47] independently of AngII-induced blood pressure changes [48]. Focal cerebral ischemia increases expression and responsiveness of the angiotensin type 1 (AT1) receptors in the vasculature, whereas pharmacologic inhibition of AT1 receptors improves cerebral perfusion after focal ischemia and cognitive dysfunction in an experimental model of Alzheimer's disease [49].

Matrix metalloproteinases

Matrix metalloproteinases (MMPs) consist of enzymes, regulated at the transcriptional level, exerting proteolytic activity on the extracellular matrix. MMPs are activated in vascular smooth muscle cells and whole arteries exposed to longitudinal tension and steady or cyclic stretch [50]. MMP-2 activity in the arterial wall of rodents and nonhuman primates has been demonstrated to increase with aging, representing an important mechanism for arterial matrix remodeling and stiffening [51]. In the brain, MMP-2, MMP-3, and MMP-9 are present and are induced by hypoxic hypoperfusion in white matter, and transient hypoxia/ischemia is more potent than chronic hypoxia in activating MMP signaling. Indeed, immunohistochemistry of necroscopic brain tissue shows increased MMP expression in white matter from subjects with vascular cognitive impairment, particularly around blood vessels in regions with loss of myelin (see [52] for review).

β-Amyloid

β-Amyloid (Aβ) is a prominent potential candidate that supports the "common soil" hypothesis. Aβ is toxic to vascular endothelium and neurons. In dementia, vasoconstriction or vasodilation can be observed in response to ischemia [53]. Transgenic mice overexpressing the amyloid precursor protein (APP) have reduced CBF and an attenuated cerebrovascular vasodilatory response [54] compared to those without amyloid plaques or amyloid angiopathy, when mice are still behaviorally normal. Acute application of Aβ1–40 to the cerebral cortex of normal mice reproduces the cerebrovascular effects observed in APP mice. Therefore, Aβ may contribute to impaired cerebrovascular regulation, and thus, may result in an impaired clearance and accumulation of Aβ in neurons and cerebral small arteries, and an overall progression of cognitive decline.

Amyloid-induced expression of MMPs

Amyloid-induced expression of MMPs in brain in blood vessels, astrocytes, and microglia [55] participates in the formation and clearance of the Aβ [56, 57]. The higher perfusion pressure required to perfuse white matter in the setting of arterial aging might also decrease Aβ clearance from perivascular spaces [58].

At present, we cannot clearly state whether any of the above factors represent a cause–effect relationship in the pathophysiology of arterial aging and microvascular brain damage, nor prove that the "common soil" hypothesis of arterial and brain aging is more than a conceptual construct. Investigation of these factors holds promise to lead to advances to decrease the rate of arterial aging and the onset of VCI and its progression.

Conclusions

Arterial aging may represent a key pathophysiologic factor in the progressive mismatch of the cross-talk between large and small arteries that is critical for the occurrence of microvascular brain damage and the onset and progression of cognitive dysfunction. Detection and reduction of arterial aging, easily measurable in a noninvasive manner in the clinical setting, may lead to a strategy for the prevention of cerebral small vessel disease and cognitive dysfunction in older persons. This approach is highly relevant given that no specific treatments have proven successful for vascular cognitive impairment.

References

1. Chobanian AV, Bakris GL, Black HR, et al. The Seventh Report of the Joint National Committee on Prevention, Detection, Evaluation, and Treatment of High Blood Pressure: the JNC 7 report. *JAMA*;289:2560–2572.
2. O'Rourke MF, Safar ME. Relationship between aortic stiffening and microvascular disease in brain and kidney: cause and logic of therapy. *Hypertension* 2005;46:200–204.
3. Scuteri A, Sgorbini L, Leggio F, Brancati AM. Aortic correlates of clinical markers of large artery structure and function. Effects of aging and hypertension. *Aging Clin Exp Res* 2006;18:452–461.
4. Scuteri A, Chen CH, Yin FCP, et al. Functional correlates of central arterial geometric phenotypes. *Hypertension* 2001;38:1471–1475.
5. Scuteri A, Manolio TA, Marino EK, Arnold AM, Lakatta EG. Prevalence of specific variant carotid geometric patterns and incidence of cardiovascular events in older persons. The Cardiovascular Health Study. *J Am Coll Cardiol* 2004;43:187–193.
6. Fornieri C, Quaglino D, Mori G. Role of the extracellular matrix in age-related modifications of the rat aorta. *Arterioscler Thromb* 1992;12:1008–1016.
7. Rosenquist TH, Beall AC, Modis L, Fishman R. Impaired elastic matrix development in the great arteries after ablation of the cardiac neural crest. *Anat Rec* 1990;226:347–359.
8. Davidson JM, Hill KE, Mason ML, Giro MG. Longitudinal gradients of collagen and elastin gene expression in the porcine aorta. *J Biol Chem* 1985;260:1901–1908.
9. Barton M, Cosentino F, Brandes RF, et al. Anatomic heterogeneity of vascular aging. Role of nitric oxide and endothelin. *Hypertension* 1997;30:817–824.
10. Najjar SS, Scuteri A, Lakatta EG. Arterial aging: is it an immutable cardiovascular risk factor? *Hypertension* 2005;46:454–462.
11. Scuteri A, Nilsson PM, Tzourio C, Redon J, Laurent S. Microvascular brain damage with aging and hypertension: pathophysiological consideration and clinical implications. *J Hypertens* 2011;29:1469–1477.
12. Gorelick PB, Scuteri A, Black SE, et al. Vascular contributions to cognitive impairment and dementia. A statement for healthcare professionals from the American Heart Association/ American Stroke Association. *Stroke* 2011;42:2672–2713.
13. Chen S, Li G, Zhang W, et al. Ischemia-induced brain damage is enhanced in human renin and angiotensinogen double-transgenic mice. *Am J Physiol Regul Integr Comp Physiol* 2009;297:R1526–R1531.
14. Pantoni L, Garcia JH. Pathogenesis of leukoaraiosis: a review. *Stroke* 1997;28:652–659.
15. Mulvany MJ. Small artery structure: time to take note? *Am J Hypertens* 2007;20:853–854.
16. Baumbach GL. Effects of increased pulse pressure on cerebral arterioles. *Hypertension* 1996;27:159–167.
17. James MA, Watt PA, Potter JF, Thurston H, Swales JD. Pulse pressure and resistance artery structure in the elderly. *Hypertension* 1996;26:301–306.
18. Joutel A, Monet-Lepretre M, Gosele C, et al. Cerebrovascular dysfunction and microcirculation rarefaction precede white matter lesions in a mouse genetic model of cerebral ischemic small vessel disease. *J Clin Invest* 2010;120:433–445.
19. Scuteri A, Modestino A, Frattari A, Di Daniele N, Tesauro M. Occurrence of hypotension in older participants. Which 24-hour ABPM parameter better correlates? *J Gerontol A Biol Sci Med Sci* 2012;67:804–810.
20. Fernando MS, Simpson JE, Matthews F, et al. White matter lesions in an unselected cohort of the elderly: molecular pathology suggests origin from chronic hypoperfusion injury. *Stroke* 2006;37:1391–1398.
21. Pantoni L. Cerebral small vessel disease: from pathogenesis and clinical characteristics to therapeutic challenges. *Lancet Neurol* 2010;9:689–697.
22. Scuteri A, Brancati AM, Gianni W, Assisi A, Volpe M. Arterial stiffness is an independent risk factor for cognitive impairment in the elderly: a pilot study. *J Hypertens* 2005;23:1211–1216.
23. Poels MM, van Oijen M, Mattace-Raso FU, et al. Arterial stiffness, cognitive decline, and risk of dementia: the Rotterdam Study. *Stroke* 2007;38:888–892.
24. Scuteri A, Tesauro M, Appolloni S, et al. Arterial stiffness as an independent predictor of longitudinal changes in cognitive function in the older individual. *J Hypertens* 2007;25:1035–1040.
25. Waldstein SR, Rice SC, Thayer JF, et al. Pulse pressure and pulse wave velocity are related to cognitive decline in the Baltimore Longitudinal Study of Aging. *Hypertension* 2008;51:99–104.
26. Muller M, van der Graaf Y, Visseren FL, et al. Blood pressure, cerebral blood flow, and brain volumes. The SMART–MR study. *J Hypertens* 2010;28:1498–1505.
27. Kim CK, Lee S-H, Kim BJ, Ryu W-S, Yoon B-W. Age-independent association of pulse pressure with cerebral white matter lesions in asymptomatic elderly individuals. *J Hypertension* 2011;29:325–329.
28. Nagai M, Hoshide S, Ishikawa J, Shimada K, Kario K. Visit-to-visit

blood pressure variations: new independent determinants for cognitive function in the elderly at high risk of cardiovascular disease. *J Hypertension* 2012;30:1556–1563.

29. Kearney-Schwartz A, Rossignol P, Bracard S, et al. Vascular structure and function is correlated to cognitive performance and white matter hyperintensities in older hypertensive patients with subjective memory complaints. *Stroke* 2009;40:1229–1236.
30. Scuteri A, Cacciafesta M, Di Bernardo MG, et al. Pulsatile versus steady-state component of blood pressure in elderly females: an independent risk factor for cardiovascular disease? *J Hypertens* 1995;13:185–191.
31. Parati G, Pomidossi G, Albini F, Malaspina D, Mancia G. Relationship of 24-hour blood pressure mean and variability to severity of target organ damage in hypertension. *J Hypertens* 1987;5:93–98.
32. Scuteri A, Coluccia R, Castello L, et al. Left ventricular mass increase is associated with cognitive decline and dementia in the elderly independently of blood pressure. *Eur Heart J* 2009;30:1525–1529.
33. Henskens LH, Kroon AA, van Oostenbrugge RJ, et al. Associations of ambulatory blood pressure levels with white matter hyperintensity volumes in hypertensive patients. *J Hypertension* 2009;27:1446–1452.
34. Henskens LH, Kroon AA, van Oostenbrugge RJ, et al. Increased aortic pulse wave velocity is associated with silent cerebral small-vessel disease in hypertensive patients. *Hypertension* 2008;52:1120–1126.
35. Scuteri A, Tesauro M, Guglini L et al. Aortic stiffness and hypotension episodes are associated with impaired cognitive function in older subjects with subjective complains of memory loss. *Int J Cardiol* 2013;169:371–377.
36. Stern MP. Diabetes and cardiovascular disease. The "common soil" hypothesis. *Diabetes* 1995;44:369–374.
37. Gould DB, Phalan FC, van Mil SE, et al. Role of COL4A1 in small-vessel disease and hemorrhagic stroke. *N Engl J Med* 2006;354:1489–1496.
38. Tarasov KV, Sanna S, Scuteri A, et al. COL4A1 is associated with arterial stiffness by genome-wide association scan. *Circ Cardiovasc Genet* 2009;2:151–158.
39. Scuteri A, Tesauro M, Rizza S, et al. Endothelial function and arterial stiffness in normotensive normoglycemic first-degree relatives of diabetic patients are independent of the metabolic syndrome. *Nutr Metab Cardiovasc Dis* 2008;18:349–356.
40. Modrick ML, Didion SP, Sigmund CD, Faraci FM. Role of oxidative stress and AT1 receptors in cerebral vascular dysfunction with aging. *Am J Physiol Heart Circ Physiol* 2009;296:H1914–H1919.
41. Niwa, K. et al. Aβ1–40 related reduction in functional hyperemia in mouse neocortex during somatosensory activation. *Proc Natl Acad Sci USA* 2000;97:9735–9740.
42. Lazarov O, Mattson MP, Peterson DA, Pimplikar SW, van Praag H. When neurogenesis encounters aging and disease. *Trends Neurosci* 2010;33:569–579.
43. Austin SA, Santhanam AV, Katusic ZS. Endothelial nitric oxide modulates expression and processing of amyloid precursor protein. *Circ Res* 2010;107:1498–1502.
44. Wang M, Khazan B, Lakatta EG. Central arterial aging and angiotensin II signaling. *Curr Hypertens Rev* 2010;6:266–281.
45. Basso N, Cini Pietrelli AR, Ferder L, Terragno NA, Inserra F. Protective effect of long-term angiotensin II inhibition. *Am J Physiol Heart Circ Physiol* 2007;293:H1351–H1358.
46. Miller AA, Drummond GR, Schmidt HH, Sobey CG. NADPH oxidase activity and function are profoundly greater in cerebral versus systemic arteries. *Circ Res* 2005;97:1055–1062.
47. Chen S, Li G, Zhang W, et al. Ischemia-induced brain damage is enhanced in human renin and angiotensinogen double-transgenic mice. *Am J Physiol Regul Integr Comp Physiol* 2009;297:R1526–R1531.
48. Capone C, Faraco G, Park L, et al. The cerebrovascular dysfunction induced by slow pressor doses of angiotensin II precedes the development of hypertension. *Am J Physiol Heart Circ Physiol* 2011;300:H397–H407.
49. Takeda S, Sato N, Takeuchi D, et al. Angiotensin receptor blocker prevented β-amyloid induced cognitive impairment associated with recovery of neurovascular coupling. *Hypertension* 2009;54:1345–1352.
50. Asanuma K, Magid R, Johnson C, Nerem RM, Galis ZS. Uniaxial strain upregulates matrix-degrading enzymes produced by human vascular smooth muscle cells. *Am J Physiol Heart Circ Physiol* 2003;284:H1778–1784.
51. Wang M, Takagi G, Asai K, et al. Aging increases aortic MMP-2 activity and angiotensin II in nonhuman primates. *Hypertension* 2003;41:1308–1316.
52. Rosenberg GA. Matrix metalloproteinases and their multiple roles in neurodegenerative diseases. *Lancet Neurol* 2009;8:205–216.
53. Chow N, Bell RD, Deane R, et al. Serum response factor and myocardin mediate arterial hypercontractility and cerebral

blood flow dysregulation in Alzheimer's phenotype. *Proc Natl Acad Sci USA* 2007; 104:823–828.

54. Iadecola C. Neurovascular regulation in the normal brain and in Alzheimer's disease. *Nat Rev Neurosci* 2004; 5:347–360.
55. Yan P, Hu X, Song H, et al. Matrix metalloproteinase-9 degrades amyloid-β fibrils in vitro and compact plaques in situ. *J Biol Chem* 2006;281:24566–24574.
56. Yin KJ, Cirrito JR, Yan P, et al. Matrix metalloproteinases expressed by astrocytes mediate extracellular amyloid-β peptide catabolism. *J Neurosci* 2006;26:10939–10948.
57. Backstrom JR, Lim GP, Cullen MJ, Tokes ZA. Matrix metalloproteinase-9 (MMP-9) is synthesized in neurons of the human hippocampus and is capable of degrading the amyloid-β peptide (1–40). *J Neurosci* 1996;16: 7910–7919.
58. Thore CR, Anstrom JA, Moody DM, et al. Morphometric analysis of arteriolar tortuosity in human cerebral white matter of preterm, young, and aged subjects. *J Neuropathol Exp Neurol* 2007;66:337–345.

Chapter 10

The neurovascular unit and possible influences on cerebral small vessel disease

Gregory J. del Zoppo, Yoshikane Izawa, and Brian T. Hawkins

Introduction

Small vessel disease (SVD) is reflected by injury to the microvasculature. Once thought to be inert immobile conduits of blood flow in the central nervous system (CNS), cerebral microvessels have since been shown to be structures of considerable complexity, with dynamic functional responses as rapid as those of neurons. Defined as cerebral vessels less than 100 μm diameter, microvessels represent one limb of the neurovascular unit. There is a meager hold of information about the cerebral microvasculature beyond their ultrastructure and histology.

SVD manifests in a variety of disorders of varying etiology, typified by lacunes, microhemorrhages, vascular cognitive impairment, and other conditions affecting microvessels and larger CNS vessels [1]. The precise targets for the initial injury may be obscured in the history of the tissue. Furthermore, there are significant limitations in our understanding of the molecular initiators of SVD, in part due to limitations in the resolution of the techniques at hand. However, considerations of the better-characterized acute and early alterations in the microvasculature evident during ischemia may be informative to the topic of SVD.

Experimental model systems have demonstrated alterations in cerebral endothelial cell reactivity, increased inflammatory responses at the endothelium, altered vascular reactivity, permeability barrier changes, and ultrastructural alterations of the microvessel components. Conditions of experimental focal ischemia in the nonhuman primate demonstrate that these events occur in the regions of neuron injury, with simultaneous evidence of microvessel and neuron injury beginning shortly after ischemia onset. This chapter will discuss a combination of experimental and clinical observations, to give a basic impression of some of the changes in the microvasculature initiated within hours of ischemia onset in the context of the "neurovascular unit," a theoretical construct linking microvessel and neuron responses to injury, and how they could apply to clinically apparent SVD.

Cerebral microvasculature

The cerebral microvasculature responds locally and regionally to maintain cerebral blood flow (CBF) and perfusion, and in the face of regional and systemic events, including focal ischemia and systemic inflammatory conditions. The microvascular beds of the CNS are tethered by large vessels. Penetrating vessels of the cortex are bounded by Virchow–Robin spaces, both a real and a virtual space (at the capillary level) that appears to involve the apposition of matrix sheaths of both the endothelial and neuropil compartments. This *glia limitans* also has functional properties. Despite the apparently static histology of the microvasculature under normoxia, ischemia and inflammation cause rapid molecular responses that occur at the matrix boundary. Inherent and unique to the microvasculature is the permeability barrier. Loss of the barrier properties begins rapidly following focal ischemia onset with transmigration of plasma components, edema formation, and hemorrhagic transformation. These events necessarily involve breach of the *glia limitans* of the microvasculature. In the context of SVD it may be hypothesized that microvessel events, as those that occur in discrete areas (lesions), could affect few or many microvessels and their neurons. Conversely, injury to microvessels may be scattered as in vascular dementias. Here we consider the processes associated with regions of focal

Cerebral Small Vessel Disease, ed. Leonardo Pantoni and Philip B. Gorelick. Published by Cambridge University Press.

ischemia as an example. One characteristic of these observations is that they occur heterogeneously in the microvasculature [2].

Microvessel beds

Microvessel density, collateral circuitry, and flow in the CNS are highly inter-related. The microvessel structure and characteristics in the CNS are remarkably preserved across species. Bär and colleagues [3–6] demonstrated a series of cascading interconnected hexagonal arrays of vessels and branching microvessels penetrating orthogonally from the pial surface through levels I–VI of the cortex to the white matter in the rat. The cortical gray matter contains a higher density of microvessels than the subtending white matter. The structure of the corpus striatum in human and nonhuman primate species appears nearly identical, but has not been definitively mapped. The organization of white matter tracks in the corpus striatum of lower species differs from that of humans and primates. In the primate striatum, the branch points for capillaries are approximately 30–40 μm distance from one another [7]. This difference in microvessel array, by location, accords with differences in regional CBF (rCBF) with location. Fenstermacher et al. [8] demonstrated a significantly lower rCBF in the corpus striatum than in the cortex. That is, in the striatum the flow is closer to ischemic threshold, as defined by positron emission tomography (PET) and other techniques [9–11]. Occlusion of the middle cerebral artery (MCA) M1 segment causes reduction of flow of the lenticulostriate arteries (LSA), which are the origin of this *globular* microvascular organization of the basal ganglia.

The circle of Willis supplies both the cortex and the deep structures via the MCA and the LSA, the anterior cerebral artery (ACA), and the posterior cerebral artery (PCA). The form of the circle of Willis is also species-dependent, but in those in whom the circle is complete, flow is distributed to both hemispheres. The cortical arteriolar supplies and venular outflows of the cortex have been mapped in rodent and primate species and in humans [4–6]. Little is known about the venous outflow of the corpus striatum, however.

Collateral system and protection

The CNS arterial supply serves a low-pressure high-flow vascular system that is reflected in the microvascular beds. Whereas sustained occlusion or low

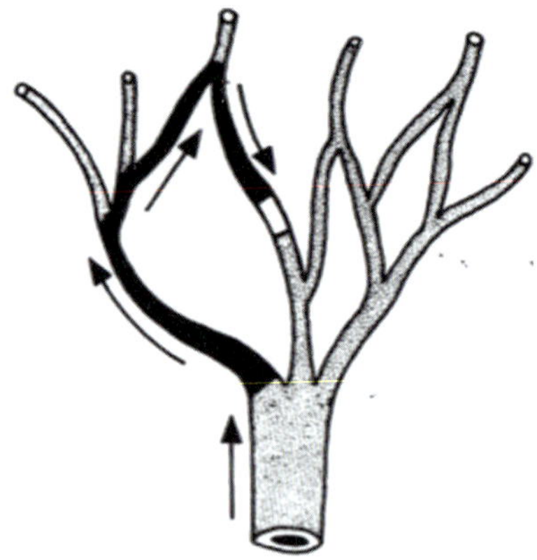

Figure 10.1 Interconnections within the cerebral vascular bed, allowing reversal of flow in the low-pressure high-flow system (after Zülch [12]). A similar arrangement is evident in the microvascular beds of the corpus striatum in the primate.

flow in a microvessel-supplying arterial branch leads to ischemic injury downstream, ordinarily the interconnections of the capillaries allow reversal of flow though their branches (e.g., striatum) [12]. Zülch [12] described this general principle in 1985 (Figure 10.1). This form of protection seems reiterated at all levels of the CNS vasculature. One implication of this observation is that for small changes in flow, where the autoregulatory system is capable of managing the flow-through, this system of protection works very well. However, with prolonged reduction or cessation in flow, the evolving injury may overtake this protective system. Furthermore, where inflammation is initiated (e.g., focal ischemia), reduction in microvessel patency, further reduced flow, and injury extension are expected in the region. That concept refers to the processes described below. Another implication is that the forms of the vascular and downstream microvessel beds in different territories (i.e., cortex, white matter, and striatum) differ. For instance, the expression and distribution of specific cell matrix-adhesion receptors within the microvasculature are location-dependent.

Collateral protection for the vascular beds of the CNS includes the circle of Willis and the pial anastomoses across the cortical surface. Preservation of flow through these systems reduces ischemic injury. The pial arteriolar and venular arrays on the cortical surface provide a functional anastomotic collateral system, which protects the cortex from flow obstruction in any vertical segment. With ascending phylogeny, branching of the leptomeningeal (pial) anastomoses shows increasing complexity, and there is increasing microvessel density [13]. With increasing cortical complexity, the branching of the pial vasculature also increases. However, the known relationships of microvessels to the neurons they supply are rather fixed in the regional structure.

In human stroke, the patency and flow/supply through the collateral circuits are important to the extent of ischemic injury. This involves a maintenance of flow through the microvascular beds supplied by the occluded artery(ies). Unfortunately, the contributions of the collateral system to microvessel integrity have not been easy to study in small animal systems. Curiously, the removal of collateral vessels present in the native cerebral vasculature has been necessary to provide reproducible lesions [14].

Neurovascular unit: relationship of microvessels to neurons

The position of the microvasculature in relationship to the neurons it serves within the cortex and the striatum is of current interest. Migration of neurons from the subventricular zone (SVZ) during development occurs along vascular tracts, which in turn follow matrix pathways [15]. One formulation that takes into account the known anatomic relationships between neurons and the microvasculature has been termed the "neurovascular unit" [3, 16, 17]. The neurovascular unit consists of microvessels (endothelium, basal lamina, and astrocyte end-feet), intervening astrocytes, the neurons, and their axons (Figure 10.2 [18]). Other cells, including pericytes, mast cells and microglia, and oligodendroglia, participate in the maintenance and responses of the neurovascular unit [16]. Within the striatum of the nonhuman primate, a strict distance relationship exists between the microvessel and its neighboring (closest) neuron. Mabuchi et al. [7] demonstrated that this relationship is highly ordered and immutable. It suggests that under conditions of normoxia there is little heterogeneity in the distance relationship in the structure.

Elements of the microvasculature

Cerebral microvessels are a necessary component of the neurovascular unit. Within the microvessel wall, pericytes, vessel wall histiocytes, and/or cells of the monocyte/macrophage lineage are located, or transit through. The endothelium, extracellular matrix (ECM), and astrocytes of cerebral microvessels each comprise separate element-specific networks that interact with each other.

Endothelium

Cerebral microvascular endothelial cells are bounded on the abluminal side by the basal lamina ECM. The endothelium provides an antithrombotic milieu, and protects the vascular wall and neuropil from plasma substances known to be toxic. Importantly, the endothelium contributes to and maintains (with its astrocyte counterparts) the subjacent basal lamina matrix. Location-dependent functional differences have been observed in the endothelium throughout the microvascular tree in the CNS [19–22]. For instance, relative differences in glucose transport and glucose metabolism under conditions of normoxia and experimental ischemia have been seen in isolated cortical microvessels [20]. Transcriptional profiling of endothelial cells derived from brain capillaries and venules shows that considerable heterogeneity also exists along different segments of the microvasculature [23]. This implies potential differences in reactivity to a given insult.

The endothelium is attached to specific matrix ligands within the basal lamina by integrins [24–26]. The distribution of integrin immunoreactivity among brain microvessels appears to depend upon microvessel diameter, cell type, and the distribution of specific ECM proteins [24]. For example, in the primate brain, integrin β_1 is expressed throughout the microvascular tree together with integrin subunits α_1 and α_6, in a manner that parallels expression of β_1-matrix ligands laminin, collagen IV, and fibronectin. Integrin α_3, which also forms dimers with β_1, is found in a subset of capillaries, and α_2, α_4, α_5, α_v, and β_3 subunits are expressed in noncapillary microvessels [24, 27]. These adhesion receptors are in turn linked via their cytoplasmic domains (COOH-termini) to elements of the actin cytoskeleton and complexes of signaling molecules, indicating that matrix adhesion is essential to both structural and functional integrity of the microvasculature.

A hallmark of the endothelium in cerebral microvessels is the presence of epithelial-like tight junction (TJ) complexes. TJ proteins that form interendothelial adhesive interactions, including claudin-5, occludin, and zonula occludens (ZO), are essential contributors to the permeability (blood–brain) barrier [28]. ZO-1 and ZO-2 are attached to the actin cytoskeleton. The intact cytoskeleton, formed by actin, microtubules, and intermediate filaments, is necessary to maintain the function of permeability barrier by providing

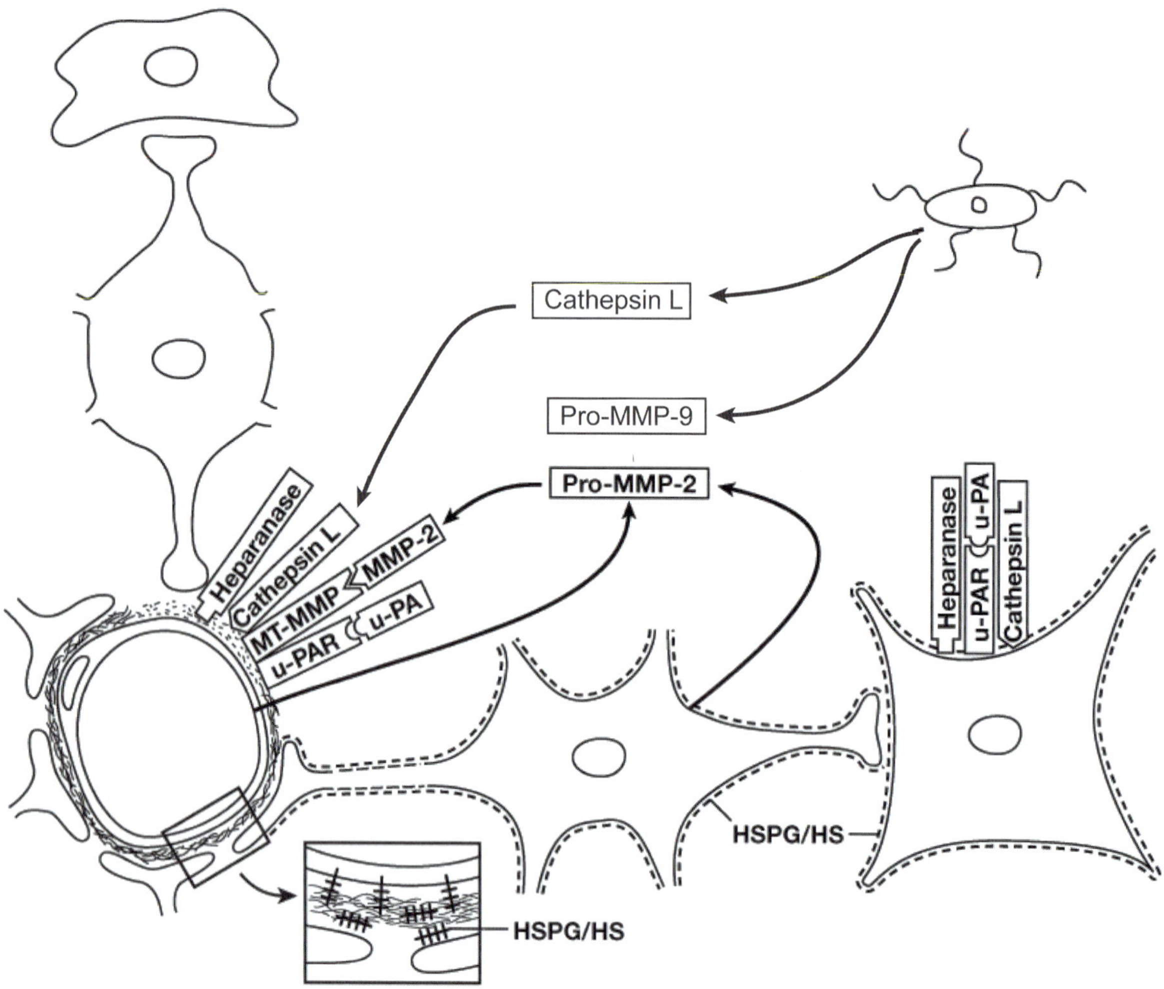

Figure 10.2 A formulation of the basic elements of the neurovascular unit, displaying the sources of matrix proteases generated following focal ischemia (in the primate). Note the interposition of astrocytes as a component of the microvessels and their contact to neurons they serve. HS, heparan sulfate; HSPG, heparan sulfate proteoglycan; MMP, matrix metalloproteinase; u-PA, urokinase; u-PAR, urokinase-type plasminogen activator receptor. From del Zoppo [18], reproduced with permission.

anchoring points for the TJ proteins. These contribute to the integrity of the barrier. Interactions of the TJ–actin–β_1 integrin complex are central to the integrity of the endothelial cell component of the permeability barrier [29].

Adherence junctions also contain vascular endothelial-cadherin (VE-cadherin) and the adapter proteins β-catenin, p120, and plakoglobin. These contribute to and maintain a looser adhesion between adjacent endothelial cells. VE-cadherin, β-catenin, and associated proteins interact with the actin cytoskeleton and may be involved in signal transduction [30]. Platelet endothelial adhesion molecule (PECAM) also contributes to inter-endothelial cell binding through homophilic cohesive interactions.

In terms of the transport of substances required to maintain neuron function across the permeability barrier, the cerebral endothelium actively regulates the passage of glucose, amino acids, and monocarboxylic acids into the cerebral parenchyma through glucose transporter-1 (Glut-1), the L-type amino-acid transporter-1 (LAT-1), and monocarboxylate transporter-1 (MCT-1), respectively. These and other transporters have a specific polarity of expression and transport directionality [31].

The intact endothelium maintains an antithrombotic milieu through the expression of heparan sulfates (HS) on its surface, and the generation of prostacyclin (PGI_2), adenosine, nitric oxide (NO), thrombomodulin (as a participant in protein C activation), and the availability of antithrombin activities. In the setting of active thrombosis, the endothelium releases tissue plasminogen activator (t-PA), urokinase (u-PA), and plasminogen activator inhibitor (PAI)-1 to maintain active antithrombotic conditions locally. This appears to depend upon the quantity of free t-PA and u-PA released, in relation to PAI-1 release.

The endothelium is also the interface for peripheral inflammation through the expression of the polymorphonuclear leukocyte adhesion receptors P-selectin, intercellular adhesion molecule 1 (ICAM-1), and E-selectin [16]. Focal ischemia initiates the luminal surface expression of these receptors [32, 33].

ECM (matrix)

In cerebral microvessels, the ECM is interposed between the endothelium and the astrocyte end-feet. The major components of the microvessel basal lamina matrix (including the laminins, type IV collagen, and fibronectin [of cellular origin]) form a biologically active carpet in which the heparan sulfate proteoglycan (HSPG) perlecan, nidogen, entactin, and other minor components reside [16].

The basal lamina ECM provides ligands for the adhesion receptors, including select integrins and $\alpha\beta$-dystroglycan, by which endothelial cells and astrocytes bind to the matrix. Furthermore, the ECM provides a depot for growth factors (e.g., fibroblast growth factor [FGF]-β) and inactive matrix proteases.

The linkage between endothelial cells and astrocytes via basal lamina adhesion contributes the *vertical* component to the permeability barrier [27, 29]. The ECM allows the close proximity of the two cell networks (compartments) to be preserved, so that interactions between endothelial cells and astrocytes maintain the permeability barrier and solute transport systems (see below). The ECM also provides a physical barrier to cellular transmigration from the plasma to the neuropil, impeding the egress of erythrocytes and leukocytes. The *horizontal* connections afforded by TJs contribute to the impermeability of the barrier [34–36].

Subject to specific insults (e.g., local thrombin generation) the endothelium can generate and release increased amounts of matrix proteins [37].

Astrocytes and their end-feet

Capillaries are surrounded by the end-feet of astrocytes, which seem to completely envelope the basal lamina matrix [38, 39]. Astrocytes link neurons to their supply microvessels and contact neurons through more than 1×10^5 synapses per neuron, playing necessary roles in trafficking, absorption, and secretion of nutrients and essential substances for neuron function [40]. Adjacent astrocytes form syncytia connected by gap junctions that allow Ca^{2+} [2] transients for communication. This form of communication is under study [38, 39, 41].

Integrins $\alpha_1\beta_1$ and $\alpha_6\beta_4$, and $\alpha\beta$-dystroglycan are expressed on astrocyte end-feet. The distributions of integrin $\alpha_6\beta_4$ and $\alpha\beta$-dystroglycan expression depend upon the diameter and location of the microvessels. For instance, $\alpha\beta$-dystroglycan is expressed throughout the microvessel tree in both gray and white matter, while integrin $\alpha_6\beta_4$ is found on larger non-capillary microvessels, in the periphery of the tissue region [25, 42]. Integrin $\alpha_6\beta_4$ is a component of hemidesmosomes that attach epithelial cells to the ECM [42], suggesting that this complex acts also to tether the microvessel bed within the tissue.

A functional aspect of astrocytes is their regulation of blood flow in response to neuron activity, by modulating the diameter of precapillary arterioles. Hence, astrocytes are thought to be involved in functional hyperemia [43], but the exact mechanisms have not been clarified. It has also been suggested that the control of capillary blood flow in response to neuronal activity is integrated at the level of the arterioles that supply the capillaries [44].

Astrocytes are also responsible – in conjunction with the endothelial permeability barrier – for maintaining the composition of the extracellular fluid in the brain within the narrow range of ion concentrations necessary for proper neuronal function. Ion channels and water channels (e.g., aquaporins) are highly expressed in astrocyte end-feet, enabling them to rapidly absorb water and swell in response to local increases in extracellular potassium ion (K^+) [45]. The functional water transport apparatus in astrocytes has recently been shown to depend on matrix adhesion via dystroglycan [46].

Pericytes

Pericytes are pluripotential cells that reside within the microvessel wall, encased in basal lamina that is sandwiched between the endothelial cells and astrocytes.

The known functional characteristics of pericytes have been discussed by Dore-Duffy et al. [47], who have shown that primary pericytes can differentiate into astrocytes, neurons, and oligodendrocytes. Capillary pericytes appear able to contract microvessels modestly in response to vasoconstrictive stimulation [48], and may contribute to modest dilation. These capabilities suggest that pericytes might regulate flow locally by changing microvessel diameter. Pericytes also contribute to the integrity of the permeability barrier, and mediate vascular wall events [49, 50]. Under conditions of ischemia, these cells become activated and can migrate and differentiate.

Although intercellular communication among pericytes and other cells comprising the neurovascular unit has been reported [51], including maintenance of permeability barrier integrity, their precise roles in the CNS are largely unknown. This is due, in part, to the low density of the pericytes in cerebral tissue and difficulties in their identification.

Mast cells

Mast cells reside in the CNS in perivascular locations [52]. Mast cell granules contain histamine, serotonin, heparin, chymase, tryptase, and cathepsin G [53]. Histamine can alter local flow conditions. The secretion of these granules is relevant to the disruption of the blood–brain barrier in ischemic and hemorrhagic stroke. Strbian and colleagues demonstrated roles of mast cells in barrier disruption following focal cerebral ischemia [54] and in experimental intracerebral hemorrhage in the rat [55]. Although the precise mechanisms of barrier disruption and basal lamina degradation induced by mast cells under ischemic and hemorrhagic stroke have not been elucidated completely, chymase and tryptase could account for the degradation [56, 57].

Microglia

Microglia play a number of roles in the inflammatory responses of the CNS to ischemia. These cells have Fc receptors, receptors for complement, and respond to a panorama of cytokines [58, 59]. Microglia also generate cytokines, including tumor necrosis factor (TNF)-α and interleukin-1β (IL-1β), and are known to regulate T-cell-mediated immune processes. Meanwhile activated microglia display shape changes, and express markers of inflammation, following exposure to ischemia [16, 60]. The activated cells can release proteases with matrix-degrading capabilities including pro-matrix metalloproteinase (MMP)-9, cathepsin L, and others [61–63]. Whether they can indeed alter microvessel integrity is under study.

Permeability barrier

The cerebral microvasculature constitutes a "blood–brain" permeability barrier to the passage of large (>1000 Da) molecules as well as to smaller, polar solutes from the circulation to the neuropil. Although originally thought to be formed by the close apposition of astrocyte end-feet to and ensheathment of the capillary endothelium, Reese and Karnovsky [64] demonstrated that the endothelium itself serves as the primary diffusion barrier to solutes. Brain capillary endothelial cells are nonfenestrated, marked by a paucity of endocytotic vesicles, and express high-resistance epithelial type TJs responsible for restricting diffusion through the paracellular space [28]. In addition, brain capillaries also express an array of multispecific xenobiotic efflux transporters that prevent more lipophilic organic molecules from entering the brain. Metabolic enzymes that rapidly degrade certain potentially neurotoxic compounds are enriched within the endothelium itself. The expressions of efflux transporters and metabolic enzymes are coordinated, and are inducible by many stimuli, including environmental toxicants and inflammatory mediators [65].

The "barrier phenotype" of the cerebral microvessel endothelium derives from its interaction with neural tissue, as demonstrated by xenograft studies [66]. The interaction of astrocytes with the endothelium is important; selective oblation of astrocytes in vivo leads to a loss of barrier integrity [67], and contact co-culture of primary brain endothelial cells with astrocytes decreases permeability, increases expression of claudin-5, and induces activity of the efflux transporter p-glycoprotein [68]. However, the permeability barrier to macromolecules is established prior to the genesis of astrocytes in developing brain [69], indicating that other cells – likely pericytes – are involved in barrier induction during development and maintenance [70]. Endothelial cell–astrocyte and endothelial cell–pericyte interactions in permeability barrier dysfunction during ischemic brain injury are not well understood.

An extremely interesting course of investigation regards the ability of neurons to alter microvessel permeability. This has some basis in experimental observation. For example, it has long been known that noradrenergic projections from the locus coeruleus innervate brain microvessels [71]. Chemical lesions of noradrenergic neurons lead to significant reductions in TJ protein expressions [72]. Finally, electrical stimulation of the sphenopalatine ganglion leads to an acute, transient opening of the barrier in the rat [73].

Neuron–vascular coupling and vessel–neuron communication

Local cerebral blood flow is under paracrine control by nitric oxide (NO) (endothelium-derived relaxing factor [EDRF]) and by neuron–vascular coupled processes, through a variety of routes. Neurons can regulate distant regional flow through interneurons [74]. Examples involve innervations of the large brain-supplying arteries, including the MCA. Precapillary arterioles control downstream flow [44]. Neurons also control microvascular flow via intervening astrocytes. This represents the efferent limb of the "neurovascular unit" [16, 75]. A number of laboratories have demonstrated the ability of stimulated neurons to generate local alterations in microvessel diameter. Iadecola has shown the role of COX-2 generation in astrocyte end-feet in muscular contraction [76].

The proximity between the endothelium and astrocytes suggests: (1) communication between the compartments to preserve microvessel integrity; and (2) that intramicrovascular events may be transmitted to the neuropil [77, 78]. Obstruction of small vessels (and presumably downstream microvessels) in lacunar disease results in neuronal dysfunction, manifest by neurologic deficits.

Cerebral microvessels under conditions of focal ischemia

The components of the neurovascular unit are variably vulnerable to oxygen and nutrient deprivation. The cerebral microvasculature is less sensitive to ischemic injury than the components of the neuropil. Within two hours of MCA occlusion in the nonhuman primate >80% of cells with evidence of DNA scission are neurons, whereas by 24 hours after MCA occlusion ~1.8% of the cells are endothelial cells [79]. In vitro, it would appear that astrocytes are more vulnerable to experimental ischemia than the endothelium [26].

Ultrastructural changes

The microvasculature displays rapid dynamic responses to focal ischemia. Garcia et al. have described histologic changes in the setting of extended ischemic injury, in the nonhuman primate [80]. In time, following ischemia onset cerebral capillaries expand and rupture [81]. These changes within the microvasculature of the ischemic territory have suggested that structural changes take place as a consequence of the ischemic event itself.

In the early moments following occlusion of a brain-supplying artery, astrocytes swell and appear to detach from the capillary basal lamina. On the luminal side of the microvessel, endothelial cell swelling has been noted, but this is probably artifactual (see below). Generally, the ultrastructural organization of the endothelium is maintained intact for some time. The group of Heo et al. [82, 83] demonstrated the loss of electron density of the microvessel ECM during focal ischemia in vivo. This accords with significant reduction in the basal lamina content of immunoreactive laminin, collagen type IV, and fibronectin (of cellular origin), observed in the nonhuman primate [84, 85]. These events occur heterogeneously within the ischemic territory.

Inflammation (both peripheral and innate) occurs within the ischemic regions, and is associated with thrombosis. Following the onset of focal ischemia, polymorphonuclear leukocyte (PMN) adhesion receptors appear on the endothelium of post-capillary venules within the ischemic territory in sequence, beginning with P-selectin (90 min), ICAM-1, and then E-selectin in the unanesthetized nonhuman primate [32, 33]. PMN leukocytes infiltrate the ischemic territory within hours of the onset of focal ischemia, followed by monocyte/macrophage infiltration [77, 86]. In addition, several groups have observed the appearance of myeloperoxidase (MPO) in the ischemic territory following MCA occlusion in the anesthetized rodent [87]. This has been attributed to transmigration and trafficking of PMN leukocytes, which shed MPO. However, it could also refer to microglial activation, and the instigation of innate inflammation. The impact of both PMN leukocyte activation in the acute phase, and the responses to the activation of innate inflammation on microvessel integrity and remodeling, have received little attention (see below). Furthermore, their presence in the events leading to neuronal necrosis, neuron nuclear pyknosis, and cytoplasmic changes, as well as significant alterations in other cell components of the neuropil, are poorly understood.

Microvessel–neuron relationships

Given the well-ordered arrangement of neurons relative to their supply microvessels, selective neuron injury within the ischemic bed could be directly related to the local supply. Mabuchi et al. [7] determined that, within a 30 μm envelope from microvessels within the primate corpus striatum, within two hours from MCA occlusion, neurons most distant from their proximate microvessels display injury (DNA scission). The finding was highly significant, occurring at a time when there was little cytoarchitectural distortion. The Krogh hypothesis suggests that the fall-off in oxygen content would be insufficient to explain the neuron injury: injury of essential components of the neurovascular unit (e.g., astrocytes) might be involved. In any event, selective neuron subtypes were found to exhibit consistent vulnerability [7, 88]. The basis for this relationship could include altered signal transduction through astrocytes and/or selective injury to astrocytes disrupting neuron function.

Alterations in matrix adhesion

Focal ischemia results in rapid profound changes to the ECM-related structural interactions within cerebral microvessels.

Adhesion receptors

The contacts between endothelial cells and astrocytes are lost in the acute phase of ischemia [25, 26, 89]. The immunoreactivity of β_1 integrins on endothelial cells and the matrix adhesion receptors integrin β_1, integrin $\alpha_6\beta_4$, and αβ-dystroglycan that link astrocytes to the basal lamina decreases shortly after ischemia onset [82, 83, 90]. The alterations are associated with detachment of astrocyte end-feet and cell swelling [82]. The losses of matrix-adhesion receptors that accompany microvessel ECM degradation lead to disruption of the neurovascular unit, and neuron injury occurs in the same time frame and in the same subregions of ischemic injury.

Matrix

Studies in the nonhuman primate model of focal ischemia and in rodents show a progressive loss of the ECM antigens laminin, fibronectin, and collagen IV from brain microvessels following MCA occlusion with reperfusion [62, 84]. Heo et al. [61, 82] have shown the loss of electron density of the basal lamina in cerebral microvessels under ischemic condition, and that this loss relates to the appearance of pro-MMP-9.

Matrix proteases

Enzymes with matrix protease specificity, including select MMPs, cathepsin L, and the serine protease u-PA, are generated and released in the ischemic cerebral tissue within a few hours after MCA occlusion [61–63]. The active forms of these proteases are hypothesized to degrade matrix substrates, including type IV collagen, laminins, and fibronectin, as well as the minor HSPG perlecan, to disturb the horizontal and vertical interactions of the normal permeability barrier within the neurovascular unit [62]. Heparanase is also released acutely, and is associated with the loss of HS side chains [62]. The appearance of certain matrix proteases, especially (pro-)MMP-9, is associated with hemorrhagic transformation during focal ischemia in the nonhuman primate [91–93]. The activation of pro-MMP-9 has not been unequivocally proven in this setting. Plasma MMP-9 levels have been associated with the appearance of hyperintensities [94], as well as with subsequent hemorrhagic transformation [95]. Technical issues are relevant to the isolation of the activity in small animal models. However, the simultaneous presence of the inactive moieties, and the loss of specific basal lamina matrix substrates in the same territory, suggest that the two observations are connected. The generation of certain matrix proteases also may reflect the reactivity of innate inflammation [16, 96, 97].

Permeability barrier

Disruption of the permeability barrier occurs very early in focal ischemia, as demonstrated by the leakage of fluid and solutes into the neuropil. In stroke patients this is visualized by gadolinium hyperintensity on magnetic resonance imaging (MRI) scan and high attenuation lesions by computed tomography (CT). The precise initiator(s) of permeability barrier disruption are not known.

Increased microvessel permeability is reflected in disruption of the TJ complex. Downregulation, degradation, and post-translational modifications of TJ proteins have been described in focal ischemia and in-vitro hypoxia models [98]. ECM degradation and loss of adhesion receptors may also contribute to destabilization of the TJ complex. For example, integrin β_1 contributes to barrier integrity via stabilization of the TJ protein claudin-5 [29]. With the loss of immunoreactive β_1-integrins from endothelial cells early during focal ischemia, it is plausible that this change contributes to changes in the endothelial portion of the permeability barrier, although this is an untested hypothesis [29, 90]. Furthermore, loss of the basal lamina structure may also lead to extravasation of erythrocytes and plasma during hemorrhagic transformation [85].

Neuron–vascular coupling and vessel–neuron communication

During focal ischemia, the changes in neuron–vascular coupling are elusive. Processes of central and peripheral neurons modulate cerebral blood flow [99]. Meanwhile, Raichle et al. [100] showed evidence that central noradrenergic terminals modulate the permeability of the blood–brain barrier. Considered together, disruption of neuron–vascular coupling resulting from ischemia might alter rCBF, leading to post-ischemic hyperemia, or focal hypoperfusion, including crossed cerebellar diaschisis (CCD). With the generation of cerebral edema, a vicious cycle could result in terms of microvascular circulation in the affected areas.

Furthermore, the loss of cell–matrix adhesion and the alterations in TJ expression with their structural consequences support the notion that vessel–neuron communication is disrupted during focal ischemia.

Clinically relevant microvessel effects during focal ischemia

Edema formation

Edema develops in the regions of ischemic injury, largely associated with increased microvessel permeability (vasogenic edema) within two to three hours of ischemia onset [77, 101]. Loss of blood flow in the brain leads to rapid depletion of adenosine triphosphate (ATP) and subsequent failure of energy-dependent ion transporters that maintain normal gradients of ions. In astrocytes, this results in sodium ion (Na^+) accumulation, as well as chloride ion (Cl^-), and water (H_2O) that flows along the osmotic gradient, resulting in cell swelling. Transcriptional upregulation of ion channels, including the sulfonylurea receptor-1 (SUR1)-regulated NC_{CA-ATP} channel, further contributes to the entry of ions and H_2O into the cells. However, this does not lead to a net accumulation of water in the brain. This occurs due the combination of the osmotic gradient created by depletion of water from the extracellular space and disruption of the permeability barrier [102].

Hemorrhagic transformation

Clinical studies of acute plasminogen activator administration suggest tissue signatures of cerebral hemorrhage risk. Hemorrhagic infarctions occur following degradation of the basal lamina matrix within the ischemic lesions, and have been attributed to the microvasculature. These are typified clinically as petechial hemorrhage or microhemorrhages on imaging studies, occurring in ~65% of individuals with focal ischemia [103]. They also appear in animal models of focal ischemia, in a stochastic fashion [61, 101]. Parenchymal hemorrhages are typified by large space-occupying collections of blood in the cerebral tissue visible as confluent hemorrhagic events on imaging, attributed to arterial leakage or rupture. Microhemorrhages can also occur spontaneously in the settings of uncontrolled hypertension and amyloid angiopathy (amyloid deposition) [104].

A hypothesis that accounts for the relationship between microvessel basal lamina degradation and hemorrhagic transformation invokes the acute appearance of several families of matrix proteases following MCA occlusion [61, 62, 84]. Although attractive, to date this hypothesis has not been strictly proven, although observations in a number of models are compatible with the possibility that matrix protease generation can be associated with hemorrhagic transformation. Technical and methodological limitations of many experimental studies weaken the assertion [61, 63, 105–110]. Montaner and colleagues [95, 111–113] have attributed separately a number of clinical consequences of stroke to MMP-9 activity, including hemorrhagic transformation, edema formation, and ischemic stroke. However, the extravasation of plasma (as edema and hemorrhage) into the neuropil can activate microglia, which release pro-MMP-9. Whether the appearance of (pro-)MMP-9 alone in plasma or in ischemic cerebral tissues is primarily responsible for hemorrhagic transformation is not settled [97].

For ischemic stroke, the risk of detectable hemorrhage increases under the condition of anticoagulation, antiplatelet agent exposure, hypertension, diabetes mellitus, and advanced age. The risk factors for cerebral hemorrhage in the setting of recombinant tissue-type plasminogen activator (rt-PA) administration include excessive time from the onset of ischemia, low body mass index, hypertension, and older age. The appearances of "early CT sign," which suggest large infarction due to embolism, are also associated with increased risk of hemorrhagic infarction. All of these factors target the arterioles, precapillary arterioles, and their microvasculature.

Focal "no-reflow"

Early-on following the onset of focal ischemia reduction in downstream microvessel patency occurs. While attributed in part to external compression by swollen astrocytes, alterations in flow could result from these intravascular processes. Histologic studies have suggested that endothelial cells could also undergo swelling, and produce luminal tags. However, these may reflect artifactual conditions, dependent upon: (1) inappropriate perfusion techniques; and (2) inappropriate osmolalities of the perfusion fluids. In experiments in which the osmolality of the perfusion fluids has been adjusted to plasma equivalence, and particular fixation techniques have been applied, these endothelial cell events have not been observed [101].

Ames et al. [114] described the significant reduction in the patency of microvascular beds following global cerebral ischemia as the "no-reflow" phenomenon, and demonstrated this obstruction by the use of carbon black tracer techniques. Sundt et al. [115] suggested this might also take place in global ischemia in large animals, while del Zoppo et al. [77] demonstrated the focal "no-reflow" phenomenon in the non-human primate subject to M1 segment MCA occlusion and perfused with carbon black tracer. In a series of experiments, that laboratory demonstrated that the microvasculature could be obstructed with PMN leukocytes, activated platelets, and/or fibrin deposition (Figure 10.3 [77]). The adhesion of PMN leukocytes accorded with the inability of carbon tracer to perfuse capillary and microvessel segments (Figure 10.4) [77, 116]. The obstruction of those microvessels accorded with the timing of the appearance of the endothelial cell leukocyte adhesion receptor expression in post-capillary venules, including P-selectin, ICAM-1, and E-selectin [33]. Furthermore, evidence was acquired demonstrating that platelet activation and deposition could occur intraluminally in the ischemic territories [32]. Finally, Okada [78] demonstrated the deposition of fibrin in the microvessel segments in the ischemic territory, and in the

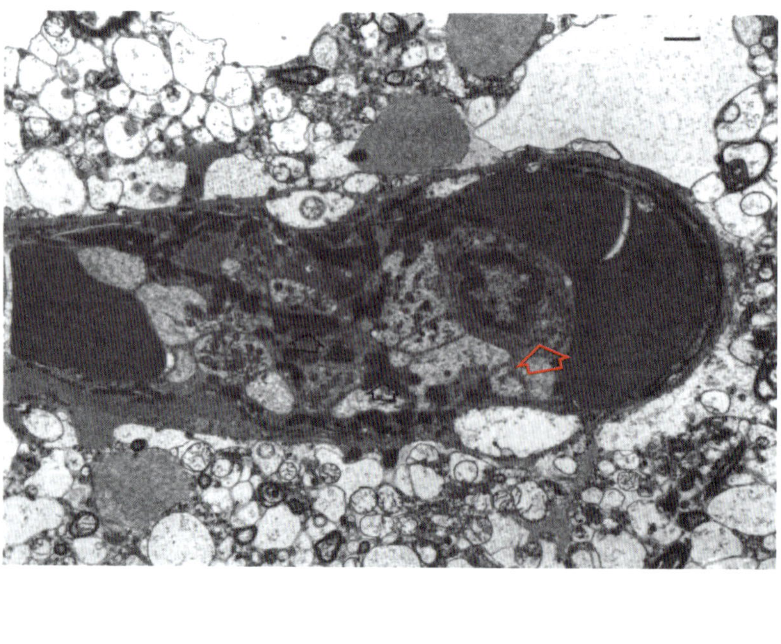

Figure 10.3 Occlusion of a microvessel with polymorphonuclear leukocyte (large open arrow), fibrin (small open arrows), and degraulated platelets following three-hour middle cerebral artery occlusion and one-hour reperfusion in the nonhuman primate striatum. Note fibrin in vessel wall. Magnification bar = 1 μm. From del Zoppo et al. [77], reproduced with permission.

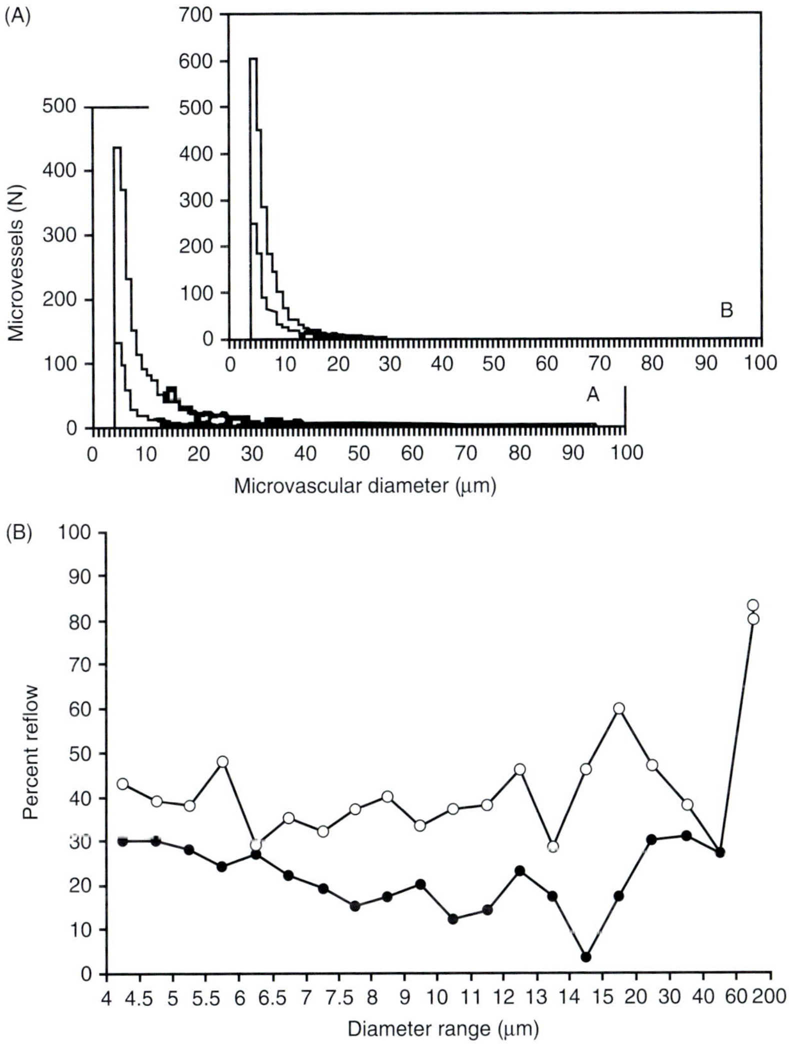

Figure 10.4 Loss of patency (focal "no-reflow") within the striatum with conditions of Figure 10.3. (A) Relative distribution of patent microvessels in two patency experiments. Note upper curves from nonischemic striatum and lower curves from ipsilateral ischemic striatum (indicating occlusion of the bed) in subjects A and B. (B) Percentage reflow in the two subjects by microvessel size class. Subject A = closed circle, subject B = open circle. Note that microvessels >60 μm diameter are completely patent.

microvessel wall. The deposition was tissue-factor dependent, suggesting that increased permeability of the microvasculature at the sites of fibrin deposition was, in part, responsible [117]. Interventions have been applied that increased microvessel patency in these territories by inhibiting PMN leukocyte adhesion [77, 116], platelet–fibrin interactions [78, 118], and fibrin deposition (through inhibition of tissue factor (TF) : factor VIIa activity) [78, 117]. Furthermore, conditions have been described in which inhibition of platelet–fibrinogen interactions in a murine model of focal cerebral ischemia decreased ischemic injury and improved neurologic outcome in that model [118, 119]. This experience and experiments with genetic constructs are consistent with the view that prevention of these microvessel events significantly reduces neuron injury from focal ischemia.

SVD and the neurovascular unit

The theoretical construct described by the neurovascular unit is suitable for considerations of microvessel–neuron interactions in the CNS (Figure 10.5). If the mean microvessel–neuron distance is ~30 μm (in the striatum) [7], then a 2 mm cerebral lesion notable on a MRI scan would contain ~1×10^5 neurovascular units. Hence, injuries that rise to the level of being radiographically detectable must involve a field of many units. Conversely injuries (e.g., amyloid angiopathy) that do not yet rise to the threshold of detectability can also affect numerous units.

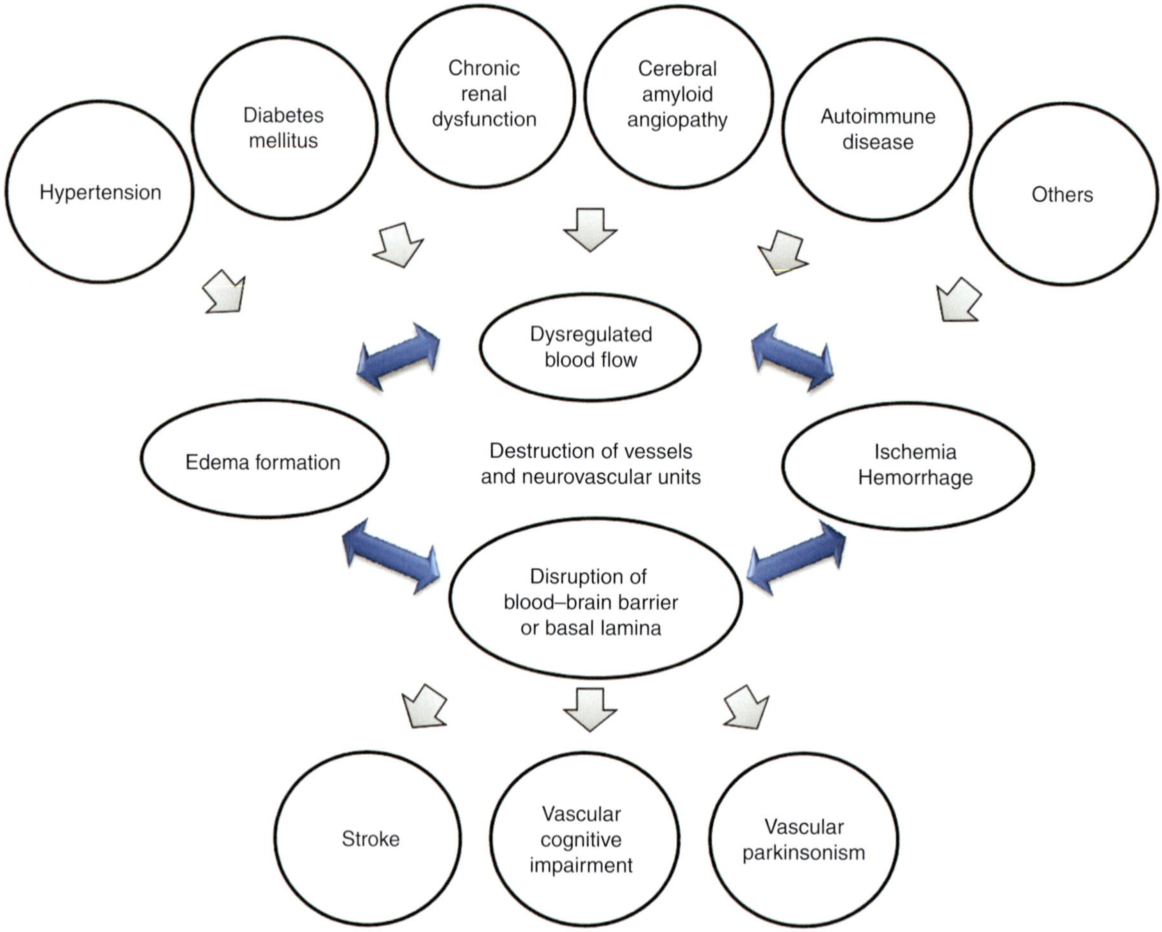

Figure 10.5 A formulation describing the potential relationships of processes causing small vessel injury to their impact on the downstream microvessels and their neurovascular units. Chronic processes (e.g., hypotension, diabetes mellitus, chronic renal dysfunction, amyloid deposition disease, autoimmune disorders, and other injurious processes) directly impact small vessels and the downstream microvasculature. Effects on the latter also disrupt the integrity of the respective neurovascular units. Dysregulated blood flow locally, ischemia, hemorrhage, disruption of the blood–brain barrier and matrix, and edema formation occur due to injury to the microvessels and their neurovascular units. This may lead to a vicious cycle of increased injury as inflammatory processes are initiated, leading to recruitment of neurovascular units into the injured pool. While clinically silent early, in time clinical manifestations of stroke, vascular cognitive impairment, and vascular parkinsonism appear. The microvascular injury and neurovascular unit loss (see Figure 10.2) increase the risk of these events. It is conceivable that injury to the neurovascular units affects the small vessels upstream. Finally, small vessels may remain patent, by virtue of the characteristics indicated in Figures 10.1 and 10.4, while the downstream microvessel beds become occluded.

Injury to one or more elements of a unit (e.g., the microvessels or their components) is likely to affect the other elements of that unit (e.g., neurons). Where a group of units interacts (whether through the endothelium, astrocyte, or neuron networks) injury to any one of the networks is likely to affect the others. However, the appropriateness of this surmise to the effects of SVD is speculative, in part because of the plethora of disorders and etiologies classified as SVD [1]. The term cerebral SVD encompasses pathologic processes that affect the small vessels of the brain, including not only small arteries and arterioles but also capillaries and venules [1]. These include lacunar infarction, Binswanger's disease, leukoaraiosis, cerebral amyloid angiopathy, microhemorrhages of various etiologies, and others. Pathologic changes of SVD, including atherosclerosis, fibrinoid necrosis, and lipohyalinosis of small arteries and arteriolosclerosis are commonly observed. But, these changes are the findings also observed in the patients with chronic hypertension or diabetes mellitus, and underlying pathologic change observed in small arteries and arterioles could also be found variously in cerebral SVD. So, clinically, it makes sense that the lesion(s) observed can represent the end-stage of multiple processes affecting various elements in a single neurovascular unit or among units. This implies that the earliest stages of the disorder are undetectable, and could involve alterations in endothelial cell integrity, intravascular thrombosis, matrix adhesion and matrix integrity, the permeability barrier, edema formation, hemorrhage, and other effects observed commonly as a result of ischemic injury.

Hence, it is conceivable that blood–brain barrier failure and the disruption of microvessel structure (and function) observed in focal ischemia are also common among certain cerebral SVDs. Whether microvessel permeability barrier dysfunction is secondary to upstream events, or is a direct result of disease processes targeting the microvasculature is uncertain. Microvessel occlusions, chronic hypoperfusion, inflammation in the vessel walls, innate inflammation, and other factors could cause the destruction of basal lamina and alterations of the permeability barrier. These events together with altered autoregulation of rCBF could lead to hemorrhage, the loss of microvessels, and a vicious cycle of decompensated hypoperfusion/nonperfusion and destruction of many neurovascular units. Moreover, these microscopic structural changes may start some years before the first symptoms of cerebral SVD appear and clinical evidence represented by physiologic and psychological symptoms [120].

Although SVD may be asymptomatic, it is associated with a high probability of stroke recurrence, cognitive impairment, and gait disturbance (so-called vascular parkinsonism). Therefore, the elucidation of the mechanisms for development and worsening of cerebral SVD is essential to avoid physical and psychological disabilities. Meanwhile, although some surveys have suggested that the control of hypertension prevents white matter lesions [121], interventions that could resolve this progression are not yet available. Hence, interventions to curb the vicious cycle leading to neurovascular unit destruction are needed, as well as remedies against the risk factors for small vessel and microvessel injury. This requires detailed elucidation of the molecular, structural, and functional mechanisms and consequences of injury to the neurovascular unit.

Acknowledgements

The authors are grateful for the support of the NIH through the grants R01 NS026745, NS038710, and NS053716, and for the support of the Uehara Memorial Foundation.

We wish to warmly thank Ms. Greta Berg for her help in formulating this manuscript.

References

1. Pantoni L. Cerebral small vessel disease: from pathogenesis and clinical characteristics to therapeutic challenges. *Lancet Neurol* 2010;9:689–701.
2. Del Zoppo GJ, Sharp FR, Heiss W-D, Albers GW. Heterogeneity in the penumbra. *J Cereb Blood Flow Metab* 2011;31:1836–1851.
3. del Zoppo GJ. The neurovascular unit in the setting of stroke. *J Intern Med* 2010;267:156–171.
4. Bär T. The vascular system of the cerebral cortex. *Adv Anat Embryol Cell Biol* 1980;59:1–62.
5. Bär T. Morphometric evaluation of capillaries in different laminae of rat cerebral cortex by automatic image analysis: changes during development and aging. In Cervos-Navarro J, ed. *Advances in Neurology*, 20th edn. New York, NY: Raven Press; 1978: pp. 1–9.
6. Bär T. Patterns of vascularization in the developing cerebral cortex. In Nugent J and O'Connor M., eds. *Ciba Foundation Symposium 100 – Development of the Vascular System.* Chichester, UK: John Wiley and Sons; 2008: pp. 20–36.
7. Mabuchi T, Lucero J, Feng A, Koziol JA, del Zoppo GJ. Focal cerebral ischemia preferentially affects neurons distant from their neighboring microvessels. *J Cereb Blood Flow Metab* 2005;25:257–266.
8. Fenstermacher J, Nakata H, Tajima A, et al. Functional variations in parenchymal microvascular systems within the brain. *Magn Reson Med* 1991;19:217–220.
9. Heiss WD. Ischemic penumbra: evidence from functional imaging in man. *J Cereb Blood Flow Metab* 2000;20:1276–1293.
10. Heiss WD. Experimental evidence of ischemic thresholds and functional recovery. *Stroke* 1992;23:1668–1672.
11. Heiss WD, Graf R, Wienhard K, et al. Dynamic penumbra demonstrated by sequential multitracer PET after middle cerebral artery occlusion in cats. *J Cereb Blood Flow Metab* 1994;14:892–902.
12. Zülch K-J. *The Cerebral Infarct: Pathology, Pathogenesis, and*

Computed Tomography. Berlin: Springer-Verlag; 1985: pp. 4–5.

13. Edvinsson L, MacKenzie ET, McCulloch J. General and comparative anatomy of the cerebral circulation. In Edvinsson L, MacKenzie ET, McCulloch J, eds. *Cerebral Blood Flow and Metabolism*. New York, NY: Raven Press; 1993: pp. 3–39.
14. Edvinsson L, MacKenzie ET, McCulloch J. *Cerebral Blood Flow and Metabolism*. New York, NY: Raven Press; 1993.
15. Garcion E, Halilagic A, Faissner A, French-Constant C. Generation of an environmental niche for neural stem cell development by the extracellular matrix molecule tenascin C. *Development* 2004;131:3423–3432.
16. del Zoppo GJ. Inflammation and the neurovascular unit in the setting of focal cerebral ischemia. *Neuroscience* 2009; 158:972–982.
17. del Zoppo GJ. The neurovascular unit, matrix proteases, and innate inflammation. *Ann NY Acad Sci* 2010;1207:46–49.
18. del Zoppo GJ. Toward the neurovascular unit: a journey in clinical translation. 2012 Thomas Willis lecture. *Stroke* 2013;44:263–269.
19. Spatz M, Bacic F, McCarron RM, et al. Human cerebromicrovascular endothelium: studies in vitro. *J Cereb Blood Flow Metab* 1989;9: S393.
20. Spatz M, Micic D, Mrsulja BB, Klatzo I. Cerebral microvessels as mediators of cerebral transport. *Adv Neurol* 1978;20:189–196.
21. Micic D, Swink M, Micic J, Klatzo I, Spatz M. The ischemic and postischemic effect on the uptake of neutral amino acids in isolated cerebral capillaries. *Experientia* 1993;15:625–626.
22. McCarron RM, Merkel N, Bembry J, Spatz M. Cerebrovascular endothelium in vitro: studies related to blood–brain barrier function. *Proceedings of the XIst International Congress of Neuropathy* 1991; (Suppl. 4):785–787.
23. Macdonald JA, Murugesan N, Pachter JS. Endothelial cell heterogeneity of blood–brain barrier gene expression along the cerebral microvasculature. *J Neurosci Res* 2010; 88:1457–1474.
24. Haring H-P, Akamine P, Habermann R, Koziol JA, del Zoppo GJ. Distribution of integrin-like immunoreactivity on primate brain microvasculature. *J Neuropathol Exp Neurol* 1996;55:236–245.
25. Milner R, Hung S, Wang X, Spatz M, del Zoppo GJ. The rapid decrease in astrocyte-associated dystroglycan expression by focal cerebral ischemia is protease-dependent. *J Cereb Blood Flow Metab* 2008;28:812–823.
26. Milner R, Hung S, Wang X, et al. Responses of endothelial cell and astrocyte matrix-integrin receptors to ischemia mimic those observed in the neurovascular unit. *Stroke* 2008;39:191–197.
27. del Zoppo GJ, Milner R. Integrin–matrix interactions in the cerebral microvasculature. *Arterioscler Thromb Vasc Biol* 2006;26:1966–1975.
28. Hawkins BT, Davis TP. The blood–brain barrier/ neurovascular unit in health and disease. *Pharmacol Rev* 2005;57:173–185.
29. Osada T, Gu Y-H, Kanazawa M, et al. Interendothelial claudin-5 expression depends upon cerebral endothelial cell–matrix adhesion by β_1-integrins. *J Cereb Blood Flow Metab* 2011;31:1972–1985.
30. Dejana E, Orsenigo F, Lampugnani MG. The role of adherens junctions and VE-cadherin in the control of vascular permeability. *J Cell Sci* 2008;121:2115–2122.
31. Pardridge WM. *Introduction to the Blood–Brain Barrier. Methodology, Biology and Pathology*. Cambridge: Cambridge University Press; 1998.
32. Okada Y, Copeland BR, Mori E, et al. P-selectin and intercellular adhesion molecule-1 expression after focal brain ischemia and reperfusion. *Stroke* 1994;25:202–211.
33. Haring H-P, Berg EL, Tsurushita N, Tagaya M, del Zoppo GJ. E-selectin appears in non-ischemic tissue during experimental focal cerebral ischemia. *Stroke* 1996;27:1386–1392.
34. Bernstein JJ, Getz R, Jefferson M, Kelemen M. Astrocytes secrete basal lamina after hemisection of rat spinal cord. *Brain Res* 1985;327:135–141.
35. Hurwitz AA, Berman JW, Rashbaum WK, Lyman WD. Human fetal astrocytes induce the expression of blood–brain barrier specific proteins by autologous endothelial cells. *Brain Res* 1993;625:238–243.
36. Webersinke G, Bauer H, Amberger A, Zach O, Bauer HC. Comparison of gene expression of extracellular matrix molecules in brain microvascular endothelial cells and astrocytes. *Biochem Biophys Res Commun* 1992;189:877–884.
37. Kaizuka M, Yamabe H, Osawa H, Okumura K, Fujimoto N. Thrombin stimulates synthesis of type IV collagen and tissue inhibitor of metalloproteinase-1 by cultured human mesangial cells. *J Am Soc Nephrol* 1999;10:1516–1523.
38. Takano T, Tian GF, Peng W, et al. Astrocyte-mediated control of cerebral blood flow. *Nat Neurosci* 2006;9:260–267.
39. Oberheim NA, Wang X, Goldman S, Nedergaard M. Astrocytic complexity distinguishes the human brain. *Trends Neurosci* 2006;29:547–553.

40. Panickar KS, Norenberg MD. Astrocytes in cerebral ischemic injury: morphological and general considerations. *GLIA* 2005;50:287–298.

41. Anderson CM, Nedergaard M. Astrocyte-mediated control of cerebral microcirculation. *Trends Neurosci* 2003;26:340–344.

42. Wagner S, Tagaya M, Koziol JA, Quaranta V, del Zoppo GJ. Rapid disruption of an astrocyte interaction with the extracellular matrix mediated by integrin $\alpha_6\beta_4$ during focal cerebral ischemia/reperfusion. *Stroke* 1997;28:858–865.

43. Koehler RC, Roman RJ, Harder DR. Astrocytes and the regulation of cerebral blood flow. *Trends Neurosci* 2009;32:160–169.

44. Itoh Y, Suzuki N. Control of brain capillary blood flow. *J Cereb Blood Flow Metab* 2012;32:1167–1176.

45. Simard M, Nedergaard M. The neurobiology of glia in the context of water and ion homeostasis. *Neuroscience* 2004;129:877–896.

46. Hawkins BT, Gu YH, Izawa Y, del Zoppo GJ. Disruption of dystroglycan–laminin interactions modulates water uptake by astrocytes. *Brain Res* 2013.

47. Dore-Duffy P, Katychev A, Wang X, Van BE. CNS microvascular pericytes exhibit multipotential stem cell activity. *J Cereb Blood Flow Metab* 2006;26:613–624.

48. Peppiatt CM, Howarth C, Mobbs P, Attwell D. Bidirectional control of CNS capillary diameter by pericytes. *Nature* 2006;443:700–704.

49. Zozulya A, Weidenfeller C, Galla HJ. Pericyte–endothelial cell interaction increases MMP-9 secretion at the blood–brain barrier in vitro. *Brain Res* 2008;1189:1–11.

50. Thanabalasundaram G, Pieper C, Lischper M, Galla HJ. Regulation of the blood–brain barrier integrity by pericytes via matrix metalloproteinases mediated activation of vascular endothelial growth factor in vitro. *Brain Res* 2010;1347:1–10.

51. Fisher M. Pericyte signaling in the neurovascular unit. *Stroke* 2009;40:S13–S15.

52. Silver R, Silverman AJ, Vitkovic L, Lederhendler I. Mast cells in the brain: evidence and functional significance. *Trends Neurosci* 1996;19:25–31.

53. Strbian D, Kovanen PT, Karjalainen-Lindsberg ML, Tatlisumak T, Lindsberg PJ. An emerging role of mast cells in cerebral ischemia and hemorrhage. *Ann Med* 2009;41:438–450.

54. Strbian D, Karjalainen-Lindsberg ML, Tatlisumak T, Lindsberg PJ. Cerebral mast cells regulate early ischemic brain swelling and neutrophil accumulation. *J Cereb Blood Flow Metab* 2006;26:605–612.

55. Strbian D, Tatlisumak T, Ramadan UA, Lindsberg PJ. Mast cell blocking reduces brain edema and hematoma volume and improves outcome after experimental intracerebral hemorrhage. *J Cereb Blood Flow Metab* 2007;27:795–802.

56. Tchougounova E, Lundequist A, Fajardo I, et al. A key role for mast cell chymase in the activation of pro-matrix metalloprotease-9 and pro-matrix metalloprotease-2. *J Biol Chem* 2005;280:9291–9296.

57. Lohi J, Harvima I, Keski-Oja J. Pericellular substrates of human mast cell tryptase: 72 000 dalton gelatinase and fibronectin. *J Cell Biochem* 1992;50:337–349.

58. Aloisi F, Ambrosini E, Columba-Cabezas S, Magliozzi R, Serafini B. Intracerebral regulation of immune responses. *Ann Med* 2001;33:510–515.

59. Aloisi F. Immune function of microglia. *GLIA* 2001;36:165–179.

60. Mabuchi T, Kitagawa K, Ohtsuki T, et al. Contribution of microglia/macrophages to expansion of infarction and response of oligodendrocytes after focal cerebral ischemia in rats. *Stroke* 2000;31:1735–1743.

61. Heo JH, Lucero J, Abumiya T, et al. Matrix metalloproteinases increase very early during experimental focal cerebral ischemia. *J Cereb Blood Flow Metab* 1999;19:624–633.

62. Fukuda S, Fini CA, Mabuchi T, et al. Focal cerebral ischemia induces active proteases that degrade microvascular matrix. *Stroke* 2004;35:998–1004.

63. Chang DI, Hosomi N, Lucero J, et al. Activation systems for latent matrix metalloproteinase-2 are upregulated immediately after focal cerebral ischemia. *J Cereb Blood Flow Metab* 2003;23:1408–1419.

64. Reese TS, Karnovsky MJ. Fine structural localization of a blood–brain barrier to exogenous peroxidase. *J Cell Biol* 1967;34:207–217.

65. Miller DS. Regulation of P-glycoprotein and other ABC drug transporters at the blood–brain barrier. *Trends Pharmacol Sci* 2010;31:246–254.

66. Stewart PA, Wiley MJ. Developing nervous tissue induces formation of blood–brain barrier characteristics in invading endothelial cells: a study using quail–chicken transplantation chimeras. *Dev Biol* 1981;84:183–192.

67. Willis CL, Leach L, Clarke GJ, Nolan CC, Ray DE. Reversible disruption of tight junction complexes in the rat blood–brain barrier, following transitory focal astrocyte loss. *GLIA* 2004;48:1–13.

68. Cohen-Kashi Malina K, Cooper I, Teichberg VI. Closing the gap between the in-vivo and in-vitro blood–brain barrier tightness. *Brain Res* 2009;1284:12–21.

69. Saunders NR, Knott GW, Dziegielewska KM. Barriers in the immature brain. *Cell Mol Neurobiol* 2000;20:29–40.

70. Daneman R, Zhou L, Kebede AA, Barres BA. Pericytes are required for blood–brain barrier integrity during embryogenesis. *Nature* 2010;468:562–566.

71. Kalaria RN, Stockmeier CA, Harik SI. Brain microvessels are innervated by locus ceruleus noradrenergic neurons. *Neurosci Lett* 1989;97:203–208.

72. Kalinin S, Feinstein DL, Xu HL, et al. Degeneration of noradrenergic fibres from the locus coeruleus causes tight-junction disorganisation in the rat brain. *Eur J Neurosci* 2006;24:3393–3400.

73. Yarnitsky D, Gross Y, Lorian A, et al. Blood–brain barrier opened by stimulation of the parasympathetic sphenopalatine ganglion: a new method for macromolecule delivery to the brain. *J Neurosurg* 2004;101:303–309.

74. Iadecola C. Neurovascular regulation in the normal brain and in Alzheimer's disease. *Nat Rev Neurosci* 2004;5:347–360.

75. del Zoppo GJ. Stroke and neurovascular protection. *N Engl J Med* 2006;354:553–555.

76. Iadecola C, Nedergaard M. Glial regulation of the cerebral microvasculature. *Nat Neurosci* 2007;10:1369–1376.

77. del Zoppo GJ, Schmid-Schönbein GW, Mori E, Copeland BR, Chang CM. Polymorphonuclear leukocytes occlude capillaries following middle cerebral artery occlusion and reperfusion in baboons. *Stroke* 1991;22:1276–1283.

78. Okada Y, Copeland BR, Fitridge R, Koziol JA, del Zoppo GJ. Fibrin contributes to microvascular obstructions and parenchymal changes during early focal cerebral ischemia and reperfusion. *Stroke* 1994;25:1847–1853.

79. Tagaya M, Liu KF, Copeland B, et al. DNA scission after focal brain ischemia. Temporal differences in two species. *Stroke* 1997;28:1245–1254.

80. Garcia JH, Conger KA. Light and electron-microscopic features of brain ischemia. In Wood JH, ed. *Cerebral Blood Flow. Physiologic and Clinical Aspects.* New York, NY: McGraw-Hill; 1987: pp. 75–91.

81. Garcia JH, Lowry SL, Briggs L, et al. Brain capillaries expand and rupture in areas of ischemia and reperfusion. In Reivich M, Hurtig HI, eds. *Cerebrovascular Diseases.* New York, NY: Raven Press; 1983: pp. 169–182.

82. Kwon I, Kim EH, del Zoppo GJ, Heo JH. Ultrastructural and temporal changes of the microvascular basement membrane and astrocyte interface following focal cerebral ischemia. *J Neurosci Res* 2009;87:668–676.

83. Heo JH, Han SW, Lee SK. Free radicals as triggers of brain edema formation after stroke. *Free Radic Biol Med* 2005;39:51–70.

84. Hamann GF, Okada Y, Fitridge R, del Zoppo GJ. Microvascular basal lamina antigens disappear during cerebral ischemia and reperfusion. *Stroke* 1995;26:2120–2126.

85. Hamann GF, Okada Y, del Zoppo GJ. Hemorrhagic transformation and microvascular integrity during focal cerebral ischemia/reperfusion. *J Cereb Blood Flow Metab* 1996;16:1373–1378.

86. Garcia JH, Liu KF, Yoshida Y, et al. Influx of leukocytes and platelets in an evolving brain infarct (Wistar rat). *Am J Pathol* 1994;144:188–199.

87. Wang X, Yue T-L, Barone FC, et al. Concomitant cortical expression of TNF-α and IL-1β mRNA following transient focal ischemia. *Mol Chem Neuropathol* 1994;23:103–114.

88. Quistorff B, Chance B, Hunding A. An experimental model of the Krogh tissue cylinder: two dimensional quantitation of the oxygen gradient. *Adv Exp Med Biol* 1977;94:127–136.

89. del Zoppo GJ. Relationship of neurovascular elements to neuron injury during ischemia. *Cerebrovasc Dis* 2009; 27(Suppl 1):65–76.

90. Tagaya M, Haring H-P, Stuiver I, et al. Rapid loss of microvascular integrin expression during focal brain ischemia reflects neuron injury. *J Cereb Blood Flow Metab* 2001;21:835–846.

91. Asahi M, Wang X, Mori T, et al. Effects of matrix metalloproteinase-9 gene knock-out on the proteolysis of blood–brain barrier and white matter components after cerebral ischemia. *J Neurosci* 2001;21:7724–7732.

92. Cheng T, Petraglia AL, Li Z, et al. Activated protein C inhibits tissue plasminogen activator-induced brain hemorrhage. *Nat Med* 2006;12:1278–1285.

93. Yamashita T, Kamiya T, Deguchi K, et al. Dissociation and protection of the neurovascular unit after thrombolysis and reperfusion in ischemic rat brain. *J Cereb Blood Flow Metab* 2009;29:715–725.

94. Barr TL, Latour LL, Lee KY, et al. Blood–brain barrier disruption in humans is independently associated with increased matrix metalloproteinase-9. *Stroke* 2010;41:e123–e128.

95. Montaner J, Alvarez-Sabin J, Molina CA, et al. Matrix metalloproteinase expression is related to hemorrhagic transformation after cardioembolic stroke. *Stroke* 2001;32:2762–2667.

96. del Zoppo GJ, Milner R, Mabuchi T, et al. Microglial activation and matrix protease generation during focal cerebral ischemia. *Stroke* 2007;38:646–651.

97. del Zoppo GJ, Frankowski H, Gu YH, et al. Microglial cell activation is a source of metalloproteinase generation during hemorrhagic transformation. *J Cereb Blood Flow Metab* 2012;32:919–932.

98. Luissint AC, Artus C, Glacial F, Ganeshamoorthy K, Couraud PO. Tight junctions at the blood brain barrier: physiological architecture and disease-associated dysregulation. *Fluids Barriers CNS* 2012;9:23.

99. Iadecola C. Neurogenic control of the cerebral microcirculation: is dopamine minding the store? *Nat Neurosci* 1998;1:263–265.

100. Raichle ME, Hartman BK, Eichling JO, Sharpe LG. Central noradrenergic regulation of cerebral blood flow and vascular permeability. *Proc Natl Acad Sci USA* 1975;72:3726–3730.

101. del Zoppo GJ, Copeland BR, Harker LA, et al. Experimental acute thrombotic stroke in baboons. *Stroke* 1986;17:1254–1265.

102. Kahle KT, Simard JM, Staley KJ, et al. Molecular mechanisms of ischemic cerebral edema: role of electroneutral ion transport. *Physiology (Bethesda)* 2009;24:257–265.

103. del Zoppo GJ, Poeck K, Pessin MS, et al. Recombinant tissue plasminogen activator in acute thrombotic and embolic stroke. *Ann Neurol* 1992;32:78–86.

104. del Zoppo GJ. Bleeding in the brain: amyloid-β may keep clots away. *Nat Med* 2009;15:1132–1133.

105. Yu F, Kamada H, Niizuma K, Endo H, Chan PH. Induction of MMP-9 expression and endothelial injury by oxidative stress after spinal cord injury. *J Neurotrauma* 2008;25:184–195.

106. Dencoff JE, Rosenberg GA, Harry GJ. Trimethyltin induces gelatinase B and urokinase in rat brain. *Neurosci Lett* 1997;228:147–150.

107. Katsu M, Niizuma K, Yoshioka H, et al. Hemoglobin-induced oxidative stress contributes to matrix metalloproteinase activation and blood–brain barrier dysfunction in vivo. *J Cereb Blood Flow Metab* 2010;30:1939–1950.

108. Copin JC, Merlani P, Sugawara T, Chan PH, Gasche Y. Delayed matrix metalloproteinase inhibition reduces intracerebral hemorrhage after embolic stroke in rats. *Exp Neurol* 2008;213:196–201.

109. Kamada H, Yu F, Nito C, Chan PH. Influence of hyperglycemia on oxidative stress and matrix metalloproteinase-9 activation after focal cerebral ischemia/reperfusion in rats: relation to blood–brain barrier dysfunction. *Stroke* 2007;38:1044–1049.

110. Walker EJ, Rosenberg GA. Divergent role for MMP-2 in myelin breakdown and oligodendrocyte death following transient global ischemia. *J Neurosci Res* 2010;88:764–773.

111. Abilleira S, Montaner J, Molina CA, et al. Matrix metalloproteinase-9 concentration after spontaneous intracerebral hemorrhage. *J Neurosurg* 2003;99:65–70.

112. Rosell A, Ortega-Aznar A, Alvarez-Sabin J, et al. Increased brain expression of matrix metalloproteinase-9 after ischemic and hemorrhagic human stroke. *Stroke* 2006;37:1399–1406.

113. Montaner J, Molina CA, Monasterio J, et al. Matrix metalloproteinase-9 pretreatment level predicts intracranial hemorrhagic complications after thrombolysis in human stroke. *Circulation* 2003;107:598–603.

114. Ames A, Wright LW, Kowada M, Thurston JM, Majors G. Cerebral ischemia. II. The no-reflow phenomenon. *Am J Pathol* 1968;52:437–453.

115. Sundt TM, Jr., Grant WC, Garcia JH. Restoration of middle cerebral artery flow in experimental infarction. *J Neurosurg* 1969;31:311–322.

116. Mori E, del Zoppo GJ, Chambers JD, Copeland BR, Arfors KE. Inhibition of polymorphonuclear leukocyte adherence suppresses no-reflow after focal cerebral ischemia in baboons. *Stroke* 1992;23:712–718.

117. Thomas WS, Mori E, Copeland BR, et al. Tissue factor contributes to microvascular defects following cerebral ischemia. *Stroke* 1993;24:847–853.

118. Abumiya T, Fitridge R, Mazur C, et al. Integrin α(IIb)β(3) inhibitor preserves microvascular patency in experimental acute focal cerebral ischemia. *Stroke* 2000;31:1402–1410.

119. Bostwick JS, Kasiewski CJ, Chu V, et al. Anti-thrombotic activity of RG13965, a novel platelet fibrinogen receptor antagonist. *Thromb Res* 1996;82:495–507.

120. Wardlaw JM. Blood–brain barrier and cerebral small vessel disease. *J Neurol Sci* 2010; 299:66–71.

121. Chobanian AV, Bakris GL, Black HR, et al. The seventh report of the Joint National Committee on Prevention, Detection, Evaluation, and Treatment of High Blood Pressure: the JNC 7 report. *JAMA* 2003;289:2560–2572.

Chapter 11

Conventional brain imaging of white matter lesions

Franz Fazekas, Christian Enzinger, Stefan Ropele, and Reinhold Schmidt

Introduction

Over the past decades brain imaging has significantly contributed to the notion of cerebral damage related to small vessel disease (SVD) as a quite broad and diverse spectrum of morphological changes. While lacunar infarction and especially deep intracerebral hemorrhage are readily associated with SVD, it has taken some time to also appreciate more diffuse damage to the white matter as one of the hallmarks of cerebral microangiopathy. To some extent this is surprising, as the recognition of rather diffuse brain damage from arteriosclerosis dates back to at least Otto Binswanger and Alois Alzheimer in the late nineteenth century. Describing the pathologic findings of what they considered as "arteriosclerotic brain degeneration" they stated: "In the immediate vicinity of the vessels even macroscopically one can see the brain substance colored lightly gray to reddish brown and slightly sunken in many places on the cortex and medulla (white matter), especially in the area of the stem (basal ganglia) and the inner capsule." They also noted that "High-degree atheromatously degenerated vessels are to be found at the midpoint of the focal changes in the medulla as in the cortex" [1]. More than 60 years later, in 1962, Jerzy Olszewski attempted to redefine the pathologic features of then called *subcortical arteriosclerotic encephalopathy* or *Binswanger's disease* noting that: "Arteriosclerotic changes affected predominantly the perforating vessels to the subcortical gray substance and white matter, leading to multiple small areas of infarction with diffuse areas of demyelination in the latter and there was a relative sparing of the subcortical arcuate fibers and of the cortex" [2, 3]. These observations received new attention when the first computed tomography (CT) scanners showed profound white matter changes together with lacunar infarcts in individuals with neuropsychiatric deficits consistent with those described by Binswanger [4, 5]. With improving resolution of scanner technology the number of individuals with some white matter changes increased, and Vladimir C. Hachinski rightly concluded that this was not evidence for an epidemic of "Binswanger's disease" but rather the consequence of more sensitive images of the brain [6]. Similarly, focal areas of signal abnormality in the white matter of elderly individuals and especially of those with vascular risk factors suddenly became an almost common incidental finding when the introduction of magnetic resonance imaging (MRI) led to a further increase in sensitivity for white matter alterations [7, 8]. From that point onward it took several years to further clarify the emerging spectrum and clinical significance of white matter lesions (WMLs). These efforts confirmed more extensive WMLs as a hallmark of SVD-related brain damage and also showed that not all incidental WMLs are clearly attributable to microangiopathy [9, 10]. Furthermore it has been shown that WMLs of presumed vascular origin can be relatively well separated from other white matter disorders. This was especially important in developing the differential diagnosis from and for multiple sclerosis (MS) [11, 12]. Thus, we subsequently will review and illustrate the characteristics of SVD-related (incidental) WMLs as seen on conventional imaging by CT and MRI. We will also address their measurement based on conventional brain imaging to allow an estimation of their extent and severity. Advanced MRI sequences can be employed to further investigate the extent of structural abnormalities within WMLs and also of the white matter which appears normal on conventional sequences [13].

Cerebral Small Vessel Disease, ed. Leonardo Pantoni and Philip B. Gorelick. Published by Cambridge University Press.

CT characteristics

SVD-related white matter changes become apparent on CT by a decrease of X-ray attenuation, which causes more or less pronounced hypodensity but, however, never approaches that of cerebrospinal fluid (CSF), as this would indicate complete tissue destruction. Pathologically such areas are characterized primarily by loss of myelin and axons [14]. More extensive tissue destruction of the white matter has been equated with "incomplete infarction" by some [15]. The rarefaction of tissue also led to the creation of the term leukoaraiosis derived from the Greek words *"leuko-"* for "white" and *"araios"* for "rarefied" [6]. More recently suggested terms for CT visible WMLs to parallel MRI terminology and remain descriptive are "white matter hypoattenuation" or "white matter hypodensities."

SVD-related WMLs tend to be symmetrically distributed throughout the brain with a preference for the periventricular and deep white matter. These lesions are usually ill-defined and characteristically spare the subcortical U-fibers (Figure 11.1). Thus WMLs can be quite reliably separated from infarctions and moderate to substantial agreement has been reported for presence or absence of leukoaraiosis and of infarcts based on these characteristics (Table 11.1) [16]. Other problems in differential diagnosis are rare. Small acute infarcts within a territory of leukoaraiosis, however, can be ruled out neither by CT nor conventional MRI, i.e., without diffusion-weighted imaging (DWI) (see below and Figure 11.2), and more discrete white matter changes are also missed by CT (Figure 11.3). Otherwise SVD-related WMLs and leukoaraiosis call attention to the possible presence of microangiopathy and causative factors when incidentally seen in patients evaluated for neurologic or neuropsychiatric disorders, and provide strong evidence for a microangiopathy-related etiology when found in the context of lacunar infarction or intracerebral bleeding.

MRI characteristics

WMLs appear bright on T2-weighted MRI. For this reason they were at first termed unidentified bright objects (UBOs) by some [17]. More commonly, WMLs of presumed vascular origin are now called white matter hyperintensities (WMHs). Unfortunately T2-signal hyperintensity is associated with many types of tissue damage, and, thus, is an insufficient characteristic for allowing assignment of a specific etiology, or even the association with SVD to such areas of signal abnormality within the white matter. It is, therefore, rather a combination of signal characteristics and the pattern of lesion distribution that need to be considered when attempting to define the MRI features of SVD-related WMLs. As already noted with CT, WMLs by definition are assumed to represent areas of only subtle tissue damage in contrast to frank infarction or other types of complete destruction of brain parenchyma. This implies that WMLs should have a signal distinctly different from CSF on all sequences (Figure 11.4). They are bright on proton DWIs (which show ideally a low signal of CSF) and remain high in signal intensity on T2-weighted sequences which suppress the signal of CSF, e.g., the fluid-attenuated inversion recovery (FLAIR) sequence. On T1-weighted images, SVD-related WMLs are not or only faintly seen unless one employs heavy T1-weighting, such as by using an inversion recovery sequence. This makes SVD-related WMLs clearly different from areas of more extensive white matter destruction due to multiple sclerosis, which may turn into dark, well-circumscribed lesions, commonly also termed "black holes" [18]. The difference in the severity of demyelination that is underlying the different signal characteristics of SVD and MS-related WMLs has also been substantiated by quantitative MRI measures such as magnetization transfer imaging [19].

SVD-related WMLs occur preferentially in the deep white matter and close to the lateral ventricles, but spare the subcortical arcuate fibers as described above for leukoaraiosis seen on CT. This distributional pattern has been also confirmed by the use of lesion probability mapping [20] (Figure 11.5). The size of WMLs is variable and in the deep white matter ranges from punctuate over patchy to large confluent lesions [21, 22] (Figure 11.3). Lesion borders are mostly indistinct and irregular.

There exist signal hyperintensities directly abutting the lateral ventricles which have a shape that is in part different from deep WMLs as it is oriented along the ventricles (Figure 11.6). The often quite distinct borders then lead to the impression of a lining of the lateral ventricles. The thickness, i.e., transverse axis of these hyperintensities, ranges from pencil-thin to a smooth halo of several millimeters in width [22–24]. A further characteristic and more focal type of periventricular WMLs are caps of signal hyperintensity around the ventricular horns [25]. Finally, irregular

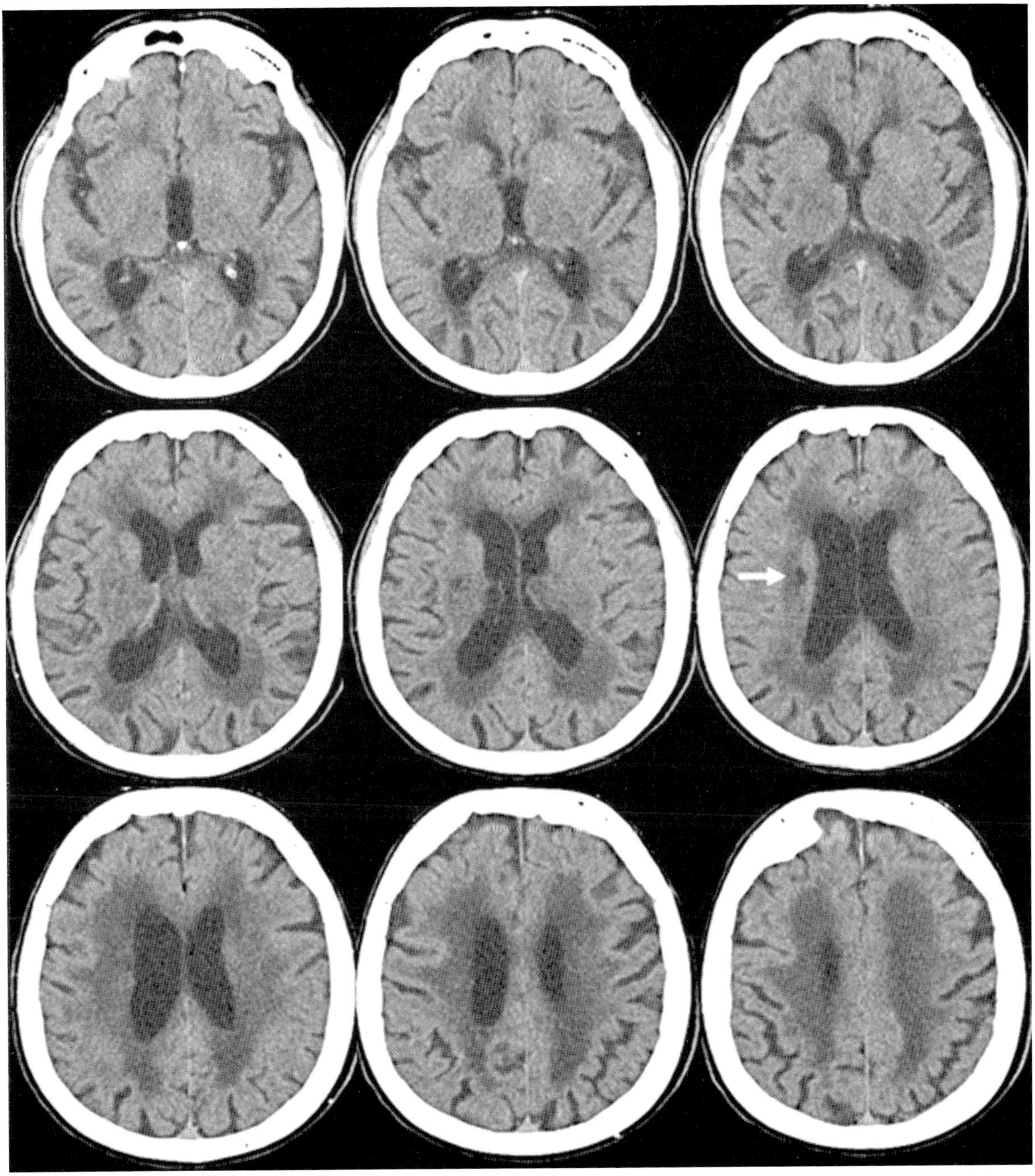

Figure 11.1 Computed tomography (CT) shows diffuse mild-to-moderate hypodensity throughout large parts of the white matter including the periventricular region. Note a sparing of the arcuate fibers. A small old lacunar infarction is seen in the right putamen (arrow).

foci of signal hyperintensity may also border the lateral ventricles and extend into the deep white matter blurring a distinction between periventricular and deep WMLs [22]. It has thus been debated, and is not yet fully clear, if strictly periventricular signal hyperintensities have the same etiology and clinical significance as WMLs in the deep white matter or if they represent a different category of abnormalities. This includes the question of whether periventricular and deep WMLs should be assessed separately.

Table 11.1 CT criteria for distinguishing infarcts and leukoaraiosis

Infarct	Leukoaraiosis
Well demarcated	Ill-defined, patchy, diffuse
Wedge-shaped	White matter only, without extension to cortex
Usually cortical extension	Ventricle and sulcus unchanged locally
Follows specific vascular territory	
Internal capsule, basal ganglia, or thalamus may be involved	
Enlargement of ipsilateral ventricle or sulcus	

From Steingart et al. [16], reproduced with permission.
CT, computed tomography.

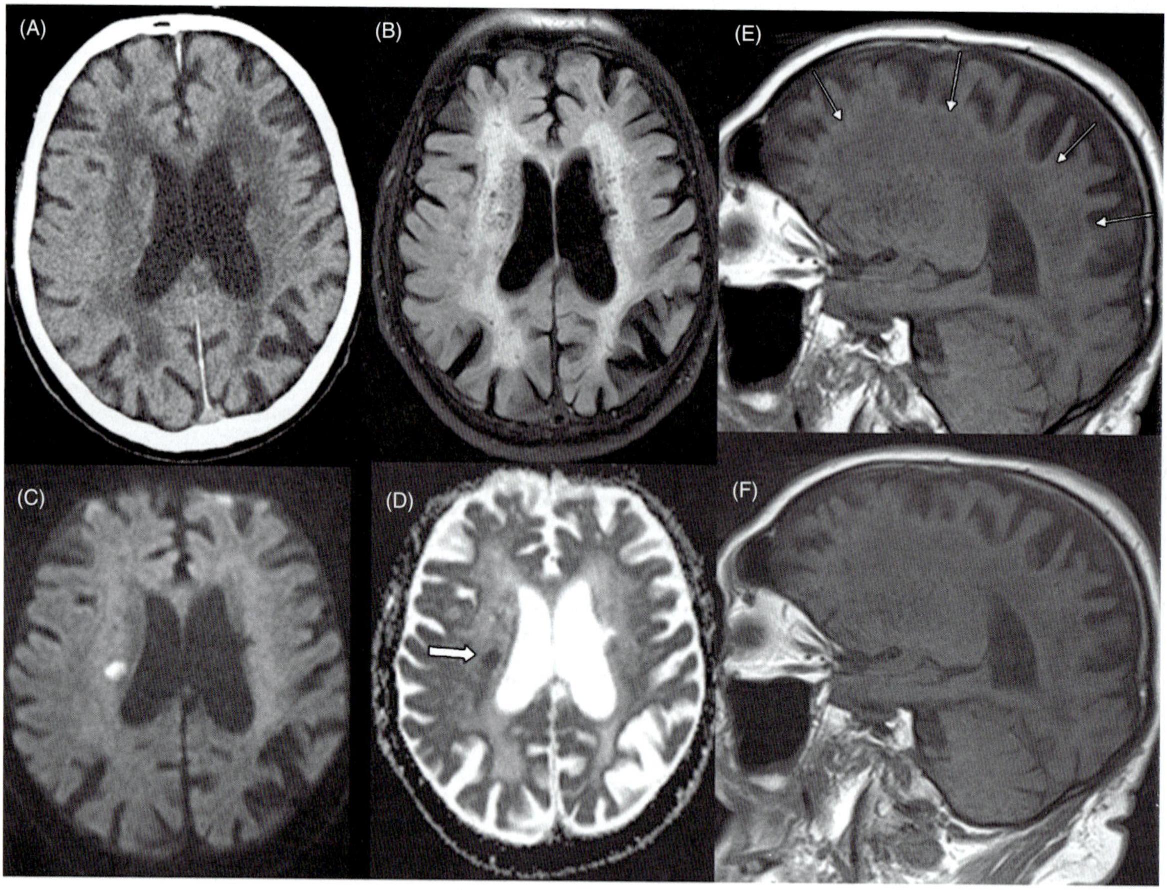

Figure 11.2 Extensive white matter lesions on (A) computed tomography (CT) and (B) magentic resonance imaging (MRI) with a small acute infarct in the right centrum semiovale seen only on (C) diffusion-weighted MRI. Restricted diffusion on the apparent diffusion coefficient map (D) confirms acute ischemia (broad arrow). Note the mild reduction in signal intensity throughout almost the entire white matter on sagittal T1-weighted scans, which spares the arcuate fibers (arrows) (E, F).

Investigations on this issue have come to different results and opinions are split [26, 27].

Histopathologic data suggest that the underlying morphological substrates – at least in part – differ between certain types of periventricular and deep WMLs [9, 10]. There is quite good evidence that a smooth hyperintense lining of the lateral ventricles is probably a consequence of increased transependymal

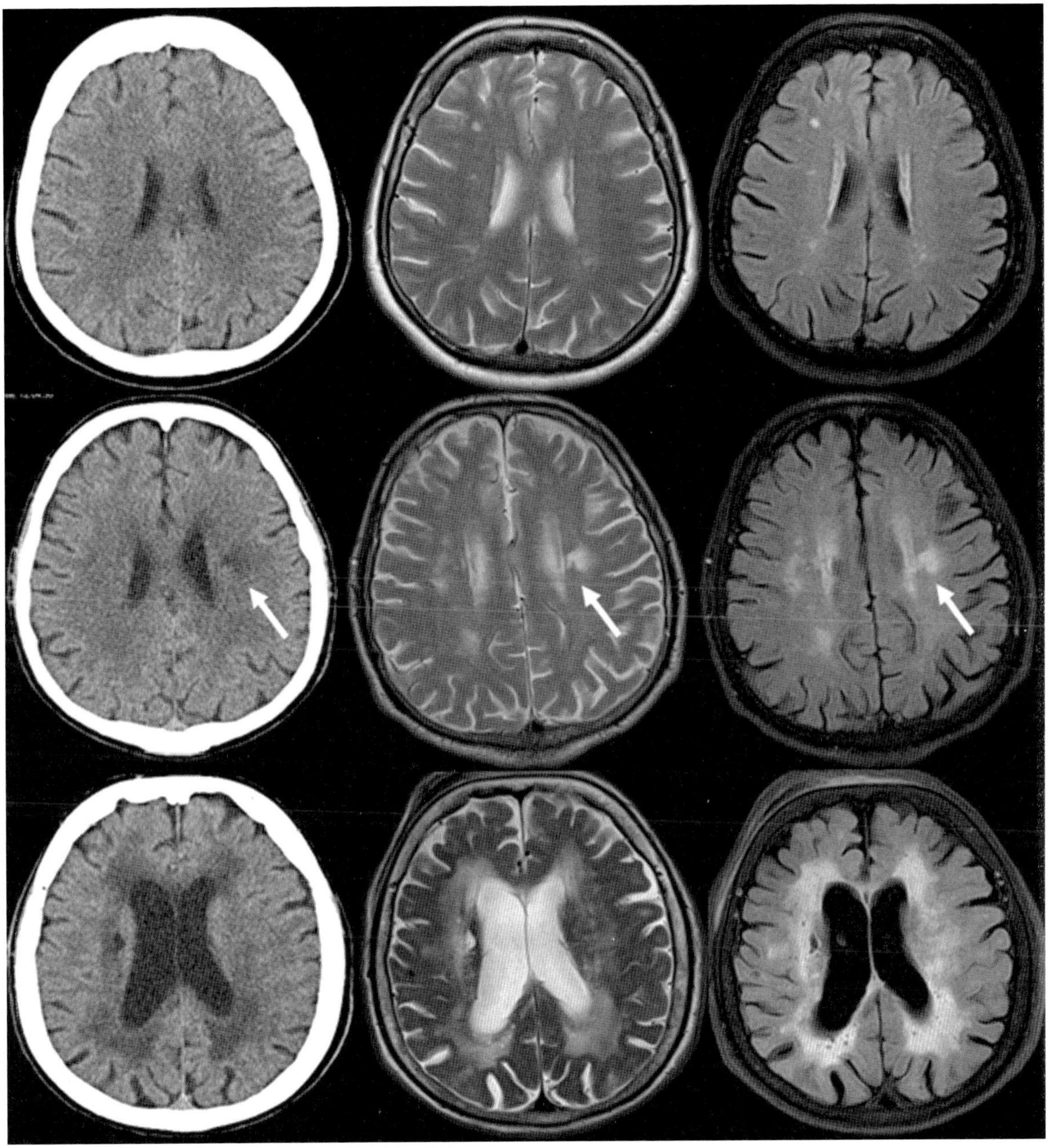

Figure 11.3 Different extents of deep white matter lesions (WMLs) (from left to right: computed tomography [CT]/T2-weighted magnetic resonance imaging/fluid-attenuated inversion recovery [MRI/FLAIR]). Punctate (upper panel) and early confluent WMLs (middle panel) are primarily seen on MRI but not CT except for an area of obviously more extensive tissue destruction in the left centrum semiovale next to an old lacune (arrow; middle panel). The lower panel shows confluent WMLs (and a paraventricular lacune).

passage of CSF [28, 29], and accumulation of interstitial fluid may also be responsible for the periventricular caps, while some kind of ischemic damage has been implicated in more extensive WMLs of the deep white matter [30, 31]. In line with these findings, most recent work on different types of periventricular WMLs seen in a large cohort of nondemented community-dwelling subjects supports the assumption that all kinds of periventricular signal hyperintensities are true abnormalities [32]. It also indicates that the

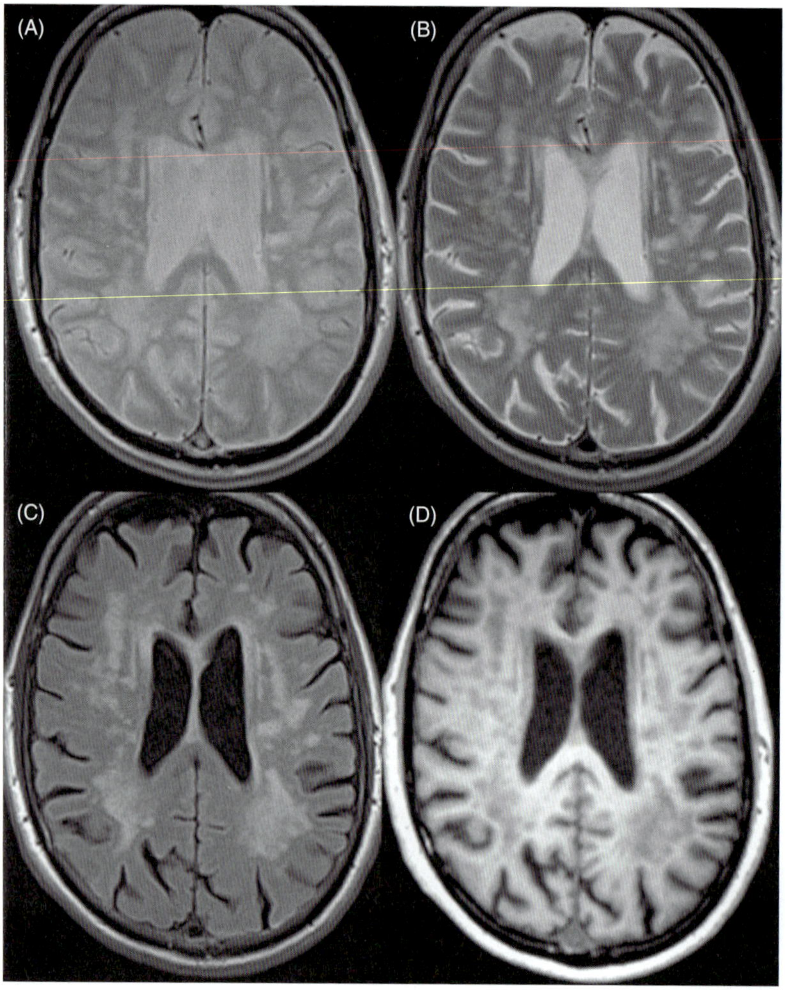

Figure 11.4 Confluent white matter lesions (WMLs) on different magnetic resonance imaging (MRI) sequences: (A) proton-density weighted; (B) T2-weighted; (C) fluid-attenuated inversion recovery (FLAIR); (D) T1-weighted. (Note that almost all WMLs are clearly seen as slightly hypointense lesions on this heavily T1-weighted image, which is different from their appearance on other T1-weighted scans – for example, Figure 11.3 – but have a signal intensity that is clearly higher than cerebrospinal fluid.)

prevalence of hypertension, hypercholesterolemia, and neuroradiologic evidence of stroke increases from individuals with a thin white line of periventricular hyperintensity over those with a thick hyperintense rim to subjects with periventricular hyperintensity penetrating towards or confluent with deep WMLs, which to some extent mirrors histopathologic findings. This work also confirms a quite close association between the extent of WMLs in the deep and periventricular white matter, which, however, does not necessarily exclude different pathologic mechanisms triggered by the same disorder.

Above described appearances of WMLs associated with SVD also help in the separation from other white matter changes. Strong emphasis in this regard has been given especially to the separation from MS [33–36]. In MS, lesions are usually much better circumscribed, rounded, or ovoid in appearance, and often quite focally border the lateral ventricles or the cortex with involvement of the subcortical white matter, i.e., they occur in a juxtacortical location. While SVD-related WMLs commonly spare the temporal white matter and the cerebellum, these are quite frequently involved in MS. Tissue destruction often is also much more prominent with MS lesions, which gives the appearance of so-called "black holes," than in SVD-related WMLs. Table 11.2 summarizes the differences in appearance between SVD-related WMLs and MS lesions.

Signal abnormalities related to SVD may not only occur in the hemispheric deep or periventricular white matter but may also be seen in the brainstem. As for supratentorial WMLs they appear rather ill defined, mostly involve the central portions of the brainstem, and are not associated with visible tissue destruction on T1-weighted images (Figure 11.7).

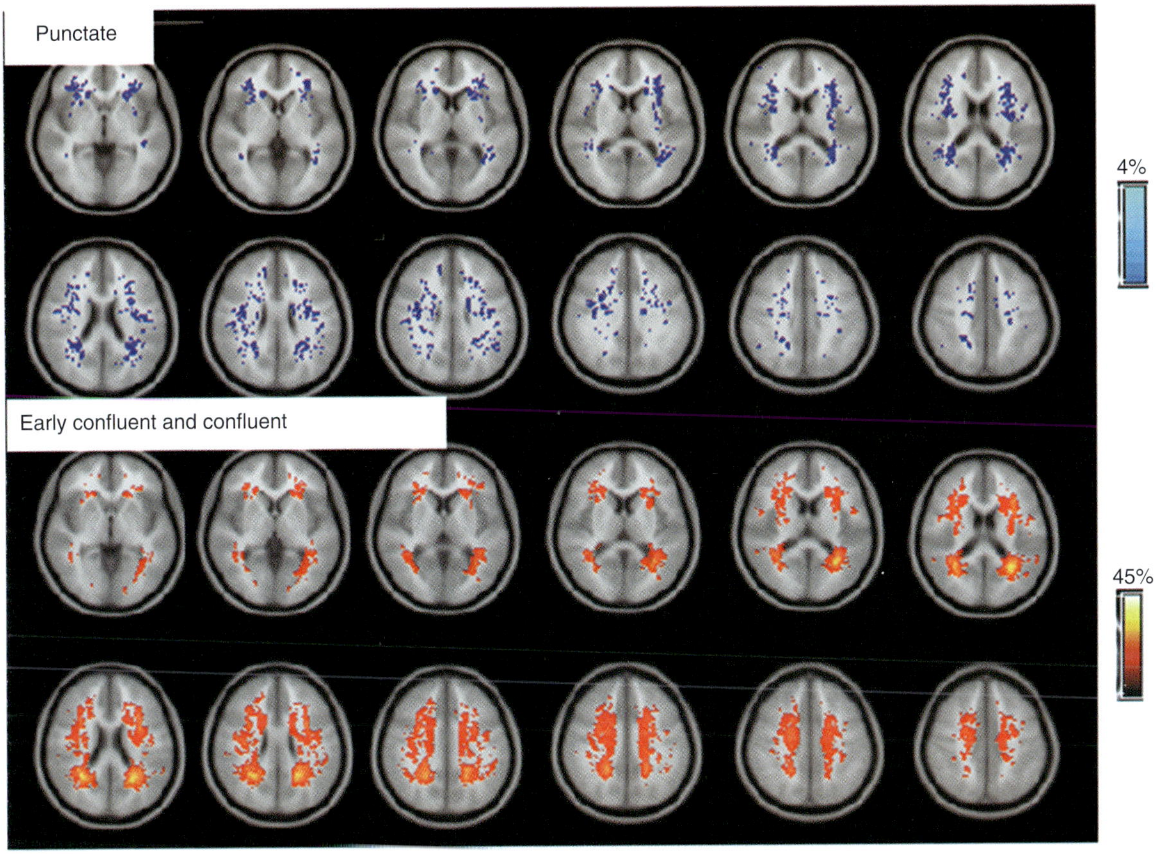

Figure 11.5 Lesion probability maps of white matter lesions (WMLs) indicate a quite similar distributional pattern for punctate and early confluent to confluent WMLs with a preference for the deep and periventricular white matter. From Enzinger et al. [20], reproduced with permission.

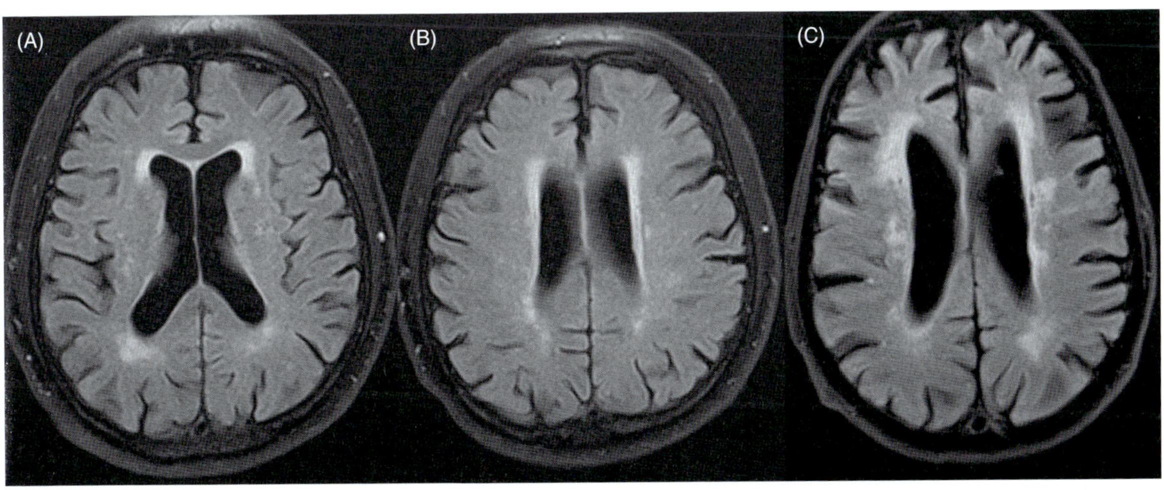

Figure 11.6 Fluid-attenuated inversion recovery (FLAIR) images show different types of periventricular white matter lesions. (A) Caps of signal hyperintensity around the frontal horns; (B) band-like periventricular signal hyperintensity; (C) focal/irregular periventricular lesions extending into the deep white matter.

Table 11.2 Comparison of imaging characteristics of SVD-related WMLs versus MS lesions

	SVD-related WMLs	MS lesions
Shape of lesions	Patchy	Ovoid (rounded)
Outer contour	Ill defined	Relatively clear margins
Typical lesion location	Deep white matter, spares temporal lobes (except for CADASIL) and cerebellum	Periventricular, juxtacortical, infratentorial
Lesion pattern	Rather symmetric	Random, asymmetric
Tissue destruction	No significant/visible tissue destruction	Variable, interspersed; "black holes" frequent
Contrast enhancement	None	Frequent

CADASIL, cerebral autosomal dominant arteriopathy with subcortical infarcts and leukoencephalopathy; MS, multiple sclerosis; SVD, small vessel disease; WMLs, white matter lesions.

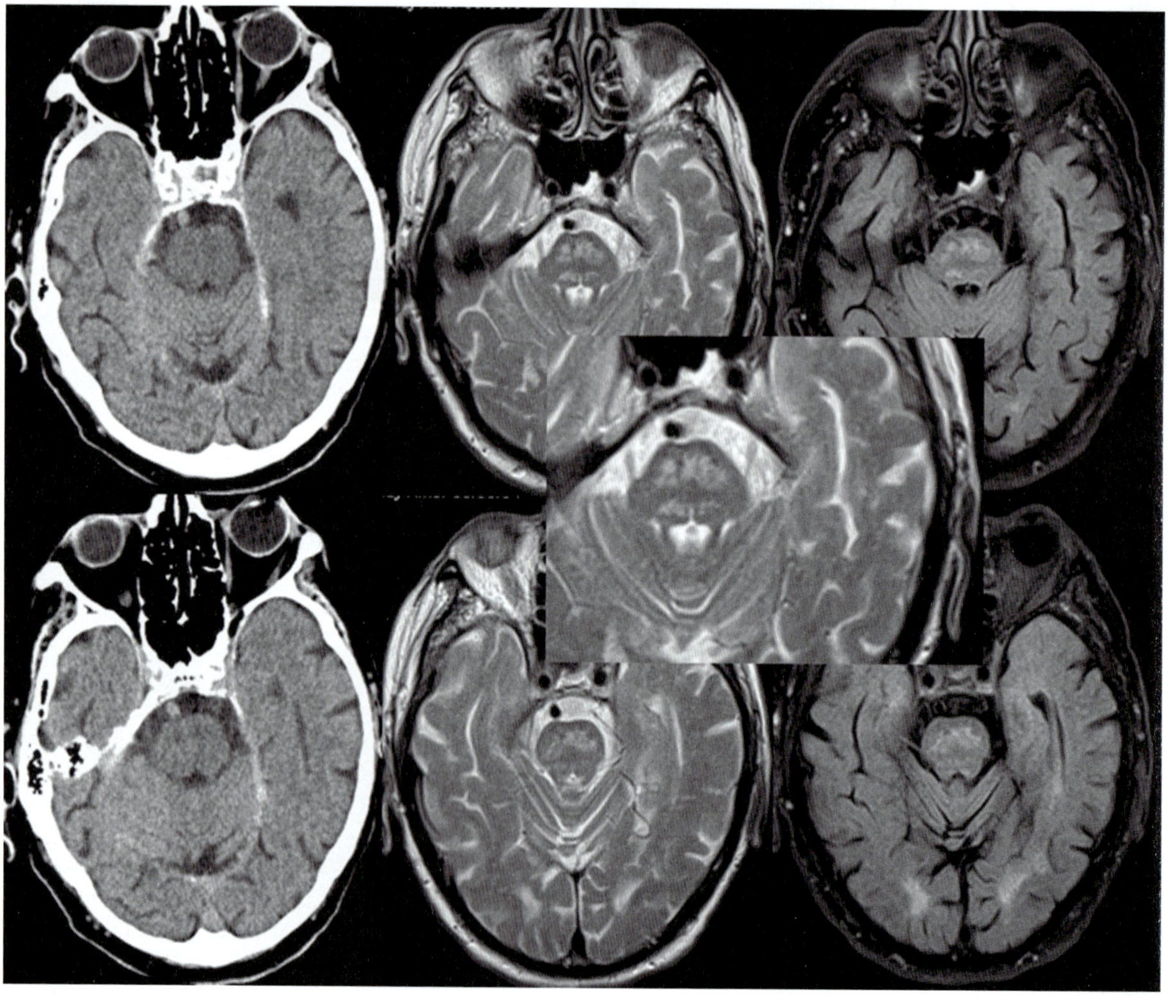

Figure 11.7 Patchy/irregular signal hyperintensity in the pons likely related to small vessel disease. Changes are not seen on computed tomography (CT).

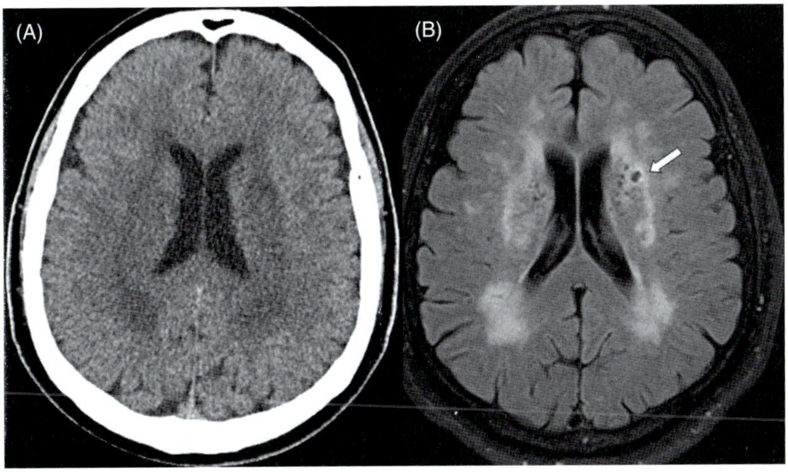

Figure 11.8 (A) Computed tomography (CT) hypodensity and (B) magnetic resonance imaging (MRI) hyperintensity on fluid-attenuated inversion recovery (FLAIR) in the deep and periventricular white matter and in the basal ganglia. (B) MRI also shows areas of cerebrospinal fluid signal intensity in the basal ganglia, probably corresponding to enlarged Virchow–Robin spaces and an old lacunar infarct (arrow).

Usually they are assumed to be associated with rather severe SVD [37]. Accordingly, they are often associated with more extensive deep or periventricular WMLs, but they may also prevail on their own. The reasons for the latter are unknown. The absence of associated specific neurologic or clinical findings facilitates the differential diagnosis from other disorders involving the brainstem besides described imaging characteristics.

Importantly, focal signal hyperintensities similar to – and possibly identical with – SVD-related WMLs also may be seen in the basal ganglia and thalami (Figure 11.8). There the separation from truly focal ischemic defects, i.e., residues of infarctions, is even more difficult than in the white matter. It has been argued that white matter tracts are also coursing through the basal ganglia and may undergo signal changes that justify the term WMLs. On the other hand, the extent to which such signal abnormalities will involve gray matter primarily, or in addition to white matter tracts, cannot be defined on conventional MRI, which suggests that hyperintense lesions in the deep gray matter should be assessed separately. Another option would be the use of a unifying term "subcortical hyperintensities" for both WMLs and signal hyperintensities in the basal ganglia and thalami.

Some specific small vessel disorders are associated with quite characteristic patterns of WML distribution that differ from those commonly seen. An example of this is cerebral autosomal dominant arteriopathy with subcortical infarcts and leukoencephalopathy (CADASIL) [38]. In this disorder, WMLs typically occur in the temporopolar region, the external capsule, and infratentorially (Figure 11.9). Likewise, other hereditary SVDs may also associate with specific lesion patterns [39].

Quantitation of WML burden

For investigational purposes, and also in the clinical context, it is necessary and desirable to obtain some measure of the total burden of SVD-related WMLs. Visual assessment on conventional imaging is a fast and relatively simple way. Thus, several rating scales have been developed, which provided different grades of refinement and, in part, also aimed to be applicable to both CT and MRI. Overall these scales demonstrated good inter-rater agreement and correlated sufficiently with the volume of white matter damage derived from fully quantitative measurements [40–42]. Nevertheless it became apparent that some of observed differences in the relation of WMLs with clinical findings and vascular risk factors were – at least in part – attributable to the employed scoring system rather than evidence for a true difference [43]. This and the nonlinearity of scoring systems are clearly in favor of true volumetric measurements. However, fully quantitative techniques also suffer from several pitfalls, including changes in signal intensity of the aging brain and of WMLs themselves [44]. Furthermore, mild increases in signal intensity appear to precede WML evolution, which attests to their commonly insidious development but also complicates the clear separation of abnormal from normal white matter [45, 46]. These problems usually become aggravated in a multicenter setting with the use of several MR scanners that cannot

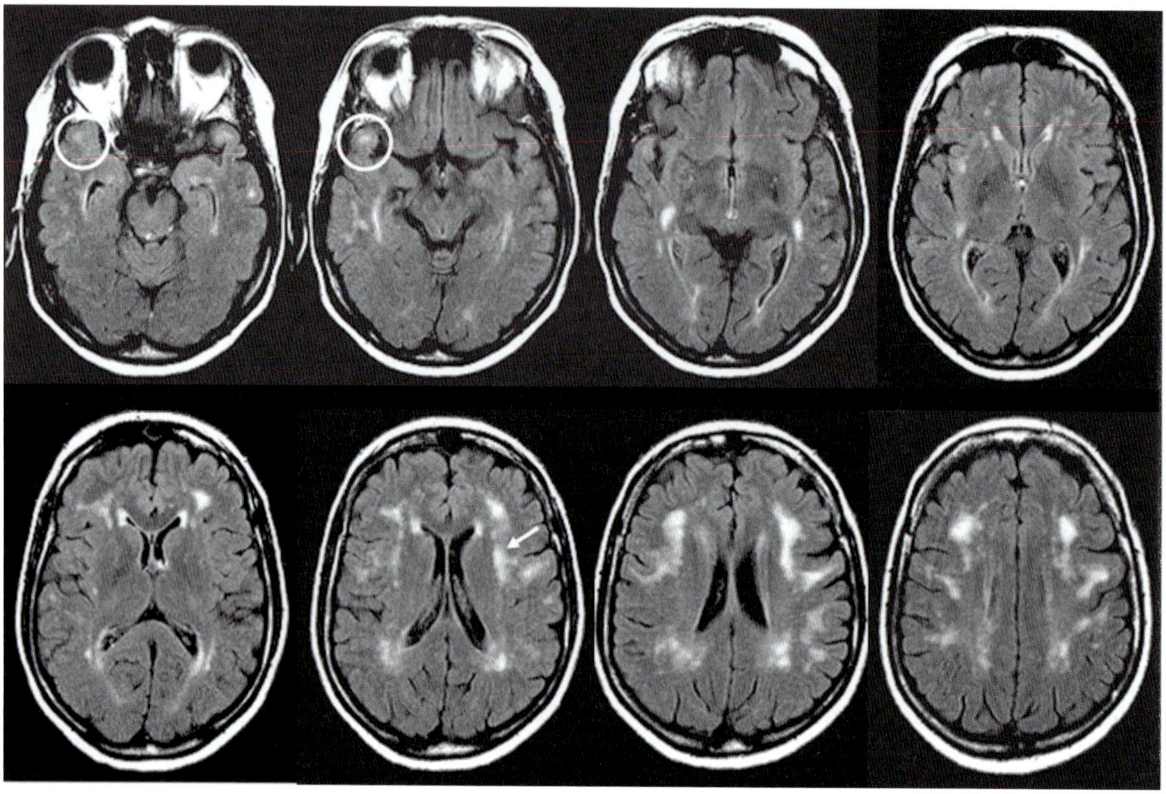

Figure 11.9 Pattern of white matter lesions (WMLs) suspicious for CADASIL. WMLs also involve the temporal pole (white rings) and the external capsule (arrow).

provide completely identical image sequences. It is reassuring, therefore, that studies have shown similar associations of WML burden with clinical findings irrespective of their assessment by scoring or in a volumetric manner [47]. Measuring progression of WML burden is yet a further challenge, as reviewed elsewhere [48].

Conclusions

Conventional brain imaging – especially with the advent of MRI – has served to identify WMLs as an important component of SVD-related brain damage. They appear as ill-defined hypodensities on CT and bright on T2-weighted MRI. WMLs range from punctate to confluent lesions in the deep white matter and can parallel the border of the lateral ventricles in a longitudinal manner. While the different appearances and extent of WMLs seen on conventional MRI give a quite good appreciation of the overall severity of white matter involvement, WMLs are nevertheless just the "tip of the iceberg" of white matter damage related to SVD as shown by nonconventional imaging [13, 49]. Furthermore the origin and etiology of a single WML often remains elusive despite the overall rather characteristic imaging appearance of SVD-related WMLs in general. Apart from differential diagnosis, CT has no further role in the scientific or even clinical evaluation for WMLs.

References

1. Roman GC. A historical review of the concept of vascular dementia: lessons from the past for the future. *Alzheimer Dis Assoc Disord* 1999;13(Suppl 3):S4–S8.

2. Olszewski J. Subcortical arteriosclerotic encephalopathy. Review of the literature on the so-called Binswanger's disease and presentation of two cases. *World Neurol* 1962;3: 359–375.

3. Loizou L, Kendall B, Marshall J. Subcortical arteriosclerotic encephalopathy: a clinical and radiological investigation. *J Neurol Neurosurg Psychiatry* 1981; 44:294–304.

4. Rosenberg GA, Kornfeld M, Stovring J, Bicknell JM. Subcortical arteriosclerotic encephalopathy (Binswanger): computerized tomography. *Neurology* 1979;29:1102–1106.
5. Zeumer H, Schonsky B, Sturm K. Predominant white matter involvement in subcortical arteriosclerotic encephalopathy (Binswanger disease). *J Comput Assist Tomogr* 1980;4:14–19.
6. Hachinski V, Potter P, Merskey H. Leuko-araiosis. *Arch Neurol* 1987;44:21–23.
7. Bradley W, Waluch V, Brant-Zawadzki M, Yadley R, Wycoff R. Patchy periventricular white matter lesions in the elderly: a common observation during NMR imaging. *Noninv Med Imag* 1984;1:35–41.
8. Awad I, Spetzler R, Hodak J, Awad C, Carey R. Incidental subcortical lesions identified on magnetic resonance imaging in the elderly. I. Correlation with age and cerebrovascular risk factors. *Stroke* 1986;17:1084–1089
9. Gouw AA, Seewann A, van der Flier WM, et al. Heterogeneity of small vessel disease: a systematic review of MRI and histopathology correlations. *J Neurol Neurosurg Psychiatry* 2011;82:126–135.
10. Schmidt R, Schmidt H, Haybaeck J, et al. Heterogeneity in age-related white matter changes. *Acta Neuropathol* 2011;122:171–185.
11. Fazekas F, Barkhof F, Filippi M, et al. The contribution of magnetic resonance imaging to the diagnosis of multiple sclerosis. *Neurology* 1999;53:448–456.
12. Polman CH, Reingold SC, Banwell B, et al. Diagnostic criteria for multiple sclerosis: 2010 revisions to the McDonald criteria. *Ann Neurol* 69:292–302.
13. Ropele S, Seewann A, Gouw AA, et al. Quantitation of brain tissue changes associated with white matter hyperintensities by diffusion-weighted and magnetization transfer imaging: the LADIS (Leukoaraiosis And DISability in the elderly) study. *J Magn Reson Imaging* 2009;29:268–274.
14. Janota I, Mirsen T, Hachinski V, Lee D, Merskey H. Neuropathologic correlates of leuko-araiosis. *Arch Neurol* 1989;46:1124–1128.
15. Brun A, Englund E. A white matter disorder in dementia of the Alzheimer type: a pathoanatomical study. *Ann Neurol* 1986;19:253–262.
16. Steingart A, Hachinski V, Lau C, et al. Cognitive and neurological findings in subjects with diffuse white matter lucencies on computed tomographic scan (leuko-araiosis). *Arch Neurol* 1987;44:32–33.
17. Kertesz A, Black S, Tokar G, et al. Periventricular and subcortical hyperintensities on magnetic resonance imaging. “Rims, caps, and unidentified bright objects.” *Arch Neurol* 1988;45:404–408.
18. Truyen L, van Waesberghe JH, van Walderveen MA, et al. Accumulation of hypointense lesions (“black holes”) on T1 spin-echo MRI correlates with disease progression in multiple sclerosis. *Neurology* 1996;47:1469–1476.
19. Fazekas F, Ropele S, Enzinger C, et al. MTI of white matter hyperintensities. *Brain* 2005;128:2926–2932.
20. Enzinger C, Smith S, Fazekas F, et al. Lesion probability maps of white matter hyperintensities in elderly individuals: results of the Austrian Stroke Prevention Study. *J Neurol* 2006;253:1064–1070.
21. Brant-Zawadzki M, Fein G, Van Dyke C, et al. MR imaging of the aging brain: patchy white-matter lesions and dementia. *AJNR Am J Neuroradiol* 1985;6:675–682.
22. Fazekas F, Chawluk J, Alavi A, Hurtig H, Zimmerman R. MRI signal abnormalities at 1.5 T in Alzheimer’s dementia and normal aging. *AJNR Am J Neuroradiol* 1987;8:421–426.
23. Zimmerman RD, Fleming C, Lee B, Saint-Louis L, Deck M. Periventricular hyperintensity as seen by magnetic resonance: prevalence and significance. *AJNR Am J Neuroradiol* 1986;7:13–20.
24. Fazekas F, Kapeller P, Schmidt R, et al. The relation of cerebral magnetic resonance signal hyperintensities to Alzheimer’s disease. *J Neurol Sci* 1996;142:121–125.
25. Sze G, De Armond S, Brant-Zawadzki M, et al. Foci of MRI signal (pseudo lesions) anterior to the frontal horns: histologic correlations of a normal finding. *AJNR Am J Neuroradiol* 1986;17:381–387.
26. DeCarli C, Fletcher E, Ramey V, Harvey D, Jagust WJ. Anatomical mapping of white matter hyperintensities (WMH): exploring the relationships between periventricular WMH, deep WMH, and total WMH burden. *Stroke* 2005;36:50–55.
27. Sachdev P, Wen W. Should we distinguish between periventricular and deep white matter hyperintensities? *Stroke* 2005;36:2342–2343; author reply 2343–2344.
28. Fazekas F, Kleinert R, Offenbacher H, et al. Pathologic correlates of incidental MRI white matter signal hyperintensities. *Neurology* 1993;43:1683–1689.
29. Scheltens P, Barkhof F, Leys D, et al. Histopathologic correlates of white matter changes on MRI in Alzheimer’s disease and normal aging. *Neurol* 1995;45:883–888.
30. Marshall V, Bradley WJ, Marshall C, Bhoopat T, Rhodes R. Deep white matter infarction: correlation of MR imaging and histopathologic findings. *Radiology* 1988;167:517–522.

31. Braffman B, Zimmerman R, Trojanowski J, et al. Brain MR: pathologic correlation with gross and histopathology. 2. Hyperintense-white matter foci in the elderly. *AJNR Am J Neuroradiol* 1988;9:629–636.

32. Wardlaw J. Morphological, distributional, volumetric and intensity characterisation of periventricular hyperintensities. *AJNR Am J Neuroradiol* 2013, Dec 12 [Epub ahead of print].

33. Paty DW, Kastrukoff LF, Hashimoto SA, et al. MRI in the diagnosis of MS: a prospective study with comparison of clinical evaluation, evoked potentials, oligoclonal banding, and CT. *Neurology* 1988;38:180–185.

34. Fazekas F, Offenbacher H, Fuchs S, et al. Criteria for an increased specificity of MRI interpretation in elderly subjects with suspected multiple sclerosis. *Neurology* 1988;38:1822–1825.

35. Offenbacher H, Fazekas F, Schmidt R, et al. Assessment of MRI criteria for a diagnosis of MS. *Neurology* 1993;43: 905–909.

36. Barkhof F, Filippi M, Miller D, et al. Comparison of MRI criteria at first presentation to predict conversion to clinically definite multiple sclerosis. *Brain* 1997;120:2059–2069.

37. Pullicino P, Ostrow P, Miller L, Snyder W, Munschauer F. Pontine ischemic rarefaction. *Ann Neurol* 1995;37:460–466.

38. Auer DP, Putz B, Gossl C, et al. Differential lesion patterns in CADASIL and sporadic subcortical arteriosclerotic encephalopathy: MR imaging study with statistical parametric group comparison. *Radiology* 2001;218:443–451.

39. Ding XQ, Hagel C, Ringelstein EB, et al. MRI features of pontine autosomal dominant microangiopathy and leukoencephalopathy (PADMAL). *J Neuroimaging* 2010;20:134–140.

40. Kapeller P, Barber R, Vermeulen RJ, et al. Visual rating of age-related white matter changes on magnetic resonance imaging: scale comparison, interrater agreement, and correlations with quantitative measurements. *Stroke* 2003;34:441–445.

41. Van Straaten EC, Fazekas F, Rostrup E, et al. Impact of white matter hyperintensities scoring method on correlations with clinical data: the LADIS study. *Stroke* 2006;37:836–840.

42. Valdes Hernandez Mdel C, Morris Z, Dickie DA, et al. Close correlation between quantitative and qualitative assessments of white matter lesions. *Neuroepidemiology* 2013;40: 13–22.

43. Mäntylä R, Erkinjuntti T, Salonen O, et al. Variable agreement between visual rating scales for white matter hyperintensities on MRI. Comparison of 13 rating scales in a poststroke cohort. *Stroke* 1997;28:1614–1623.

44. Olsson E, Klasson N, Berge J, et al. White matter lesion assessment in patients with cognitive impairment and healthy controls: reliability comparisons between visual rating, a manual, and an automatic volumetrical MRI method – the Gothenburg MCI study. *J Aging Res* 2013 (2013):198471.

45. De Groot M, Verhaaren BF, de Boer R, et al. Changes in normal-appearing white matter precede development of white matter lesions. *Stroke* 2013;44:1037–1042.

46. Fazekas F, Wardlaw JM. The origin of white matter lesions: a further piece to the puzzle. *Stroke* 2013;44:951–952.

47. Inzitari D, Pracucci G, Poggesi A, et al. Changes in white matter as determinant of global functional decline in older independent outpatients: three year follow-up of LADIS (Leukoaraiosis And DISability) study cohort. *BMJ* 2009;339:2477.

48. Schmidt R, Petrovic K, Ropele S, Enzinger C, Fazekas F. Progression of leukoaraiosis and cognition. *Stroke* 2007;38:2619–2625.

49. Vernooij MW, Ikram MA, Vrooman HA, et al. White matter microstructural integrity and cognitive function in a general elderly population. *Arch Gen Psychiatry* 2009;66:545–553.

Chapter 12

Conventional imaging of lacunar infarcts

Eric Jouvent and Hugues Chabriat

Introduction

Lacunar infarcts represent one of the most important magnetic resonance imaging (MRI) markers of small vessel disease (SVD) of the brain. Yet, their definition remains highly variable among neurologists, even among those who are highly specialized in cerebrovascular disorders [1]. The term "lacunar infarct" may stand for an acute small deep brain infarct, be it or not, revealed by a stroke, or describe a small cavity in deep brain areas observed remote from an acute symptomatic ischemic event. A lacunar infarct may also be discovered by chance on brain imaging in a patient who never experienced stroke symptoms [2].

This ambiguous terminology originates in the nineteenth century. The term *lacune* ("hole" in Latin) was first used by French neurologists in the initial part of the nineteenth century, Dechambre [3] and Durand-Fardel [4], who described small cavities within the brain parenchyma on pathologic examination. These lesions were afterwards attributed to ischemia [5]. More than one century later, in his seminal work reported in the 1960s, C. Miller Fisher proposed the "lacunar hypothesis" [6]. Lesions of the vascular wall, distinct from classical atheroma, would be responsible for specific alterations of small vessels within the brain that can potentially lead to the occlusion of a single long perforating artery. Thus, a small deep infarct occurs and is revealed by one of the different lacunar syndromes described during the same period [7, 8]. Years later, with the development of computed tomography (CT) scans and the advent of MRI, lacunar infarcts are routinely detected on brain MRI, even in patients who never experienced a stroke.

Recent imaging studies allowed refining these initial concepts and terminology to which we refer in this chapter. The occlusion of a single long perforator can lead to the occurrence of an acute small deep infarct inconsistently associated with clinical manifestations depending on whether the lesion lies in a "symptomatic" pathway (motor, sensory, etc.) or not. Eventually, the lesion evolves progressively leading to the formation of a cavity, the lacunar infarct per se, which may be discovered by chance on brain imaging in the absence of clinical manifestations (silent lacunar infarct). We will avoid, when possible, the use of the term "lacunar syndrome" in this chapter because it lacks specificity as it can be revealed by cortical infarcts [9] or even brain hemorrhages [10]. In our opinion, this term also has the disadvantage of mixing clinical, radiologic, and pathologic concepts.

The identification of small ischemic lesions with brain imaging is necessarily a challenging task. Both the imaging modality (CT scan or MRI) and within a single modality itself, the parameters used (type of acquisition, type of contrast, slice thickness, etc.) can impact the potential to identify acute small deep infarcts or lacunar infarcts. The differential diagnosis of lacunar infarcts with other cavities located inside the cerebral parenchyma represents another major issue, particularly their differentiation from dilated perivascular spaces (i.e., Virchow–Robin spaces).

In this chapter, the diagnosis of acute small deep infarcts and lacunar infarcts, silent or not, using conventional imaging is reviewed. Importantly, adequate imaging techniques play a key role in the diagnosis and the longitudinal study of such lesions.

Conventional imaging of acute small deep infarcts

Imaging of acute small deep infarcts (ASDIs) has been studied using both MRI and CT scan.

Cerebral Small Vessel Disease, ed. Leonardo Pantoni and Philip B. Gorelick. Published by Cambridge University Press.

On CT scan, ASDIs, when visible, appear as punctuate areas of low attenuation. The sensitivity of CT scan to ASDIs is low, particularly in the first hours, and when they are located in the posterior fossa [11]. The first studies performed in the 1980s using CT scan showed that lesions were detectable within 10 days of clinical symptom onset in up to 55% of ASDIs [12]. In a study of 37 patients presenting with classical lacunar syndromes, repeated CT scans allowed the detection of ASDIs in 18 patients (49%), while CT scan was normal in 13 (35%), and large-sized strokes were observed in six others [13]. Other studies of pure motor stroke found higher detection rates [14]. It is important to note that these detection rates were probably overestimated as only strokes revealed by classical lacunar syndrome, described by Fisher and suggestive of hemispheric lesions, were included in those studies, restricting the potential risk to miss the smallest lesions, particularly in posterior fossa [15]. Finally, CT scanning does not allow differentiating lesions according to their age, unless exams are repeated and show a lesion for which absence on previous exams allows one to precisely date its occurrence [13].

Thereafter, MRI proved to be of higher sensitivity. The assessment of 31 patients with strokes suggestive of ASDIs using both MRI (before the advent of diffusion imaging) and CT scan showed that ASDIs could be detected in 23 of 31 cases (74%) using MRI, compared to 4 of 26 cases (15%) using CT scan. None of the 10 patients imaged within 5 days after stroke onset had visible recent lesions on CT scan, versus 7 of 12 (58%) on MRI [16]. Subsequent studies showed the diagnostic value of different MRI sequences for the detection of ASDIs with T2-weighted sequences appearing superior to T1-weighted ones. In a series of 22 patients with stroke suggestive of ASDIs, T1-weighted sequence was positive in 42% of cases, close to CT scan results (35%), while T2-weighted sequence detected an ASDI in 98% of cases [17]. This detection rate for T2-weighted sequences now appears over optimistic. This may be due to the inclusion of patients with classical lacunar syndromes only, suggestive of hemispheric rather than smaller posterior fossa lesions, or to the detection of older lesions not responsible for the actual acute symptoms. In general, T2-weighted imaging was indeed shown inferior to diffusion-weighted imaging (DWI) sequences for the detection of acute stroke [18]. A recent study comparing MRI with DWI and CT scan in the acute phase of stroke showed a sensitivity of MRI of 83% for acute ischemic stroke versus 16% for CT scan, and a specificity of 96% for MRI and 98% for CT scan. Details were not given, however, according to stroke subtypes in this study [19].

On MRI, ASDIs appear as hyperintense lesions on DWI sequences together with restricted diffusion on apparent diffusion coefficient (ADC) maps. In the first few hours, ASDIs may be only visible on DWI and absent on T2 or fluid-attenuated inversion recovery (FLAIR) sequences, as it has been reported for acute stroke in general [18]. Later, ASDIs will be visible as an hyperintense lesion on DWI, T2, and FLAIR sequences for several days [20]. The hyperintense aspect on DWI usually disappears within 14 days [21]. When several lesions are visible on T2 or FLAIR imaging, the hyperintensity on DWI together with the area of restricted diffusion on ADC maps allow differentiation of acute from older lesions [22]. The association of clinical symptoms and typical MRI image findings is nearly specific for a lesion of ischemic origin, but some exceptions exist. Indeed, acute inflammatory lesions may on occasion appear as DWI hyperintense lesions with restricted ADC, mimicking ASDIs [23]. Despite the obvious advantages of MRI over CT scan for the detection of small ischemic lesions, some authors reported high rates of DWI-negative ASDIs; up to 20% in the context of minor strokes [24]. These results remain difficult to interpret, however, in the absence of other means of diagnosis for minor strokes when conventional MRI is normal at baseline and remains normal at follow-up, even in cases in which there is high clinical confidence for the diagnosis of stroke. With the common use of MRI in the context of SVD, ASDIs not associated with a stroke are now reported in various circumstances. For example, ASDIs were observed remote to an acute brain hemorrhage in 15 of 114 patients in a recent study [25]. Further studies are needed to better understand the mechanisms and consequences of ASDIs when discovered by chance on MRI.

Several additional points about MRI in the setting of ASDIs are worth discussing. For example, the effect of magnetic field strength on the detection of ASDIs has not been assessed thus far. This is a challenging issue as already reported for all types of acute stroke. Indeed, DWI reported on 3 Tesla may be less sensitive than on 1.5 Tesla for identification of acute ischemic lesions in the context of stroke [26]. Also, optimal MRI parameters remain to be determined.

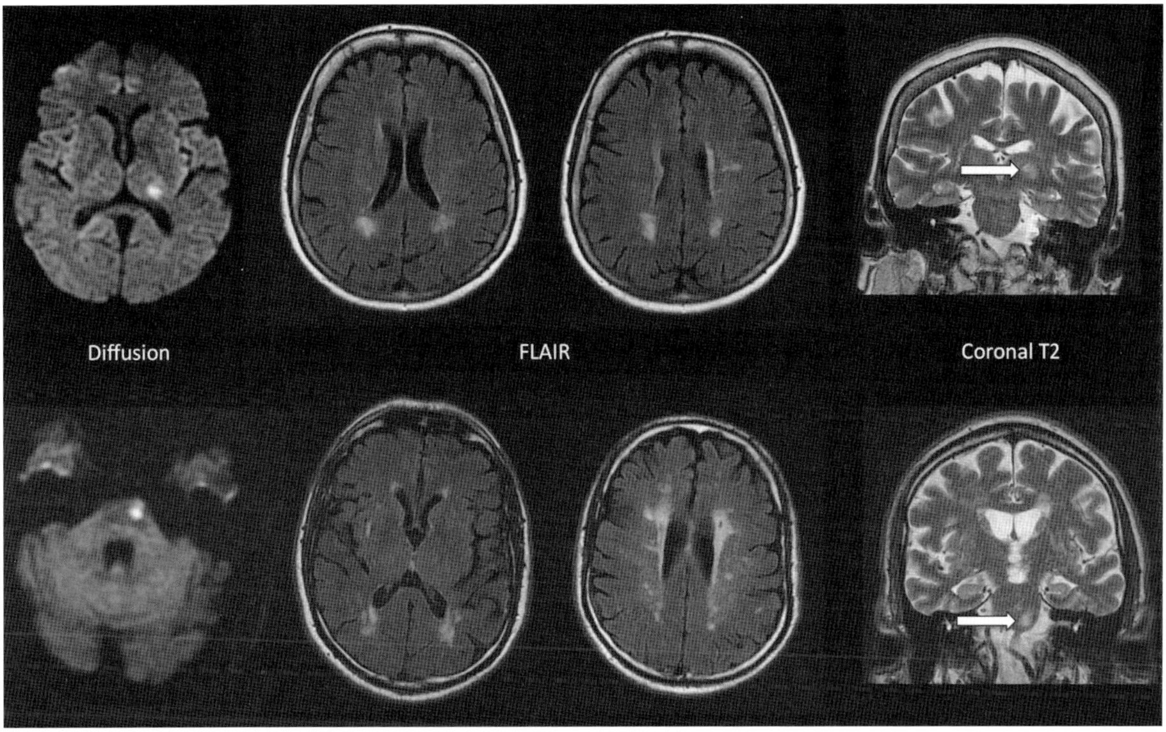

Figure 12.1 Examples of acute small deep infarcts in the context of small vessel disease in two individuals. Top row: small deep infarct affecting the left thalamus, accompanied by an acute sensory loss of right side of the body, in a 69-year-old hypertensive woman. Note the size of the lesion, less than 15 mm in both axial and coronal planes, as well as the associated signs of small vessel disease on fluid-attenuated inversion recovery (FLAIR) sequences. Bottom row: acute small deep infarct in the pons accompanied by acute right hemiplegia and left peripheral facial palsy in a 64-year-old hypertensive individual. Here again, note the size of the lesion in both axial and coronal planes, as well as the signs of small vessel disease on FLAIR sequence. From Jouvent et al. [30], reproduced with permission.

Particularly, the minimal detectable lesion size largely depends on the slice thickness (usually 5 mm) and on the intraslice resolution, but to our knowledge, no specific study has focused primarily on this subject thus far.

The identification of ASDIs on brain MRI requires differentiation of other types of ischemic lesions that can mimic their appearance. Size is the main criterion used to distinguish ASDIs from more proximal sources of ischemia. According to Fisher, the maximal size of an ischemic lesion due to the occlusion of a single perforating artery should be 15 mm [27]. Using this threshold criterion will probably exclude actual ASDIs, as shown in a recent study [28]. When taking into account the swelling observed in the acute phase, a threshold of 20 mm appears more reliable. This threshold should be taken into account both in the axial and coronal planes to exclude capsule–lenticular infarcts [29, 30] (Figures 12.1 and 12.2).

After the occurrence of ASDIs, the lesions begin to cavitate, leading to a lacunar infarct per se [31]. The exact timing and extent of cavitation after the occurrence of ASDIs remain incompletely understood (Figure 12.3). Among 55 patients with an ASDI confirmed by MRI, 25% of lesions had cavitated after 30 days on FLAIR and T2 sequences, compared to 53% on T1 sequence. After 90 days, cavitation was observed in 76% of cases on FLAIR, 80% on T2, and 94% on T1 [31]. Similar results were obtained in a two-year follow-up study [32]. The detection of such a cavity is strongly related to the imaging modality itself, i.e., the use of high-resolution three-dimensional (3D)-T1 acquisitions. Indeed, high-resolution 3D acquisitions can provide high resolution and contrast together with the possibility to reformat all images in any plane, which is needed to detect small cavitated lesions and to evaluate precisely the shape of lesions (Figure 12.4). The lesions that do not cavitate may take part in the formation of white matter

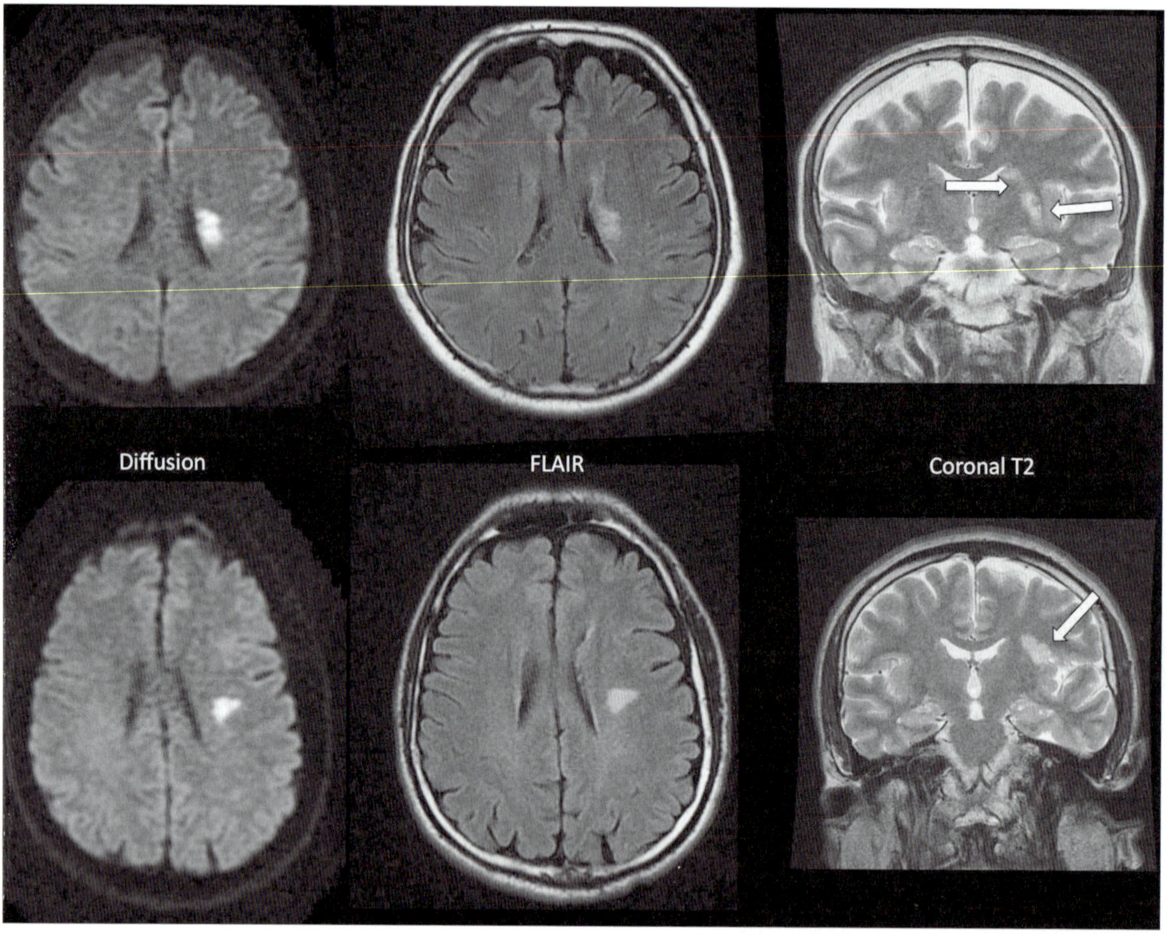

Figure 12.2 Mimics of small deep infarcts. Top row: acute deep ischemic stroke presenting as a right hemiparesis in a 57-year-old non-hypertensive individual. Note the size of the lesion, about 15 mm on diffusion in the axial plane, but which exceeds this size on coronal T2 sequences, corresponding to disease of the proximal lenticulostriate arteries. Also note the absence of markers of small vessel disease (SVD) on fluid-attenuated inversion recovery (FLAIR) sequence. Bottom row: acute deep ischemic stroke presenting as a right upper arm paresis in a 61-year-old nonhypertensive individual. Note that the lesion, potentially related to SVD, in fact corresponds to proximal occlusion of a penetrating artery on T2 coronal sequence. Also, note the absence of SVD markers on FLAIR sequence. From Jouvent et al. [30], reproduced with permission.

hyperintensities on T2/FLAIR sequences. Some authors report a very low degree of cavitation, and ASDIs become white matter hyperintensities in up to four of five cases [33]. However, in this study, the follow-up interval was short and used both CT scan and MRI as imaging modalities. These results should be interpreted with caution. It is also important to note that when cavitation is not present initially, up to 9% of ASDIs may disappear on follow-up MRI depending on the imaging protocol used, particularly if 3D-T1 millimetric acquisitions are not routinely performed [32]. When located in "silent areas," the cavity can be detected on CT or MRI. The detection of such cavities on imaging in patients who have never experienced stroke has led to the concept of silent lacunar infarcts [34].

Conventional imaging of silent lacunar infarcts

Silent infarcts were reported in early studies using CT scan [35]. Criteria used to define silent infarcts in CT-scan studies were rarely detailed and appear very vague. For example, in the Asymptomatic Carotid Artery Study, a randomized control trial comparing medical treatment and surgery (carotid

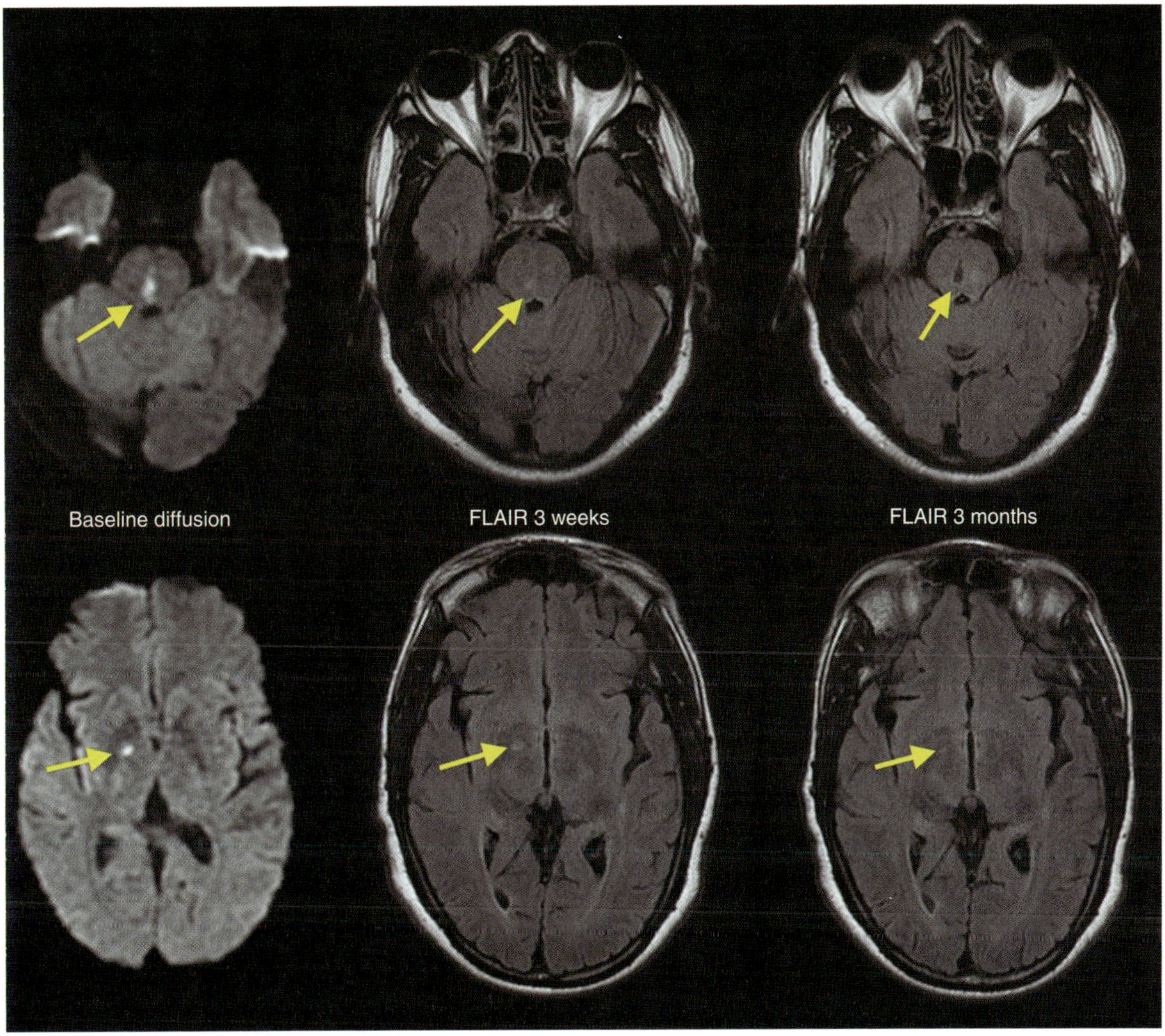

Figure 12.3 Illustration of the cavitation process in two cases of acute small deep infarcts (ASDIs). Top row: ASDI in the pons revealed by isolated ophthalmoplegia. Note that cavitation occurs between three weeks and three months in this case. Bottom row: ASDIs not presenting as a stroke. Note the absence of cavitation and near-complete disappearance of the lesion on follow-up scans.

endarterectomy) versus medical treatment alone in high-grade asymptomatic carotid artery stenosis, silent infarcts were defined as "any circumscribed area of low attenuation consistent with cerebral infarction" [36]. Generally, the detection of silent brain infarcts in those studies mostly relied on radiologic identification [37]. There was no set of criteria at this stage to differentiate silent lacunar infarcts from the other types of infarcts, or to differentiate ischemic cavitated lesions from the other types of cavities [38].

With the advent of MRI, the detection of silent lacunar infarcts became a diagnostic challenge. Different criteria were proposed to capture the main MRI features of lacunar infarcts, among which signal intensity and size were the most strongly investigated. The MRI criteria used for the definition of silent lacunar infarcts on a signal basis are highly variable. These lesions are defined as hyperintense T2 and hypointense T1 lesions in some studies [39, 40]; as lesions with cerebrospinal fluid (CSF) signal on all sequences in others [41, 42]; or sometimes with distinct definitions for lesions in gray or in white matter [43–45]. The size limit appears less the subject of debate in the literature. Three millimeters is most

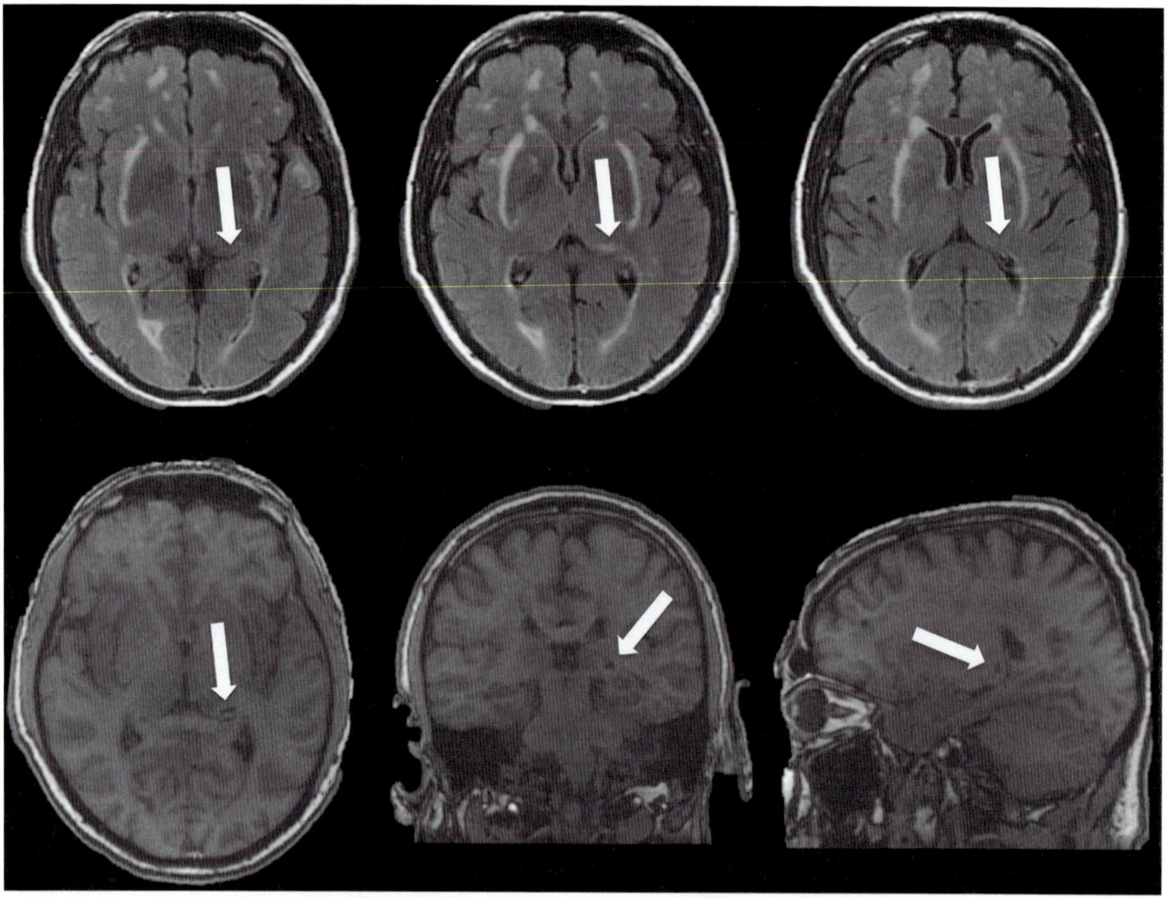

Figure 12.4 Impact of sequence type on identification of cavitation. Top row: consecutive axial slices, fluid-attenuated inversion recovery (FLAIR) sequence, slice thickness 5.5 mm; hyperintense lesion in the posterior part of the left thalamus, only visible on the middle slice. Bottom row: corresponding axial, coronal, and sagittal T1 slices from three-dimensional T1-millimetric acquisitions showing a small cavity at the exact corresponding location of the hyperintense lesion on FLAIR sequence.

often recognized as the minimal size of lacunar infarcts, although some authors chose 5 mm as the minimal diameter [46, 47]. The vast majority of authors adopted the 15-mm limit proposed by Fisher for the maximal diameter of the lesion [47]. It remains unclear whether the lower limit of 3 mm is linked to pathologic data or if it just represents the minimally detectable lesion size on conventional MRI. The second hypothesis seems more probable in light of recent works that emphasize the potential importance of smaller lacunar infarcts, not detectable on conventional MRI [48, 49]. Recent studies have shown that the cavitation process, demonstrated by a CSF-like appearance of the lesion on all sequences, is probably the best hint to identify a lacunar infarct [31] (see above). By contrast, a threshold for size may not allow a correct discrimination between lacunar infarcts and perivascular spaces [47]. For this purpose, more elaborate methods to reconstruct the 3D shape of lacunar infarcts may be helpful in the future [50, 51].

Globally, silent brain infarcts are observed in one quarter of individuals 65 years of age or older in the general population, with a linear increase of their frequency with age, from 5% by around 65 years up to 40% by around 85 years [52]. Most studies have not excluded lesions of more than 15 mm or those lying in cortical–subcortical areas. This probably leads to an overestimation by about 15% of the number of silent lacunar infarcts [44, 45]. On the other hand, it has been shown that some true lacunar infarcts do not evolve toward cavitation and remain undistinguishable from white matter lesions [28]. Despite the high heterogeneity in these different studies, reported prevalence of silent infarcts seems comparable between studies, suggesting that the different sources of variability roughly cancel out one another [47].

Differentiation of silent lacunar infarcts from other types of cavities within the brain

When penetrating through the brain, arteries and arterioles are accompanied to a various extent by meningeal layers filled with CSF, called Virchow–Robin or perivascular spaces. Most of these spaces are not visible on imaging, except the largest ones, frequently called dilated or enlarged Virchow–Robin spaces (dVRS). When large, the dVRS may mimic lacunar infarcts, particularly when they are observed on axial imaging slices. As dVRS are thought not to have clinical pertinence, the differentiation of dVRS from lacunar infarcts is of importance.

The first correlative studies between postmortem MRI and neuropathology showed a high frequency of dVRS and emphasized their relationships with lacunar lesions, as well as the limitations of CT scanning for differentiation of these imaging findings [53]. During the same time period, some authors reported symptoms attributed to lacunar infarcts [54], which were in fact probably dVRS, as revealed by MRI [55]. Actually, when dilated, distinction between lacunar infarcts and perivascular spaces may be difficult [47]. In many studies, size is used as the main diagnostic criterion to distinguish lacunar lesions (cavities of more than 3 mm in diameter) from dVRS (those of 3 mm or less) [47]. Although helpful, the threshold of 3 mm may be inadequate since dVRS of diameter greater than 3 mm are not uncommon, and lacunar infarcts of diameter less than 3 mm may occur [48, 56]. In a recent population-based study, a prevalence of 33.2% of large dVRS (>3 mm) was reported using 3D-T1 millimetric imaging in 1818 elderly subjects aged between 65 and 80 years [57]. Additionally, small infarcts of less than 3 mm in diameter do exist but are difficult to identify on conventional MRI due to insufficient resolution and the need for refined techniques for diagnosis [49]. Location has also been used as a differentiation criterion (presence of dVRS along perforating or medullary arteries or in the lower third of the basal ganglia) [47]. Various authors have stressed the

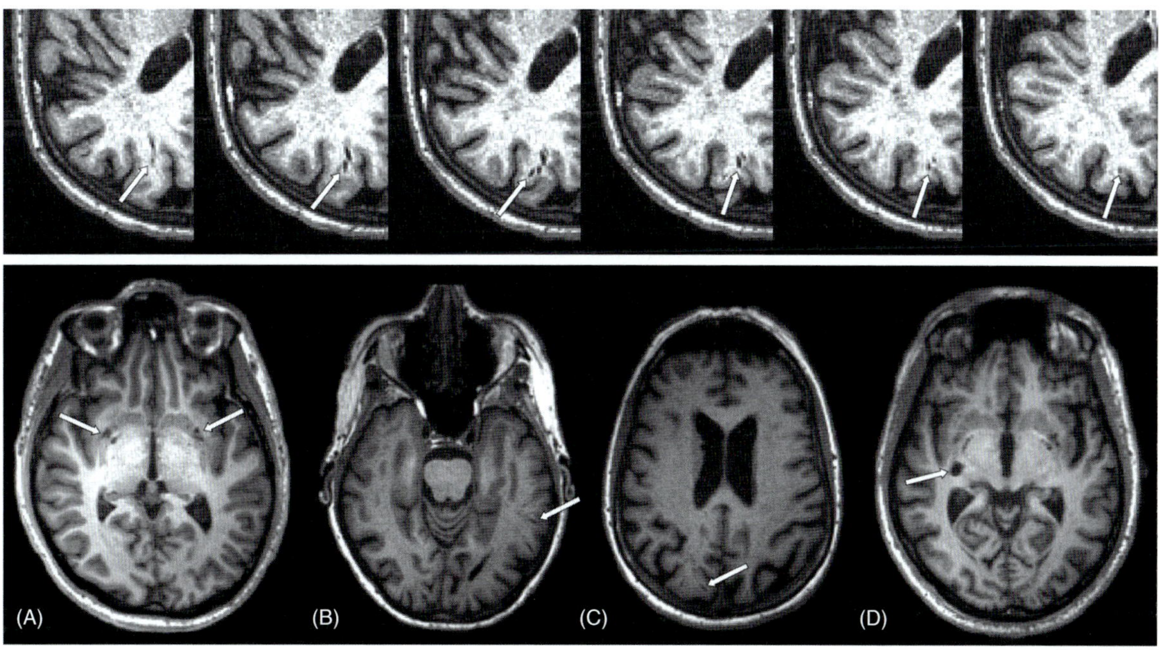

Figure 12.5 High-resolution magnetic resonance imaging of dilated perivascular spaces. Top row: contiguous slices of zoomed axial three-dimensional T1-weighted images, in the occipital lobe. Note the linear shape of these cavitary lesions, following the trajectory of penetrating vessels, corresponding to dilated perivascular spaces. Bottom row: (A) usual location of dilated perivascular spaces, in the anterior perforated substance, lower third of basal ganglia; (B) and (C) examples of in-plane appearance of dilated perivascular spaces; (D) extra-large perivascular space in a healthy individual.

importance of a peri-lesional rim of hyperintense signal on FLAIR sequences that would be specific for a lesion of ischemic origin [58, 59]. Here again, this criterion may not be adapted since astrocytic gliosis has been repeatedly observed postmortem around large dVRS and can be responsible for a hyperintense rim on FLAIR images [60, 61]. The imaging analysis of the shape of cavities was recently shown to be crucial for discriminating dVRS from lacunar infarcts [62]. Here again, shape analysis requires high-resolution MRI and 3D image analyses, which were not used in most previous studies of silent brain infarcts [47] (Figure 12.5).

Finally, lacunar infarcts should also be differentiated from other types of cavities of vascular origin, particularly the cavities related to hemorrhagic scars. Gradient echo T2 (or T2*) sequences are helpful for this purpose by showing the dark border of the lesion in the case of hemorrhage. However, this does not allow making the differentiation between a remote ASDI that would have bled during its natural history and an actual hemorrhagic lesion. To our knowledge, these aspects have not been clarified in specific studies thus far.

Conclusion

Despite the importance of lacunar infarcts in the setting of SVD, their imaging diagnostic criteria remain often imprecise in the literature. In addition, there is now a need to adopt a specific terminology for the different concepts formerly referred to as "lacunar infarct." We propose to use the term "acute small deep infarcts" to describe acute ischemic brain lesions related to SVD, either symptomatic or detected incidentally on MRI [63]. The term "lacunar infarct" should be used only to describe a cavity occurring after an acute small deep infarct. Among patients who did not experience a stroke compatible with the corresponding lesion site, the term silent lacunar infarct should be used. This will eventually help neuroscientists to harmonize their methodologies and render their results comparable. The term "lacunar syndrome" should probably be abandoned because of the inefficient mixing of clinical, radiologic, and pathologic concepts related to this term.

MRI has definitely shown its superiority compared to CT scan for identification of SVD markers [64]. Imaging modalities are of key importance for detection of lesions such as microbleeds whose number may change in proportion to slice thickness, field strength, or use of susceptibility-weighted imaging [65]. They are also crucial for detection and differential diagnosis of lesions of small size such as dVRS or lacunar infarcts. In the future, there is an obvious need to determine the minimum prerequisites for imaging lacunar infarcts and to harmonize their imaging diagnostic criteria [66].

References

1. Potter GM, Marlborough FJ, Wardlaw JM. Wide variation in definition, detection, and description of lacunar lesions on imaging. *Stroke* 2011;42:359–366.
2. Wardlaw JM. What is a lacune? *Stroke* 2008;39:2921–2922.
3. Dechambre A. [Mémoire sur la curabilité du ramollissement cérébral.] *Gaz Med Paris* 1838;6:305–314 [in French].
4. Durand-Fardel M. [Mémoire sur une altération particulière de la substance cérébrale.] *Gaz Med Paris* 1842;10:23–38 [in French].
5. Marie P. [Des foyers lacunaires de désintégration et de différents autres états cavitaires du cerveau.] *Rev Med Paris* 1901;21:281–298 [in French].
6. Fisher CM. The arterial lesions underlying lacunes. *Acta Neuropathol* 1968;12: 1–15.
7. Fisher CM. A lacunar stroke. The dysarthria–clumsy hand syndrome. *Neurology* 1967;17:614–617.
8. Fisher CM, Curry HB. Pure motor hemiplegia of vascular origin. *Arch Neurol* 1965;13: 30–44.
9. Gan R, Sacco RL, Kargman DE, et al. Testing the validity of the lacunar hypothesis: the Northern Manhattan Stroke Study experience. *Neurology* 1997;48:1204–1211.
10. Arboix A, Garcia-Eroles L, Massons J, Oliveres M, Targa C. Hemorrhagic lacunar stroke. *Cerebrovasc Dis* 2000;10:229–234.
11. Alcala H, Gado M, Torack RM. The effect of size, histologic elements, and water content on the visualization of cerebral infarcts. *Arch Neurol* 1978;35:1–7.
12. Donnan GA, Tress BM, Bladin PF. A prospective study of lacunar infarction using computerized tomography. *Neurology* 1982;32:49–56.
13. Nelson RF, Pullicino P, Kendall BE, Marshall J. Computed tomography in patients presenting

with lacunar syndromes. *Stroke* 1980;11:256–261.

14. Rascol A, Clanet M, Manelfe C, Guiraud B, Bonafe A. Pure motor hemiplegia: CT study of 30 cases. *Stroke* 1982;13:11–17.
15. Huang C, Woo E, Yu YL, Chan FL. Lacunar syndromes due to brainstem infarct and haemorrhage. *J Neurol Neurosurg Psychiatry* 1988;51:509–515.
16. Rothrock JF, Lyden PD, Hesselink JR, Brown JJ, Healy ME. Brain magnetic resonance imaging in the evaluation of lacunar stroke. *Stroke* 1987;18:781–786.
17. Brown JJ, Hesselink JR, Rothrock JF. MR and CT of lacunar infarcts. *AJR Am J Roentgenol* 1988;151:367–372.
18. Van Everdingen KJ, van der Grond J, Kappelle LJ, Ramos LM, Mali WP. Diffusion-weighted magnetic resonance imaging in acute stroke. *Stroke* 1998;29: 1783–1790.
19. Chalela JA, Kidwell CS, Nentwich LM, et al. Magnetic resonance imaging and computed tomography in emergency assessment of patients with suspected acute stroke: a prospective comparison. *Lancet* 2007;369:293–298.
20. Augustin M, Bammer R, Simbrunner J, et al. Diffusion-weighted imaging of patients with subacute cerebral ischemia: comparison with conventional and contrast-enhanced MR imaging. *AJNR Am J Neuroradiol* 2000;21:1596–1602.
21. Burdette JH, Ricci PE, Petitti N, Elster AD. Cerebral infarction: time course of signal intensity changes on diffusion-weighted MR images. *AJR Am J Roentgenol* 1998;171:791–795.
22. Singer MB, Chong J, Lu D, et al. Diffusion-weighted MRI in acute subcortical infarction. *Stroke* 1998;29:133–136.
23. Rosso C, Remy P, Creange A, et al. Diffusion-weighted MR imaging characteristics of an acute strokelike form of multiple sclerosis. *AJNR Am J Neuroradiol* 2006;27:1006–1008.
24. Doubal FN, Dennis MS, Wardlaw JM. Characteristics of patients with minor ischaemic strokes and negative MRI: a cross-sectional study. *J Neurol Neurosurg Psychiatry* 2011;82:540–542.
25. Charidimou A, Gregoire SM, Werring DJ. Letter by Charidimou et al. regarding article, "Blood pressure reduction, decreased diffusion on MRI, and outcomes after intracerebral hemorrhage." *Stroke* 2012;43:e34; author reply e35.
26. Rosso C, Drier A, Lacroix D, et al. Diffusion-weighted MRI in acute stroke within the first 6 hours: 1.5 or 3.0 Tesla? *Neurology* 2010;74:1946–1953.
27. Fisher CM. Lacunar strokes and infarcts: a review. *Neurology* 1982;32:871–876.
28. Koch S, McClendon MS, Bhatia R. Imaging evolution of acute lacunar infarction: leukoariosis or lacune? *Neurology* 2011;77: 1091–1095.
29. Donnan GA, Bladin PF, Berkovic SF, et al. The stroke syndrome of striatocapsular infarction. *Brain* 1991;114(Pt 1A):51–70.
30. Jouvent E, Hervé D, Chabriat H. Partie 1: Maladies des petites artères cérébrales liées à l'âge et à l'hypertension. *Pratique Neurologique-FMC*, 2012;3: 197–205.
31. Moreau F, Patel S, Lauzon ML, et al. Cavitation after acute symptomatic lacunar stroke depends on time, location, and MRI sequence. *Stroke* 2012;43:1837–1842.
32. Loos CMJ, Staals J, Wardlaw JM, van Oostenbrugge RJ. Cavitation of deep lacunar infarcts in patients with first-ever lacunar stroke: a two-year follow-up study with MR 2012;43:2245–2247.
33. Potter GM, Doubal FN, Jackson CA, et al. Counting cavitating lacunes underestimates the burden of lacunar infarction. *Stroke* 2010;41:267–272.
34. Vermeer SE, Prins ND, den Heijer T, et al. Silent brain infarcts and the risk of dementia and cognitive decline. *New Engl J Med* 2003;348:1215–1222.
35. Davis PH, Clarke WR, Bendixen BH, et al. Silent cerebral infarction in patients enrolled in the TOAST study. *Neurology* 1996; 46:942–948.
36. Brott T, Tomsick T, Feinberg W, et al. Baseline silent cerebral infarction in the asymptomatic carotid atherosclerosis study. *Stroke* 1994;25:1122–1129.
37. Boon A, Lodder J, Heuts-van Raak L, Kessels F. Silent brain infarcts in 755 consecutive patients with a first-ever supratentorial ischemic stroke. Relationship with index-stroke subtype, vascular risk factors, and mortality. *Stroke* 1994;25:2384–2390.
38. Ricci S, Celani MG, La Rosa F, et al. Silent brain infarctions in patients with first-ever stroke. A community-based study in Umbria, Italy. *Stroke* 1993;24:647–651.
39. Putaala J, Kurkinen M, Tarvos V, et al. Silent brain infarcts and leukoaraiosis in young adults with first-ever ischemic stroke. *Neurology* 2009;72:1823–1829.
40. Kanai A, Kawamura T, Umemura T, et al. Association between future events of brain infarction and soluble levels of intercellular adhesion molecule-1 and C-reactive protein in patients with type 2 diabetes mellitus. *Diabetes Res Clin Pract* 2008; 82:157–164.
41. Das RR, Seshadri S, Beiser AS, et al. Prevalence and correlates of silent cerebral infarcts in the

Framingham Offspring Study. *Stroke* 2008;39:2929–2935.

42. Wright CB, Festa JR, Paik MC, et al. White matter hyperintensities and subclinical infarction: associations with psychomotor speed and cognitive flexibility. *Stroke* 2008;39: 800–805.
43. Vermeer SE, Koudstaal PJ, Oudkerk M, Hofman A, Breteler MM. Prevalence and risk factors of silent brain infarcts in the population-based Rotterdam Scan Study. *Stroke* 2002;33:21–25.
44. Bryan RN, Cai J, Burke G, et al. Prevalence and anatomic characteristics of infarct-like lesions on MR images of middle-aged adults: the atherosclerosis risk in communities study. *AJNR Am J Neuroradiol* 1999; 20:1273–1280.
45. Price TR, Manolio TA, Kronmal RA, et al. Silent brain infarction on magnetic resonance imaging and neurological abnormalities in community-dwelling older adults. The Cardiovascular Health Study. CHS Collaborative Research Group. *Stroke* 1997;28:1158–1164.
46. Bokura H, Kobayashi S, Yamaguchi S. Distinguishing silent lacunar infarction from enlarged Virchow–Robin spaces: a magnetic resonance imaging and pathological study. *J Neurol* 1998;245:116–122.
47. Zhu YC, Dufouil C, Tzourio C, Chabriat H. Silent brain infarcts: a review of MRI diagnostic criteria. *Stroke* 2011;42:1140–1145.
48. Smith EE, Schneider JA, Wardlaw JM, Greenberg SM. Cerebral microinfarcts: the invisible lesions. *Lancet Neurol* 2012;11:272–282.
49. Jouvent E, Poupon C, Gray F, et al. Intracortical infarcts in small vessel disease: a combined 7-T postmortem MRI and neuropathological case study in cerebral autosomal-dominant arteriopathy with subcortical infarcts and leukoencephalopathy. *Stroke* 2011;42:E27–E30.
50. Herve D, Mangin JF, Molko N, Bousser MG, Chabriat H. Shape and volume of lacunar infarcts: a 3D MRI study in cerebral autosomal dominant arteriopathy with subcortical infarcts and leukoencephalopathy. *Stroke* 2005;36:2384–2388.
51. Hervé D, Godin O, Dufouil C, et al. Three-dimensional MRI analysis of individual volume of lacunes in CADASIL. *Stroke* 2009;40:124–128.
52. Vermeer SE, Longstreth WT, Koudstaal PJ. Silent brain infarcts: a systematic review. *Lancet Neurol* 2007;6:611–619.
53. Braffman BH, Zimmerman RA, Trojanowski JQ, et al. Brain MR: pathologic correlation with gross and histopathology. 1. Lacunar infarction and Virchow–Robin spaces. *AJR Am J Roentgenol* 1988;151:551–558.
54. Mayo J, Arias M, Leno C, Berciano J. Vascular parkinsonism and periarteritis nodosa. *Neurology* 1986;36: 874–875.
55. Pullicino PM, Miller LL, Alexandrov AV, Ostrow PT. Infraputaminal "lacunes." Clinical and pathological correlations. *Stroke* 1995;26:1598–1602.
56. Lammie GA. Hypertensive cerebral small vessel disease and stroke. *Brain Pathol* 2002;12: 358–370.
57. Zhu YC, Dufouil C, Mazoyer B, et al. Frequency and location of dilated Virchow–Robin spaces in elderly people: a population-based 3D MR imaging study. *AJNR Am J Neuroradiol* 2011; 32:709–713.
58. Nomura K, Hamamoto Y, Takahara S, et al. Relationship between carotid intima-media thickness and silent cerebral infarction in Japanese subjects with type 2 diabetes. *Diabetes Care* 2010;33:168–170.
59. Kwon HM, Kim BJ, Park JH, et al. Significant association of metabolic syndrome with silent brain infarction in elderly people. *J Neurol* 2009;256:1825–1831.
60. Lammie GA, Brannan F, Wardlaw JM. Incomplete lacunar infarction (type IB lacunes). *Acta Neuropathol* 1998;96:163–171.
61. Benhaiem-Sigaux N, Gray F, Gherardi R, Roucayrol AM, Poirier J. Expanding cerebellar lacunes due to dilatation of the perivascular space associated with Binswanger's subcortical arteriosclerotic encephalopathy. *Stroke* 1987;18:1087–1092.
62. Groeschel S, Chong WK, Surtees R, Hanefeld F. Virchow–Robin spaces on magnetic resonance images: normative data, their dilatation, and a review of the literature. *Neuroradiology* 2006;48:745–754.
63. Auriel E, Gurol ME, Ayres A, et al. Characteristic distributions of intracerebral hemorrhage-associated diffusion-weighted lesions. *Neurology* 2012;79: 2335–2341.
64. Fazekas F, Kleinert R, Roob G, et al. Histopathologic analysis of foci of signal loss on gradient-echo T2*-weighted MR images in patients with spontaneous intracerebral hemorrhage: evidence of microangiopathy-related microbleeds. *AJNR Am J Neuroradiol* 1999;20:637–642.
65. Greenberg SM, Vernooij MW, Cordonnier C, et al. Cerebral microbleeds: a guide to detection and interpretation. *Lancet Neurol* 2009;8:165–174.
66. Wardlaw JM, Smith EE, Biessels G, et al. Neuroimaging standards for research into small vessel disease and its contributions to ageing and neurodegeneration. *Lancet Neurol* 2013;12:822–838.

Chapter 13

Imaging of hemorrhagic cerebral small vessel diseases

Jennifer Linn, Steven Greenberg, and Anand Viswanathan

Introduction

Hemorrhagic cerebral small vessel diseases (CSVDs) are defined in this chapter as small vessel diseases presenting with predominately hemorrhagic intracranial manifestations. Although hemorrhagic lesions are a component of many cerebral microangiopathies, there are no "pure" hemorrhagic CSVDs. Indeed, all the hemorrhagic CSVDs discussed here may also have ischemic intracranial lesions as part of their clinical presentation. The first part of this chapter discusses the characteristic imaging manifestations in CSVD in general with a focus on the hemorrhagic manifestations, while the second part of the chapter details specific imaging presentations of the most important disease entities.

Imaging findings in hemorrhagic CSVDs: general aspects

Cerebral macrohemorrhages

Large, symptomatic intracerebral hemorrhages (ICHs) constitute the most clinically devastating acute complications of hemorrhagic CSVDs. The two most common sporadic cerebral microangiopathies (i.e., hypertension-related microangiopathy and cerebral amyloid angiopathy [CAA]) together account for the vast majority of nontraumatic ICHs [1–3]. ICHs caused by CSVD are commonly referred to as "primary" ICHs, in contrast to so-called "secondary" ICHs, which have many etiologies, including vascular malformations, cavernomas, hemorrhagic tumors, coagulopathies, sinus and venous thromboses, and secondary hemorrhagic transformation of ischemic strokes [3, 4].

The specific imaging findings in hypertension-related microangiopathy- and CAA-related ICHs are detailed in the respective paragraphs below. This section focuses on general computed tomography (CT) and magnetic resonance (MR) characteristics of ICHs and on the differential diagnosis between primary (i.e., microangiopathic) and secondary bleeding causes.

Computed tomography

Nonenhanced cranial CT findings in ICHs

Nonenhanced cranial CT is still the first choice of imaging modality in the emergency setting in most clinical departments, and therefore plays a major role in the detection of acute ICHs. An acute ICH typically presents as a hyperdense parenchymal mass with Hounsfield Units (HU) of 50 to 70 (Figure 13.1A). In rare instances – for example in patients with low hemoglobin values (<8–10 g/dl) or bleeding disorders – an acute ICH might be isodense to the brain parenchyma on initial CT. Fluid–fluid levels within an acute ICH are often found in patients with underlying coagulopathies or after thrombolytic therapy. The initially high attenuation of an ICH typically decreases by approximately 1.5 HU per day, and becomes isodense to the brain parenchyma within 1–6 weeks (= "subacute" ICH). A "chronic" ICH (>6 weeks) is delineated as a hypodense parenchymal defect. Depending on the size and configuration of the initial hemorrhage, variable residua can be found after an ICH on nonenhanced CT. In up to 30% of cases virtually no residua are visible, while hypodense areas can be depicted in about 40%, slit-like lesions in about 25%, and calcifications in approximately 10% of cases [3, 5].

Cerebral Small Vessel Disease, ed. Leonardo Pantoni and Philip B. Gorelick. Published by Cambridge University Press.

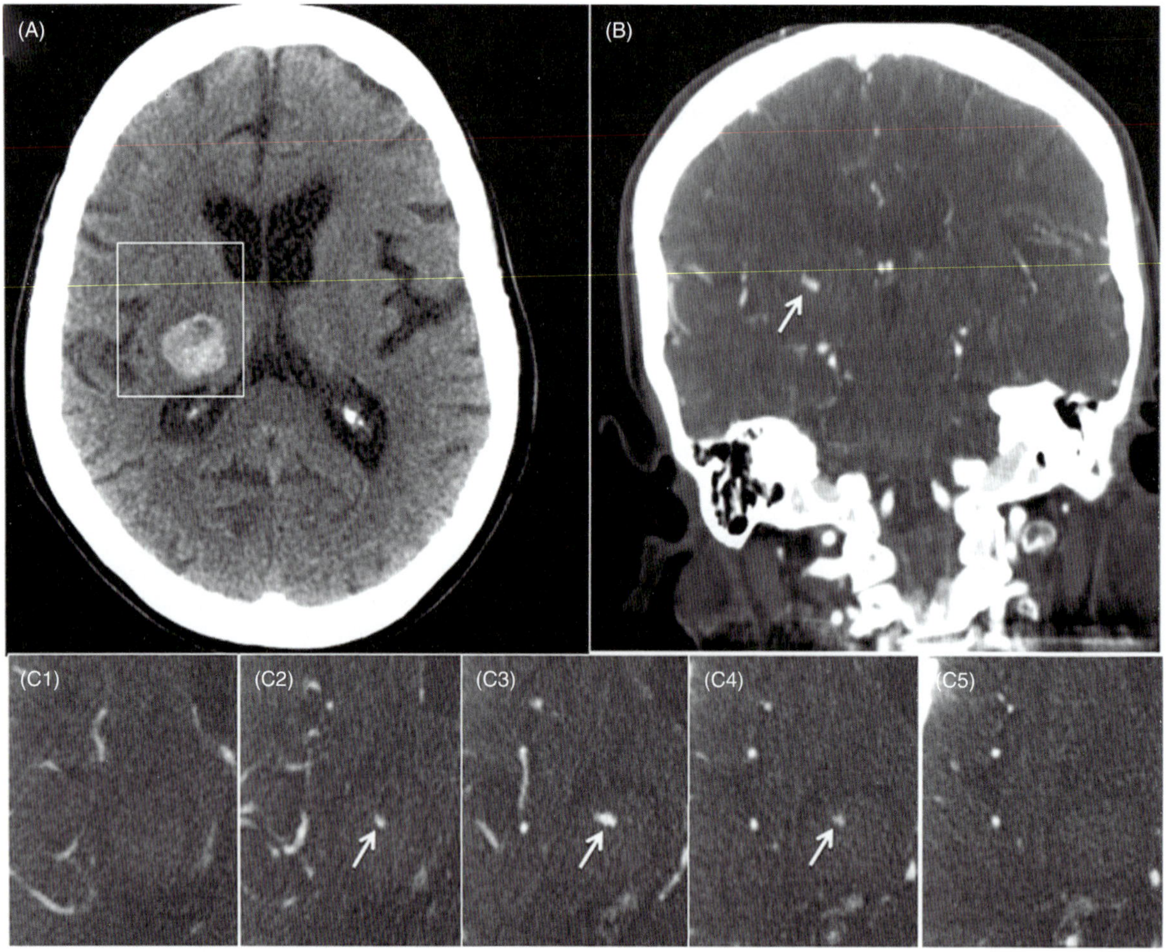

Figure 13.1 Compute tomography (CT) and CT angiography (CTA) findings in acute intracerebral hemorrhages. A 63-year-old patient with an acute left-sided hemiparesis. (A) Unenhanced CT at presentation reveals an acute intracerebral macrohemorrhage in the right thalamus. The area marked by white rectangle in (A) is shown at higher magnification in (C1–C5). Coronal reconstruction (B) and axial source images (C1–C5) of the CTA show a so-called "spot sign" (arrows), which reflects active extravasation of contrast agent and, thus, indicates active bleeding.

Diagnostic yield of CT angiography (CTA) in acute ICHs

Contrast-enhanced CT and particularly CTA can provide valuable additional differential diagnostic information in acute ICHs [6]. Contrast-enhanced CT can reveal contrast-enhancing areas indicative of an underlying neoplasm as secondary bleeding cause. However, magnetic resonance imaging (MRI) is superior to contrast-enhanced CT in this regard and one has to be aware of the fact that subacute and chronic ICH can show a peripheral "ring" enhancement on contrast-enhanced CT, which can be present up to six months and should not be misinterpreted as tumor.

One major role of CTA is the detection or exclusion of macroangiopathic ICH causes (e.g., aneurysms, arteriovenous malformations, or sinus or venous thrombosis). It has, for example, been demonstrated that CTA reveals underlying macrovascular lesions as the bleeding cause in up to 4% of patients with typical "hypertensive" ICHs within the deep gray nuclei [6–9].

Furthermore, there is a growing body of evidence for a considerable role of CTA in predicting clinical outcome after acute ICHs. The presence of a so-called "spot sign" on CTA or contrast-enhanced CT has been shown to be an independent predictor of subsequent hematoma growth and mortality [10–12]. The CT "spot sign" is caused by active extravasation of contrast agent and thus reflects active bleeding (Figure 13.1B). To improve spot sign detection, it has been recommended to perform both early and late scans after intravenous contrast injection. A recent study found that CT perfusion was more sensitive in detecting a spot sign compared to CTA and could circumvent the need for early and late scans due to dynamic acquisition of repeated slices during intravenous injection of a contrast bolus. The study found a peak spot attenuation at a median time of 50 seconds after contrast bolus injection [13].

Magnetic resonance imaging

The role of MRI in the diagnostic work-up of ICH has considerably increased within the last several years. So-called susceptibility-sensitive sequences are considered equivalent to nonenhanced CT for the identification or exclusion of acute ICHs [14, 15]. Furthermore, MRI is of particular additional value in the differential diagnosis of both primary and secondary bleeding causes compared to CT, including CTA [16].

Sequence- and stage-dependent MRI signal characteristics of ICHs

Due to variable signal characteristics of the different blood degradation products oxyhemoglobin, deoxyhemoglobin, methemoglobin, hemosiderin, and ferritin MR signal characteristics of ICHs considerably depend on the age of the respective ICH and on the MR sequence used [3]. Therefore, up to six different stages of ICHs can be distinguished based on MRI at field strengths of 1.0 Tesla or higher: a hyperacute stage (<6 hours), an acute stage (7 hours up to 3 days), an early subacute stage (4–7 days), a late subacute stage (1–4 weeks), an early chronic stage (months), and a late chronic stage (months to years) [3, 17–19] (Figure 13.2). Table 13.1 summarizes the typical signal characteristics of those different ICH stages on common MRI sequences including the respective blood degradation products, which are responsible for the MR presentation.

While a considerable number of 1.5-Tesla MRI studies on the signal characteristics of the different ICH stages exist, data on the influence of higher field strength (3 Tesla and more) are considerably sparser [20, 21]. Available studies suggest that 3-Tesla MRI allows the determination of acute to late subacute ICH stages comparably to 1.5-Tesla studies, but with significantly more profound hypointense signal in all parts of acute and early subacute ICHs at 3 Tesla [20, 21]. At very low field strengths (0.02–0.50 Tesla), some characteristic features of ICHs, such as the central hypointense central area in acute lesions and the parenchymal hypointense rim in late to chronic lesions on T2-weighted images, cannot be observed [22].

Diagnostic yield of MRI for the detection of primary versus secondary bleeding causes

MRI not only allows the determination of ICH stage but is of particular diagnostic value for the differentiation of primary versus secondary bleeding causes [16]. In primary ICHs, MRI is clearly superior to CT, including CTA, and undoubtedly represents the noninvasive gold standard to detect concomitant imaging findings, as for example cerebral microbleeds (CMBs), which may be indicative of the respective underlying CSVD (see below).

At the same time, MRI is of considerable diagnostic yield if secondary bleeding causes are suspected. It is the ideal imaging method to detect underlying hemorrhagic tumors, sinus and venous thrombosis, and secondary hemorrhagic transformation of ischemic strokes. Although invasive digital subtraction angiography (DSA) is still the diagnostic gold standard for the detection and pretherapeutic evaluation of vascular malformations, recent advances in MR-sequence technology have considerably increased its value in the detection of pial arteriovenous malformations and dural arteriovenous fistulas as secondary ICH causes [23–25]. In addition, these techniques yield very promising results for the classification of these vascular malformations [26].

Digital subtraction angiography

In CSVD, DSA – analogous to CTA and MRA – typically yields negative results. As the diameter of affected vessels in CSVD is within the submillimeter range, even the high spatial resolution of DSA is not sufficient to visualize the pathologic changes. Thus, DSA is not indicated if noninvasive imaging and clinical findings unequivocally argue for a primary ICH. Yet, as it still represents the gold standard for the detection and evaluation of vascular malformations, DSA is strongly recommended in the diagnostic work-up of ICHs if noninvasive imaging modalities yield equivocal results concerning the underlying

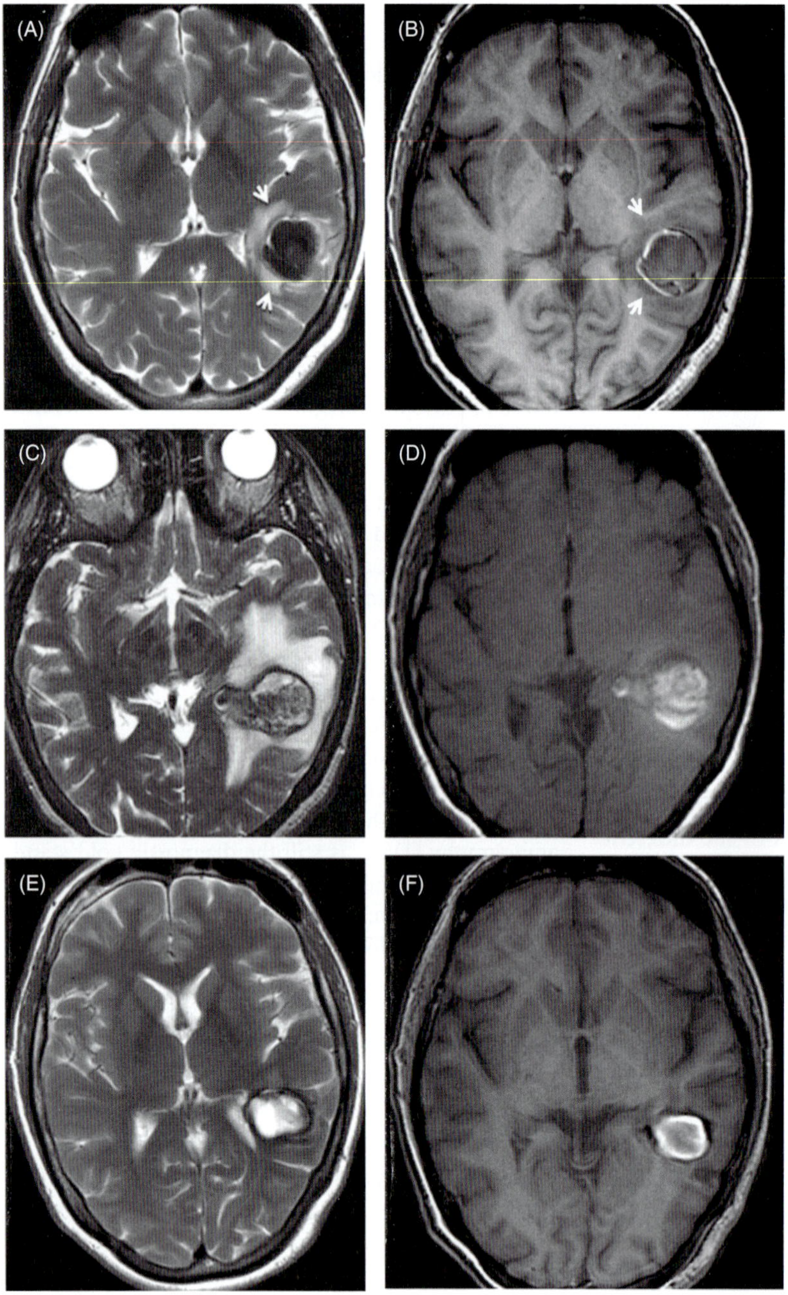

Figure 13.2 Magnetic resonance imaging (MRI) findings in acute intracerebral hemorrhage (ICH). A 49-year-old patient with von Willebrand disease. The initial MRI performed 24 hours after symptom onset (A,B) reveals an acute left temporal cerebral macrohemorrhage (ICH). In the acute stage the ICH shows a profoundly hypointense signal on T2-weighted imaging (A), while it is isointense with a very subtle hyperintense rim on T1-weighted imaging (B). Arrows in (A) and (B) indicate perifocal edema. Follow-up MRI after five days (early subacute stage, C,D) and after eight weeks (early chronic stage, E,F) shows the typical stage-dependent MRI signal characteristics of ICHs on T2-weighted (C,E) and T1-weighted sequences (D,F) as detailed in Table 13.1.

bleeding cause, especially in young, normotensive patients [23, 27, 28].

Cerebral microbleeds

Within the past decade, scientific interest regarding the clinical significance of CMBs has grown substantially. There is evidence that the presence of CMBs is an independent risk factor for cognitive impairment [29]. While their role as potential risk factor for future ICHs in different patient populations is still a matter of debate, their importance as MRI surrogate parameters for hemorrhagic CSVDs is undoubted [30, 31]. The anatomic localization of CMBs plays a substantial role in the imaging differential diagnoses of these diseases [31]. CMBs must be differentiated from

Table 13.1 Stage-dependent MRI signal characteristics of ICHs

ICH stage	Time from onset	Hemoglobin state/ blood degradation product	MR signal intensity		
			T1w	T2w	T2*-GRE
Hyperacute	<6 hours	Intracellular oyxhemoglobin	Isointense	Hyperintense (may have hypointense rim)	Hypointense
Acute	7 hours to 3 days	Intracellular deoxyhemoglobin	Isointense	Hypointense	Profoundly hypointense
Early subacute	4–7 days	Intracellular methemoglobin	Hyperintense	Hypointense	Profoundly hypointense
Late subacute	1–4 weeks	Extracellular methemoglobin	Hyperintense	Hyperintense	Profoundly hypointense
Early chronic	Months	Extracellular methemoglobin + ferritin/hemosiderin wall	Hyperintense	Hyperintense with pronounced low signal rim	Profoundly hypointense
Late chronic	Months to years	Hemosiderin	Isointense	Hypointense	Profoundly hypointense

ICH, intracerebral hemorrhage; MR, magentic resonance; MRI, magnetic resonance imaging; T1w, T1-weighted sequence; T2w, T2-weighted sequence; T2*-GRE, T2*-weighted gradient-recalled echo sequence.

so-called "mimics," that is, other entities with a similar MR appearance (see Differential diagnosis of CMBs section, below).

Imaging-based definition and typical imaging findings

CMBs are defined as small foci of chronic blood products (hemosiderin) which are surrounded by normal or near normal brain tissue [31, 32] (Figure 13.3A). They were first described in a neuroradiologic paper by Offenbacher et al. [32] in 1996 as "focal areas of signal loss" consisting of "homogeneous, rounded lesions with diameters of 2–5 mm" on blood-sensitive, T2*-weighted gradient-recalled echo (T2*-GRE) MRI sequences (Figure 13.3). Although CMBs primarily constitute a radiologic construct, they correlate with specific histopathologic findings, namely perivascular collections of hemosiderin deposits that represent foci of past hemorrhages [32, 33] (Figure 13.3).

On MRI, CMBs are identified by the following imaging characteristics: (1) size (small); (2) shape (e.g., ovoid, spherical, round or dot-like); and (3) MRI signal (profoundly hypointense on T2*-weighted images and causing marked susceptibility artifacts in these sequences) (Figure 13.3). However, since their initial description in 1996, the criteria used to identify CMBs on MRI have varied in the literature, making comparability between studies difficult [34].

In an effort to solve this problem, an Expert Group suggested standardized procedural guidelines for CMB identification on MRI [31]. According to these consensus criteria, CMBs are defined as small, rounded, or ovoid lesions (rather than linear or curvilinear lesions), that are homogeneously hypointense on T2*-GRE and related MRI sequences that are sensitive for susceptibility effects.

The areas of low signal intensity seen on T2*-weighted MRI are significantly larger in diameter compared to the corresponding hemosiderin deposits detected on histopathologic examinations (Figure 13.3). The extent of this so-called "blooming effect," and thus the diameter of CMBs on T2*-GRE sequences, varies significantly depending on the MRI parameters that are used to image CMBs (such as field strength and pulse sequence; for details see below), and not only on the actual amount of deposited hemosiderin [31, 35]. It has been shown that CMBs and ICHs seem not to represent a continuum regarding their size, but rather have a distinctly bimodal size distribution, with separated and widely spaced peaks for diameters of CMBs versus ICHs [36]. Based on these data, the Consensus Group has

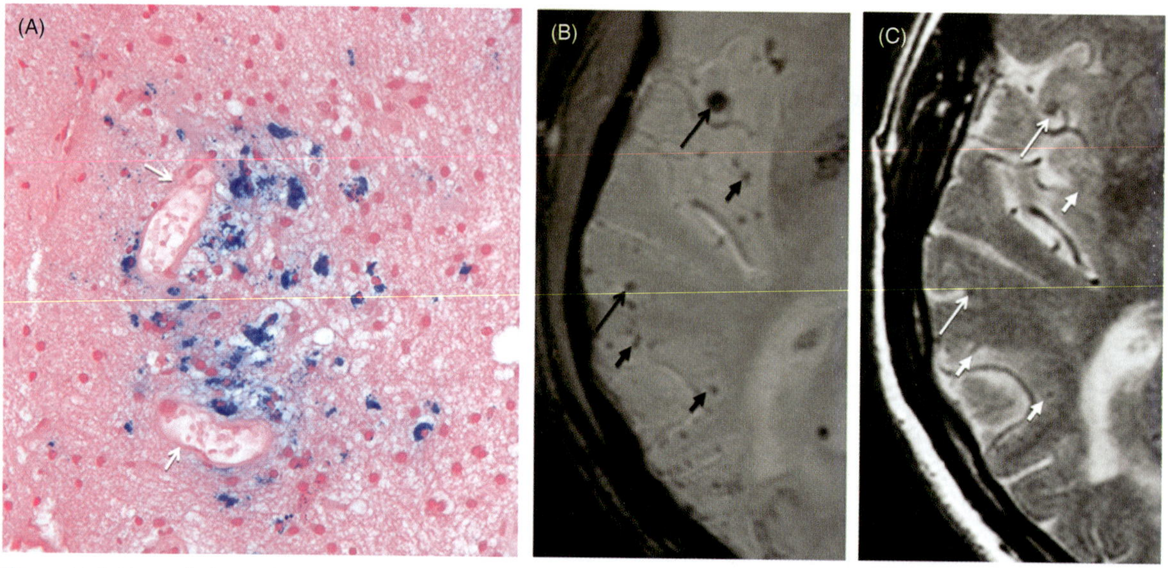

Figure 13.3 Histopathological findings and magnetic resonance imaging (MRI) in cerebral microbleeds (CMBs). These are defined as small foci of chronic blood products (hemosiderin), which are surrounded by normal or near normal brain tissue. (A) Prussian blue stain of an old CMB shows two small cortical vessels (arrows) with hemosiderin-loaded perivascular macrophages (stained in blue), indicating previous perivascular bleedings. (Courtesy of Prof. Dr. Armin Giese, Zentrum für Neuropathologie und Prionforschung, Ludwig-Maximilians-University, Munich, Germany.) (B) T2*-gradient-recalled echo (GRE) sequence depicts multiple CMBs as profoundly hypointense, small dots in a patient with probable cerebral amyloid angiopathy. Due to the so-called "blooming effect," the diameter of the low signal intensity spots on T2*-GRE is larger compared to the actual hemosiderin deposits, which can be detected on histopathological examination. (C) On T2-spin-echo-MR sequence some CMBs cause subtle hypointensities (e.g., long white arrows in C), while smaller CMBs cannot be detected on this sequence (e.g., short white arrows in C).

recommended using an upper-size limit ranging from 5 to 10 mm for CMBs on standard T2*-GRE MRI sequences [31, 34, 37, 38].

The definition provided by the Consensus Group means to distinguish CMBs from ICHs, subarachnoid hemorrhages (SAHs), and superficial siderosis, as well as from cavernous malformations, residues from ICHs due to so-called secondary bleeding (e.g., arteriovenous malformations or tumors), and nonhemorrhagic causes of hypointense signal on T2*-GRE MRI (e.g., calcifications or air–bone susceptibility-related signal loss) [31, 39].

Methodological considerations

Since the first description of CMBs, considerable advances in both MRI soft- and hardware have resulted in a substantial increase in its sensitivity to detect CMBs. The striking effect of methodological aspects on the delineation of CMBs is well reflected in the wide range of their reported prevalence in population-based studies ([40–46]; see below). There is currently no consensus regarding optimal MR parameters for CMB identification, despite their strong influence on the sensitivity of CMB detection. CMBs are best detected on MR sequences that are highly sensitive for susceptibility effects.

As discussed above, the diameter of signal hypointensities seen as CMBs on susceptibility-sensitive sequences is, as a rule, considerably larger than the actual size of the corresponding hemosiderin deposits seen in histopathologic tissue examination (Figure 13.3). The blooming phenomenon is caused by dephased protons adjacent to the blood residues [33, 47, 48]. Based on a recent histopathologic–imaging correlation study, blooming results in a 1.57 ± 0.75-fold larger diameter of CMBs delineated on MRI compared to the physical diameter of the hemosiderin deposit detected on tissue examination [49]. The extent of the blooming on T2*-GRE is not necessarily proportional to the physical diameter of the hemosiderin deposit but rather depends on the actual amount of paramagnetic material present (i.e., the iron content).

In addition, the blooming effect strongly depends on the MRI parameters used, especially on magnetic field strength, echo time (TE), spatial resolution, and image post-processing techniques [31, 35, 50–55]. The impact of these influencing factors on the demarcation of CMBs is detailed in the following paragraphs.

Role of magnetic field strength

The susceptibility effect which is caused by paramagnetic substances increases in proportion to the strength of the static magnetic field of the MR scanner. Thus, the use of higher magnetic field strengths – e.g., 3 Tesla versus 1.5 Tesla – enhances the blooming effect caused by the same amount of hemosiderin and results in an increased CMB diameter on susceptibility-sensitive sequences. In addition, higher field strength also results in a higher contrast to noise ratio [35].

As a consequence of both phenomena, more CMBs are delineated at higher field strength compared to 1.5 Tesla [35, 53, 56, 57] (Figure 13.4A,B). Besides this effect on the number of CMBs, it has also been shown that ultra-high field MRI (7 Tesla) also enhances the reliability of CMB detection compared to standard field strength [57].

The advantages of higher field strengths are to some extent counteracted by the fact that the stronger susceptibility effect results not only in a better CMB delineation but also in an increase of the susceptibility artifacts in other areas with profound magnetic field inhomogeneities, particularly at air–bone interfaces such as the basal forebrain.

Echo time

As regarding the MRI sequence parameters, the TE is of particular interest in the visualization of CMBs. This parameter determines the time interval between excitation pulse and sampling of the MR signal. In studies on CMBs, TEs between 25 and 50 ms are typically used. The longer the TE, the more time for the spins to dephase is available, and thus the stronger the susceptibility effect. Therefore, the length of TE is critical for the sensitivity of T2*-GRE sequences for CMBs [31]. For example, a lengthening of TE from 40 to 60 ms results in a substantial increase in total number of CMBs detected [52]. This modification goes along with a certain loss of image quality, as one of the results is more pronounced susceptibility artifact adjacent to other magnetic field inhomogeneities; for example, air–tissue interfaces or near the skull base. Thus, the use of longer TEs can lead to an increased uncertainty in the differentiation between CMBs and their "mimics" [52]. The optimal TE depends on the magnetic field strength. At higher field strengths, a shorter TE can be used [35, 53].

Spatial resolution

Given the small size of CMBs and the even smaller diameter of the underlying hemoglobin deposits, the spatial resolution of the MR sequences plays a crucial role in CMB detection. In general, the signal provided by a specific voxel is an average of the signal intensities of all objects within the respected voxel. Due to this so-called partial-volume averaging, the actual signal of objects that are smaller than the voxel size is underestimated. In-plane resolution of routine brain MRI sequences is within the acceptable range for CMB detection, while the spatial resolution in z-direction in routine MRI is significantly lower at typical slice thicknesses of 5 or 6 mm. This limits CMB detection due to the above-mentioned partial volume effects. On the other hand, a higher spatial resolution will cause a significant loss of MR signal because a reduction of voxel size by a factor of two will decrease the MR signal provided by each voxel by a factor of four. To overcome this drawback, a three-dimensional Fourier transform technique with parallel imaging has been used to acquire a high-resolution T2*-GRE sequence with a submillimeter spatial resolution (reconstructed voxel size of $0.5 \times 0.5 \times 0.8$ mm^3) and a relatively high signal to noise ratio [55]. On thin-sliced reconstructions of this sequence more CMBs could be detected compared to a conventional two-dimensional T2*-GRE sequence [55]. Furthermore, a reduction of the slice thickness not only reveals a higher number of CMBs, but also facilitates the detection of individual CMBs by reducing the partial volume effect. For example, it has been shown that individual CMBs are detected with a higher contrast index on 1.5 mm thin slices compared to 5 mm slices (5 mm) [35].

Susceptibility-weighted imaging

As detailed above, all T2*-weighted MR sequences are very sensitive to susceptibility effects. In recent years, different approaches have been used to further enhance this effect using two different methods. The most popular approach combines both magnitude and phase information of the MRI signal using adequate post-processing steps. This is known as susceptibility-weighted imaging (SWI) [58–60]. The second method applies multiple TEs (centered around

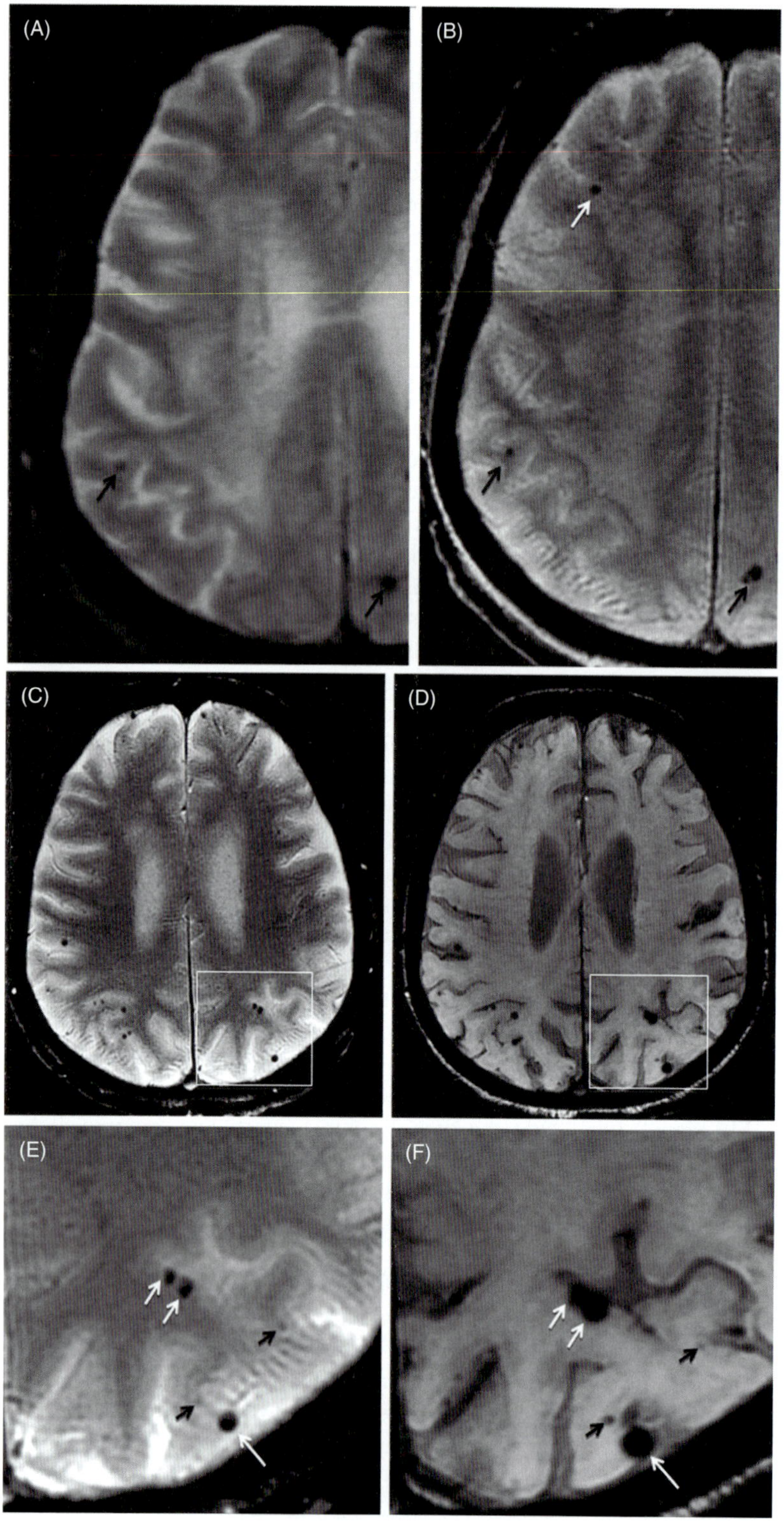

Figure 13.4 Magnetic resonance imaging (MRI) of cerebral microbleeds (CMBs) – methodological considerations. (A,B) Influence of magnetic field strength on the detection of CMBs. An 80-year-old male patient with probable cerebral amyloid angiopathy (CAA) and several CMBs in cortical and subcortical localization (arrows). T2*-gradient-recalled echo (GRE) sequences performed on a 1.5 Tesla (A) and on a 3 Tesla scanner (B) (slice thickness = 5 mm). At 3 Tesla, CMBs are detected with a higher contrast to noise ratio, and an additional CMB in the right frontal lobe can be detected compared to 1.5 Tesla (white arrow in B). (C–F) Susceptibility-weighted imaging (SWI) (D,F) improves CMB detection compared to conventional T2*-GRE MRI (C, E). A 73-year-old patient with probable CAA and multiple CMBs. Due to the enhanced susceptibility effect, CMBs (white arrows in E and F) show a more pronounced hypointense signal and a larger diameter on SWI (D,F) compared to standard T2*-GRE imaging (C,E). In addition, SWI detects more and smaller CMBs (black arrows in E and F). The areas marked by white rectangles in (C) and (D) are shown at higher magnification in (E) and (F), respectively.

25 ms), thereby taking advantage of the positive influence of longer TEs on susceptibility, but reducing the geometric distortion and artifacts of single-echo long TE scans. The latter approach is called T2-star-weighted angiography (SWAN) [61]. Though systematic comparative studies are lacking, the visual aspects of SWI and SWAN are very similar [62], suggesting that the two approaches may yield comparable results in CMB detection.

Compared to the multiecho approach, SWI using magnitude and phase information distinguishes true CMBs from some of their "mimics," such as from calcifications (for details, see Differential diagnosis of CMBs section, below).

SWI currently appears to be the most sensitive in vivo method for CMB detection and analysis [50, 59]. It not only detects significantly more CMBs, but also smaller CMBs (1 mm or even smaller in diameter, Figure 13.4C–F) [50], which might shed new light on the significance of subtle pericapillary hemosiderin deposits recently found in some histologic studies [63–66].

Although the superiority of SWI compared to conventional T2*-GRE sequences concerning improved CMB detection is evident, the advantage in matters of clinical relevance is not yet clear. The full potential of SWI, i.e., its reliability, sensitivity, specificity, and "added value" in the diagnostic work-up of CSVD must still be determined in detail [31, 67, 68].

Prevalence of CMBs in population-based studies

Large population-based studies detected CMBs in a high percentage of clinically asymptomatic volunteers. The reported CMB prevalence in the general population varies on a wide scale from 6.4 to 23.5%. This discrepancy is explained by the different MR sequence parameters and spatial resolution that were used in the different studies [40, 41, 43–45]. The differences further emphasize the need for standardized MR sequence parameters and reporting criteria to allow comparison between studies on the clinical significance of CMBs.

The population-based data suggest a significant overlap between normal aging and asymptomatic stages of age-related hemorrhagic CSVD, particularly CAA and hypertension-related microangiopathy [46, 68]. Recent follow-up data from the population-based Rotterdam Scan Study indicate that improved CMB detection might be helpful to identify individuals with asymptomatic CSVD [68, 69]. The risk profile of participants with CMBs on high-resolution but not conventional T2*-GRE was more similar to those with CMBs on conventional T2*-GRE than to those without any CMBs on either sequence [68, 69]. Furthermore, these individuals had a higher risk for new CMBs during follow-up (25.0% vs. 5.9%) compared to those without any CMBs. Although these findings suggest an additional value of SWI compared to conventional T2*-GRE, more studies are needed to definitively determine the impact of SWI in the diagnostic work-up of CSVDs.

Differential diagnosis of CMBs

All paramagnetic substances induce susceptibility artifacts on T2*-GRE MRI resulting in a hypointense signal on these sequences. Depending on the size and configuration of these lesions they can strongly resemble CMBs. Therefore, a set of criteria has been introduced to differentiate these so called "mimics" (including artifacts) from true CMBs [31, 39]. Two major types of CMB mimics can be distinguished: lesions containing blood or blood degradation products (e.g., cavernous malformations and vessels) and lesions without blood residues (e.g., calcifications).

Key imaging aspects to differentiate genuine CMBs from their mimics and from artifacts are:

1. The geometry of the lesion (size and shape).
2. The lesion's signal intensity on other MR sequences (e.g., T1-weighted and T2-weighted spin-echo sequences) and on CT.
3. The anatomical localization of the lesion [31, 39].

Depending on the topographic localization of the respective lesion, other differential diagnoses become more likely. Typical CMB mimics in cortical or immediate subcortical localization are vascular flow voids resulting from small cortical vessels as well as partial volume artifacts. In basal ganglia and thalami, calcifications or deposits of other minerals and flow voids from deep perforating vessels must be considered as likely diagnoses. Yet, some CMB mimics (e.g., cavernomas) can be found in any anatomic localization.

Vascular flow voids

The flow void induced by small arteries with oxygenated blood does not cause a significant blooming effect on susceptibility-sensitive sequences. On the contrary, due to the oxyhemoglobin arteries typically

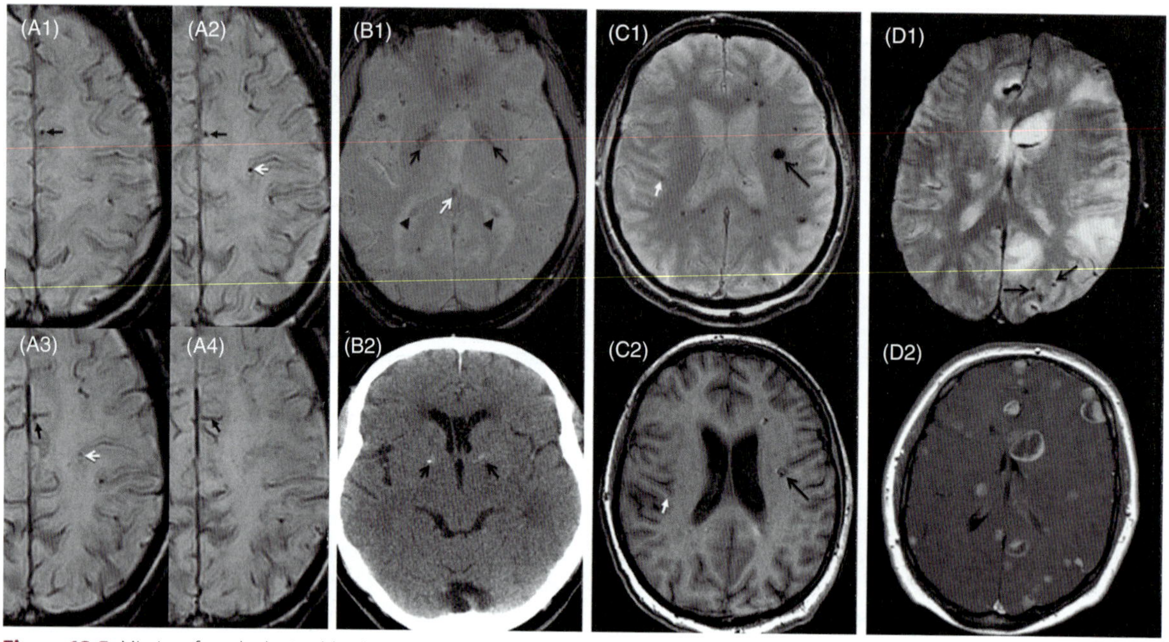

Figure 13.5 Mimics of cerebral microbleeds (CMBs) on susceptibility-sensitive sequences. Besides CMBs, all paramagnetic substances induce susceptibility artifacts on T2*-gradient-recalled echo (GRE) sequences, which result in a hypointense signal on these sequences and can mimic CMBs. (A) Vascular flow voids mimicking CMBs. SWI of a 67-year-old patient with a single CMB in the left lobe (white arrows in A2 and A3). Small veins running perpendicular to the imaging plane appear quite similar to a CMB on single slices (black arrow in A2). However, the different three-dimensional extent of vessels and CMBs allows their differentiation by inspection of adjacent slices. While the CMB is only delineated in two continuous slices (A2 and A3, white arrows), the vessel can be followed over more than three slices (A1–A4, black arrows). (B) Calcifications mimicking CMBs. A 76-year-old patient with cerebral amyloid angiopathy (CAA) and multiple CMBs in cortical and subcortical localization. In addition to the CMBs, T2*-GRE shows hypointensities bilaterally in the anterior part of the globus pallidus (black arrows in B1) and the pineal region (white arrow in B1). Those correspond to calcifications in typical anatomic localizations, as proven by their hyperdensity on unenhanced computed tomography (CT) (e.g., black arrows in B2 indicate calcifications bilaterally in the anterior part of the globus pallidus). (C) Cavernomas mimicking CMBs. A 53-year-old patient with multiple cavernomas. In contrast to CMBs, cavernomas (e.g., black arrows in C1 and C2) are usually not only detectable on T2*-GRE sequences (C1) but also on T1-weighted sequences (C2). However, very tiny cavernomas (e.g., white arrows in C1 and C2) are only detected on T2*-GRE, and, thus, can be indistinguishable from CMBs. (D) Melanoma metastasis as mimics of CMBs. A 49-year-old patient with cerebral metastases from malignant melanoma. On T2*-GRE sequence (D1) the metastases present as multiple, round, hypointense lesions. Larger and middle-sized metastasis can be easily differentiated from CMBs by the presence of perifocal edema, and contrast enhancement on contrast-enhanced T1-weighted sequences (D2). However, small melanotic metastases (e.g., arrows in D1) might be difficult to distinguish from CMBs.

present with a hyperintense signal on SWI [62]. Thus, they can be quite easily distinguished from CMBs. In contrast, differentiation between CMBs and small veins is considerably more challenging because of the high deoxyhemoglobin fraction of the venous blood. Deoxyhemoglobin is paramagnetic and therefore causes a sizable blooming effect on susceptibility-sensitive sequences, especially on SWI [50]. In particular, small veins running perpendicular to the imaging plane appear quite similar to CMBs on single slices (Figure 13.5A). However, the different three-dimensional extent of both entities allows their differentiation. The linear configuration of the small vessels can be best appreciated and distinguished from the round to ovoid shape of CMBs by careful inspection of adjacent slices. Depending on the slice thickness, a single CMB is delineated in a maximum of two or three continuous slices (e.g., at a slice thickness of 2 mm), while a vessel running perpendicular to the image plane can be typically followed over more than three slices (Figure 13.5A).

The susceptibility-related contrast of SWI images can be amplified by post-processing techniques; for example, minimum-intensity projection images [60]. In questionable cases, the additional three-dimensional information provided by these reconstructions can be helpful to distinguish CMBs from vessels.

Cavernous malformations

Cavernous malformations (also termed cavernomas) are benign vascular hamartomas containing a mass of dilated immature blood vessels with single layers of endothelium that lie immediately side by side, without any neuronal tissue in between. These thin-walled vessels resemble sinusoidal cavities filled with stagnant blood, and appear as a "mulberry-like" nodule on gross pathologic examination. Cavernomas are found with an overall prevalence of approximately 0.5%, and a recent large population-based study on incidental findings on cerebral MRI reported a prevalence of 0.4% for asymptomatic cavernomas in the general population [50]. Symptomatic cavernomas typically present with seizures (30–50% of patients) or ICHs (20–25% of patients, [70]). In up to 25% of patients multiple cavernomas are present. While most cavernomas are sporadic, familial (multiple) cavernous malformation syndromes are also known. An autosomal dominant hereditary disorder with variable penetrance is described in Americans of Hispanic origin [71].

The intralesional MR signal characteristics of cavernous malformations depend on their size and on the presence or absence of different blood degradation products, calcifications, partially thrombosed areas, and blood flow within the caverns. Typically, CMs show a hyperintense or mixed signal within their center on both T1- and T2-weighted sequences, and a hypointense rim, due to hemosiderin deposits (Figure 13.5B). Important differential diagnoses of larger cavernomas include thrombosed aneurysms, residues of primary ICH, as well as secondary intratumoral ICHs [72]. Medium to large cavernomas can nonetheless be quite easily diagnosed on MRI due to their characteristic "mulberry-like" appearance (Figure 13.5B). On the other hand, very small cavernomas can be indistinguishable from CMBs on T2*-GRE. In such cases, the best differential diagnostic clue is the lesion's signal characteristics on T2- and T1-weighted MR sequences. While classical CMBs are typically not detected on these sequences because of the very tiny physical diameter of the underlying hemosiderin deposit, small cavernomas can usually be identified by their hyperintense or mixed signal on these sequences. In some cases, unenhanced CT might be helpful to detect calcifications that are present in 40–60% of cavernomas, while they are not found in CMBs. In analogy to the detection of CMBs, the use of SWI or higher magnetic-field strength enhances the number of cavernomas that can be found compared to conventional T2*-GRE MRI [70]. Thus their actual prevalence might be even higher than reported.

Calcifications

Like ferrous deposits, calcium results in areas of hypointense signal on T2*-GRE. Intracranial calcifications are typically found, for example, bilaterally in the anterior part of the globus pallidus, in the choroid plexus, and in the pineal gland (Figure 13.5C). Identifying this characteristic topographic distribution of calcifications helps in the differential diagnosis versus CMBs. Calcium deposits in uncommon localizations e.g., cortical or subcortical, can be indistinguishable from CMBs on conventional T2*-GRE, while SWI, which uses both magnitude and phase information, allows discrimination between the two types of lesions. Because of their diamagnetic characteristics, calcifications show a *hyperintense* signal in phase images, as opposed to the paramagnetic iron within CMBs, which is hypointense on both magnitude and phase images [73]. If SWI is not available, nonenhanced CT may be helpful, since calcifications appear as profoundly hyperdense areas (Figure 13.5C).

Cerebral metastasis from malignant melanoma

Due to their melanin content on the one hand and their tendency to bleed on the other, cerebral metastases from malignant melanoma can also present as (multiple) round hypointense lesions on T2*-GRE. Usually they can be differentiated from actual CMBs by the presence of perifocal edema, concomitant hyperintense signal on T1-weighted sequences caused by the melanin, and their variable size (Figure 13.5D). Nevertheless, in exceptional cases, small melanotic metastases might be indistinguishable from CMBs [31, 74].

Cerebral microhemorrhages caused by underlying diseases other than CSVD

Besides the different CMB mimics, one should be aware of a variety of causes and diseases other than CSVD as potential causes of (multiple) small hemorrhagic lesions. Those "secondary" microhemorrhages might not be distinguishable from "primary," SVD-related CMBs based on their imaging appearance alone.

Head trauma constitutes one important cause of such secondary cerebral microhemorrhages. In particular, traumatic microbleeds are an imaging hallmark of diffuse axonal injury [75]. This specific trauma sequel is typically caused by shear-strain forces to the head resulting in lesions at the interface between different tissues, such as, for example, the junctions between gray and white matter. Besides the clinical history, the localization of these "tissue-tear hemorrhages," which often involve the corpus callosum, allows their differentiation from "primary" CMBs [75]. Concomitant imaging findings in head trauma comprise parenchymal, sub-, and epidural, and SAHs, as well as T2- and fluid-attenuated inversion recovery (FLAIR) hyperintensities and areas of restricted diffusion indicative of underlying focal cytotoxic edema at the side of the sheer injuries [76]. Another important disease entity that must be mentioned in this regard is infectious endocarditis, which can also manifest with multiple CMBs [77, 78].

Any entity resulting in a generalized hemorrhagic prone state, such as hematologic disorders, can lead to cerebral micro- (or macro-) hemorrhages. As an example, CMBs were found in over 10% of young, neurologically asymptomatic patients (mean age: 20.5 years) with newly diagnosed aplastic anemia [79]. However, data on the role of CMBs in hematologic disorders are extremely sparse to date.

Focal SAHs and supratentorial superficial siderosis

Focal subarachnoid hemorrhages (fSAHs) and supratentorial superficial siderosis (SS) have recently been recognized as additional typical imaging findings in a specific subtype of CSVD, namely CAA [80–83]. The value of these findings as in vivo biomarkers of this disease is detailed in the Sporadic CAA section, below. This section focuses on their imaging characteristics, on differential diagnoses, and mimics.

Imaging-based definition and imaging characteristics of fSAH and SS

fSAHs are defined as acute, nontraumatic SCHs within a restricted number of sulci of the hemispheric convexities [82, 83]. In general, CT and MRI are equally sensitive in the detection of acute SAHs. On nonenhanced CT, fSAHs are delineated as linear hyperdense areas in one or more cortical sulci. With regard to MRI, FLAIR- and proton-density-weighted sequences are best suited to detect acute and subacute SAHs as linear hyperintense signal within the subarachnoid space [84, 85]. The interpretation of the subarachnoid space on FLAIR images can be obscured by the presence of marked artifacts due to pulsations of the cerebrospinal fluid (CSF). This drawback of FLAIR can be overcome by the use of three-dimensional FLAIR sequences, or so-called PROPELLER or BLADE sequences [86]. The latter techniques reduce artifacts by using an alternative way of sampling k-space. However, as these pulsation artifacts mainly occur in the basal cisterns and the ventricles, they usually do not hamper the detection of fSAHs in the convexities. Proton-density-weighted sequences are much less prone to CSF pulsation artifacts compared to FLAIR. They are very sensitive to detect fresh subarachnoid blood provided that the sequence parameters are optimized in such a way that normal CSF is hypo- or isointense, i.e., the repetition time (TR) must not be too long (e.g., 2200 ms) [87].

A distinguishing feature of fSAHs compared to most aneurysmal SAHs is their limited extent. Although they can affect several adjacent sulci, they are often restricted to one sulcus or even to a small part of one sulcus. Therefore, suspicion must be high and images must be carefully analyzed in order not to miss a subtle fSAH. Thin-sliced multiplanar reconstructions of nonenhanced CT datasets might be helpful in questionable cases (L. Ertl, D. Morhard, M. Deckert-Schmitz, et al. [unpubl. obs.])

Supratentorial SS is defined as linear deposits of hemosiderin within the subarachnoid space and the superficial cortical layers of the sulci and gyri of the cerebral convexities [80, 81, 88]. It can be either focal (restricted to up to three cortical sulci) or disseminated (involving four or more sulci) [81] (Figure 13.6). Analogous to CMBs, the underlying hemosiderin in SS causes a significant blooming effect on susceptibility-sensitive sequences, i.e., on T2*-GRE and especially on SWI (Figure 13.6). Thus, the methodological considerations regarding MR sequence parameters discussed for CMBs basically also apply for SS (Figure 13.6). Depending on the exact localization of the hemosiderin (see Pathophysiology of supratentorial SS section, below), SS is delineated on these sequences either as a single linear hypointensity within the subarachnoid space or as two almost parallel, bilinear hypointensities within the superficial cortical layers (Figure 13.6). This "track-like" appearance on axial sections is caused by the relatively high signal intensity of the normal-appearing subarachnoid space in the middle, which is bordered bilaterally by hypointense linear deposits of hemosiderin in the superficial layers of the adjacent cortex [80] (Figure 13.6).

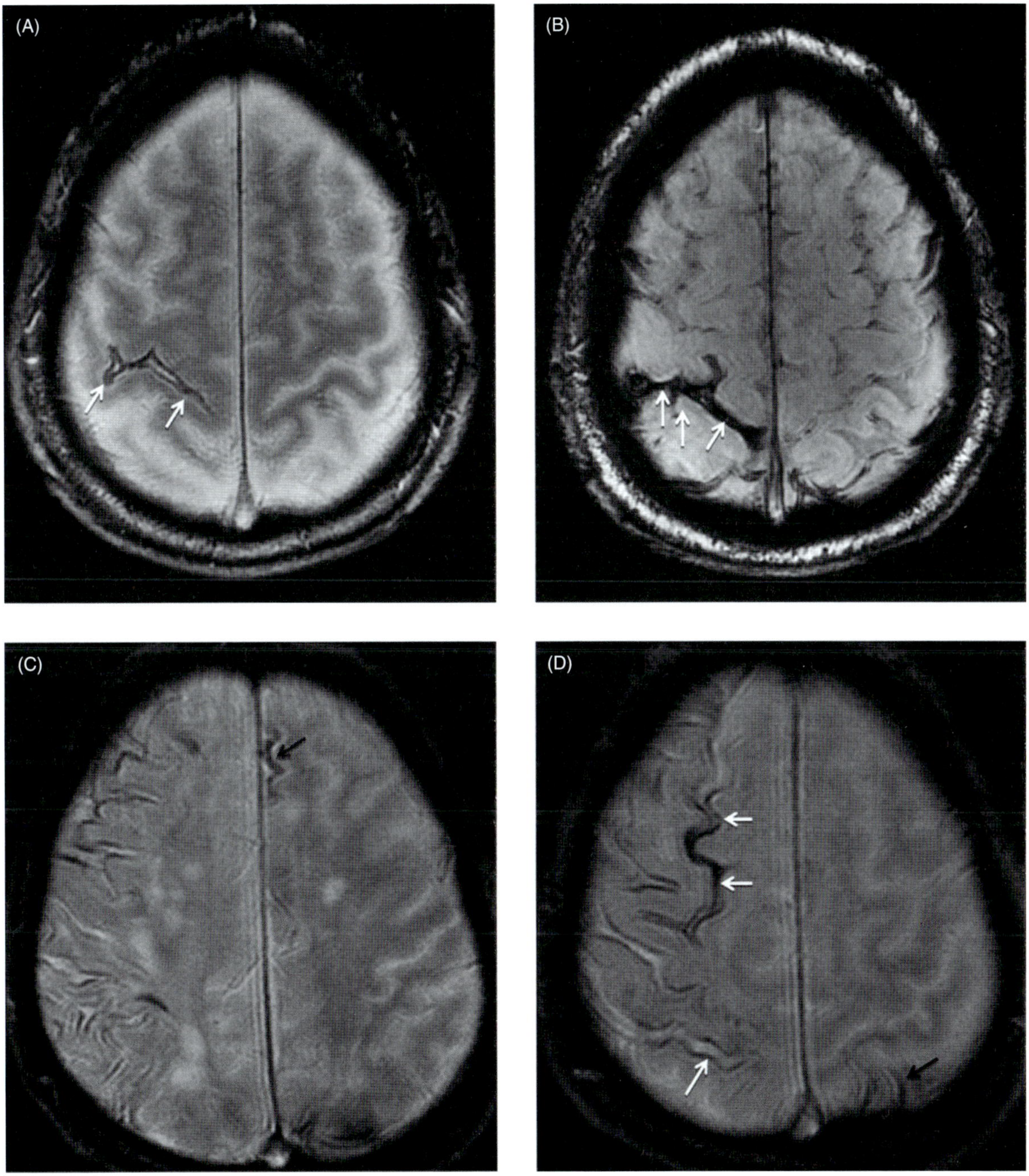

Figure 13.6 Magnetic resonance imaging (MRI) findings in supratentorial superficial siderosis (SS). Two different patients with possible cerebral amyloid angiopathy according to the modified Boston criteria (see Table 13.3) and focal (patient 1, A,B) and disseminated (patient 2, C,D) supratentorial SS (see, e.g., arrows). Depending on the exact localization of the hemosiderin, SS is delineated on T2*-gradient-recalled echo (GRE) (A,C,D) and susceptibility-weighted imaging (SWI) (B), either as a single linear hypointensity within the subarachnoid space, or as two almost parallel, bilinear hypointensities within the superficial cortical layers. This "track-like" appearance on axial sections is caused by the relatively high signal intensity of the normal-appearing subarachnoid space in the middle, which is bordered bilaterally by hypointense linear deposits of hemosiderin in the superficial layers of the adjacent cortex (e.g., arrows in A). Note that SS shows a more pronounced hypointense signal on SWI (B) compared to conventional T2*-GRE (A).

Pathophysiology of supratentorial SS

Two distinct etiologic types of intracranial SS should be distinguished. SS related to CSVD – more precisely to CAA – typically affects predominately and almost exclusively the supratentorial sulci and gyri of the cerebral convexity, whereas a second type of siderosis, namely the classical "SS of the central nervous system" primarily affects the *infratentorial* compartment (posterior fossa, brainstem, basal cisterns, and spinal cord) and is typically a feature of processes other than CSVD [88].

Although the two types of SS differ significantly with regard to their etiologies and clinical presentation, the pathomechanism underlying siderosis formation is similar. Both manifestations constitute residues of previous SAHs, deposited primarily in the form of hemosiderin-laden macrophages [80, 89]. While CSVD-related SS is formed by degradation of acute, restricted fSAHs, which can be either clinically silent or symptomatic (see Sporadic CAA section, below), infratentorial siderosis is caused by clinically inapparent *persistent* small bleedings into the subarachnoid space [88, 89]. These intermittent or continuous hemorrhages in infratentorial siderosis result from different underlying pathologies, such as CNS tumors, trauma, or head or spinal surgery [88]. Independent of the bleeding cause, this type of siderosis presents with rather invariant imaging findings and typical symptoms: slowly progressive gait ataxia, cerebellar dysarthria, sensorineural hearing impairment, and myelopathic signs [88], symptoms that are not found in CSVD-related SS.

Mimics of fSAHs and SS

To avoid misinterpretation, one has to be aware of potential mimics of fSAHs and SS. Besides fSAHs, sulcal hyperintensities on FLAIR-weighted images can be found in inflammatory and neoplastic meningeal diseases [90, 91], after intra-arterial administration of iodinated contrast media [92], and as a consequence of administration of oxygen during MRI due to the T1 shortening effect of the gas [93]. Furthermore, metal structures, as for example dental braces, can hamper fluid suppression and thus result in artificial hyperintense sulci on FLAIR [94]. On nonenhanced CT, partial volume effects caused by the adjacent bone might mimic or obscure fSAHs. In questionable cases, MRI might be indicated to prove or exclude fSAHs in such cases.

Important mimics of SS on T2*-GRE likewise include linear cortical or superficial calcifications, but also cortical vein thrombosis and normal cerebral vessels (especially veins). The calcifications can best be differentiated from SS on CT, based on their higher density. In cortical vein thrombosis, the intravascular clot usually causes a more pronounced blooming effect compared to SS on susceptibility-sensitive sequences, resulting in a tubular aspect on slices parallel to the lesion, and a round-to-oval cross-section on slices perpendicular to the lesion [81, 95]. In addition, the affected cortical veins, which do not run within the cortical sulci, but at the surface of the cerebral convexities, enables the differentiation between venous clot and SS. Analogous to thrombosed veins, normal cerebral veins can be distinguished from SS due to their different anatomic course.

Non-CSVD-related causes of fSAHs and SS: differential diagnosis

A wide variety of possible etiologies of nontraumatic fSAHs has been described in case reports or single-case series within the last decade [83, 96, 97]. However, recent studies show that CAA and reversible cerebral vasoconstriction syndrome (RCVS) constitute by far the most common causes of fSAHs, with CAA being responsible for most fSAHs in elderly patients (>60 years of age), and RCVS being the most likely etiology in younger patients [81, 82, 96–98].

Rare fSAH etiologies include primary angiitis of the central nervous system, secondary hyperperfusion syndrome, for example after carotid endarterectomy or carotid stenting, and cortical venous thrombosis [99–102].

All of the above fSAH causes can also result in SS, as a residuum of the acute hemorrhage, and thus have to be considered as potential differential diagnoses.

Imaging of hemorrhagic CSVDs: specific entities

Sporadic CAA

Sporadic CAA is defined as the deposition of β-amyloid (Aβ) in the walls of the cortical and leptomeningeal cerebral vessels [103–105]. CAA predominately presents with hemorrhagic manifestations, although concomitant ischemic lesions are also found (e.g., white matter lesions [WMLs], microinfarctions) [106]. Current in vivo diagnostic criteria for CAA rely primarily on the presence of hemorrhagic lesions [81, 107].

CAA pathology is very common in the elderly population, with prevalence rates of over 60% in the very old, and is associated with Alzheimer's disease pathology [103–105]. The Aβ deposits in sporadic CAA are predominately found in the occipital lobes, followed by the frontal, temporal, and parietal lobes [108–111]. In advanced stages of the disease, the cerebellum can also be affected, while the deep gray nuclei, the white matter, and the brainstem are typically spared [112]. This characteristic topographic distribution of the vascular amyloid deposits mirrors the anatomic localization of the parenchymal hemorrhagic lesions in the disease. On tissue examination, vascular amyloid typically shows a patchy pattern, with foci of severely affected vessels found adjacent to areas with mild or absent vascular Aβ deposition [108].

One of the most devastating consequences of CAA is symptomatic, lobar ICH [113]. A lobar ICH is defined as a macrohemorrhage in cortical and/or subcortical localization (i.e., at the gray–white matter interface) – as opposed to deep ICHs in hypertension-related microangiopathy, which are typically located in the deep gray nuclei or brainstem (Figure 13.7). Lobar hemorrhages are more commonly located in the posterior regions (occipital and posterior temporal lobes). Patients who have suffered a lobar ICH are at high risk of recurrence, and these hemorrhages are important sources of morbidity and mortality in the disease [108, 110, 113, 114]. Sporadic CAA accounts for 15–20% of all "primary" ICHs in patients older than 60 years, and thus constitutes a major risk factor for ICH in elderly patients. CAA should be considered as cause of a nontraumatic ICH in any patient older than 55 years who presents with at least one lobar parenchymal hemorrhage. With a recurrence rate of approximately 10% per year in elderly cohorts, survivors of lobar ICH are at higher risk of ICH recurrence compared to patients with non-CAA-related deep ICHs [108, 113, 115–117]. Recurrent ICHs in CAA patients often affect the same lobe as the initial hemorrhage [113]. On T2*-GRE imaging, residues of smaller, clinically inapparent previous ICHs might be detected in patients presenting with an acute lobar ICH. The main known risk factors for recurrence of CAA-related ICH are apolipoprotein E (APOE) ε2 or ε4 alleles, previous ICHs, and CMBs on follow-up imaging [116, 118].

In addition to acute lobar ICHs, characteristic MRI biomarkers of CAA include:

- (Multiple) CMBs
- Acute fSAHs
- Supratentorial SS
- Patchy or confluent microangiopathic WMLs (mWMLs), and
- Silent acute, cerebral microinfarcts.

Analogous to large symptomatic ICHs, CAA-related CMBs typically show a lobar, cortical–subcortical distribution, with a predilection for posterior lobar regions [113, 119], while basal ganglia, thalami, and brainstem are spared (Figure 13.8). The burden of

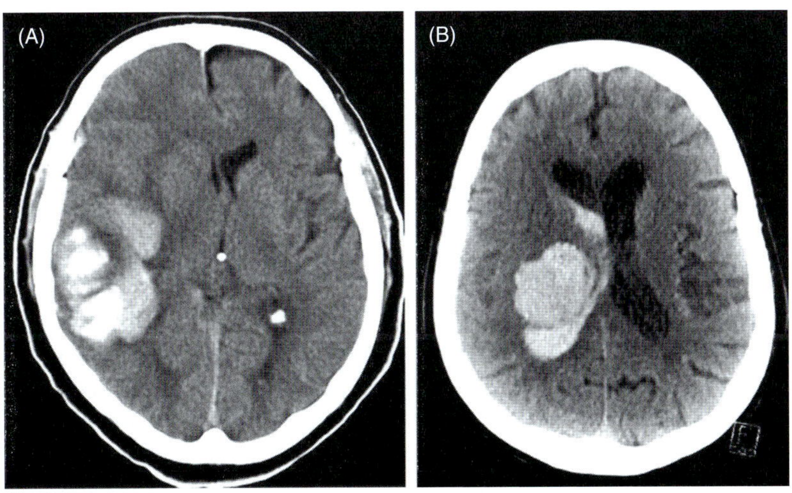

Figure 13.7 Lobar versus deep intracerebral hemorrhages (ICHs). (A) Unenhanced computed tomography (CT) in a patient with probable cerebral amyloid angiopathy (CAA) according to the modified Boston criteria (see Table 13.3) and an acute lobar ICH in the right temporal lobe. Note the characteristic cortical and/or subcortical localization of CAA-related lobar ICHs. (B) Unenhanced CT in a patient with hypertension-related microangiopathy and an acute, deep ICH in the right thalamus, which has ruptured into the lateral ventricle.

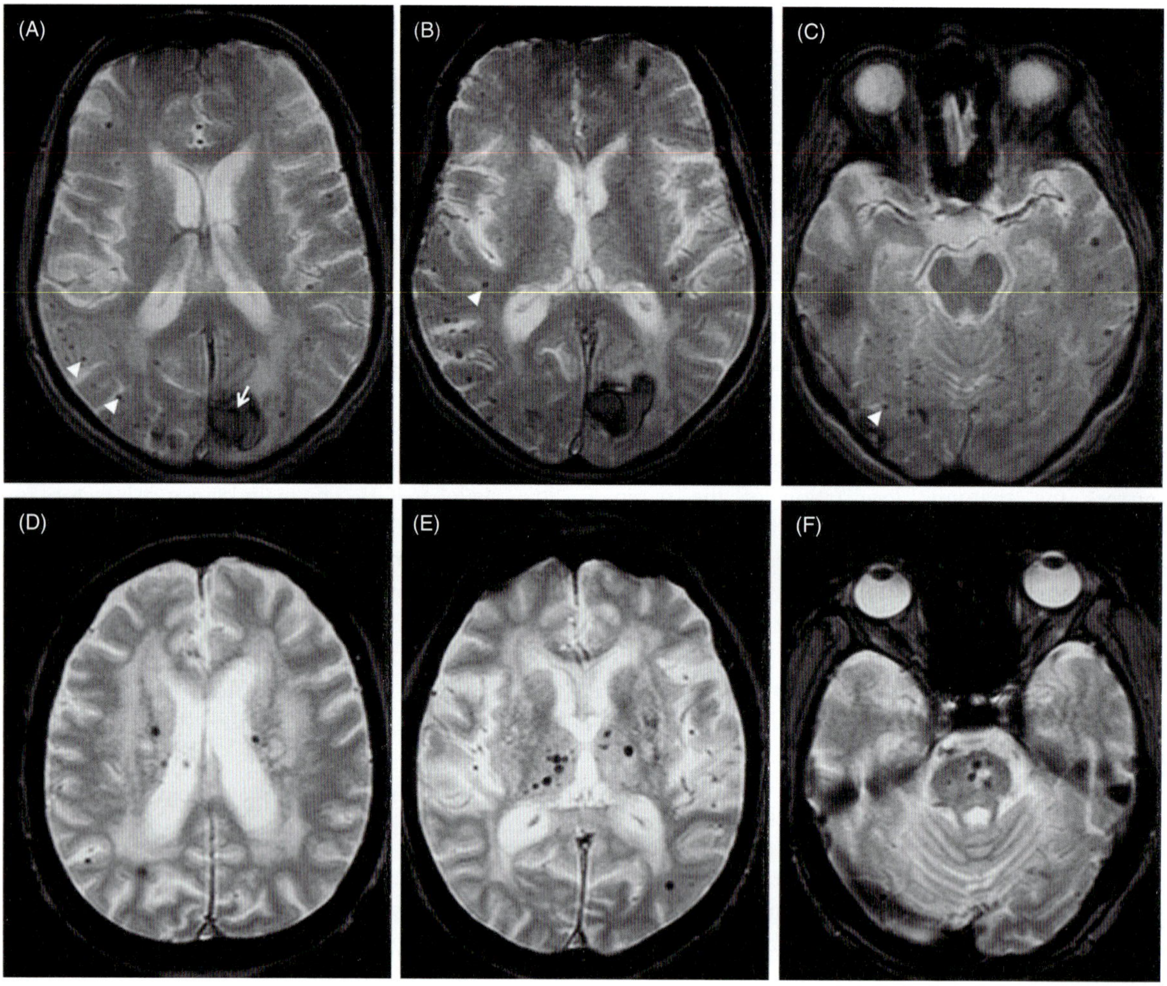

Figure 13.8 Different localization of cerebral microbleeds (CMBs) in cerebral amyloid angiopathy (CAA) and hypertension-related microangiopathy. (A–C) A 69-year-old patient with probable CAA according to the Boston criteria (see Table 13.3). T2*-gradient-recalled echo (GRE) images show multiple CAA-related CMBs in a lobar, cortical–subcortical distribution (e.g., arrow heads in A–C), and a recent lobar intracerebral macrohemorrhage (normal arrow in A). Note that CAA-related CMBs typically spare the basal ganglia, the thalami, and the brainstem. (D–F) An 84-year-old patient with hypertension-related microangiopathy and multiple deep CMBs, which are particularly located in the thalami and the pons.

CMBs correlates with the risk of recurrent lobar ICH [116], which indicates not only a diagnostic, but also a prognostic role for CMBs in CAA. By combining T2*-GRE MRI and noninvasive Pittsburgh Compound B (PiB) amyloid imaging, a cross-sectional study demonstrated increased PiB retention at the location of CMBs compared to simulated control lesions. This association was also seen in a longitudinal study examining the relationship of PiB to the location of new CMBs in CAA [120]. These findings indicate that CAA-related CMBs occur preferentially in local regions of concentrated amyloid [121].

Several large community-dwelling studies have found strictly lobar CMBs in a considerable percentage of the elderly general population (range: 6.4–23.5%) [40, 41, 43–45]. Strictly lobar CMBs were also strongly associated with the APOE ε4 allele, an important risk factor for sporadic CAA, in these study populations [122]. These findings strongly indicate that strictly lobar CMBs might be a marker of subclinical CAA. If the significance of strictly lobar CMBs as preclinical indicators of CAA can be validated in further studies, they might serve as important biomarkers to identify presymptomatic individuals who could benefit from new therapeutic agents.

In recent years, acute fSAHs and SS, as residues of previous fSAHs, have been recognized as new important imaging biomarkers of CAA [80–83, 98] (Figure 13.6). In a cohort with histologically proven sporadic CAA, focal or disseminated SS was found with a prevalence of >60% [81].

Based on several case reports and small case series, it is hypothesized that fSAHs and SS may be responsible for the transient neurologic symptoms observed in CAA patients [83, 123–126]. These deficits are often stereotypical (transient hemiparesis or hemihypesthesia) and have been described by different authors as "transient-ischemic-attack-like," "aura-like," "migraineous," or as "focal seizures" [124, 125, 127, 128]. The fSAHs detected in these patients most commonly affect the central sulcus [124, 125, 127, 128]. However, T2*-GRE MRI in these patients often reveals a disseminated SS that involves other parts of the cerebral convexities as well [125]. This observation implies that symptomatic, acute fSAHs might only represent the "tip of the iceberg," while SAHs in other, less eloquent cortical regions might be clinically asymptomatic and go unimaged in the acute phase. Systematic prospective data on the prevalence and incidence of acute CAA-related fSAHs are lacking.

In addition to their relevance as a presumptive cause of transient neurologic symptoms in CAA patients, fSAHs and SS might be of prognostic value in CAA patients. During a median follow-up time period of 35.3 months, a recent study on 51 patients with SS and possible or probable CAA according to the modified Boston criteria observed any new ICHs in 35.3% of patients. In 25.5% of cases, ICH on follow-up was located immediately adjacent to the pre-existing SS [129]. These retrospective data may suggest that patients with SS are at high risk for subsequent ICH at the site of pre-existing SS, and that SS might be considered as a warning sign for future ICH at its location. However, the precise anatomic relationships between amyloid burden, fSAH, and SS, as well as the clinical and prognostic significance of these findings in CAA, still need to be determined in larger, prospective studies.

Patchy-to-confluent periventricular and deep mWMLs are another very common finding in CAA. While some studies found no major difference between CAA-related mWMLs and mWMLs due to hypertension-related microangiopathy [130, 131], others found a preferential involvement of the posterior regions [131, 132] (Figure 13.9). There is evidence that CAA-related mWMLs might be caused by chronic hypoperfusion of the periventricular white matter and disruption of the blood–brain barrier secondary to amyloid deposits in the cortical small vessels [133–135], or might result from accumulation of silent ischemic lesions [136–138].

While asymptomatic ischemic infarcts are a well-known histopathological finding in advanced stages of CAA [139–143], these lesions have only recently

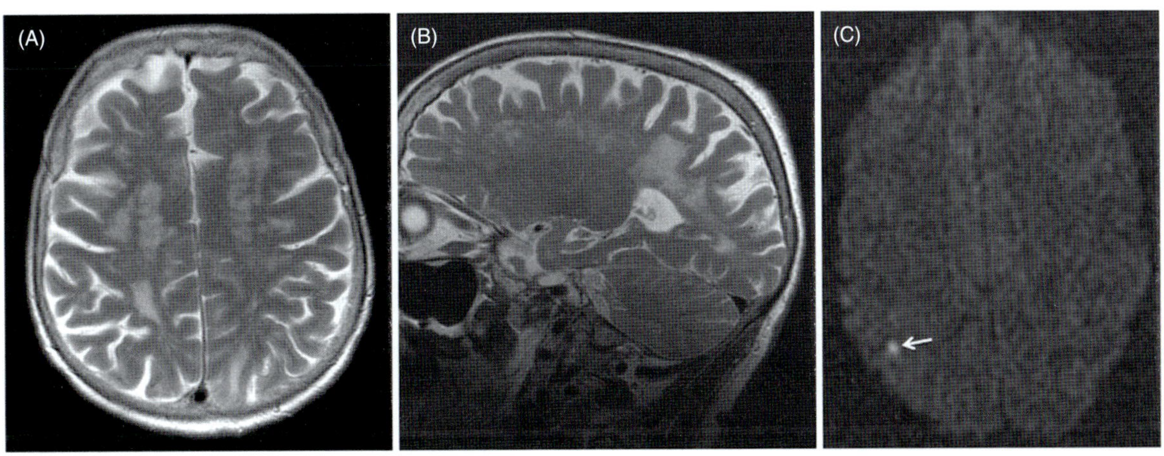

Figure 13.9 Examples of non-hemorrhagic lesions in cerebral amyloid angiopathy (CAA). A 69-year-old patient with probable CAA according to the Boston criteria (see Table 13.3). Axial (A) and sagittal (B) views reveal patchy to confluent periventricular and microangiopathic white matter lesions, with a preferential involvement of the posterior regions (i.e. the parietal white matter). Diffusion-weighted magnetic resonance imaging (MRI) (C) detects a silent cortical microinfarct in the right parietal lobe, which shows a hyperintense signal on diffusion-weighted imaging due to diffusion-restriction (arrows in C).

been recognized as a frequent imaging finding in this disease [136, 144]. Diffusion-weighted imaging, as the most sensitive method for the detection of acute ischemic lesions, reveals a high prevalence of asymptomatic ("silent") acute ischemic lesions in patients with advanced CAA. These lesions are associated with mWML severity and CMB burden and are frequently found after recent ICHs [137, 145, 146].

A distinct clinical and imaging manifestation, characterized by subacute cognitive decline, seizures, and diffuse hyperintensities attributed to vasogenic edema, has been observed in a subset of CAA patients. This acute presentation of CAA is associated with evidence of vasculitis or perivascular inflammation on histopathologic tissue examination, and thus referred to as CAA-related inflammation (CAA-RI) [147–152]. It is important to be aware of this specific entity because it represents a potentially treatable cause of rapid cognitive decline, and because a favorable response to immunosuppressive therapy such as corticosteroids is common. Typical imaging findings include patchy or confluent, asymmetric white matter hyperintensities, which can present with a local mass effect resembling a tumor [152, 153], but likely reflect vasogenic edema. Patchy leptomeningeal or parenchymal contrast enhancement have been reported in some cases, and concomitant CMBs are found in the wide majority of patients (Figure 13.10). DSA might reveal subtle irregularities of the distal branches of the cerebral arteries in a subset of patients, but is normal in most cases [152]. In 2011, Chung et al. [152] proposed diagnostic criteria for CAA-RI based on the clinical and imaging findings in published cases (Table 13.2). The major differential diagnoses of CAA-RI include posterior reversible encephalopathy syndrome (PRES), infectious diseases (particularly progressive multifocal leukoencephalopathy), acute disseminated encephalomyelitis, and neoplastic disorders (e.g., primary central nervous system lymphoma and gliomatosis cerebri) [152].

The underlying pathomechanism of CAA-RI is not yet completely understood. However, presence of autoantibodies to Aβ40 and Aβ42 in the CSF of affected patients suggests an immune response against vascular Aβ deposits as a potential cause [81]. Interestingly, imaging and clinical findings of CAA-RI are strikingly similar to parenchymal changes observed as an adverse event in clinical Alzheimer therapy trials with bapineuzumab, an Aβ42 antibody [154]. These changes predominantly occurred in patients receiving higher antibody doses and in APOE ε4 allele carriers, supporting a role of anti-Aβ antibodies and APOE ε4 alleles in the pathomechanism of spontaneous CAA-RI.

To date, there exists no diagnostic test that allows the definite diagnosis of CAA during life. The "classical" and the "modified" Boston criteria estimate the likelihood of the presence of CAA in vivo, with categories of possible and probable CAA based on the pattern of intracranial hemorrhagic lesions on neuroimaging studies [81, 107]. The "classical" Boston criteria require the presence of one or more hemorrhages restricted to lobar, cortical, or corticosubcortical regions, including cerebellar hemorrhages in patients over 55 years of age, for the diagnosis of possible or probable CAA, respectively [107] (Table 13.3). The initial criteria do not comment on the size of the lobar hemorrhages; however, it has been shown recently that inclusion of corticosubcortical CMBs as "hemorrhages" in terms of the criteria

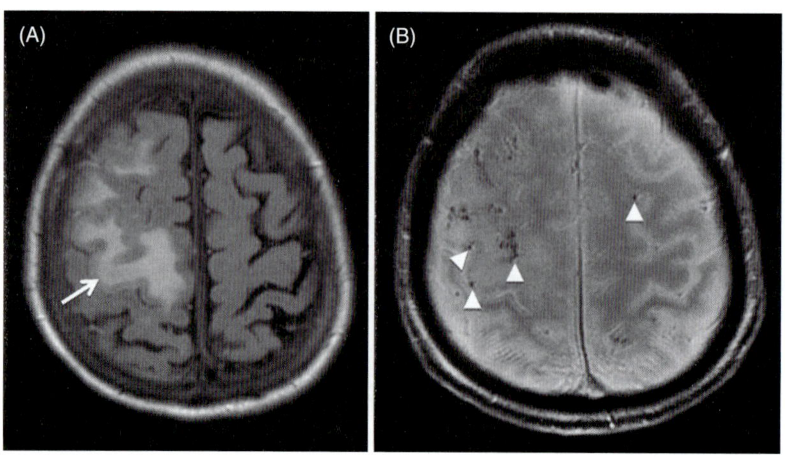

Figure 13.10 Inflammatory subtype of cerebral amyloid angiopathy (CAA-RI). A 78-year-old patient with histologically proven inflammatory subtype of cerebral amyloid angiopathy (CAA-I). (A) Fluid-attenuated inversion recovery (FLAIR)-weighted sequence shows confluent, asymmetric leukencephalopathic changes with a subtle local mass effect in the right frontal white matter with involvement of the subcortical U-fibers (e.g., arrow in A). (B) T2*-gradient-recalled echo (GRE) reveals multiple associated cerebral microbleeds in cortical and subcortical localization (e.g., arrowheads in B).

Table 13.2 Diagnostic criteria for CAA-I*

Probable CAA-I

All of the following:

- Acute or subacute onset of symptoms
- 40 years of age or older
- At least one of the following clinical features: headache, mental status or behavioral change, focal neurologic signs, and seizure
- MRI shows patchy or confluent T2 or FLAIR hyperintensity which is:
    - usually asymmetric
    - with or without mass effect
    - with or without leptomeningeal or parenchymal enhancement
- Evidence of pre-existing CAA on susceptibility-weighted MRI sequences:
    - multiple cortical and subcortical hemorrhages or microhemorrhages and/or
    - recent or past lobar hemorrhage
- Absence of neoplastic, infectious, or other cause

Definite CAA-I

All of the above plus histopathologic confirmation with:

- Perivascular, transmural, and/or intramural inflammation
- Amyloid deposition within vessels of affected area in the cortex and leptomeninges

* As proposed by Chung et al. [152].

CAA, cerebral amyloid angiopathy; CAA-I, inflammatory subtype of cerebral amyloid angiopathy; FLAIR, fluid-attenuated inversion recovery; MRI, magnetic resonance imaging.

increases their sensitivity [155]. Based on the finding that SS can be the only pathologic MRI finding in patients with histologically proven CAA, "modified" Boston criteria including SS as an imaging sign of CAA have been proposed [81] (Table 13.3). This modification increases the sensitivity of these criteria without limiting their specificity [81].

As detailed above, T2*-GRE and SWI are very sensitive for acute, subacute, and chronic blood products, and thus are ideally suited to detect the variety of hemorrhagic manifestations in CAA (ICH, CMBs, SS, and fSAH). To detect or exclude acute fSAHs and CAA-related mWMLs, the MRI protocol in suspected CAA should also include FLAIR- and/or proton-density- or T2-weighted sequences. In addition, diffusion-weighted imaging is recommended to detect subclinical small microinfarcts. CTA, MRA, and DSA are typically normal in patients with CAA. The potential additive value of recently developed positron emission tomography (PET) amyloid tracers for in vivo detection of intracranial amyloid deposits in CAA is discussed below.

Hypertension-related microangiopathy

This very common sporadic form of CSVD has been variously termed degenerative microangiopathy, hypertensive microangiopathy, or arteriolosclerosis in the literature [133, 156–158]. Advanced age, arterial hypertension, diabetes mellitus, and additional risk factors (e.g., nicotine, hypercholesteremia) [133, 157, 159] result in chronic microangiopathic changes of the deep perforating arteries originating from the middle, anterior, or posterior cerebral arteries, or from the basilar artery.

Histopathologically, severe arteriolosclerosis and thickening of the vessel walls due to lipohyalinotic changes (known as lipohyalinosis, plasmatic vascular destruction, and acute hypertensive fibrinoid necrosis) as well as pseudoaneurysms, indicating a degeneration of the media and smooth vessels, are observed [158, 160–164]. These microvascular changes presumably lead to a reduced compliance of the vessel walls, and thus to an impaired vasoreactivity [160]. As a consequence, both ischemic and hemorrhagic parenchymal lesions are found in the vascular territories of the affected deep penetrating arteries.

Patchy-to-confluent hypertension-related mWMLs typically affect the deep and periventricular white matter and the pons, and usually spare the subcortical U-fibers, the external capsule, and the corpus callosum. In addition to mWMLs, lacunar infarcts in the deep gray nuclei (basal ganglia and thalami), the internal capsule, the brainstem, and the deep and

Table 13.3 Classic and modified Boston criteria for CAA-related hemorrhage

	Classic Boston criteria	Modified Boston criteria
Definite CAA	*Full postmortem examination demonstrating:* • Lobar, cortical, or corticosubcortical hemorrhage • Severe CAA with vasculopathy • Absence of other diagnostic lesion	No modification
Probable CAA with supporting pathology	*Clinical data and pathologic tissue (evacuated hematoma or cortical biopsy) demonstrating:* • Lobar, cortical, or corticosubcortical hemorrhage • Some degree of CAA in specimen • Absence of other diagnostic lesion	No modification
Probable CAA	*Clinical data and MRI or CT demonstrating:* • Multiple hemorrhages restricted to lobar, cortical, cortical or corticosubcortical regions • Age ≥55 years • Absence of other cause of hemorrhage	*Clinical data and MRI or CT demonstrating:* • Multiple hemorrhages restricted to lobar, or corticosubcortical regions (cerebellar hemorrhage allowed) or • Single lobar, cortical, or corticosubcortical hemorrhage *and* focal* or disseminated† superficial siderosis • Age ≥55 years • Absence of other cause of hemorrhage or superficial siderosis
Possible CAA	*Clinical data and MRI or CT demonstrating:* • Single lobar, cortical, or corticosubcortical hemorrhage • Age ≥55 years • Absence of other cause of hemorrhage	*Clinical data and MRI or CT demonstrating:* • Single lobar, cortical, or corticosubcortical hemorrhage *or* • Focal* or disseminated† superficial siderosis • Age ≥55 years • Absence of other cause of hemorrhage or superficial siderosis

See Linn et al. [81] and Knudsen et al. [107].
* Siderosis restricted to three or fewer sulci.
† Siderosis affecting at least four sulci.
CAA, cerebral amyloid angiopathy; CT, computed tomography; MRI, magnetic resonance imaging.

perivascular white matter are an imaging hallmark of hypertension-related microangiopathy. The lacunar infarcts within the basal ganglia and thalami are most probably due to chronic lipohyalinosis and atheromatous changes, while arteriolosclerosis is thought to be predominately responsible for mWMLs and white matter lacunar infarcts [158]. Multiple CMBs in basal ganglia, thalami, brainstem, and cerebellum are found in approximately 1–5% of all cases with hypertension-related microangiopathy and are regularly present in advanced disease stages [163, 164] (Figure 13.8D–F). Recently, dilated perivascular spaces in deep areas have been considered as an additional imaging marker of hypertension-related microangiopathy, but further studies are needed to determine their diagnostic relevance for this disease [165–167].

Acute ICHs constitute the most devastating complication of hypertension-related microangiopathy, and are due to fibrinoid necrosis. Analogous to CMBs and lacunar strokes, acute hypertension-related ICHs are most commonly found in the basal ganglia (60–65%) and the thalamus (15–25%) (brain areas that are supplied by small perforating arteries from the middle and posterior cerebral arteries, Figure 13.7B). The pons and the cerebellum are affected in 10% of cases, while lobar ICHs are rare in hypertension-related microangiopathy. Although secondary intraventricular hemorrhages can occur in any ICHs, thalamic hemorrhages are especially prone to rupture into the ventricles. Intraventricular hemorrhages can result in hydrocephalus due to impairment of CSF circulation resulting from blood clots within the foramina or the aqueduct and this represents a risk factor for poor outcome [168].

MRA, CTA, and DSA might show an elongation of the intracranial vessels in patients with hypertension-related microangiopathy, which reflects secondary changes due to long-standing severe arterial hypertension, but are otherwise typically normal.

Uncommon causes of hemorrhagic CSVD

Hereditary CAA

Besides the very common sporadic form of CAA, a wide variety of rare, hereditary forms of CAA have been recognized and genetically characterized [169–172]. Although they are very rare diseases that tend to present in the form of autosomal-dominant disorders in selected families, they have served as important disease models for the common sporadic forms [169–172]. Hereditary subtypes of CAA include both Aβ and non-Aβ forms of vascular deposits. Lobar ICHs are characteristic of the Aβ-forms and of the non-Aβ–Icelandic type [173].

Hereditary cerebral hemorrhage with amyloidosis–Dutch type (HCHWA-D), initially described in families from two villages in the Netherlands, is the most thoroughly characterized hereditary CAA. It is caused by a single base mutation (G for C nucleotide change) at codon 693 of the amyloid precursor protein gene on chromosome 21 [174], and presents clinically with strokes (predominately of the hemorrhagic type) and cognitive impairment [155, 175]. MR findings in HCHWA-D are rather similar to sporadic CAA and include ICHs, CMBs, SS, and mWMLs [155]. Analogous to sporadic CAA, ICHs and CMBs are found in exclusively lobar and cortico-subcortical localizations or the cerebellum, while basal ganglia, thalamus, and brainstem are spared [155]. CMBs are regularly found in symptomatic patients, but can also be present in asymptomatic mutation carriers [176, 177].

COL4A1-related CSVD

In recent years, mutations in the *COL4A1* gene encoding the type IV collagen alpha-1 chain have been recognized as a further monogenic cause of SVD [178]. This familial vasculopathy can have ischemic and hemorrhagic manifestations in both children and adults. Infantile hemiparesis or congenital porencephaly (likely due to perinatal hemorrhages) are the most common pediatric manifestations of the disease. Brain MRI findings are not specific and include diffuse mWMLs (63.5%), deep and subcortical CMBs (52.9%), lacunar strokes (13.5%), and dilated perivascular spaces (19.2%). In addition, intracranial aneurysms are found in over 40% of subjects (255), and patients can suffer from symptomatic ICHs [179–183]. Additionally, marked tortuosity of medium and small retinal arterioles (without capillary abnormalities, vessel tortuosity, retinal ischemic changes, or visual loss) has been associated with the mutation. These retinal arteriole abnormalities appear to be either asymptomatic or responsible for retinal hemorrhages and transient visual loss in the disease [183].

New approaches in the imaging of CSVD

Functional MRI

Functional MRI (fMRI) enables the indirect in vivo visualization of brain function both in resting state and in response to external tasks. fMRI studies on patients with specific hemorrhagic CSVD are sparse, but might provide further insight into their underlying pathomechanisms and the link between vascular damage and brain function. As an example, a recent fMRI study in patients with probable CAA identified significant differences in the response to visual stimulation in patients with advanced CAA compared to controls, suggesting impaired vascular reactivity to physiologic stimuli [184].

Molecular in vivo imaging of vascular amyloid

While MRI abnormalities reflect the consequences of Aβ deposition in the brain, the recent development of amyloid-specific PET radioligands for the first time enabled its direct in vivo detection. The most widely studied amyloid tracer to date is ^{11}C-Pittsburgh Compound B (^{11}C-PiB), which binds to parenchymal and vascular Aβ in the brain. CAA patients show an increased global PiB uptake compared to healthy elderly controls, with an occipital predominance of PiB retention in CAA compared to those patients with Alzheimer's disease [185, 186]. As discussed above, analysis of the spatial relationship between CMBs and amyloid deposits as revealed by PiB retention indicates that CMBs are preferentially located in regions with concentrated amyloid [121]. In addition, Aβ deposition in asymptomatic elderly subjects correlated significantly with presence of lobar CMBs [187]. These data suggest that amyloid PET might allow the definite detection of CAA in vivo, even in asymptomatic stages of the disease, and thus might be of important value with regard to disease monitoring and future treatment strategies. However, it has to be taken into account that ^{11}C-PiB and other amyloid tracers label not only vascular but also senile plaque amyloid, which limits their specificity for the diagnosis of CAA. Recently, the phenoxazine derivate resorufin has been reported to bind preferentially to vascular amyloid in transgenic mice, and thus might have potential as a CAA-specific amyloid tracer [188].

Ultra-high field MRI

Ultra-high field MRI at field strengths of 7 Tesla or more provides another very promising method for in vivo diagnosis of CSVDs, by enhancing both spatial resolution and susceptibility effect (see also Role of magnetic field strength section, above). Ultra-high field MRI would be expected to have higher sensitivity for parenchymal blood products, and thus might have important impact on early diagnosis of hemorrhagic cerebral microangiopathies [189]. In addition to its potential improvement regarding the delineation of the classical MRI signs of CSVD, ultra-high field MRI might also detect abnormalities which cannot be revealed at standard field strength. A postmortem study on formalin-fixed brain samples found hypointense foci in all specimens with histologic evidence of cerebral amyloid deposition, but not in controls. The authors hypothesized that their findings might open up the possibility for direct MRI visualization of amyloid deposition [190]. Further studies are needed to determine the additive value of ultra-high field MRI for the diagnostic evaluation of CSVD.

References

1. Fewel ME, Thompson BG Jr, Hoff JT. Spontaneous intracerebral hemorrhage: a review. *Neurosurg Focus* 2003;15:1–16.
2. Qureshi AI, Tuhrim S, Broderick JP, et al. Spontaneous intracerebral hemorrhage. *N Engl J Med* 2001;344:1450–1460.
3. Linn J, Brückmann H. Differential diagnosis of nontraumatic intracerebral hemorrhage. *Klin Neuroradiol* 2009;19:45–61.
4. Foulkes MA, Wolf PA, Price TR, Mohr JP, Hier DB. The Stroke Data Bank: design, methods, and baseline characteristics. *Stroke* 1988;19:547–554.
5. Parizel PM, Makkat S, van Miert E, et al. Intracranial hemorrhage: principles of CT and MRI interpretation. *Eur Radiol* 2001;11:1770–1783.
6. Khosravani H, Mayer SA, Demchuk A, et al. Emergency noninvasive angiography for acute intracerebral hemorrhage. *AJNR Am J Neuroradiol* 2013; 34:1481–1487.
7. Delgado Almandoz JE, Schaefer PW, Forero NP, et al. Diagnostic accuracy and yield of multidetector CT angiography in the evaluation of spontaneous intraparenchymal cerebral hemorrhage. *AJNR Am J Neuroradiol* 2009;30:1213–1221.
8. Yeung R, Ahmad T, Aviv RI, et al. Comparison of CTA to DSA in determining the etiology of spontaneous ICH. *Can J Neurol Sci* 2009;36:176–180.
9. Zhu XL, Chan MS, Poon WS. Spontaneous intracranial hemorrhage: which patients need diagnostic cerebral angiography? A prospective study of 206 cases and review of the literature. *Stroke* 1997;28:1406–1409.
10. Kim J, Smith A, Hemphill JC, 3rd, et al. Contrast extravasation on CT predicts mortality in primary intracerebral hemorrhage. *AJNR Am J Neuroradiol* 2008; 29:520–525.
11. Wada R, Aviv RI, Fox AJ. CT angiography "spot sign" predicts hematoma expansion in acute intracerebral hemorrhage. *Stroke* 2007;38:1257–1262.
12. Demchuk AM, Dowlatshahi D, Rodriguez-Luna D, et al. PREDICT/Sunnybrook ICH CTA Study Group. Prediction of haematoma growth and outcome in patients with intracerebral haemorrhage using the CT-angiography spot sign (PREDICT): a prospective observational study. *Lancet Neurol* 2012;11:307–314.
13. Koculym A, Huynh TJ, Jakubovic R, Zhang L, Aviv RI. CT perfusion spot sign improves sensitivity for prediction of outcome compared with CTA and postcontrast CT. *AJNR Am J Neuroradiol* 2013;34:965–970.
14. Fiebach JB, Schellinger PD, Gass A, et al. Stroke magnetic

resonance imaging is accurate in hyperacute intracerebral hemorrhage: a multicenter study on the validity of stroke imaging. *Stroke* 2004;35:502–506.

15. Kidwell CS, Chalela JA, Saver JL, et al. Comparison of MRI and CT for detection of acute intracerebral hemorrhage. *JAMA* 2004;292:1823–1830.
16. Lummel N, Lutz J, Brückmann H, Linn J. The value of magnetic resonance imaging for the detection of the bleeding source in non-traumatic intracerebral haemorrhages: a comparison with conventional digital subtraction angiography. *Neuroradiology* 2012;54:673–680.
17. Bradley WG Jr. MR appearance of hemorrhage in the brain. *Radiology* 1993;189:15–26.
18. Hayman LA, Taber KH, Ford JJ, Bryan RN. Mechanisms of MR signal alteration by acute intracerebral blood: old concepts and new theories. *AJNR Am J Neuroradiol* 1991;12:899–907.
19. Linn J, Wiesmann M, Brückmann H, eds. [*Atlas Klinische Neuroradiologie.*] Berlin: Springer-Verlag; 2011 [in German].
20. Allkemper T, Tombach B, Schwindt W, et al. Acute and subacute intracerebral hemorrhages: comparison of MR imaging at 1.5 and 3.0 T – initial experience. *Radiology* 2004;232:874–881.
21. Sohn CH, Baik SK, Lee HJ, et al. MR imaging of hyperacute subarachnoid and intraventricular hemorrhage at 3T: a preliminary report of gradient echo T2*-weighted sequences. *AJNR Am J Neuroradiol* 2005;26:662–665.
22. Seidenwurm D, Meng TK, Kowalski H, Weinreb JC, Kricheff II. Intracranial hemorrhagic lesions: evaluation with spinecho and gradient-refocused MR imaging at 0.5 and 1.5 T. *Radiology* 1989;172:189–194.
23. Hadizadeh DR, Falkenhausen M von, Gieske J, et al. Cerebral arteriovenous malformation: Spetzler–Martin classification at subsecond-temporal-resolution four-dimensional MR angiography compared with that at DSA. *Radiology* 2008;246: 205–213.
24. Unlu E, Temizoz O, Albayram S, et al. Contrast-enhanced MR 3D angiography in the assessment of brain AVMs. *Eur J Radiol* 2006;60:367–368.
25. Taschner CA, Gieseke J, Le Thuc V, et al. Intracranial arteriovenous malformations: time-resolved contrast-enhanced MR angiography with combination of parallel imaging, keyhole acquisition, and k-space sampling techniques at 1.5 T. *Radiology* 2008;246:871–879.
26. Meckel S, Maier M, Ruiz DS, et al. MR angiography of dural arteriovenous fistulas: diagnosis and follow-up after treatment using a time-resolved 3D contrast-enhanced technique. *AJNR Am J Neuroradiol* 2007;28:877–884.
27. Fasulakis S, Andronikou S. Comparison of MR angiography and conventional angiography in the investigation of intracranial arteriovenous malformations and aneurysms in children. *Pediatr Radiol* 2003;33:378–384.
28. Wintermark M, Dillon WP. Advanced CT and MR imaging techniques: an academic whim or a clinical standard in the making? *AJNR Am J Neuroradiol* 2006;27:1257.
29. Werring DJ, Frazer DW, Coward LJ, et al. Cognitive dysfunction in patients with cerebral microbleeds on T2*-weighted gradient-echo MRI. *Brain* 2004;127:2265–2275.
30. Cordonnier C. Brain microbleeds: more evidence, but still a clinical dilemma. *Curr Opin Neurol* 2011;24:69–74.
31. Greenberg SM, Vernooij MW, Cordonnier C, et al. Microbleed Study Group. Cerebral microbleeds: a guide to detection and interpretation. *Lancet Neurol* 2009;8:165–174.
32. Offenbacher H, Fazekas F, Schmidt R, et al. MR of cerebral abnormalities concomitant with primary intracerebral hematomas. *AJNR Am J Neuroradiol* 1996;17:573–578.
33. Fazekas F, Kleinert R, Roob G, et al. Histopathologic analysis of foci of signal loss on gradient-echo T2*-weighted MR images in patients with spontaneous intracerebral hemorrhage: evidence of microangiopathy-related microbleeds. *AJNR Am J Neuroradiol* 1999;20: 637–642.
34. Cordonnier C, Al-Shahi Salman R, Wardlaw J. Spontaneous brain microbleeds: systematic review, subgroup analyses and standards for study design and reporting. *Brain* 2007;130:1988–2003.
35. Nandigam RN, Viswanathan A, Delgado P, et al. MR imaging detection of cerebral microbleeds: effect of susceptibility-weighted imaging, section thickness, and field strength. *AJNR Am J Neuroradiol* 2009;30:338–43.
36. Greenberg SM, Nandigam RN, Delgado P, et al. Microbleeds versus macrobleeds: evidence for distinct entities. *Stroke* 2009;40:2382–2386.
37. Koennecke HC. Cerebral microbleeds on MRI: prevalence, associations, and potential clinical implications. *Neurology* 2006;66:165–171.
38. Viswanathan A, Chabriat H. Cerebral microhemorrhage. *Stroke* 2006;37:550–555.
39. Fiehler J. Cerebral microbleeds: old leaks and new haemorrhages. *Int J Stroke* 2006;1:122–130.
40. Horita Y, Imaizumi T, Niwa J, et al. [Analysis of dot-like hemosiderin spots using brain dock system.] *No Shinkei Geka* 2003;31:263–267 [in Japanese].

41. Jeerakathil T, Wolf PA, Beiser A, et al. Cerebral microbleeds: prevalence and associations with cardiovascular risk factors in the Framingham study. *Stroke* 2004;35:1831–1835.

42. Poels MM, Vernooij MW, Ikram MA, et al. Prevalence and risk factors of cerebral microbleeds: an update of the Rotterdam Scan Study. *Stroke* 2010;41(Suppl 10): S103–S106.

43. Roob G, Schmidt R, Kapeller P, et al. MRI evidence of past cerebral microbleeds in a healthy elderly population. *Neurology* 1999;52:991–994.

44. Sveinbjornsdottir S, Sigurdsson S, Aspelund T, et al. Cerebral microbleeds in the population based AGES Reykjavik Study: prevalence and location. *J Neurol Neurosurg Psychiatry* 2008;79:1002–1006.

45. Tsushima Y, Tanizaki Y, Aoki J, Endo K. MR detection of microhemorrhages in neurologically healthy adults. *Neuroradiology* 2002;44: 31–36.

46. Vernooij MW, van der Lugt A, Ikram MA, et al. Prevalence and risk factors of cerebral microbleeds: the Rotterdam Scan Study. *Neurology* 2008;70: 1208–1214.

47. Shoamanesh A, Kwok CS, Benavente O. Cerebral microbleeds: histopathological correlation of neuroimaging. *Cerebrovasc Dis* 2011;32:528–534.

48. Tanaka A, Ueno Y, Nakayama Y, Takano K, Takebayashi S. Small chronic hemorrhages and ischemic lesions in association with spontaneous intracerebral hematomas. *Stroke* 1999;30: 1637–1642.

49. Schrag M, McAuley G, Pomakian J, et al. Correlation of hypointensities in susceptibility-weighted images to tissue histology in dementia patients with cerebral amyloid angiopathy: a postmortem MRI study. *Acta Neuropathol* 2010;119: 291–302.

50. Ayaz M, Boikov AS, Haacke EM, et al. Imaging cerebral microbleeds using susceptibility weighted imaging: one step toward detecting vascular dementia. *J Magn Reson Imaging* 2010;31:142–148.

51. Conijn MM, Geerlings MI, Luijten PR, et al. Visualization of cerebral microbleeds with dual-echo T2*-weighted magnetic resonance imaging at 7.0 T. *J Magn Reson Imaging* 2010;32:52–59.

52. Gregoire SM, Jäger HR, Yousry TA, et al. Brain microbleeds as a potential risk factor for antiplatelet-related intracerebral haemorrhage: hospital-based, case-control study. *J Neurol Neurosurg Psychiatry* 2010;81:679–684.

53. Stehling C, Wersching H, Kloska SP, et al. Detection of asymptomatic cerebral microbleeds: a comparative study at 1.5 and 3.0 T. *Acad Radiol* 2008;15:895–900.

54. Tatsumi S, Ayaki T, Shinohara M, Yamamoto T. Type of gradient recalled-echo sequence results in size and number change of cerebral microbleeds. *AJNR Am J Neuroradiol* 2008;29:e13.

55. Vernooij MW, Ikram MA, Wielopolski PA, et al. Cerebral microbleeds: accelerated 3D T2*-weighted GRE MR imaging versus conventional 2D T2*-weighted GRE MR imaging for detection. *Radiology* 2008;248:272–277.

56. Scheid R, Ott DV, Roth H, Schroeter ML, von Cramon DY. Comparative magnetic resonance imaging at 1.5 and 3 Tesla for the evaluation of traumatic microbleeds. *J Neurotrauma* 2007;24:1811–1816.

57. Conijn MM, Geerlings MI, Biessels GJ, et al. Cerebral microbleeds on MR imaging: comparison between 1.5 and 7T. *AJNR Am J Neuroradiol* 2011;32:1043–1049.

58. Haacke EM, Xu Y, Cheng YC, Reichenbach JR. Susceptibility weighted imaging (SWI). *Magn Reson Med* 2004;52:612–618.

59. Mittal S, Wu Z, Neelavalli J, Haacke EM. Susceptibility-weighted imaging: technical aspects and clinical applications, part 2. *AJNR Am J Neuroradiol* 2009;30:232–252.

60. Sehgal V, Delproposto Z, Haacke EM, et al. Clinical applications of neuroimaging with susceptibility-weighted imaging. *J Magn Reson Imaging* 2005;22:439–450.

61. Kunimatsu A, Suzuki Y, Hagiwara K, et al. Clinical value of 3D T2*-weighted imaging with multi-echo acquisition: comparison with conventional 2D T2*-weighted imaging and 3D phase-sensitive MR imaging. *Magn Reson Med Sci* 2012;11:205–211.

62. Boeckh-Behrens T, Lutz J, Lummel N, et al. Susceptibility-weighted angiography (SWAN) of cerebral veins and arteries compared to TOF-MRA. *Eur J Radiol* 2012;81:1238–1245.

63. Yakushiji Y, Nishiyama M, Yakushiji S, et al. Brain microbleeds and global cognitive function in adults without neurological disorder. *Stroke* 2008;39:3323–3328.

64. Charidimou A, Werring DJ. Cerebral microbleeds and cognition in cerebrovascular disease: an update. *J Neurol Sci* 2012;322:50–55.

65. De Reuck J, Auger F, Cordonnier C, et al. Comparison of 7.0-T T2*-magnetic resonance imaging of cerebral bleeds in postmortem brain sections of Alzheimer patients with their neuropathological correlates. *Cerebrovasc Dis* 2011;31:511–517.

66. Fisher M, French S, Ji P, Kim RC. Cerebral microbleeds in the elderly: a pathological analysis. *Stroke* 2010;41:2782–2785.

67. Goos JD, van der Flier WM, Knol DL, et al. Clinical relevance of improved microbleed detection by susceptibility-weighted magnetic resonance imaging. *Stroke* 2011;42:1894–1900.

68. Poels MM, Ikram MA, van der Lugt A, et al. Cerebral microbleeds are associated with worse cognitive function: the Rotterdam Scan Study. *Neurology* 2012.78:326–333.

69. Poels MM, Ikram MA, Vernooij MW. Improved MR imaging detection of cerebral microbleeds more accurately identifies persons with vasculopathy. *AJNR Am J Neuroradiol* 2012;33:1553–1556.

70. Vernooij MW, Ikram MA, Tanghe HL, et al. Incidental findings on brain MRI in the general population. *N Engl J Med* 2007;357:1821–1828.

71. Zabramski JM, Wascher TM, Spetzler RF, et al. The natural history of familial cavernous malformations: results of an ongoing study. *J Neurosurg* 1994;80:422–432.

72. Rigamonti D, Drayer BP, Johnson PC, et al. The MRI appearance of cavernous malformations (angiomas). *J Neurosurg* 1987;67:518–524.

73. Wu Z, Mittal S, Kish K, et al. Identification of calcification with MRI using susceptibility-weighted imaging: a case study. *J Magn Reson Imaging* 2009;29:177–182.

74. Gaviani P, Mullins ME, Braga TA, et al. Improved detection of metastatic melanoma by T2*-weighted imaging. *AJNR Am J Neuroradiol* 2006;27:605–608.

75. Scheid R, Preul C, Gruber O, Wiggins C, von Cramon DY. Diffuse axonal injury associated with chronic traumatic brain injury: evidence from T2*-weighted gradient-echo imaging at 3 T. *AJNR Am J Neuroradiol* 2003;24:1049–1056.

76. Li XY, Feng DF. Diffuse axonal injury: novel insights into detection and treatment. *J Clin Neurosci* 2009;16:614–619.

77. Okazaki S, Sakaguchi M, Hyun B, et al. Cerebral microbleeds predict impending intracranial hemorrhage in infective endocarditis. *Cerebrovasc Dis* 2011;32:483–488.

78. Klein I, Iung B, Labreuche J, et al; IMAGE Study Group. Cerebral microbleeds are frequent in infective endocarditis: a case-control study. *Stroke* 2009;40:3461–3465.

79. Sharma S, Malhotra P, Lal V, et al. Asymptomatic cerebral bleeds in patients with aplastic anemia. *Ann Hematol* 2012;91:1187–1191.

80. Linn J, Herms J, Dichgans M, et al. Subarachnoid hemosiderosis and superficial cortical hemosiderosis in cerebral amyloid angiopathy. *AJNR Am J Neuroradiol* 2008;29:184–186.

81. Linn J, Halpin A, Demaerel P, et al. Prevalence of superficial siderosis in patients with cerebral amyloid angiopathy. *Neurology* 2010;74:1346–1350.

82. Kumar S, Goddeau RP Jr, Selim MH, et al. Atraumatic convexal subarachnoid hemorrhage: clinical presentation, imaging patterns and etiologies. *Neurology* 2010;74:893–899.

83. Raposo N, Viguier A, Cuvinciuc V, et al. Cortical subarachnoid haemorrhage in the elderly: a recurrent event probably related to cerebral amyloid angiopathy. *Eur J Neurol* 2011;18:597–603.

84. Yuan MK, Lai PH, Chen JY, et al. Detection of subarachnoid hemorrhage at acute and subacute/chronic stages: comparison of four magnetic resonance imaging pulse sequences and computed tomography. *J Chin Med Assoc* 2005;68:131–137.

85. Noguchi K, Ogawa T, Seto H, et al. Subacute and chronic subarachnoid hemorrhage: diagnosis with fluid-attenuated inversion-recovery MR imaging. *Radiology* 1997;203:257–262.

86. Lummel N, Schoepf V, Burke M, Brueckmann H, Linn J. 3D fluid-attenuated inversion recovery imaging: reduced CSF artifacts and enhanced sensitivity and specificity for subarachnoid hemorrhage. *AJNR Am J Neuroradiol* 2011;32:2054–2060.

87. Wiesmann M, Mayer TE, Yousry I, et al. Detection of hyperacute subarachnoid hemorrhage of the brain by using magnetic resonance imaging. *J Neurosurg* 2002;96:684–689.

88. Kumar N, Cohen-Gadol AA, Wright RA, et al. Superficial siderosis. *Neurology* 2006;66:1144–1152.

89. Koeppen AH, Michael SC, Li D, et al. The pathology of superficial siderosis of the central nervous system. *Acta Neuropathol* 2008;116:371–382.

90. Maeda M, Yagishita A, Yamamoto T, Sakuma H, Takeda K. Abnormal hyperintensity within the subarachnoid space evaluated by fluid-attenuated inversion-recovery MR imaging: a spectrum of central nervous system diseases. *Eur Radiol* 2003;13(Suppl 4):L192–L201.

91. Tha KK, Terae S, Kudo K, Miyasaka K. Differential diagnosis of hyperintense cerebrospinal fluid on fluid-attenuated inversion recovery images of the brain. Part I: pathological conditions. *Br J Radiol* 2009;82:426–434.

92. Kim EY, Kim SS, Na DG, et al. Sulcal hyperintensity on fluid-attenuated inversion recovery imaging in acute ischemic stroke patients treated with intra-arterial thrombolysis: iodinated contrast media as its possible cause and the association with hemorrhagic transformation. *J Comput Assist Tomogr* 2005;29:264–269.

93. Anzai Y, Ishikawa M, Shaw DW, et al. Paramagnetic effect of supplemental oxygen on CSF

hyperintensity on fluid-attenuated inversion recovery MR images. *AJNR Am J Neuroradiol* 2004;25:274–279.

94. Tha KK, Terae S, Kudo K, Miyasaka K. Differential diagnosis of hyperintense cerebrospinal fluid on fluid-attenuated inversion recovery images of the brain. Part II: non-pathological conditions. *Br J Radiol* 2009;82:610–614.

95. Linn J, Michl S, Katja B, et al. Cortical vein thrombosis: the diagnostic value of different imaging modalities. *Neuroradiology* 2010;52:899–911.

96. Ducros A, Fiedler U, Porcher R, et al. Hemorrhagic manifestations of reversible cerebral vasoconstriction syndrome: frequency, features, and risk factors. *Stroke* 2010;41:2505–2511.

97. Ducros A, Boukobza M, Porcher R, et al. The clinical and radiological spectrum of reversible cerebral vasoconstriction syndrome. A prospective series of 67 patients. *Brain* 2007; 130:3091–3101.

98. Beitzke M, Gattringer T, Enzinger C, et al. Clinical presentation, etiology, and long-term prognosis in patients with nontraumatic convexal subarachnoid hemorrhage. *Stroke* 2011;42:3055–3060.

99. Cuvinciuc V, Viguier A, Calviere L, et al. Isolated acute nontraumatic cortical subarachnoid hemorrhage. *AJNR Am J Neuroradiol* 2010; 31:1355–1362.

100. Panda S, Prashantha DK, Shankar SR, Nagaraja D. Localized convexity subarachnoid haemorrhage – a sign of early cerebral venous sinus thrombosis. *Eur J Neurol* 2010;17:1249–1258.

101. Field DK, Kleinig TJ. Aura attacks from acute convexity subarachnoid haemorrhage not due to cerebral amyloid angiopathy. *Cephalalgia* 2011;31:368–371.

102. Bodenant M, Leys D, Lucas C. Isolated subarachnoidal hemorrhage following carotid endarterectomy. *Case Rep Neurol* 2010;2:80–84.

103. Viswanathan A, Greenberg SM. Cerebral amyloid angiopathy in the elderly. *Ann Neurol* 2011;70:871–880.

104. Auriel E, Greenberg SM. The pathophysiology and clinical presentation of cerebral amyloid angiopathy. *Curr Atheroscler Rep* 2012;14:343–350.

105. Charidimou A, Gang Q, Werring DJ. Sporadic cerebral amyloid angiopathy revisited: recent insights into pathophysiology and clinical spectrum. *J Neurol Neurosurg Psychiatry* 2012;83:124–137.

106. Viswanathan A, Greenberg SM. Cerebral amyloid angiopathy in the elderly. *Ann Neurol* 2011;70:871–880.

107. Knudsen KA, Rosand J, Karluk D, Greenberg SM. Clinical diagnosis of cerebral amyloid angiopathy: validation of the Boston criteria. *Neurology* 2001;27;56:537–539.

108. Vinters HV. Cerebral amyloid angiopathy. A critical review. *Stroke* 1987;18:311–324.

109. Attems J, Jellinger K, Thal DR, et al. Review: sporadic cerebral amyloid angiopathy. *Neuropathol Appl Neurobiol* 2011;37:75–93.

110. Vinters HV, Gilbert JJ. Cerebral amyloid angiopathy: incidence and complications in the aging brain. II. The distribution of amyloid vascular changes. *Stroke* 1983;14:924–928.

111. Attems J, Quass M, Jellinger KA, Lintner F. Topographical distribution of cerebral amyloid angiopathy and its effect on cognitive decline are influenced by Alzheimer disease pathology. *J Neurol Sci* 2007;257:49–55.

112. Attems J. Sporadic cerebral amyloid angiopathy: pathology, clinical implications, and possible pathomechanisms. *Acta Neuropathol* 2005;110:345–359.

113. Rosand J, Muzikansky A, Kumar A, et al. Spatial clustering of hemorrhages in probable cerebral amyloid angiopathy. *Ann Neurol* 2005;58:459–462.

114. Samarasekera N, Smith C, Al-Shahi Salman R. The association between cerebral amyloid angiopathy and intracerebral haemorrhage: systematic review and meta-analysis. *J Neurol Neurosurg Psychiatry* 2012;83:275–281.

115. Passero S, Burgalassi L, D'Andrea P, Battistini N. Recurrence of bleeding in patients with primary intracerebral hemorrhage. *Stroke* 1995;26:1189–1192.

116. Greenberg SM, Eng JA, Ning M, Smith EE, Rosand J. Hemorrhage burden predicts recurrent intracerebral hemorrhage after lobar hemorrhage. *Stroke* 2004;35:1415–1420.

117. Viswanathan A, Rakich SM, Engel C, et al. Antiplatelet use after intracerebral hemorrhage. *Neurology* 2006;66:206–209.

118. Biffi A, Sonni A, Anderson CD, et al. Variants at APOE influence risk of deep and lobar intracerebral hemorrhage. *Ann Neurol* 2010:68:934–943.

119. Schrag M, McAuley G, Pomakian J, et al. Correlation of hypointensities in susceptibility-weighted images to tissue histology in dementia patients with cerebral amyloid angiopathy: a postmortem MRI study. *Acta Neuropathol* 2010;119: 291–302.

120. Gurol ME, Dierksen G, Betensky R, et al. Predicting sites of new hemorrhage with amyloid imaging in cerebral amyloid angiopathy. *Neurology* 2012;79:320–326.

121. Dierksen GA, Skehan ME, Khan MA, et al. Spatial relation between microbleeds and amyloid deposits

in amyloid angiopathy. *Ann Neurol* 2010;68:545–548.

122. O'Donnell HC, Rosand J, Knudsen KA, et al. Apolipoprotein E genotype and the risk of recurrent lobar intracerebral hemorrhage. *N Engl J Med* 2000;342:240–245.

123. Maia LF, Mackenzie IR, Feldman HH. Clinical phenotypes of cerebral amyloid angiopathy. *J Neurol Sci* 2007;257:23–30.

124. Izenberg A, Aviv RI, Demaerschalk BM, et al. Crescendo transient aura attacks: a transient ischemic attack mimic caused by focal subarachnoid hemorrhage. *Stroke* 2009;40:3725–3729.

125. Brunot S, Fromont A, Ricolfi F, Moreau T, Giroud M. [Focal subarachnoid hemorrhage and cerebral amyloid angiopathy: a non-fortuitous association.] *Rev Neurol (Paris)* 2010;166:83–89 [in French].

126. Charidimou A, Peeters A, Fox Z, et al. Spectrum of transient focal neurological episodes in cerebral amyloid angiopathy: multicentre magnetic resonance imaging cohort study and meta-analysis. *Stroke* 2012;43:2324–2330.

127. Brunot S, Osseby GV, Rouaud O, et al. Transient ischaemic attack mimics revealing focal subarachnoid haemorrhage. *Cerebrovasc Dis* 2010;30:597–601.

128. Kleinig TJ, Kiley M, Thompson PD. Acute convexity subarachnoid haemorrhage: a cause of aura-like symptoms in the elderly. *Cephalalgia* 2008;28:658–663.

129. Linn J, Wollenweber FA, Lummel N, et al. Superficial siderosis is a warning sign for future intracranial hemorrhage. *J Neurol* 2013;260:176–181.

130. Holland CM, Smith EE, Csapo I, et al. Spatial distribution of white-matter hyperintensities in Alzheimer disease, cerebral amyloid angiopathy, and healthy aging. *Stroke* 2008;39:1127–1133.

131. Smith EE. Leukoaraiosis and stroke. *Stroke* 2010;41:139–143.

132. Zhu YC, Chabriat H, Godin O, et al. Distribution of white matter hyperintensity in cerebral hemorrhage and healthy aging. *J Neurol* 2012;259:530–536.

133. Pantoni L. Cerebral small vessel disease: from pathogenesis and clinical characteristics to therapeutic challenges. *Lancet Neurol* 2010;9:689–701.

134. Wardlaw JM. Blood brain barrier and cerebral small vessel disease. *J Neurol Sci* 2010;299:66–71.

135. Gouw AA, Seewann A, van der Flier WM, et al. Heterogeneity of small vessel disease: a systematic review of MRI and histopathology correlations. *J Neurol Neurosurg Psychiatry* 2010;82:126–135.

136. Kimberly WT, Gilson A, Rost NS, et al. Silent ischemic infarcts are associated with hemorrhage burden in cerebral amyloid angiopathy. *Neurology* 2009;72:1230–1235.

137. Gregoire SM, Charidimou A, Gadapa N, et al. Acute ischaemic brain lesions in intracerebral haemorrhage: multicentre cross-sectional magnetic resonance imaging study. *Brain* 2011;134:2376–2386.

138. Potter GM, Doubal FN, Jackson CA, et al. Counting cavitating lacunes underestimates the burden of lacunar infarction. *Stroke* 2010;41:267–272.

139. Okazaki H, Reagan TJ, Campbell RJ. Clinicopathologic studies of primary cerebral amyloid angiopathy. *Mayo Clin Proc* 1979;54:22–31.

140. Olichney JM, Hansen LA, Hofstetter CR, et al. Cerebral infarction in Alzheimer's disease is associated with severe amyloid angiopathy and hypertension. *Arch Neurol* 1995;52:702–708.

141. Cadavid D, Mena H, Koeller K, Frommelt RA. Cerebral β amyloid angiopathy is a risk factor for cerebral ischemic infarction. A case control study in human brain biopsies. *J Neuropathol Exp Neurol* 2000;59:768–773.

142. Haglund M, Passant U, Sjöbeck M, Ghebremedhin E, Englund E. Cerebral amyloid angiopathy and cortical microinfarcts as putative substrates of vascular dementia. *Int J Geriatr Psychiatry* 2006;21:681–687.

143. Soontornniyomkij V, Lynch MD, Mermash S, et al. Cerebral microinfarcts associated with severe cerebral β-amyloid angiopathy. *Brain Pathol* 2010;20:459–467.

144. Menon RS, Kidwell CS. Neuroimaging demonstration of evolving small vessel ischemic injury in cerebral amyloid angiopathy. *Stroke* 2009;40: e675–e677.

145. Kidwell CS, Greenberg SM. Red meets white: do microbleeds link hemorrhagic and ischemic cerebrovascular disease? *Neurology* 2009;73:1614–1615.

146. Auriel E, Gurol ME, Ayres A, et al. Characteristic distributions of intracerebral hemorrhage-associated diffusion-weighted lesions. *Neurology* 2012;79: 2335–2341.

147. Fountain NB, Eberhard DA. Primary angiitis of the central nervous system associated with cerebral amyloid angiopathy: report of two cases and review of the literature. *Neurology* 1996;46:190–197.

148. Eng JA, Frosch MP, Choi K, Rebeck GW, Greenberg SM. Clinical manifestations of cerebral amyloid angiopathy-related inflammation. *Ann Neurol* 2004;55:250–256.

149. Kinnecom C, Lev MH, Wendell L, et al. Course of cerebral amyloid angiopathy-related inflammation. *Neurology* 2007;68:1411–1416.

150. Kloppenborg RP, Richard E, Sprengers ME, et al. Steroid responsive encephalopathy in cerebral amyloid angiopathy: a case report and review of evidence for immunosuppressive treatment. *J Neuroinflammation* 2010;7:18.

151. Greenberg SM, Frosch MP. Life imitates art: anti-amyloid antibodies and inflammatory cerebral amyloid angiopathy. *Neurology* 2011;76:772–773.

152. Chung KK, Anderson NE, Hutchinson D, Synek B, Barber PA. Cerebral amyloid angiopathy related inflammation: three case reports and a review. *J Neurol Neurosurg Psychiatry* 2011;82: 20–26.

153. Harkness KA, Coles A, Pohl U, et al. Rapidly reversible dementia in cerebral amyloid inflammatory vasculopathy. *Eur J Neurol* 2004;11:59–62.

154. Salloway S, Sperling R, Gilman S, et al. Bapineuzumab 201 clinical trial investigators. A phase 2 multiple ascending dose trial of bapineuzumab in mild to moderate Alzheimer disease. *Neurology* 2009;73:2061–2070.

155. Van Rooden S, van der Grond J, van den Boom R, et al. Descriptive analysis of the Boston criteria applied to a Dutch-type cerebral amyloid angiopathy population. *Stroke* 2009;40:3022–3027.

156. Pantoni L, Garcia JH. The significance of cerebral white matter abnormalities 100 years after Binswanger´s report. *Stroke* 1995;26:1293–1301.

157. Ringelstein EB, Nabavi DG. Cerebral small vessel diseases: cerebral microangiopathies. *Curr Opin Neurol* 2005;18:179–188.

158. Lammie GA. Hypertensive cerebral small vessel disease and stroke. *Brain Pathol* 2002;12: 358–370.

159. Tuszynski MH, Petito CK, Levy DE. Risk factors and clinical manifestations of pathologically verified lacunar infarctions. *Stroke* 1989;20:990–999.

160. Lammie GA. Pathology of small vessel stroke. *Br Med Bull* 2000;56:296–306.

161. Fisher CM. Lacunar strokes and infarcts: a review. *Neurology* 1982;32:871–876.

162. Fisher CM. The arterial lesions underlying lacunes. *Acta Neuropathol* 1968;12:1–15.

163. Fisher CM. Hypertensive cerebral hemorrhage. Demonstration of the source of bleeding. *J Neuropathol Exp Neurol* 2003;62:104–147.

164. Cole FM, Yates PO. Pseudo-aneurysms in relationship to massive cerebral hemorrhage. *J Neurol Neurosurg Psychiatry* 1967;30:61–66.

165. Doubal FN, MacLullich AM, Ferguson KJ, Dennis MS, Wardlaw JM. Enlarged perivascular spaces on MRI are a feature of cerebral small vessel disease. *Stroke* 2010;41:450–454.

166. Rouhl RP, van Oostenbrugge RJ, Knottnerus IL, Staals JE, Lodder J. Virchow–Robin spaces relate to cerebral small vessel disease severity. *J Neurol* 2008;255: 692–696.

167. Martinez-Ramirez S, Pontes-Neto OM, Dumas AP, et al. Topography of dilated perivascular spaces in a memory cohort. *Neurology* 2013;80: 1551–1556.

168. Naff NJ. Intraventricular hemorrhage in adults. *Curr Treat Options Neurol* 1999;1:173–178.

169. Rost NS, Greenberg SM, Rosand J. The genetic architecture of intracerebral hemorrhage. *Stroke* 2008;39:2166–2173.

170. Biffi A, Greenberg SM. Cerebral amyloid angiopathy: a systematic review. *J Clin Neurol* 2011;7:1–9.

171. Revesz T, Holton JL, Lashley T, et al. Genetics and molecular pathogenesis of sporadic and hereditary cerebral amyloid angiopathies. *Acta Neuropathol* 2009;118:115–130.

172. Zhang-Nunes SX, Maat-Schieman ML, van Duinen SG, et al. The cerebral β-amyloid angiopathies: hereditary and sporadic. *Brain Pathol* 2006;16:30–39.

173. Levy E, Lopez-Otin C, Ghiso J, Geltner D, Frangione B. Stroke in Icelandic patients with hereditary amyloid angiopathy is related to a mutation in the cystatin C gene, an inhibitor of cysteine proteases. *J Exp Med* 1989;169:1771–1778.

174. Levy E, Carman MD, Fernandez-Madrid IJ, et al. Mutation of the Alzheimer's disease amyloid gene in hereditary cerebral hemorrhage, Dutch type. *Science* 1990;248:1124–1126.

175. Maat-Schieman ML, van Duinen SG, Bornebroek M, Haan J, Roos RA. Hereditary cerebral hemorrhage with amyloidosis–Dutch type (HCHWA-D): II. a review of histopathological aspects. *Brain Pathol* 1996;6: 115–120.

176. Van den Boom R, Bornebroek M, Behloul F, et al. Microbleeds in hereditary cerebral hemorrhage with amyloidosis – Dutch type. *Neurology* 2005;64:1288–1289.

177. Maat-Schieman M, Roos R, van Duinen S. Hereditary cerebral hemorrhage with amyloidosis-Dutch type. *Neuropathology* 2005;25:288–297.

178. Lanfranconi S, Markus HS. *COL4A1* mutations as a monogenic cause of cerebral small vessel disease: a systematic review. *Stroke* 2010;41:e513–518.

179. Weng YC, Sonni A, Labelle-Dumais C, et al. *COL4A1* mutations in patients with sporadic late-onset intracerebral hemorrhage. *Ann Neurol* 2012;71:470–477.

180. Vahedi K, Kubis N, Boukobza M, et al. *COL4A1* mutation in a

patient with sporadic, recurrent intracerebral hemorrhage. *Stroke* 2007;38:1461–1464.

181. Gould DB, Phalan FC, van Mil SE, et al. Role of *COL4A1* in small-vessel disease and hemorrhagic stroke. *N Engl J Med* 2006;354:1489–1496.

182. Vahedi K, Boukobza M, Massin P, et al. Clinical and brain MRI follow-up study of a family with *COL4A1* mutation. *Neurology* 2007;69:1564–1568.

183. Vahedi K, Alamowitch S. Clinical spectrum of type IV collagen (*COL4A1*) mutations: a novel genetic multisystem disease. *Curr Opin Neurol* 2011;24:63–68.

184. Dumas A, Dierksen GA, Gurol ME, et al. Functional magnetic resonance imaging detection of vascular reactivity in cerebral amyloid angiopathy. *Ann Neurol* 2012;72:76–81.

185. Bacskai BJ, Frosch MP, Freeman SH, et al. Molecular imaging with Pittsburgh Compound B confirmed at autopsy: a case report. *Arch Neurol* 2007;64: 431–434.

186. Johnson KA, Gregas M, Becker JA, et al. Imaging of amyloid burden and distribution in cerebral amyloid angiopathy. *Ann Neurol* 2007;62:229–234.

187. Yates PA, Sirisriro R, Villemagne VL, et al. Cerebral microhemorrhage and brain β-amyloid in aging and Alzheimer disease. *Neurology* 2011;77:48–54.

188. Han BH, Zhou ML, Vellimana AK, et al. Resorufin analogs preferentially bind cerebrovascular amyloid: potential use as imaging ligands for cerebral amyloid angiopathy. *Mol Neurodegener* 2011;6:86.

189. Theysohn JM, Kraff O, Maderwald S, et al. Seven Tesla MRI of microbleeds and white matter lesions as seen in vascular dementia. *J Magn Reson Imaging* 2011;33:782–791.

190. Van Rooden S, Maat-Schieman ML, Nabuurs RJ, et al. Cerebral amyloidosis: postmortem detection with human 7.0-T MR imaging system. *Radiology* 2009;253:788–796.

Chapter 14

Nonconventional MR techniques for imaging cerebral small vessel disease

David Nyenhuis and Glenn T. Stebbins

If neuroimaging provides a "picture" of ischemic subcortical vascular disease (ISVD), then recent structural and functional imaging innovations add clarity and depth to this picture by providing additional angles or views of the origins, pathology, and clinical implications of ISVD. This chapter focuses on four innovative imaging techniques: diffusion tensor imaging (DTI), magnetic resonance spectroscopy (MRS), functional magnetic resonance imaging (fMRI), and a specific fMRI technique, arterial spin labeling (ASL). Each section of the chapter will begin with a brief description of the technique, followed by examples of its use in the context of ISVD.

Diffusion tensor imaging

Diffusion-weighted imaging (DWI) has become one of the mainstays of MRI modalities for assessing patients with recent ischemic events (see Chapter 12). It is based on weighted differences in the decay of MRI signal that is particularly sensitive to water content. It has been used to document the advent of new lesions in patients with ischemic leukoaraiosis and cerebral autosomal dominant arteriopathy with subcortical infarcts (CADASIL) [1]. Although DWI is sensitive to manifest white matter damage, it does not provide information on three-dimensional diffusion, but instead is limited to measuring diffusion in one direction. A novel imaging technique that can measure diffusion in three dimensions is DTI. It accomplishes this multidimensional measurement by increasing the number of gradient directions to fully describe the shape of diffusion within a given volume element or voxel.

The physics of DTI is based on sensitizing the MR signal to movement of hydrogen on the order of several microns. This is accomplished through the simultaneous application of diffusion-weighted gradients in at least six noncollinear directions. The direction and magnitude of hydrogen movement is then measured on the readout [2]. The application of the noncollinear gradients allows for examination of diffusion characteristics irrespective of the orientation of the head within the bore of the magnet, and provides a full description of the diffusion motion. The gradient readouts can be represented in a 3 × 3 matrix and the three-dimensional geometry of the diffusion in a voxel can be described by a mathematical construct called a "tensor." From this tensor in each voxel, three eigenvalues (λ_1, λ_2, and λ_3) defining the magnitude of the diffusion system are derived as well as the three associated eigenvectors that describe the direction of the diffusion system. The average of the three eigenvalues represents the mean translational molecular motion (mean diffusivity [MD]) that is affected by barriers to diffusion, but does not provide information on the directionality of the diffusion. Based on the ratio of the three eigenvalues, the intravoxel direction of hydrogen diffusion can be determined. This scalar measure is fractional anisotropy (FA), and can range from 0 to 1, with 0 indicating completely random diffusion (isotropic diffusion) and 1 representing completely directional diffusion (anisotropic diffusion). The typical measures derived from DTI scans are translational diffusion (MD) and directional diffusion (FA).

Directional diffusion is determined by the anisotropy of the diffusion within a given voxel. Low anisotropy is found in regions with few barriers to diffusion (e.g., cerebrospinal fluid [CSF]) because hydrogen is free to diffuse in any direction. Brain structures with some barriers (e.g., gray matter) have varying levels

Cerebral Small Vessel Disease, ed. Leonardo Pantoni and Philip B. Gorelick. Published by Cambridge University Press.

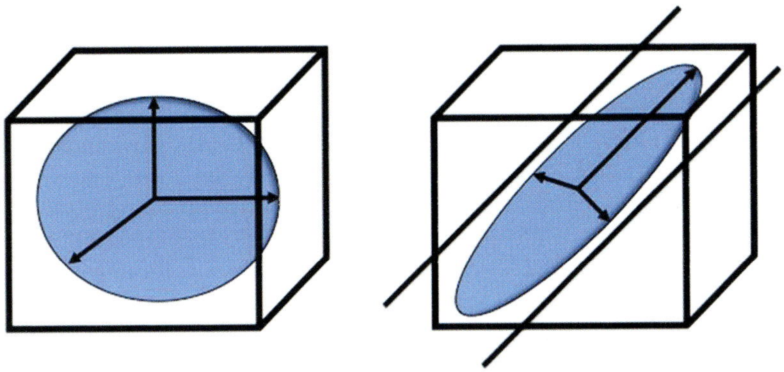

Figure 14.1 Schematic representation of diffusion patterns within individual volume elements (voxels). The voxel on the left contains few barriers to diffusion, such as would be found in regions of cerebrospinal fluid. Note that the diffusion pattern is isotropic and extends equally in all three planes for the primary, secondary, and tertiary eigenvectors. This pattern corresponds with a low fractional anisotropy value. The voxel on the right has a highly organized parallel structure, such as would be found in the axons of white matter tracts. Note that the diffusion pattern is anisotropic, with the primary eigenvector extending along the long axis of the diffusion plane and the secondary and tertiary eigenvectors extending perpendicular to the long axis of the diffusion plane. This pattern corresponds with a high fractional anisotropy value.

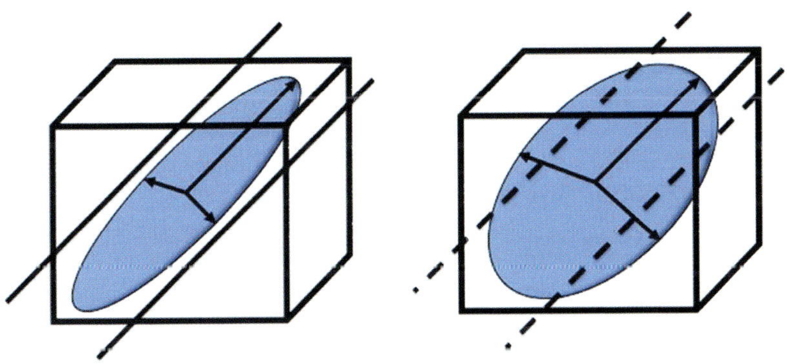

Figure 14.2 Schematic representation of diffusion patterns within two different voxels. The voxel on the left represents the high fractional anisotropy value found in highly organized parallel structure such as white matter. As the organization of the structure degrades (voxel on the right), the diffusion pattern becomes more isotropic and the fractional anisotropy value decreases.

of anisotropy because cellular structures (e.g., cell membrane, organelles) impede the free diffusion of hydrogen but do not necessarily promote organized, directional diffusion. Highly organized brain structures (e.g., white matter tracts) have high anisotropy because hydrogen diffusion is directionally constrained by the tract's cellular organization (Figure 14.1).

Because the diffusion tensor describes the direction of diffusion, in white matter intervoxel continuation of the primary eigenvalue can be used to develop models of fiber orientations, a technique termed tractography. As the similarity of eigenvectors continues across many voxels, the path of the white matter tract is described [3]. These models can be used to define intracerebral connections, and measuring the average FA and MD of the tracts can be used to infer the integrity of these various connections.

When the barriers to free diffusion of hydrogen in white matter degenerate, for example in white matter damage, mean diffusivity increases and the direction of intravoxel diffusion becomes more isotropic (Figure 14.2). Thus, one would predict increased mean translational diffusion (MD) and isotropic diffusion (decreased directional diffusion: FA) in the white matter of patients with ISVD. However, these expectations are rather simplistic, given the complexity of white matter architecture. In regions with a complex matrix of white matter organization, with crossing or other nonparallel fiber structures, DTI indicators of damage may manifest a pattern other than increased MD and decreased FA. For example, if damage occurs to a white matter region with an organizationally complex matrix with crossing fibers, increases in MD would occur due to increased translational diffusion. FA, however, would increase due to a decrease in crossing fibers or other nonparallel organization [4].

This sensitivity to the ultrastructure of white matter ought to provide additional information above that gleaned from typical MRI examinations. In one study using DTI in nine patients with ISVD with lacunar infarcts and 10 aged-matched controls [5], it was noted that both increased translational diffusion (MD) and decreased directional diffusion (FA) were associated with areas of leukoaraiosis due to the white matter damage. In addition they noted large variances in these DTI parameters across different regions of leukoaraiosis in the patients, suggesting a nonuniform disruption to white matter integrity within the lesions.

These findings were extended in a sample of patients with CADASIL, an autosomal dominant disorder of the *NOTCH3* gene resulting in ISVD with subcortical infarcts and dementia [6]. In a study of 16 CADASIL patients (divided into mild or severe disease based on cognitive function and Rankin score) and 10 age-matched control subjects, Chabriat et al. [7] examined DTI measures of translational diffusion (MD) and directional diffusion (FA) in both regions of leukoaraiosis and normal-appearing white matter (NAWM). Within regions of T2 identified hyperintensities in the CADASIL group, they found significantly increased translational diffusion and decreased anisotropic diffusion compared to control subjects. Additionally, these two measures were significantly different between the mild and severe CADASIL groups, with the more severe patients demonstrating increased translational diffusion and decreased directional diffusion compared to the mildly affected patients. The DTI measures within the white matter hyperintensities (WMHs) were strongly correlated with a measure of cognitive function as well as a measure of stroke-related disability. The results of the NAWM examination were even more striking. Even though these regions appeared normal on standard T2 radiologic examinations, significant alterations to the diffusion parameters were found. The NAWM in the CADASIL group showed significant increases in translational diffusion and significant decreases in directional diffusion compared to control subjects. There were no significant differences between the mild and severe CADASIL subgroups on these measures in the NAWM. However, the directional diffusion measure was significantly correlated with the measure of stroke disability.

In a report of 30 patients with leukoaraiosis and 17 control subjects, a different study examined whether DTI abnormalities extended beyond the areas of WMHs evident on T2 imaging in patients with ISVD but not CADASIL [8]. This study also explored the relationship between these values and behavioral measures of cognitive function in patients with ISVD. DTI measures of translational diffusion and directional diffusion were significantly altered within the lesions, with increases in MD and decreases in FA compared to control values. Additionally, in radiologically defined NAWM, there were significant disruptions to white matter integrity with increased MD and decreased FA in the patients. This difference remained significant even when the patient group was compared to hypertensive normal subjects and when gender and age were used as covariates. Perhaps the most interesting finding was the relationship between DTI measures and the behavioral assessments in the leukoaraiosis group. Directional diffusion in the anterior periventricular NAWM was significantly correlated with a measure of global cognitive function, and translational diffusion in the centrum semiovale was significantly related to executive function measures.

These studies highlight the utility of DTI in examining the effects of ISVD in white matter regions outside of the frank infarction. Other studies have investigated the application of DTI in assessing the integrity of deep gray matter structures, where lacunar infarcts often occur, in patients with CADASIL. The rationale for using DTI to assess the integrity of the relatively parallel structure of white matter is well supported, because this structure promotes anisotropic diffusion. However, gray matter has a nonparallel structure at the voxel level and the utility of assessing diffusion anisotropy is not as clearly established. One mitigating influence that provides support for the use of DTI in gray matter in stroke is that iron concentration levels have a direct effect on FA levels [9].

Alterations in DTI parameters have been reported in CADASIL patients in both normal appearing and lesioned deep gray matter. One study found both increased translational diffusion and decreased directional diffusion in the putamen and the thalamus in CADASIL patients compared to control subjects [10]. Additionally, the translational diffusion values in the thalamus were significantly negatively correlated with a measure of general cognitive function. Similar results were found in another study of CADASIL, with increased translational diffusion in basal ganglia structures (putamen and globus pallidus) and the thalamus, but reduced directional diffusion only in the thalamus [11]. Of interest in this study was the finding that the altered diffusion values were significantly related to behavioral measures of executive function, but only weakly related to measures of general cognitive function and memory, suggesting a specificity of these DTI measures to the common executive disorder seen in ISVD. The relationship of thalamic diffusion integrity to cognitive function mirrors that of thalamic volume, where decreased volume of the thalamus was found to be the most significant predictor of cognitive status in ischemic stroke patients [12].

Although a number of the previously mentioned studies have highlighted the significant relationship between DTI measures of translational and directional diffusion with cognitive performance measures in patients with ISVD, the magnitude of the relationship is often rather low. For example, in the RUN DCM (Radboud University Nijmegen Diffusion Tensor and Magnetic Resonance Cohort) study of 503 patients with ISVD, DTI parameters were found to be significantly correlated to multiple cognitive domains, including global cognitive function, speed of cognition, and cognitive shifting abilities [13]. However, the magnitude of any of the significant correlations was less than 0.2, demonstrating less than 4% shared variance between the variables. Indeed, neither NAWM nor white matter lesion translational or directional diffusion measures significantly increased the prediction of cognitive function above that obtained with traditional MRI indices in ISVD using a multivariate approach [14].

In contrast to this report, multiple studies have found a significant relationship between DTI measures and cognitive function in patients with ISVD, and have noted the superiority of DTI measures to predict cognitive function over standard MRI indicies. Although some studies have reported significant relationships between diffusion measures and global cognitive and memory function [7, 10, 15], the majority of studies have found a significant relationship between DTI measures and executive cognitive function [8, 11, 16, 17] as manifest in tests of speeded cognitive processing, attention, fluency, and abstract reasoning. The typical relationship between DTI measures and executive function is seen in decreased executive function associated with increased translational diffusion and decreased directional diffusion in both lesioned white matter as well as NAWM. It has been hypothesized that the association between DTI measures of white matter integrity and cognitive function characterizes the effect of disconnections of white matter tracts due to leukoaraiosis, lacunar infarcts, and cerebral microbleeds [18].

DTI has also been employed in longitudinal studies of patients with ISVD. In a whole-brain DTI study of 35 patients with ISVD followed for one year, significant increases in translational diffusion and decreases in directional diffusion were found [17]. There were no significant changes in other MRI measures of brain volume, lesion load, or number of lacunar infarcts. Similar increases in translational diffusion were found in a study of 14 CADASIL patients followed for approximately 21 months [19] and a study of 62 CADASIL patients followed for approximately 26 months [20]. It is important to note that these studies examined whole-brain DTI indices, including white matter, gray matter, and infarcted tissue. In a longitudinal DTI study examining NAWM in a series of 80 ischemic stroke patients with three years of follow-up, significant improvements in directional diffusion were noted [21]. The slope of change in FA suggested an improvement in NAWM integrity over the first two years, with a stabilization of that effect by the third year of follow-up (Figure 14.3).

The physiologic underpinnings of altered translational and directional diffusion as detected by DTI are not clearly known. MRS (see below) studies provide some indication of the underlying metabolic alterations associated with perturbed DTI measures. MRS derived *N*-acetylaspartate : choline ratios have been shown to be positively correlated with DTI-derived directional diffusion measures and negatively correlated with translational diffusion [22]. The relationship is thought to reflect the metabolic dysfunction or loss of axons in white matter.

One of the more recent advances in DTI is the development of models of individual patient-specific white matter tracts. Diffusion tensor tractography is ideally suited to examine the effects of ISVD on white matter tracts. The process of following the tensor directional vectors (or the primary eigenvector) across adjacent voxels allows for the development of white matter tract models [3], and effects of ISVD lesions on the integrity of these tracts can be

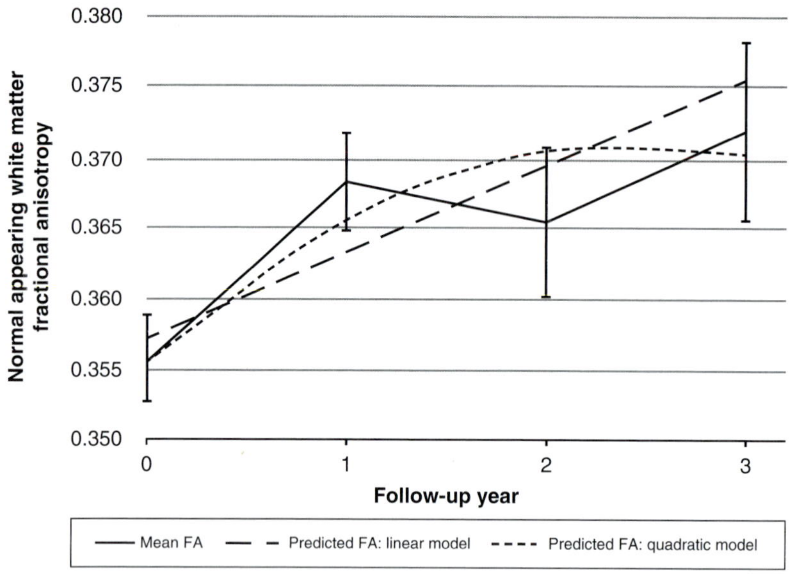

Figure 14.3 Line graph showing the change-over-time in fractional anisotropy (FA) values for normal appearing white matter in patients with ischemic stroke followed for three years. Mean FA (± standard error of mean [SEM]) is shown for each evaluation time period. The solid line represents the actual mean change over time. The long-dash line represents the estimated change in FA-based mixed-model regression linear model. The short-dashed line represents the estimated change in FA based on mixed-model regression quadratic model. Note that the quadratic model provides a better fit to the actual mean change in FA, suggesting increasing anisotropic diffusion over the first two years of follow-up followed by stabilization at year three.

described. Recent studies have used tractographic techniques to identify the proximity of infarcted tissue to major white matter tracts [23], the impact of CADASIL on major white matter tracts [24], the effects on cortical thickness of specific lesioned white matter tracts [25], and the relationship of tract-based DTI parameters on cognitive functioning in patients with ISVD. Because this is a newer development, its full impact on studies of ISVD has not been realized.

Magnetic resonance spectroscopy

Magentic resonance sprectroscopy (MRS) provides a window through which to observe the neurochemical underpinnings of ISVD. MRS is based on the unique MR spectra possessed by molecules, allowing their metabolic concentration to be identified in a region of interest (ROI). ROIs in MRS research may vary from a single voxel that is repeatedly measured to promote reliability, to an entire imaging slice or slices by way of chemical shift imaging techniques. A metabolite of specific interest is *N*-acetylaspartate (NAA), because it is only found within neurons and has been identified as a measure of general neuronal health. Decreased NAA concentrations have been noted in a variety of neurologic conditions, including multiple sclerosis, Alzheimer's disease, and traumatic brain injury. In many studies, the ratio of NAA to choline (Ch), or creatnine (Cr), is used as a marker of interest. However, because Ch and Cr concentrations may not be static in the face of neural insult, absolute NAA concentrations have also been used as markers. Some investigators report both. For example, in work that was discussed in the previous section, Nitkunan et al. [22] demonstrated correlations between MRS-attained ratios, such as NAA : Cr, and DTI values using chemical shift imaging. The group later replicated the finding using absolute metabolite values [17].

MRS studies have been useful in demonstrating ISVD pathology. For example, altered gray and white matter metabolism has been demonstrated in patients with CADASIL [26]. Structural MR markers of ISVD, such as WMHs and lacunar infarctions, have been found to be related to relative and absolute NAA levels. Capizzano et al. [27] found lower NAA in the cerebral cortex of patients with lacunes and dementia, compared with healthy, age-matched control subjects, as well as an inverse correlation between NAA in frontal cortex and both WMH volume and the number of lacunar infarcts in their patient group. Other investigators [28] found lower mean metabolite ratios for NAA : Cr, NAA : Ch, and Ch : Cr ratios in anterior versus posterior areas of the centrum semiovale of CADASIL patients, consistent with our understanding of the pattern of CADASIL-related neuropathology. Lower NAA : Cr values have also been found in corona radiata of preclinical CADASIL patients than in controls, suggesting that metabolic changes predate clinical symptoms in this patient group [29]. A more recent study by Akhvlediani et al. [30] demonstrated not only relatively decreased metabolism in the WMHs of CADASIL patients versus healthy controls, but also *increased* metabolite ratios in NAWM of CADASIL patients versus controls, suggesting potential adaptive metabolic changes in cells as a response to inferred hypoperfusion and impaired vasoreactivity.

Metabolites have also been correlated with cognitive function in patients with ISVD. Hund-Georgiadis et al. [31] found relationships between measures of attention and decreased NAA : Ch and NAA : Cr ratios. Others have measured NAA : Cr ratios from NAWM in the centrum semiovale both ipsilateral and contralateral to a single lacunar infarct located some distance away from the ROI. They found neuropsychological test scores to correlate with the metabolite ratio, with more significant correlations ipsilateral than contralateral to the infarct [32]. More recently, Gasparovic et al. [33] showed relationships between absolute concentrations of NAA and Cr and neuropsychological measures of executive function, as defined by a combined score derived from Trail Making part B, Wisconsin Card Sorting Test total errors, and Digit Span Backwards Test scores. The relationships appeared to be stronger than those between neuropsychological test scores and lesion volume, a traditional, albeit relatively weak, factor in vascular cognitive impairment (VCI) research. Another group examined NAA : Cr ratios and DTI-related factors in a sample of patients with leukoaraiosis and matched healthy controls [34]. Imaging values were obtained from ROIs in anterior and posterior periventricular regions as well as from medial regions of the thalamus. MRS and DTI values correlated with neuropsychological test scores (Mini Mental State Examination [MMSE] and tests of executive function) at roughly a similar level in the periventricular regions, while the NAA : Cr ratio score appeared to show a stronger relationship with cognitive tests than fractional anisotropy or mean diffusivity in thalamic regions. This relationship of thalamus to cognitive impairment in ISVD is consistent with previous work using voxel-based morphometric methods [12]. Other studies have not found significant metabolite–cognitive relationships. For example, Capizzano et al. [27] did not find relative or absolute NAA concentrations to correlate with MMSE scores.

In addition to work with MRS-created values used as disease markers of ISVD, investigators have looked for clues of the neuropathologic underpinnings of ISVD using MRS methods. In an earlier study, Brooks et al. [35] differentiated WMHs of normal elderly to those of patients with subcortical arteriosclerotic encephalopathy with proton MRS (1H-MRS). NAA : Cr and NAA : Ch ratios were reduced in the encephalopathic group compared to the asymptomatic subjects, even though the WMH volumes were similar in the two groups. This would suggest that not all WMH is equal in terms of its relationship to cognitive function. In addition, studies which combine MRS with DTI [17, 22] provide evidence that the lower FA and higher MD DTI values have their root in metabolically altered white matter, thus providing validation for both techniques.

Functional MRI

Blood oxygen level dependent (BOLD) functional MRI (fMRI) exploits the T2* signal sensitivity to changes in the paramagnetic state of oxygenated and deoxygenated cerebral blood. Task-related changes in cerebral activation are reflected by regional increases in oxygenated blood that are then detected by the changes in T2*. Because of the excellent spatial resolution of MRI, these changes can be localized to the activated tissue. Different tasks can be used to probe for cognitive, motor, or sensory activities. A newer development in fMRI does not depend on task-related activity, but instead investigates differences in resting-state activation.

The most common use for fMRI in stroke has been to monitor cortical activation changes in the post-stroke period, either with or without specific rehabilitative interventions (for a review see [36]). Most studies have examined the effects of discrete subcortical or cortical infarcts on motor-related cerebral activation. Although there are variations in results, there appears to be a reorganization of the activation within the affected motor cortex, with expansion and shifting of activation location [37] as well as a general increase in activation in the non-affected motor cortex [38].

fMRI studies in patients with more diffuse disease are not as well represented in the literature. It appears that in ISVD the relationship between infarcts and fMRI activation is altered in a more global manner. One study reported a 30% decrease in sensorimotor cortical activation on the side contralateral to the infarct compared to activation obtained from healthy controls [39]. An interesting finding from this study was that there was a similar diminution of BOLD activation in the sensorimotor cortex on the side ipsilateral to the stroke. The authors hypothesized that this bilateral decrease in activation was related to general changes in the cerebral vascular system.

Support for this hypothesis was found in a study of the effect of WMHs on fMRI activation during a motor task in elderly subjects [40]. In this study, a significant negative correlation was found between activation and a brain-volume normalized measure of WMH volume. Because the hyperintensities were widely distributed across white matter regions and not specifically involving the motor system, these results again suggest a nonspecific decoupling of the hemodynamic response due to white matter disruption resulting in decreased fMRI activation. Although the specific mechanisms of this decoupling are not known, it has been suggested that it is due to microvascular reactivity changes [41].

It appears that this inverse relationship between fMRI activation and ISVD may be modulated by coexistent factors [42]. In contrast to studies finding an inverse relationship between fMRI activation and ISVD severity, a positive correlation was found between motor activation and severity of leukoaraiosis in a sample of patients with mild cognitive impairment. A similar positive correlation between fMRI activation and WMHs was found in a sample of elderly patients with major depression [43]. The results of these studies suggest that the relationship between fMRI activation and ISVD is not a simple one.

Arterial spin labeling

Arterial spin labeling (ASL) is an fMRI technique used to quantitatively measure cerebral blood flow (CBF). Other imaging and ultrasound techniques, such as transcranial Doppler (TCD) techniques, have suggested a relationship between ISVD and CBF. For example, TCD studies have shown a slowing of CBF as part of the aging process [44] and linkages between slower CBF, hypertension, and WMHs [45]. Slower CBF and impaired cerebral vasomotor reactivity have also been linked to increased risk for subsequent stroke and cognitive impairment. However, TCD is limited in its spatial specificity and other techniques that measure CBF, such as computed tomography (CT), perfusion and positron emission tomography (PET), and single photon emission CT, require either ionizing radiation or an injection of a bolus of an exogenous contrast agent.

ASL uses water as an endogenous, diffusible tracer, thus dispensing with the need to inject an exogenous agent. This provides the opportunity for multiple, repeated imaging sessions, thus allowing for longitudinal designs when needed, such as when measuring disease progression or the effects of therapy. Another advantage of ASL is that it provides an absolute rather than a percentage-based CBF marker, so that flow changes can be identified in physiologically meaningful units. ASL techniques also provide greater spatial specificity than other CBF methods.

There are many ASL techniques. All of them involve an initial "labeling" of arterial water protons by inversion or saturation, using relatively short or long magnetic pulse sequences. Just downstream from the labeling, the energy that is released from the protons as they revert back to their initial state provides the CBF information. Continuous ASL (CASL) uses a relatively long (about 2 s) labeling pulse, which produces a thin labeling plane and relatively high signal to noise ratio (SNR), but also may introduce a potential confound of magnetization transfer effects in the labeled, but not the control scans. By contrast, pulsed ASL (PASL) involves brief (about 10–15 ms) pulses that invert proton spins in an "inversion slab" with adiabatic hyperbolic secant radio-frequency pulses. However, SNR is generally lower for PASL than CASL. More recent pseudo-continuous ASL (pCASL) techniques seek to improve SNR while maintaining PASL efficiency by using a rapid series of brief pulses instead of one long, continuous pulse. In a recent review of ASL techniques, Borogovac and Asllani [46] consider pCASL to be the "best choice" among ASL techniques for brain research, because of its high efficiency, multislice capability, and relative ease of use, while not overtaxing imaging hardware.

ASL has been used in a number of different ways in ISVD research. ASL techniques demonstrate relationships between CBF velocity and ISVD markers, including WMHs and lacunar infarctions. For example, using PASL, the Leukoaraiosis And DISability (LADIS) study group found CBF to be 20% slower in global flow rate in patients with confluent WMHs than in subjects with either punctiform or beginning-confluent WMHs [47]. Using within-subjects research designs, reductions in CBF have also been found in areas of identified WMHs compared with either radiologically defined NAWM or gray matter [48]. ASL has also been used to examine the possible origins of WMHs. Mandell et al. [49] investigated whether the "steal phenomenon" might be a factor in producing WMHs. The steal phenomenon hypothesizes that some areas of brain are susceptible to hypoperfusion, especially in times of high metabolic demand or vessel damage. The investigators used both blood oxygen load-dependent MRI and ASL to identify areas of reduced cerebrovascular reserve in the white matter of young, healthy volunteers. They then overlaid the maps of reduced reserve on to areas commonly associated with WMHs later in life and found significant overlap. They hypothesize that areas susceptible to WMHs might be especially vulnerable to the steal phenomenon.

Hajjar et al. [50] studied the relationship of hypertension to cerebral vasoreactivity using CASL. Understanding vasoreactivity is important because of its known relationship to gait disturbance and cognitive decline. The work followed a line of previous studies that used TCD, and defined vasoreactivity as the regression slope between end-tidal carbon dioxide and cerebral perfusion. In a sample that included some patients with a history of stroke, they found a relationship between hypertension and vasoreactivity, which remained after statistically accounting for the presence of stroke and the extent of WMHs. Moreover, taking advantage of CASL's ability to detect regional CBF, the investigators found both global and lobar (frontal, temporal, and parietal lobe) vasoreactivity. The results of the study suggest that

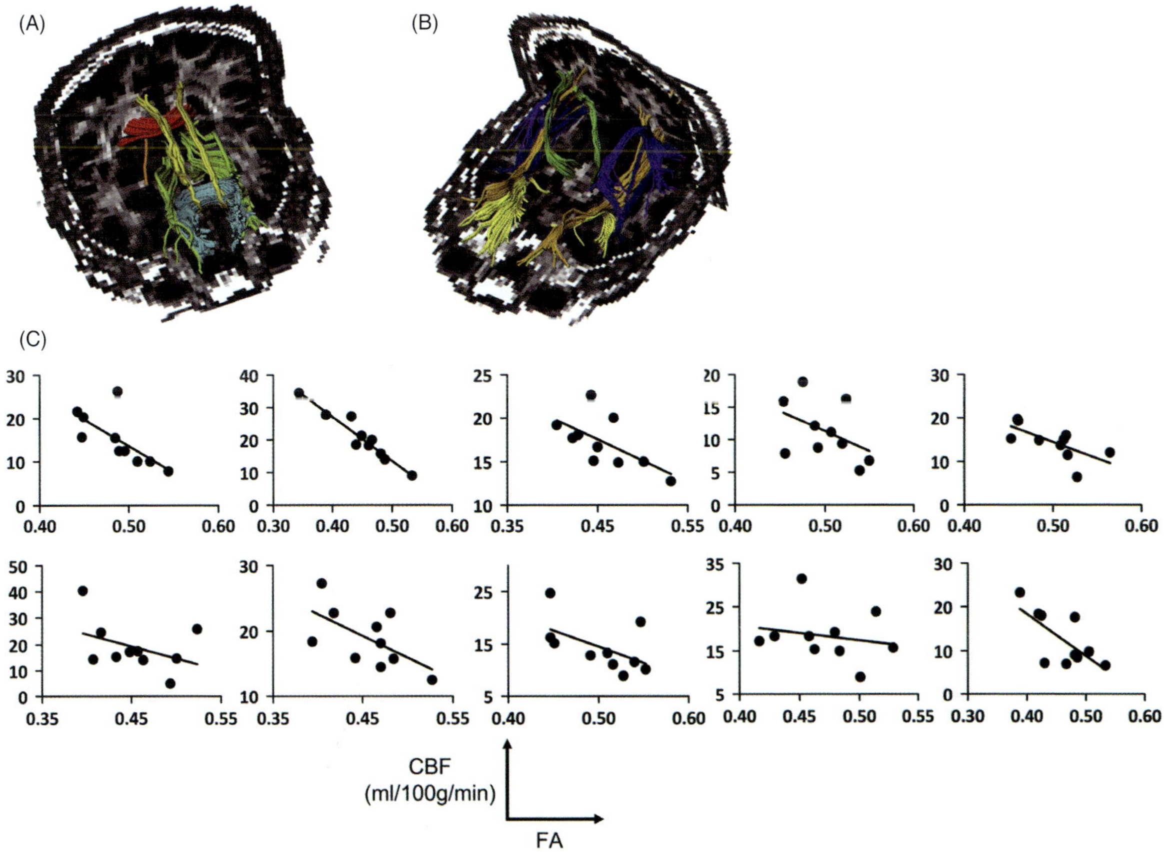

Figure 14.4 Relationship between tract-specific fractional anisotropy (FA) and cerebral blood flow (CBF). (A,B) Illustration of 10 major fiber tracts overlaid on FA maps. For clarity, five fibers are shown in (A) and five are shown in (B). The fibers in (A) are: forceps major of the corpus callosum (red), forceps minor of the corpus callosum (blue), cingulum in the cingulate cortex (yellow), cingulum to hippocampus (orange), and anterior thalamic radiation (green). The fibers in (B) are: uncinate fasciculus (yellow), corticospinal tract (green), arcuate fasciculus (pink), inferior fronto-occipital fasciculus (blue), and inferior longitudinal fasciculus (orange). (C) Scatter plots between FA and CBF across fiber tracts. Each subplot displays data from one subject. Within a subplot, different points indicate different tracts. An inverse correlation is observed in all subjects. In statistical analysis, the ml values from the subplots are combined in a meta-analysis to yield a *t* statistic. From Aslan et al. [54], reproduced with permission.

hypertension may have ongoing, deleterious effects on vessel function, both before and after stroke, and point to the need for additional research on the effects of antihypertensive agents on vasoreactivity.

ASL has also been used in conjunction with other fMRI techniques to study the effects of cerebral amyloid angiopathy (CAA) on vessel function. Dumas et al. [51] compared patients with CAA to normal controls in the response to a visual stimulus (a flashing checkerboard pattern). The patients with CAA showed reduced BOLD amplitude, prolonged time to peak, and prolonged time to baseline when compared with the normal control subjects. However, patients with CAA did not show slower resting CBF than the control group. The investigators summarized that the lack of CBF differences across the two groups increased the validity of their other findings because CBF difference may in itself alter the hemodynamic response. They also suggest that their findings may show that the primary impact of advanced CAA is to change the dynamic response to alterations in local metabolic demand rather than to slow CBF.

ASL has also been used to more accurately classify cerebral infarcts by providing additional information regarding the perfusion territories associated with the infarct location. Using ASL, Hendrikes et al. [52] reclassified 11% of cortical or border zone infarcts in a series of ischemic stroke patients that had been originally classified using standard templates. Strokes in subcortical areas, brainstem, and cerebellum did not require reclassification.

Future directions

The next wave of imaging-based innovation is multimodal MRI. Hao et al. [53] demonstrate the complementary and mutually informative methods of combining anatomic MRI, fMRI, DTI, and MRS as a means of further understanding the data that each separate method provides. Multimodal imaging has been used in samples of patient with ISVD as well, as is demonstrated by the combined use of DTI and MRS already discussed. Two other recent studies provide another example of its potential. Aslan et al. [54] combined DTI and ASL-defined CBF techniques to

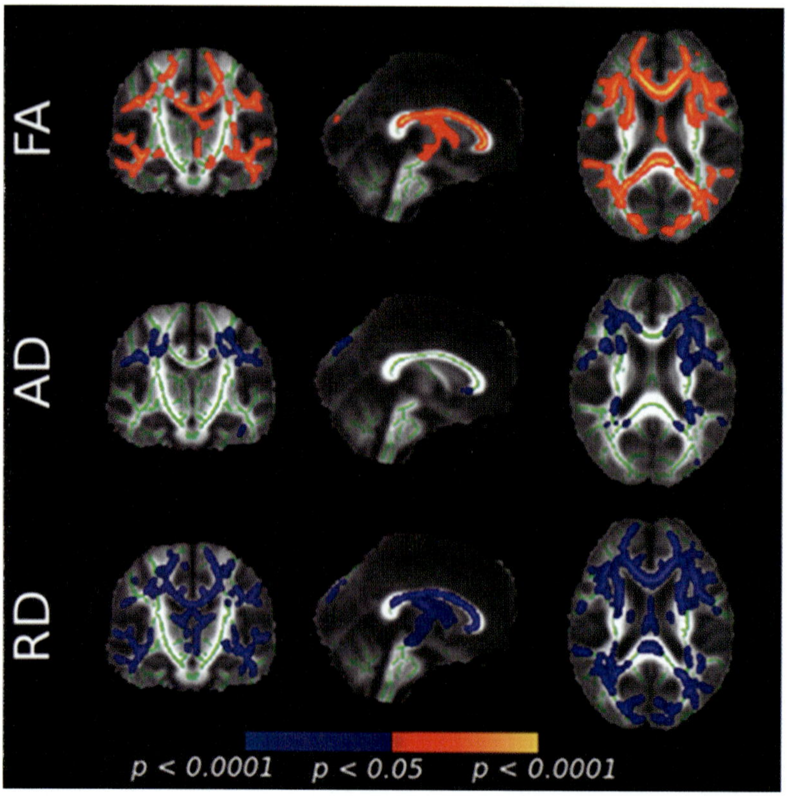

Figure 14.5 Correlations between diffusion tensor imaging parameters and mean cortical cerebral blood flow (CBF) collapsed across age. The white-matter skeleton is shown in green. Cortical CBF was positively associated with white matter fractional anisotropy (FA) (shown in red–yellow), and negatively associated with both axial and radial diffusivity (AD and RD, respectively). From Chen et al. [55], reproduced with permission.

better understand tract-specific relationships between CBF and white matter integrity. Their laboratory had previously developed a pCASL technique combined with a phase contrast sequence that permitted voxel-by-voxel CBF approximation. They slightly modified this method by using spin-echo echo planar imaging (EPI) rather than gradient echo acquisition to allow for similar image registration for ASL and DTI. The end result was the ability to measure both tract-specific CBF and white matter integrity in 10 major fiber tracts. While it was expected that there would be a positive relationship between CBF and fiber-specific white matter integrity, the opposite was found: a consistent inverse relationship between CBF and FA in each of the 10 patients tested across the 10 fiber tracts (Figure 14.4 [54]). A meta-analysis computed across all the subjects found a partial correlation of –0.66 between the two values, after factoring out the contributions of white matter probability and layer index. The authors reviewed possible explanations for this unexpected finding, including potential relationships between CBF and axonal diameter, the possibility that lower CBF reflected greater efficiency of the tract, and a potential relationship between the tightness of the fiber bundle and CBF.

Chen et al. [55] also combined ASL and DTI techniques in an examination of potential relationships between cortical CBF and subcortical white matter integrity. They imaged the brains of healthy adults aged 23–88 and found an expected inverse relationship between CBF and age. They also found a positive association between cortical CBF and subcortical white matter integrity, measured via FA. The relationship was consistent across several brain regions (Figure 14.5 [55]). The authors acknowledged the earlier finding by Aslan's group of a possible inverse relationship between CBF and white matter integrity and stated that the contradictory findings represent "alternative models of how CBF relates to neural health" and need to be reconciled.

The two studies demonstrate that innovative MR techniques will bring with them additional questions as well as answers when working the ISVD puzzle. This will likely continue as imaging techniques continue to provide different angles to the "picture" of ISVD.

References

1. O'Sullivan M, Rich PM, Barrick TR, Clark CA, Markus HS. Frequency of subclinical lucunar infarcts in ischemic leukoaraiosis and cerebral autosomal dominant arteriopathy with subcortical infarcts and leukoencephalopathy. *AJNR Am J Neuroradiol* 2003;24:1348–1354.
2. Basser PJ, Mattiello J, LeBihan D. Estimation of the effective self-diffusion tensor from the NMR spin echo, *J Magn Reson B* 1994;103:247–254.
3. Basser PJ, Pajevic S, Pierpaoli C, Duda J, Aldroubi A. In vivo fiber tractography using DT–MRI data. *Magn Reson Med* 2000; 44:625–632.
4. Stebbins GT, Smith CA, Bartt RE, et al. HIV-associated alterations in normal-appearing white matter: a voxel-wise diffusion tensor imaging study. *J Acquir Immune Defic Syndr* 2007;46: 564–573.
5. Jones DK, Lythgoe D, Horsfield MA, et al. Characterization of white matter damage in ischemic leukoaraiosis with diffusion tensor MRI. *Stroke* 1999;30:393–397.
6. Tournier-Lasserve E, Joutel A, Melki J, et al. Cerebral autosomal dominant arteriopathy with subcortical infarcts and leukoencephalopathy maps to chromosome 19q12. *Nature Genet* 1993;3:256–259.
7. Chabriat H, Pappata S, Poupon C, et al. Clinical severity in CADASIL related to ultrastructural damage in white matter: in vivo study with diffusion tensor MRI. *Stroke* 1999;30:2637–2643.
8. O'Sullivan M, Summers PE, Jones DK, et al. Normal-appearing white matter in ischemic leukoaraiosis: a diffusion tensor MRI study. *Neurology* 2001;57:2307–2310.
9. Pfefferbaum A, Adalsteinsson E, Rohlfing T, Sullivan EV. Diffusion tensor imaging of deep gray matter brain structures: effects of age and iron concentration. *Neurobiol Aging* 2010;31: 482–493.
10. Molko N, Pappata S, Mangin JF, et al. Diffusion tensor imaging study of subcortical gray matter in CADASIL. *Stroke* 2001;32: 2049–2054.
11. O'Sullivan M, Singhal S, Charlton R, Markus HS. Diffusion tensor imaging of thalamus correlates with cognitive in CADASIL without dementia. *Neurology* 2004;62:702–707.
12. Stebbins GT, Nyenhuis DL, Wang C, et al. Gray matter atrophy in patients with ischemic stroke with cognitive impairment. *Stroke* 2008;39:785–793.
13. Van Norden AG, de Laat KF, van Dijk EJ, et al. Diffusion tensor imaging and cognition in cerebral small vessel disease: the RUN DMC study. *Biochem Biophys Acta* 2012;1822:401–407.

14. Van Norden AG, van Uden IW, de Laat KF, van Dijk EJ, de Leeuw FE. Cognitive function in small vessel disease: the additional value of diffusion tensor imaging to conventional magnetic resonance imaging: the RUN DCM study. *J Alzheimers Dis* 2012;32:667–676.
15. Gons RA, van Oudheusden LJ, de Laat KF, et al. Hypertension is related to the microstructure of the corpus callosum: the RUN DMC study. *J Alzheimers Dis* 2012;32:623–631.
16. O'Sullivan M, Morris RG, Huckstep B, et al. Diffusion tensor MRI correlates with executive dysfunction in patients with ischaemic leukoaraiosis. *J Neurol Neurosurg Psychiatry* 2004;75:441–447.
17. Nitkunan A, Barrick TR, Charlton RA, Clark CA, Markus HS. Multimodal MRI in cerebral small vessel disease: its relationship with cognition and sensitivity to change over time. *Stroke* 2008;39:1999–2005.
18. O'Sullivan M. Imaging small vessel disease lesion topography, networks, and cognitive deficits investigated with MRI. *Stroke* 2010;41(Suppl 1):S154–S158.
19. Moldo N, Pappata S, Magin JF, et al. Monitoring disease progression in CADASIL with diffusion magnetic resonance imaging a study with whole brain histogram analysis. *Stroke* 2002;33:2902–2908.
20. Holtmannspotter M, Peters N, Opherk C, et al. Diffusion magnetic resonance histograms as a surrogate marker and predictor of disease progression in CADASIL: a two-year follow-up study. *Stroke* 2005;36:2559–2565.
21. Wang C, Stebbins GT, Nyenhuis DL, et al. Longitudinal changes in white matter following ischemic stroke: a three-year follow-up study. *Neurobiol Aging* 2006;27:1827–1833.
22. Nitkunan A, McIntyre JO, Barrick TR, et al. Correlations between MRS and DTI in cerebral small vessel disease. *NMR Biomed* 2006;19:610–616.
23. Yamada K, Mori S, Nakamura H, et al. Fiber-tracking method reveals sensorimotor pathway involvement in stroke patients. *Stroke* 2003;34:159–162.
24. Mascalchi M, Ginestroni A, Toschi N, et al. The burden of microstructural damage modulates cortical activation in elderly subjects with MCCI and leuko-araiosis. *Hum Brain Mapp* 2012, Dec 8 [Epub ahead of print].
25. Duering M, Righart R, Csanadi E, et al. Incident subcortical infarcts induce focal cortical thinning in connected cortical regions. *Neurology* 2012;79:2025–2028.
26. Auer DP, Schirmer T, Heidenreich JO, et al. Altered white and gray matter metabolism in CADASIL: a proton MR spectroscopy and 1H-MRSI study. *Neurology* 2001;56:635–642.
27. Capizzano AA, Schuff N, Amend DL, et al. Subcortical ischemic vascular dementia: assessment with quantitative MR imaging and 1H MR spectroscopy. *AJNR Am J Neuroradiol* 2000;21: 621–630.
28. Macrì MA, Colonnese C, Garreffa G, et al. A chemical shift imaging study on regional metabolite distribution in a CADASIL family. *Magn Reson Imaging* 2006;24:443–447.
29. Stromillo ML, Dotti MT, Battaglini M, et al. Structural and metabolic brain abnormalities in preclinical cerebral autosomal dominant arteriopathy with subcortical infarcts and leucoencephalopathy. *J Neurol Neurosurg Psychiatr* 2009; 80:41–47.
30. Akhvlediani T, Henning A, Sándor PS, Boesiger P, Jung HH. Adaptive metabolic changes in CADASIL white matter. *J Neurol* 2010;257:171–177.
31. Hund-Georgiadis M, Norris DG, Guthke T, von Cramon DY. Characterization of cerebral small vessel disease by proton spectroscopy and morphological magnetic resonance. *Cerebrovasc Dis* 2001;12:82–90.
32. Van Zandvoort MJ, van der Grond J, Kappelle LJ, de Haan EH. Cognitive deficits and changes in neurometabolites after a lacunar infarct. *J Neurol* 2005;252: 183–190.
33. Gasparovic C, Prestopnik J, Thompson J, et al. ^{1}H-MR spectroscopy metabolite levels correlate with executive function in vascular cognitive impairment. *J Neurol Neurosurg Psychiatry* 2013;84:715–721.
34. Li C, Ling X, Liu S, et al. Abnormalities of magnetic resonance spectroscopy and diffusion tensor imaging are correlated with executive dysfunction in patients with ischemic leukoaraiosis. *J Clin Neurosci* 2012;19:718–722.
35. Brooks WM, Wesley MH, Kodituwakku PW, Garry PJ, Rosenberg GA. ^{1}H-MRS differentiates white matter hyperintensities in subcortical arteriosclerotic encephalopathy from those in normal elderly. *Stroke* 1997;28:1940–1943.
36. Calautti C, Baron JC. Functional neuroimaging studies of motor recovery after stroke in adults. *Stroke* 2003;34:1553–1566.
37. Weiller C, Ramsay SC, Wise RJ, et al. Individual patterns of functional reorganization in the human cerebral cortex after capsular infarction. *Ann Neurol* 1993;33:181–189.
38. Gerloff C, Bushara K, Sailer A, et al. Multimodal imaging of brain reorganization in motor areas of the contralesional hemisphere of well recovered patients after

capsular stroke. *Brain* 2006;129:791–808.

39. Pineiro R, Pendlebury S, Johansen-Berg H, Matthews PM. Altered hemodynamic response in patients after subcortical stroke measured by functional MRI. *Stroke* 2002;33:103–109.

40. Patel MJ, Boada FE, Price JC, et al. Association of small vessel ischemic white matter changes with BOLD fMRI imaging in the elderly. *Psychiatry Res* 2012;204:117–122.

41. Rossini PM, Altamura C. Ferretti A, et al. Does cerebrovascular disease affect the coupling between neuronal activity and local haemodynamics? *Brain* 2004;127:99–110.

42. Dennis A, Bosnell R, Dawes H, et al. Cognitive context determines dorsal premotor cortical activity during hand movements in patients after stroke. *Stroke* 2011;42: 1056–1061.

43. Aizenstein HJ, Andreescu C, Edelman KL, et al. fMRI correlates of white matter hyperintensities in late-life depression. *Am J Psychiatry* 2011;168:1075–82.

44. Bakker SL, de Leeuw FE, den Heijer T, et al. Cerebral haemodynamics in the elderly: the Rotterdam Study. *Neuroepidemiology* 2004;23: 178–184.

45. Kozera GM, Dubaniewicz M, Zdrojewski T, et al. Cerebral vasomotor reactivity and extent of white matter lesions in middle-aged men with arterial hypertension: a pilot study. *Am J Hypertens* 2010; 23:1198–1203.

46. Borogovac A, Asllani I. Arterial spin labeling (ASL) fMRI: advantages, theoretical constraints, and experimental challenges in neurosciences. *Int J Biomed Imaging* 2012;2012:818456.

47. Bastos-Leite AJ, Kuijer JP, Rombouts SA, et al. Cerebral blood flow by using pulsed arterial spin-labeling in elderly subjects with white matter hyperintensities. *AJNR Am J Neuroradiol* 2008;29: 1296–1301.

48. Brickman AM, Zahra A, Muraskin J, et al. Reduction in cerebral blood flow in areas appearing as white matter hyperintensities on magnetic resonance imaging. *Psychiatry Res* 2009;172:117–120.

49. Mandell DM, Han JS, Poublanc J, et al. Selective reduction of blood flow to white matter during hypercapnia corresponds with leukoaraiosis. *Stroke* 2008;39:1993–1998.

50. Hajjar I, Zhao P, Alsop D, Novak V. Hypertension and cerebral vasoreactivity: a continuous arterial spin labeling magnetic resonance imaging study. *Hypertension* 2010;56: 859–864.

51. Dumas A, Dierksen GA, Gurol ME, et al. Functional magnetic resonance imaging detection of vascular reactivity in cerebral amyloid angiopathy. *Ann Neurol* 2012;72:76–81.

52. Hendrikes J, Petersen ET, Chèze A, et al. Relation between cerebral perfusion territories and location of cerebral infarcts. *Stroke* 2009;40:1617–1622.

53. Hao X, Xu D, Bansal R, et al. Multimodal magnetic resonance imaging: the coordinated use of multiple, mutually informative probes to understand brain structure and function. *Hum Brain Mapp* 2013;34:253–271.

54. Aslan S, Huang H, Uh J, et al. White matter cerebral blood flow is inversely correlated with structural and functional connectivity in the human brain. *Neuroimage* 2011;56:1145–1153.

55. Chen JJ, Rosas HD, Salat DH. The relationship between cortical blood flow and sub-cortical white-matter health across the adult age span. *PLoS One* 2013;8: e56733.

Chapter 15

Cerebral hemodynamics in cerebral small vessel disease

Hugh S. Markus, Charlotte L. Allan, and Klaus P. Ebmeier

Introduction

Cerebral ischemia is thought to be an important disease mechanism in cerebral small vessel disease (SVD). It has been hypothesized that acute ischemia in the territory of the perforating artery results in lacunar stroke, while chronic ischemia occurring in the distal territories of the perforating arteries results in changes to cerebral white-matter, known as leukoaraiosis. The spatial pattern of leukoaraiosis, with changes first occurring in the brain regions furthest from the origin of the perforating arteries, would be consistent with disease occurring due to hypoperfusion. This has led to the suggestion that cerebral blood flow (CBF) is reduced in SVD, and many studies have been performed to investigate this issue. In addition, cerebral arteriopathy underlying SVD may also impair the ability of small cerebral vessels to vasodilate, leading to problems maintaining perfusion in response to drops in blood pressure and perfusion pressure. Impairments of cerebral reactivity to vasodilatory stimuli [1] and of cerebral autoregulation [2] have been shown in animal models of cerebral autosomal dominant arteriopathy with subcortical infarcts and leukoencephalopathy (CADASIL), a genetic form of SVD. These processes have been investigated in patients with sporadic SVD, as well as with CADASIL.

We review the different techniques that can be used to measure CBF, cerebral reactivity, and cerebral autoregulation. We then consider recent studies investigating cerebral hemodynamics in SVD.

Methods for measurement of CBF

A number of different techniques have been used to measure CBF in SVD, although many are only semi-quantitative [3, 4]. Most measure CBF or perfusion within brain tissue; however, others measure volume flow within the major supplying arteries (Table 15.1). Measurement of blood *velocity* can be made using transcranial Doppler ultrasound of the intracranial vessels.

Cerebral tissue perfusion techniques require a tracer or contrast agent, which may be derived endogenously, as with magnetic resonance imaging (MRI), and an imaging technique to allow its concentration to be measured as it passes through the cerebral circulation [3]. Commonly used techniques include: positron emission tomography (PET), single photon emission computed tomography (SPECT), xenon-based techniques (usually using computed tomography [CT] to image concentration changes), contrast CT perfusion, and MRI perfusion studies.

Nuclear medicine methods

Nuclear medicine imaging can be divided into two main techniques: coincidence detection and single photon methods [3]. These are distinguished on the basis of the physical characteristics of the radionuclides used.

PET uses coincidence radiation employing positron-emitting radionuclides, which, after annihilation, produce two 511 keV photons traveling in opposite directions. SPECT uses lower energy photon emitting radionuclides. PET is often considered the gold standard, as it is the more sensitive method, not losing any information due to absorption in collimators (see below). The most widely used PET compound for CBF imaging is water, using positron-emitting oxygen-15 to produce $H_2{}^{15}O$. This allows accurate measurement of oxygen utilization, and therefore of the oxygen extraction fraction (OEF), through direct repeated measurements of arterial and venous

Cerebral Small Vessel Disease, ed. Leonardo Pantoni and Philip B. Gorelick. Published by Cambridge University Press.

Table 15.1 Methods of measurement of CBF

Technology	Specific method	Relevant points
Perfusion (regional CBF)		
PET	^{15}O-labeled water	Allows O_2 consumption measurement
SPECT	^{99m}Tc-HMPAO, ^{99m}Tc-ECD ^{123}I-labeled IMP	
Xenon-based methods	Stable xenon methods Intravenous xenon methods Xenon SPECT Xenon CT	
MR-based methods	Exogenous perfusion Endogenous perfusion	
CT-based techniques	Contrast perfusion imaging Xenon CT	
Volume flow (in major arteries)		
Carotid and vertebral artery ultrasound	Doppler-based techniques Non-Doppler-based techniques	
MR-based techniques		
Flow velocity techniques		
Transcranial Doppler ultrasound		Changes in velocity only parallel flow if MCA diameter remains unchanged

CBF, cerebral blood flow; CT, computed tomography; ^{123}I-IMP, *N*-isopropyl-*p*-[123I]-iodoamphetamine; MCA, middle cerebral artery; MR, magnetic resonance; O_2, oxygen; ^{15}O, oxygen-15; ^{99m}Tc-ECD, technetium-99m ethyl cysteinate dimer; ^{99m}Tc-HMPAO, technetium-99m-hexamethylpropyleneamine oxime; PET, photon emission tomography; SPECT; single photon emission computed tomography

levels of ^{15}O. Oxygen-15 needs to be produced in a cyclotron, which is not only expensive, but also has to be on site due to the short half-life of oxygen-15, which is two minutes. Therefore, PET CBF measurement is only available in a few centers. More often than oxygen-15 labeled water and O_2 (^{15}O-H_2O), fluorine-18-labeled deoxyglucose (^{18}F-FDG) is used to measure regional glucose uptake, which represents aerobic and anaerobic glucose metabolism and is largely parallel to regional CBF (rCBF) and perfusion. The production of ^{18}F-FDG only requires a desktop cyclotron, which is more widely available than the facilities required to generate $H_2{}^{15}O$.

SPECT is widely available in nuclear medicine departments. Radio-isotopes used in SPECT emit gamma rays. The source of radiation is detected by photomultiplier crystals after filtering through collimators that restrict access to the camera crystal and rotate to locate the origin of the radiation in three dimensions. The ligands used are highly lipophilic, are taken up into the brain on first pass, and are bound in the brain by metabolism into hydrophilic compounds that give a snapshot of blood flow, or better perfusion within the minute after injection (e.g., Technetium-[^{99m}Tc]-hexamethyl-propyleneamine oxime [HMPAO] and ^{99m}Tc-ethyl cysteinate diethylester [^{99m}Tc-ECD]). The most common clinical use of perfusion SPECT is in the differential diagnosis of Alzheimer's disease, but it has also been used to investigate perfusion differences in rarer types of dementia and in conditions that can affect cerebral small vessels.

Xenon-gas-based techniques in combination with CT or SPECT have been widely used for the measurement of CBF, although they have become less popular with the advent of easier to administer tracers that give three-dimensional (3D) reconstruction at a higher resolution. Xenon gas at high concentrations is an anesthetic, but at tracer concentrations can be inhaled without significant risk. It dissolves in the blood and rapidly diffuses through the blood–brain barrier. Xenon has a high atomic number relative to air and soft tissues, and, therefore, its presence can be measured by CT. A washout method is used: an initial equilibrium of xenon is reached in the tissue after which the supply is acutely discontinued, the concentration decays in an exponential fashion, and the initial decay corresponds to cerebral perfusion.

Contrast CT perfusion

Perfusion CT is widely available on modern CT scanners and involves sequential acquisition of cerebral CT sections during intravenous administration of an iodinated contrast agent. Analysis of the resultant contrast enhancement curves, according to the central volume principle, allows calculation of CBF, mean transit time (MTT), and cerebral blood volume (CBV). CT perfusion can potentially be used to calculate absolute flow values if information on arterial input and venous outflow curves are derived, although the reliability of this technique has not been fully established and there may be significant variation between different scanner processing protocols.

Magnetic resonance perfusion

MRI methods to measure perfusion fall into two categories, exogenous and endogenous techniques.

Exogenous contrast methods are the most widely used: they rely on the intravenous injection of a paramagnetic tracer, such as gadolinium, and rapid acquisition of images using echo-planar imaging techniques. As the tracer passes through the cerebral vasculature, it induces a magnetic field, leading to dephasing effects which cause reduced signal from tissue in its immediate vicinity. Since this effect is closely related to flow of tracer through the brain, it provides a measure of cerebral perfusion. This method also allows measurement of CBV and MTT. It has been suggested that absolute quantification is possible if an arterial input function is obtained by imaging through a supplying artery, although in practice it is usually treated as a semiquantitative technique.

Endogenous tracer methods in magnetic resonance (MR) perfusion imaging (arterial spin labeling [ASL]) use a model that assumes the tracer freely diffuses from the intravascular compartment into the tissue compartment. This model is similar to that used in PET and SPECT, where a tracer is administered and the regional accumulation (influenced by regional blood flow and tracer half-life) is measured [5]. Endogenous MR perfusion methods (e.g., ASL) take advantage of signal loss resulting from magnetically labeled water protons flowing into the imaging plane and exchanging with tissue water protons. Water protons within inflowing arterial blood are magnetically labeled (or "tagged") by the application of a special radio-frequency pulse designed to invert spins in a thick slab proximal to the slice of interest. By measuring signal changes between tagged images and baseline untagged images, qualitative or quantitative images of CBF can be obtained. These techniques are entirely noninvasive and can be repeated as often as desired – indeed multiple acquisitions may be required as the signal to noise ratio is low.

Volume flow methods

These techniques quantify volume flow in the major supplying arteries, rather than focusing on regional perfusion. Carotid and vertebral neck ultrasound using either Doppler-based or non-Doppler-based methods has been used to quantify flow, and more recently flow quantification has been performed by MR angiographic techniques. Flow measurements reflect total CBF in both the gray matter and white matter, and, therefore, they do not provide information on regional perfusion changes in SVD.

Transcranial Doppler ultrasound

Transcranial Doppler ultrasound (TCD) measures flow velocity in the basal intracerebral vessels. Most commonly, flow velocity is measured in the middle cerebral artery (MCA). Changes in velocity will only reflect changes in flow if the MCA diameter remains constant. This has been demonstrated when the vasodilator carbon dioxide (CO_2) is given [6]. However, some agents, particularly those affecting the nitric oxide system, can result in alterations in MCA diameter and these potentially invalidate TCD flow measurements [7]. Since TCD measures flow velocity in the large arteries, this again reflects flow in the combined gray and white matter.

The great advantage of TCD is its high temporal resolution allowing rapid changes in flow velocity to be determined. This has led to its widespread use in the estimation of cerebral reactivity and cerebral autoregulation.

Methods of measurement for cerebral autoregulation and reactivity

CBF remains relatively constant despite modest variations in perfusion pressure; for example, resulting from changes in arterial blood pressure. This phenomenon is referred to as cerebral autoregulation. It has an important protective role against the danger of hypoxia at low perfusion pressure, and the risk of brain edema at higher arterial pressure. In a healthy individual, mean arterial pressures are maintained relatively constant between 60 and 150 mmHg, but once these limits are reached, CBF increases or decreases passively with increases or decreases in perfusion pressure. This autoregulatory plateau is shifted to higher values in patients with chronic hypertension and this can lead to deleterious effects, if blood pressure is excessively reduced, when symptoms of ischemia occur at a relatively higher blood pressure [8].

"Cerebral autoregulation" can be estimated directly, or an indirect estimate can be obtained by measuring the ability of CBF to increase in response to vasodilatory stimuli. Measurement of true cerebral autoregulation can be divided into techniques measuring "static" or "dynamic" autoregulation.

During static autoregulation measurement, steady state values of CBF are determined across a range of blood pressures. A variety of methods can be used to measure CBF, and blood pressure is manipulated by the use of drugs or shifts in blood volumes; for example, by the use of tilt tables or negative pressure. To determine the full range of static autoregulation requires blood pressure to be manipulated across a wide range and, as imaging needs to be performed at each blood pressure, this is a laborious process. For this reason, the majority of more recent studies in SVD have estimated "dynamic" autoregulation. Here the rate of change in CBF, or CBV, is determined after a sudden change in arterial blood pressure. Such a technique requires measurement of CBF with a very high temporal resolution and the only technique that can provide this is TCD. Initial techniques induced a sudden large fall in blood pressure by deflating leg cuffs that had previously been inflated to above venous pressure [9]. The rate of rise of CBF velocity in the MCA is then compared with the rate of rise in blood pressure continually monitored using a non-invasive device. More recently, spontaneous fluctuations in blood pressure have been used instead of induced fluctuations [10].

Cerebral reactivity measurements determine CBF at baseline, and following administration of a cerebral vasodilator. The most commonly used vasodilator is an increased concentration of inspired CO_2. This results in a marked and rapid increase in CBF. TCD is most widely used to monitor the change in CBF although other imaging techniques including MRI techniques have also been used. Acetazolamide, a carbonic anhydrase inhibitor, can also be used as a vasodilator stimulus instead of CO_2.

It is important to appreciate that cerebral autoregulation and cerebral reactivity are different processes, although frequently impairment of one occurs in parallel with impairment of the other. In diffuse arteriopathies, such as SVD, the same disease process might be expected to impair both autoregulation and the ability of small arteries to vasodilate in response to CO_2. The mechanisms responsible for cerebral autoregulation are not fully understood, although neurogenic, myogenic, and metabolic factors have been proposed. Endothelial factors, particularly nitric oxide (NO), have been suggested as important mediators of cerebral autoregulation [4]; data from humans show that the NO synthase inhibitor L-MMNA resulted in significant impairment of dynamic autoregulation [11]. In contrast, NO synthase inhibition using the same inhibitor did not alter the hypercapnic response [12, 13].

Studies measuring resting CBF in cerebral SVD

Many studies have investigated CBF in cerebral SVD, and these are reviewed below. The majority demonstrate impaired CBF, but a number of important factors need to be taken into account in their interpretation. SVD has been used to describe different disease processes ranging from asymptomatic white matter hyperintensities (WMHs) in normal individuals, through to symptomatic disease in patients presenting with stroke but who have normal cognition, and to patients with dementia.

Many studies have looked at measurements of CBF or perfusion in different phenotypes of SVD. These have used a wide variety of the different techniques described above. To identify relevant studies, on December 6, 2012 we performed a systematic review using the terms lacunar stroke, OR leukoaraiosis, OR SVD, OR white matter hyperintensity, OR vascular dementia, AND CBF. We also searched reference lists. Studies are summarized in Table 15.2 according to the type of patient studied [14–38].

An early study using HMPAO SPECT in 17 individuals with symptomatic lacunar stroke with leukoaraiosis found decreased CBF in the periventricular region but no change in the temporal or parietal cortex [14]. A subsequent and more extensive study in a similar group of symptomatic lacunar stroke patients with leukoaraiosis used HMPAO SPECT to measure CBF and PET to measure glucose metabolism [15]. In contrast to the first study, no reduction in cortical CBF or glucose metabolism was found, even with severe white matter lesions (WMLs). The authors concluded that brain atrophy and cognitive function were the major determinants of both. They suggested that accompanying brain atrophy may confound CBF results, and that although total cortical CBF may fall, CBF per unit volume of brain tissue does not alter. Using Xenon CT, cortical CBF was found to be reduced in patients with lacunar infarcts [16], and in a further study from the same group it was lower in patients with multiple compared with single lacunar infarcts [17]. A study in 246 neurologically normal individuals using a Xenon-133 inhalation method found the presence of asymptomatic lacunar infarcts was associated with lower CBF [25]. A more recent MRI study using exogenous contrast in patients with symptomatic lacunar stroke and confluent leukoaraiosis found reduced white matter CBF, but normal gray matter CBF [19]. In contrast, a PET study in lacunar stroke patients found severe WMLs to be associated with higher CBF, higher O_2 extraction fraction, and lower oxygen metabolism in the centrum semiovale [18].

Taken together, these results suggest that lacunar stroke, particularly with leukoaraiosis, is associated with reduced CBF in the white matter and possibly also in the cortex. It may be that cortical reductions only occur with more severe disease, as in patients with dementia (see below). The presence of atrophy, which is a feature of cerebral SVD [39], is an important confound because this can result in reduced CBF if the atrophy is not controlled for.

Studies in patients with vascular dementia, predominantly due to SVD, show a reduction in CBF more consistently. CT xenon studies found reduced CBF in all regions, and frontal leukoaraiosis was correlated with reduced CBF in the subcortical gray matter [21], putamen, and thalamus [22]. A small PET study in five subjects with "Binswanger's disease" found both CBF and cerebral metabolic rate for O_2 ($CMRO_2$) were markedly reduced in the white matter and there was a reduction in the frontal and temporal cortex where no abnormalities were detected by CT or MRI [23]. A further study compared patients with lacunes and leukoaraiosis plus dementia with those with lacunar stroke without dementia. Patients with dementia had lower CBF and $CMRO_2$ with increased O_2 extraction ratio in all cerebral regions except the cerebellum [24]. Taken together, these results suggest that both white and gray matter CBF is reduced in patients with vascular dementia due to SVD.

Studies have also looked at WMHs in patients with Alzheimer's disease. Patients with Alzheimer's disease with leukoaraiosis had significantly lower bilateral perfusion in the basal ganglia, thalamus, and frontal lobes than patients with Alzheimer's disease without leukoaraiosis [27], and CBF was lower in WMH lesions in patients with Alzheimer's disease compared with normal-appearing white matter [26].

A number of studies have looked at CBF in neurologically normal individuals. The presence of WMHs has been associated with lower white matter CBF measured using xenon CT [29, 31], although studies relating asymptomatic WMHs to reduced cortical CBF have given conflicting results [30, 36]. Higher resolution imaging techniques have allowed measurement of CBF within areas of WMHs. Lower CBF has been consistently shown in areas of asymptomatic WMHs compared with normal-appearing white matter in the same subjects using a variety of techniques, including SPECT [38], exogenous contrast MRI [35], and endogenous contrast MRI [33]. A large study in 628 individuals with a mean age of 68.8 years found that WMHs were associated with lower CBF velocity, measured by TCD, and that there was a progressive reduction in CBF velocity as WMH severity increased [38]. CBF velocity was found to be a stronger risk factor for WMHs than was high blood pressure.

Most studies have been cross-sectional but two have provided longitudinal data. A substudy of the PROspective Study of Pravastatin in the Elderly at Risk (PROSPER) trial of statin therapy investigated 390 individuals with cardiovascular disease including myocardial infarction and stroke or with cardiovascular risk factors. MRI was used to measure flow volume in both the carotid and vertebral arteries [37]. There was no association between CBF and the prevalence of total, periventricular, or deep WMHs at

Table 15.2 Summary of studies looking at resting CBF in patients with various presentations of cerebral SVD

Author	Patient group	Technique	Finding
Lacunar stroke			
Reiche et al. [14]	Symptomatic lacunar stroke and leukoaraiosis (N = 17)	HMPAO SPECT	Severe leukoaraiosis (but not mild) associated with decreased periventricular CBF, but no change in temporal or parietal CBF
Sabri et al. [15]	Symptomatic lacunar stroke and leukoaraiosis (N = 57)	HMPAO SPECT, Glucose PET	No reduction in rCBF or rMRGlu even with severe WMLs. Brain atrophy and cognitive function major determinants of CBF and rMRGlu
Mochizuki et al. [16]	Symptomatic lacunar infarction (N = 10)	Xenon CT	Cortical CBF reduced in patients with lacunar infarcts
Mochizuki et al. [17]	Single (N = 15) and multiple (N = 10) lacunar infarcts	Xenon CT	Cortical CBF lower in those multiple than single lacunar infarcts
Nezu et al. [18]	Lacunar patients (N = 18)	PET $^{15}O_2$	Severe WMHs had lower CBF and higher OEF in centrum semiovale
Markus et al. [19]	Symptomatic lacunar stroke with confluent leukoaraiosis (N = 8)	Exogenous contrast MRI	Lower CBF in white matter but not in gray matter
O'Sullivan et al. [20]	Symptomatic lacunar stroke with confluent leukoaraiosis (N = 21)	Exogenous contrast MRI	CBF lowest in WMHs but lower in normal-appearing white matter (but not centrum semiovale or gray matter) than controls
Vascular dementia			
Kawamura et al. [21]	"Multi-infarct" dementia (71% lacunar) (N = 35)	Xenon CT	Putamen and thalamus CBF correlated with degree of frontal leukoaraiosis
Kawamura et al. [22]	"Multi-infarct" dementia (N = 23)	Xenon CT	CBF reduced in all regions in multi infarct dementia. Frontal leukoaraiosis correlated with reduced CBF in subcortical gray matter
Yao et al. [23]	Vascular dementia of Binswanger type (N = 5)	PET ^{15}O	CBF and $CMRO_2$ reduced in white matter, and in the parietal, frontal, and temporal cortices
De Reuck et al. [24]	Lacunes, leukoaraiosis, and dementia (N = 16)	PET ^{15}O	CBF and $rCMRO_2$ decreased with increased OER in all cerebral regions except cerebellum in subjects with dementia
Asymptomatic lacunar infarcts			
Kobayashi et al. [25]	Silent lacunar infarcts in neurologically normal adults (N = 246)	^{133}Xe inhalation	Lower CBF in those with silent lacunes
Alzheimer's disease			
Makedonov et al. [26]	Alzheimer's disease (N = 16)	^{99m}Tc-ECD SPECT	WMHs associated with lower CBF and higher OEF in all cortical and white matter regions
Starkstein et al. [27]	Alzheimer's disease (N = 46)	HMPAO SPECT	Lower CBF in basal ganglia, thalamus, and frontal lobes in Alzheimer's with leukoaraiosis
Leukoaraiosis in mixed SVD phenotypes			
Bastos-Leite et al. [28]	1. Vascular dementia; 2. Alzheimer's disease; 18 normal cognition	Endogenous contrast MRI	Reduced global, subcortical, and cortical CBF with severe WMHs compared to those with punctate or early confluent WMHs

Table 15.2 *(cont.)*

Author	Patient group	Technique	Finding
Asymptomatic WMHs			
Kobari et al. [29]	Normal individuals (N = 37, aged 18–88)	Xe CT	WMHs associated with lower white matter CBF
Kawamura et al. [30]	Normal individuals (N = 42, of different ages)	Xe CT	Severity of frontal leukoaraiosis correlated with reductions of CBF within frontal white matter and caudate nucleus
Miyazawa et al. [31]	Neurologically normal (N = 135, aged 26–89)	Xe CT	Progressive reduction in CBF in centrum semiovale with increasing degrees of WMH
Isaka et al. [32]	Asymptomatic neurologically normal with risk factors (N = 28)	IV Xe clearance	Periventricular WMHs not related to CBF
Makedonov et al. [26]	Elderly controls (N = 50)	^{99m}Tc-ECD SPECT	CBF lower in WMHs than in normal-appearing white matter
Brickman et al. [33]	Healthy older adults (N = 17, aged 61–70)	Endogenous contrast MRI	Lower CBF in WMHs compared with normal-appearing white matter
Kraut et al. [34]	Healthy elderly (N = 74)	PET ^{15}O	Prospective study: a different pattern of CBF changes was found in stable versus progressive WMHs
Marstrand et al. [35]	Healthy 85 year olds (N = 25)	Exogenous contrast MRI	Lower CBF in WMHs compared with normal-appearing white matter
Wen et al. [36]	Stroke patients (28 stroke patients and 27 controls)	Exogenous contrast MRI	Negative correlation between WMHs and cortical CBF. Thalamic and basal ganglia CBF correlated more with frontal CBF
Ten Dam et al. [37]	PROSPER study of cardiovascular disease/risk factors (N = 390, aged 70–82)	MR volume flow	Prospective study: reduced CBF associated with increased periventricular WMHs but not deep white matter WMHs
Tzourio et al. [38]	Healthy elderly (N = 628, mean age 68.8)	TCD	WMH severity negatively correlated with CBF velocity

CBF, cerebral blood flow; CMRO$_2$, cerebral metabolic rate for O$_2$; CT, computed tomography; HMPAO, hexamethylpropyleneamine oxime; IV, intravenous; MR, magnetic resonance; MRI, magnetic resonance imaging; ^{15}O, oxygen-15; OEF, oxygen extraction fraction; PET, photon emission tomography; PROSPER, PROspective Study of Pravastatin in the Elderly at Risk; rCBF, regional cerebral blood flow; rCMRO$_2$, regional cerebral metabolic rate for O$_2$; rMRGlu; regional myocardial metabolic rate of glucose; SPECT, single photon emission computed tomography; SVD, small vessel disease; TCD, transcranial Doppler; ^{99m}Tc-ECD, technetium-99m ethyl cysteinate dimer; WMH, white matter hemorrhage; Xe, xenon

baseline. Individuals were rescanned after an average interval of 33 months. Decline in CBF was not associated with any increase in total WMH. However, when the volume of WMHs was separated into periventricular and deep WMHs, for every 50 ml/M decrease in total CBF there was a 1.32 increase in risk of developing periventricular WMHs. In contrast, there was no association between a decrease in CBF and risk of developing deep WMHs. For the reasons described above, this technique of blood flow measurement measures total CBF and is unable to separate out white matter or regional flow. For this reason it may be less sensitive to more subtle changes particularly in white matter flow. This could explain the lack of association at baseline with WMHs.

A second longitudinal study, the Baltimore Longitudinal Study of Aging, evaluated MRI scans and resting H_2O PET at baseline and after an average of 7.7 years in participants without dementia [34]. Subjects were divided into two groups, one in whom WMHs progressed and the other in whom they were stable. Analysis considered changes in cortical but not white matter CBF. A different pattern of CBF changes was found in patients whose WMHs remained stable compared with those who had progression of WMHs. The group with progressive white matter abnormalities showed greater increase in CBF in the right inferior temporal gyrus/fusiform gyrus, right anterior cingulate, and the rostral aspect of the left superior temporal gyrus. Regions of greater longitudinal decrease in this group were evident in the right inferior parietal lobule and at the right occipital pole. The authors hypothesized that the longitudinal increases may reflect cortical compensation mechanisms for reduced efficacy of interregional neural communications that result from white matter deterioration.

One key question is whether any reduction in CBF is primary, or merely occurs secondary to brain damage. Due to vaso-neuronal coupling, reductions in brain metabolism are associated with reductions in blood flow. Therefore, tissue damage is associated with reduced CBF. One way of examining this is to look at CBF not only in WMLs but also in normal-appearing white matter. A study in patients with symptomatic lacunar stroke and confluent leukoaraiosis that used exogenous contrast MRI found that in the periventricular region CBF was reduced to an intermediate level between that seen in WMLs and white matter in normal controls; however, there was no such reduction detected in the deep white matter [20].

Taken together, most studies do suggest a reduction in white matter CBF across different phenotypes of SVD ranging from vascular dementia to asymptomatic WMHs. The majority, but not all, have found the reduction in CBF is greater in patients with more severe WMHs. Studies looking at cortical CBF in nondemented individuals have shown less consistent results, but in more severely affected individuals with dementia due to SVD, most have shown a reduction in both subcortical and cortical CBF. Data regarding white matter that appears normal are limited, but suggest that CBF is reduced [20]. This is consistent with a causal role of CBF in disease pathogenesis; however, it is important to note that more sensitive white matter imaging with diffusion tensor imaging (DTI) has shown subtle structural changes in normal-appearing white matter, and these could themselves be associated secondarily with minor reductions in CBF due to vaso-neuronal coupling [39, 40].

Studies measuring cerebral reactivity and autoregulation in SVD

TCD studies looking at the increase in MCA CBF velocity in response to either hypercapnia or acetazolamide have shown reduced cerebral reactivity in patients with lacunar infarcts [41–43], more marked in those with multiple compared with single infarcts [43], and a reduction in reactivity that correlated with the degree of leukoaraiosis [44]. In patients with symptomatic lacunar infarction, no difference was found between the symptomatic and asymptomatic signs, suggesting that there is a diffuse abnormality of autoregulation, rather than an abnormality related to the episode of symptomatic ischemia [43]. This is consistent with cerebral autoregulation studies presented below that show bilateral abnormalities.

As discussed above, TCD offers high temporal resolution but gives a global measure of autoregulation in the MCA territory, and does not allow regional cerebral reactivity to be assessed. This is possible using imaging techniques such as MRI and PET. Studies using xenon techniques have shown that reactivity to acetazolamide is reduced in white matter [16] and cortex, with a greater reduction seen in patients with multiple compared with single lacunes [17]. One PET study in patients with microangiopathy, lacunes, white matter changes, and dementia showed a reduction in acetozalamide vasoreactivity in all cerebral regions, although in similar patients without dementia a reduction was only seen in the thalamus [44]. This was consistent with another PET study in normotensive and hypertensive individuals, which found reduced reactivity in those with leukoaraiosis and an inverse correlation between leukoaraiosis severity and reduced reactivity [45]. Further supporting evidence comes from a *N*-isopropyl-*p*-[123I]-iodoamphetamine (^{123}I-IMP) SPECT study that showed reduced reactivity in severe leukoaraiosis compared to mild leukoaraiosis in the unaffected hemisphere of patients with a variety of neurologic diseases [46]. In contrast, another PET study found lower resting CBF in patients with lacunar stroke who had severe WMLs, compared with lacunar stroke patients with few WMHs but no reduction of reactivity [18]. Other studies in asymptomatic populations have found reduced reactivity in patients with WMHs compared with those without [32]. One using exogenous contrast MRI found a relative reduction in reactivity in WMLs themselves compared with normal white matter [35].

There have been fewer studies of cerebral autoregulation compared with reactivity. One early study of resting CBF and static autoregulation in 51 hypertensive patients with minor strokes (43 with lacunar infarcts and eight with deep basal minor hemorrhage) related measurements of cerebral autoregulation to the degree of periventricular lesions determined on CT. The argon inhalation technique was used to measure CBF, with arterial blood sampling; this allowed measurement of absolute blood flows and accurate blood pressure measurements. Autoregulation was determined by measuring CBF at different blood pressures, with the use of a tilt-table to alter blood pressure. Impaired autoregulation was more common in patients with more severe periventricular lesions, and multiple regression demonstrated that impaired autoregulation was an independent determinant of the severity of periventricular lesions [47]. Dynamic autoregulation has been shown to be impaired in SVD. One study measured dynamic autoregulation in acute stroke patients, by correlating spontaneous fluctuations in blood pressure with changes in MCA flow velocity, determined using TCD. In large artery (nonlacunar) MCA stroke unilateral reduction in autoregulation was found. In contrast, in lacunar stroke patients a bilateral reduction was found, consistent with a diffuse abnormality of dynamic autoregulation in SVD [48].

Studies in CADASIL

The above studies are in patients with "sporadic" SVD. Broadly similar findings have been published in studies of the autosomal genetic form of SVD, cerebral autosomal dominant arteriopathy with subcortical infarcts and leukoencephalopathy (CADASIL). Although the molecular pathogenesis of CADASIL is distinct, resulting from mutations in the *NOTCH3* gene, a similar pattern of small vessel involvement occurs to that seen in sporadic lacunar stroke with leukoaraiosis. Corresponding to this, CADASIL patients suffer lacunar infarcts and leukoaraiosis in both the periventricular and deep white matter regions.

An early study using exogenous contrast MRI found significant reduction in absolute and relative CBF and CBV within areas of WMHs. This reduction was more severe in patients with dementia compared to those without. No significant change in absolute CBF and CBV values was observed in the cortex of patients with CADASIL [49]. These results were confirmed in a second study also using exogenous contrast MRI, which found lower CBV within WMHs compared with normal-appearing white matter [50]. Mean CBV in the gray matter was within the normal range. Both cognitive impairment and disability showed negative correlations with CBV in subcortical WMHs, but not with CBV in the normal-appearing white matter. A similar reduction in CBF has been found using PET, with mean CBF found to be significantly lower in frontal and occipital white matter, and CBF decreased significantly with increased severity of the disease [51]. The patients had lower mean glucose metabolism than controls, although differences were not statistically significant and WMH severity scores correlated significantly with white matter CBF (but not with glucose metabolism).

Studies estimating the change in large artery flow in response to hypercapnia, either using TCD or MRI angiography, have given conflicting results in CADASIL. In 29 CADASIL subjects reactivity to CO_2 was reduced compared with controls, and the difference persisted when only nondisabled patients were included [52]. In contrast in 24 CADASIL patients without cognitive impairment, no reduction in CO_2 reactivity could be detected using the same technique [53]. It was suggested that this lack of reduction might be due to reactivity not being impaired in early disease, or that TCD may not be a sufficiently sensitive tool to detect hemodynamic changes in early disease [53]. A second study using phase-contrast MRI angiography to measure global CBF in 40 mutation positive CADASIL subjects also found no reduction in acetazolamide reactivity, although there was a reduction in resting CBF [54]. However, a second study from the same group in 25 *NOTCH3* mutation carriers found that lower reactivity at baseline predicted progression of WMHs over a seven-year follow-up period [55]. A 24-week course of acetazolamide at 250 mg daily was associated with increased CBF velocity and increased reactivity to CO_2, and the authors suggested this as a possible treatment approach [56]. In contrast, statin therapy, which has been suggested to increase reactivity, had no effect when given for eight weeks, with reactivity assessed using TCD [57].

Higher resolution techniques have looked at reactivity in different brain regions in CADASIL.

Using exogenous contrast MRI, there was a smaller increase in CBF following acetazolamide within areas of WMHs, compared with the white matter of control subjects [49]. Only one study has measured dynamic cerebral autoregulation using TCD in 24 CADASIL patients without dementia, and this found no reduction compared with normal controls [53].

Conclusions

Studies have investigated cerebral hemodynamics in a variety of clinical presentations of sporadic SVD, both symptomatic and asymptomatic, as well as in CADASIL. The results are consistent with a reduction in white matter CBF in both sporadic SVD and CADASIL. This reduction is greater within WMHs, but there also appears to be reduced flow within normal-appearing white matter. Whether cortical CBF is also reduced is less certain; it may be that it is normal in earlier stages of the disease but that reductions occur in late-stage disease, particularly with the onset of dementia.

In sporadic disease cerebral reactivity to CO_2 and acetazolamide appears to be reduced, and higher spatial resolution imaging techniques suggest this reduction is greater within WMHs. Both reactivity and autoregulation studies suggest this abnormality may be diffuse and, not just in the symptomatic territory, consistent with a diffuse arteriopathy. There are fewer data in CADASIL on reactivity and autoregulation and results have been less consistent.

References

1. Lacombe P, Oligo C, Domenga V, Tournier-Lasserve E, Joutel A. Impaired cerebral vasoreactivity in a transgenic mouse model of cerebral autosomal dominant arteriopathy with subcortical infarcts and leukoencephalopathy arteriopathy. *Stroke* 2005;36:1053–1058.
2. Joutel A, Monet-Leprêtre M, Gosele C, et al. Cerebrovascular dysfunction and microcirculation rarefaction precede white matter lesions in a mouse genetic model of cerebral ischemic small vessel disease. *J Clin Invest* 2010;120:433–445.
3. Griffiths PD, Hoggard N, Dannels WR, Wilkinson ID. In vivo measurement of cerebral blood flow: a review of methods and applications. *Vasc Med* 2001;6: 51–60.
4. Markus HS. Cerebral perfusion and stroke. *J Neurol Neurosurg Psychiatry* 2004;75:353–361.
5. Petrella JR, Provenzale JM. MR perfusion imaging of the brain techniques and applications. *AJR Am J Roentgenol* 2000;175: 207–219.
6. Huber P, Handa J. Effect of contrast material, hypercapnia, hyperventilation, hypertonic glucose and papaverine on the diameter of cerebral arteries. *Invest Radiol* 1967;2: 17–32.
7. White RP, Deane C, Hindley C, et al. The effect of the nitric oxide donor glyceryl trinitrate on global and regional cerebral blood flow in man. *J Neurol Sci* 2000;178: 23–28.
8. Paulson OB, Strandgaard S, Edvinsson L. Cerebral autoregulation. *Cerebrovasc Brain Metab Rev* 1990;2:161–192.
9. Tiecks FP, Lam AM, Aaslid R, Newell DW. Comparison of static and dynamic cerebral autoregulation measurements. *Stroke* 1995;26:1014–1019.
10. Panerai RB, White RP, Markus HS, Evans DH. Grading of cerebral dynamic autoregulation from spontaneous fluctuations in arterial blood pressure. *Stroke* 1998;29:2341–2346.
11. White RP, Vallance P, Markus HS. Effect of inhibition of nitric oxide synthase on dynamic cerebral autoregulation in humans. *Clin Sci (Lond)* 2000;99:555–560.
12. White RP, Hindley C, Bloomfield PM, et al. The effect of the nitric oxide synthase inhibitor L-NMMA on basal CBF and vasoneuronal coupling in man: a PET study. *J Cereb Blood Flow Metab* 1999;19:673–678.
13. White RP, Deane C, Vallance P, Markus HS. Nitric oxide synthase inhibition in humans reduces cerebral blood flow but not the hyperemic response to hypercapnia. *Stroke* 1998;29: 467–472.
14. Reiche W, Weiller C, Weigmann R, et al. [A comparison of MRT and SPECT findings in patients with cerebral microangiopathy.] *Nuklearmedizin* 1991;30:161–169 [in German].
15. Sabri O, Ringelstein EB, Hellwig D, et al. Neuropsychological impairment correlates with hypoperfusion and hypometabolism but not with severity of white matter lesions on MRI in patients with cerebral microangiopathy. *Stroke* 1999;30:556–566.
16. Mochizuki Y, Oishi M, Hara M, Yoshihashi H, Takasu T. Regional cerebral blood flow in lacunar infarction. *J Stroke Cerebrovasc Dis* 1997;6:137–140.
17. Mochizuki Y, Oishi M, Takasu T. Cerebral blood flow in single and multiple lacunar infarctions. *Stroke* 1997;28:1458–1460.
18. Nezu T, Yokota C, Uehara T, et al. Preserved acetazolamide reactivity

in lacunar patients with severe white-matter lesions: ^{15}O-labeled gas and H_2O positron emission tomography studies. *J Cereb Blood Flow Metab* 2012;32: 844–850.

19. Markus HS, Lythgoe DJ, Ostegaard L, O'Sullivan M, Williams SC. Reduced cerebral blood flow in white matter in ischaemic leukoaraiosis demonstrated using quantitative exogenous contrast based perfusion MRI. *J Neurol Neurosurg Psychiatry* 2000;69: 48–53.
20. O'Sullivan M, Lythgoe DJ, Pereira AC, et al. Patterns of cerebral blood flow reduction in patients with ischemic leukoaraiosis. *Neurology* 2002;59:321–326.
21. Kawamura J, Meyer JS, Terayama Y, Weathers S. Leukoaraiosis correlates with cerebral hypoperfusion in vascular dementia. *Stroke* 1991;22: 609–614.
22. Kawamura J, Meyer JS, Ichijo M, et al. Correlations of leukoaraiosis with cerebral atrophy and perfusion in elderly normal subjects and demented patients. *J Neurol Neurosurg Psychiatry* 1993;56:182–187.
23. Yao H, Sadoshima S, Kuwabara Y, Ichiya Y, Fujishima M. Cerebral blood flow and oxygen metabolism in patients with vascular dementia of the Binswanger type. *Stroke* 1990;21:1694–1699.
24. De Reuck J, Decoo D, Marchau M, et al. Positron emission tomography in vascular dementia. *J Neurol Sci* 1998;21:55–61.
25. Kobayashi S, Okada K, Yamashita K. Incidence of silent lacunar lesion in normal adults and its relation to cerebral blood flow and risk factors. *Stroke* 1991;22: 1379–1383.
26. Makedonov I, Black SE, Macintosh BJ. Cerebral small vessel disease in aging and Alzheimer's disease: a comparative study using MRI and SPECT. *Eur J Neurol* 2013;20:243–250.
27. Starkstein SE, Sabe L, Vázquez S, et al. Neuropsychological, psychiatric, and cerebral perfusion correlates of leukoaraiosis in Alzheimer's disease. *J Neurol Neurosurg Psychiatry* 1997;63: 66–73.
28. Bastos-Leite AJ, Kuijer JP, Rombouts SA, et al. Cerebral blood flow by using pulsed arterial spin-labeling in elderly subjects with white matter hyperintensities. *AJNR Am J Neuroradiol* 2008;29:1296–1301.
29. Kobari M, Meyer JS, Ichijo M. Leukoaraiosis, cerebral atrophy, and cerebral perfusion in normal aging. *Arch Neurol* 1990;47: 161–165.
30. Kawamura J, Terayama Y, Takashima S, et al. Leukoaraiosis and cerebral perfusion in normal aging. *Exp Aging Res* 1993;19: 225–240.
31. Miyazawa N, Satoh T, Hashizume K, Fukamachi A. Xenon contrast CT–CBF measurements in high-intensity foci on T2-weighted MR images in centrum semiovale of asymptomatic individuals. *Stroke* 1997;28:984–987.
32. Isaka Y, Okamoto M, Ashida K, Imaizumi M. Decreased cerebrovascular dilatory capacity in subjects with asymptomatic periventricular hyperintensities. *Stroke* 1994;25:375–381.
33. Brickman AM, Zahra A, Muraskin J, et al. Reduction in cerebral blood flow in areas appearing as white matter hyperintensities on magnetic resonance imaging. *Psychiatry Res* 2009;172:117–120.
34. Kraut MA, Beason-Held LL, Elkins WD, Resnick SM. The impact of magnetic resonance imaging-detected white matter hyperintensities on longitudinal changes in regional cerebral blood flow. *J Cereb Blood Flow Metab* 2008;28:190–197.
35. Marstrand JR, Garde E, Rostrup E, et al. Cerebral perfusion and cerebrovascular reactivity are reduced in white matter hyperintensities. *Stroke* 2002;33:972–976.
36. Wen W, Sachdev P, Shnier R, Brodaty H. Effect of white matter hyperintensities on cortical cerebral blood volume using perfusion MRI. *Neuroimage* 2004;21:1350–1356.
37. Ten Dam VH, van den Heuvel DM, de Craen AJ, et al. Decline in total cerebral blood flow is linked with increase in periventricular but not deep white matter hyperintensities. *Radiology* 2007;243:198–203.
38. Tzourio C, Lévy C, Dufouil C, et al. Low cerebral blood flow velocity and risk of white matter hyperintensities. *Ann Neurol* 2001;49:411–414.
39. Nitkunan A, Lanfranconi S, Charlton RA, Barrick TR, Markus HS. Brain atrophy and cerebral small vessel disease: a prospective follow-up study. *Stroke* 2011;42:133–138.
40. O'Sullivan M, Summers PE, Jones DK, et al. Normal-appearing white matter in ischemic leukoaraiosis: a diffusion tensor MRI study. *Neurology* 2001;57:2307–2310.
41. Molina C, Sabín JA, Montaner J, et al. Impaired cerebrovascular reactivity as a risk marker for first-ever lacunar infarction: a case-control study. *Stroke* 1999;30:2296–2301.
42. Terborg C, Gora F, Weiller C, Röther J. Reduced vasomotor reactivity in cerebral microangiopathy: a study with near-infrared spectroscopy and transcranial Doppler sonography. *Stroke* 2000;31:924–929.
43. Maeda H, Matsumoto M, Handa N, et al. Reactivity of cerebral

blood flow to carbon dioxide in various types of ischemic cerebrovascular disease: evaluation by the transcranial Doppler method. *Stroke* 1993;24:670–675.

44. De Reuck J, Decoo D, Hasenbroekx MC, et al. Acetazolamide vasoreactivity in vascular dementia: a positron emission tomographic study. *Eur Neurol* 1999;41:31–36.

45. Kuwabara Y, Ichiya Y, Sasaki M, et al. Cerebral blood flow and vascular response to hypercapnia in hypertensive patients with leukoaraiosis. *Ann Nucl Med* 1996;10:293–298.

46. Tomura N, Sasaki K, Kidani H, et al. Reduced perfusion reserve in leukoaraiosis demonstrated using acetazolamide challenge ^{123}I-IMP SPECT. *J Comput Assist Tomogr* 2007;31:884–887.

47. Matsushita K, Kuriyama Y, Nagatsuka K, et al. Periventricular white matter lucency and cerebral blood flow autoregulation in hypertensive patients. *Hypertension* 1994;23:565–568.

48. Immink RV, van Montfrans GA, Stam J, et al. Dynamic cerebral autoregulation in acute lacunar and middle cerebral artery territory ischemic stroke. *Stroke* 2005;36:2595–2600.

49. Chabriat H, Pappata S, Ostergaard L, et al. Cerebral hemodynamics in CADASIL before and after acetazolamide challenge assessed with MRI bolus tracking. *Stroke* 2000;31:1904–1912.

50. Bruening R, Dichgans M, Berchtenbreiter C, et al. Cerebral autosomal dominant arteriopathy with subcortical infarcts and leukoencephalopathy: decrease in regional cerebral blood volume in hyperintense subcortical lesions inversely correlates with disability and cognitive performance. *AJNR Am J Neuroradiol* 2001;22: 1268–1274.

51. Tuominen S, Miao Q, Kurki T, et al. Positron emission tomography examination of cerebral blood flow and glucose metabolism in young CADASIL patients. *Stroke* 2004;35: 1063–1067.

52. Pfefferkorn T, von Stuckrad-Barre S, Herzog J, et al. Reduced cerebrovascular CO_2 reactivity in CADASIL: a transcranial Doppler sonography study. *Stroke* 2001;32:17–21.

53. Singhal S, Markus HS. Cerebrovascular reactivity and dynamic autoregulation in nondemented patients with CADASIL (cerebral autosomal dominant arteriopathy with subcortical infarcts and leukoencephalopathy). *J Neurol* 2005;252:163–167.

54. Van den Boom R, Lesnik Oberstein SA, Spilt A, et al. Cerebral hemodynamics and white matter hyperintensities in CADASIL. *J Cereb Blood Flow Metab* 2003;23:599–604.

55. Liem MK, Lesnik Oberstein SA, Haan J, et al. Cerebrovascular reactivity is a main determinant of white matter hyperintensity progression in CADASIL. *AJNR Am J Neuroradiol* 2009;30: 1244–1247.

56. Huang L, Yang Q, Zhang L, et al. Acetazolamide improves cerebral hemodynamics in CADASIL. *J Neurol Sci* 2010; 292:77–80.

57. Peters N, Freilinger T, Opherk C, Pfefferkorn T, Dichgans M. Effects of short term atorvastatin treatment on cerebral hemodynamics in CADASIL. *J Neurol Sci* 2007;260:100–105.

Chapter 16

Markers of endothelial dysfunction, oxidative stress, and inflammation in cerebral small vessel disease

Francesca Pescini and Rosanna Abbate

Introduction

The hallmarks of cerebral small vessel disease (CSVD) are widespread lesions in the white matter (white matter lesions [WMLs]) and lacunar infarcts identified on neuroimaging. In the vast majority of patients, CSVD is related to aging and vascular risk factors, such as hypertension and diabetes mellitus (sporadic CSVD) [1]. Less frequently, inherited diseases can cause similar neuroimaging alterations, and among these the most studied is cerebral autosomal dominant arteriopathy with subcortical infarcts and leukoencephalopathy (CADASIL), which is considered the model of pure vascular dementia due to small vessel pathology [2].

It has been hypothesized that the brain damage is induced primarily by a chronic ischemia caused by cerebral hypoperfusion and impaired autoregulation related to the structural alterations of parenchymal small vessel walls (tunica media thickening and hyaline degeneration in the cases due to arterial hypertension [1], and genetically determined smooth muscle cell degeneration in CADASIL [3]).

Several studies using different methods, including brain positron emission tomography (PET) and magnetic resonance imaging (MRI), have shown cerebral hypoperfusion in sporadic CSVD. In particular, reduced perfusion was found within the cerebral white matter not only in conjunction with WMLs but also in MRI normal-appearing white matter [4]. This result would support a causal role of hypoperfusion in determining brain lesions, contrasting with the hypothesis that it could be a consequence of reduced demand from damaged tissue. Also, reduced resting perfusion was found in CADASIL patients [5].

However, pathophysiologic factors modulating the incidence, severity, and clinical–functional phenotype of sporadic CSVD and CADASIL are not completely understood. In fact, considering sporadic CSVD, although the association between aging, hypertension, and brain lesions is strong and consistent, it explains only partially both the occurrence and the severity of the lesions. For example, not all hypertensive patients develop WMLs, and the severity of WMLs varies from one patient to another independently of duration, severity, and treatment of hypertension. In the Northern Manhattan Stroke Study, the prevalence of hypertension and other vascular risk factors, such as diabetes mellitus, hypercholesterolemia, and smoking, did not differ between patients with lacunar infarcts and those with other stroke subtypes [6]. On the other hand, despite a highly stereotyped nature of the mutations causing CADASIL, marked phenotypic variation has been reported from the clinicoradiologic point of view both between and within families [3]. The genotype–phenotype relationship has been incompletely studied; however, data available up to now suggest that the site of the *NOTCH3* mutation has little bearing on phenotype. The genetic mutation may, then, not be the only pathogenic mechanism involved in CADASIL.

These aspects lead to hypothesizing that other factors, genetic and environmental, could play a synergistic role in modulating expressivity in sporadic CSVD and CADASIL. Among these factors, endothelial dysfunction seems to have an important role, contributing both to impaired vessel reactivity and autoregulation and to blood–brain barrier alterations with extravasation of serum proteins into the perivascular parenchyma and ensuing toxic effects [1, 7].

The endothelial layer represents a biologic and mechanical barrier between the blood components and the vascular wall. It is an indispensable organ in

Cerebral Small Vessel Disease, ed. Leonardo Pantoni and Philip B. Gorelick. Published by Cambridge University Press.

the regulation of tonicity and vascular homeostasis based on several properties: vasodilatation, inhibition of leukocyte adhesion and migration, inhibition of proliferation and migration of smooth muscular fibers, inhibition of platelet adhesion and aggregation, antioxidant and anti-inflammatory activity, and anticoagulant and profibrinolytic effects. These effects are reduced and could disappear in endothelial dysfunction.

Endothelial dysfunction can be considered the common consequence of several factors acting through different pathways and inducing a series of events leading to oxidative stress and inflammatory mechanisms that promote endothelial dysfunction itself [8, 9].

High blood pressure, oxidized low density lipoproteins, very low density lipoproteins, diabetes, smoking, infections, and hyperhomocysteinemia have a pro-oxidative effect and increase reactive oxygen species (ROS) production, exceeding the detoxification capacity of the endothelium (by means of antioxidant enzymes such as superoxide dismutase, catalase, and endothelial nitric oxide synthase [eNOS]). This leads to intracellular synthesis of peroxynitrite (OONO), which implies a situation of oxidative stress [9]. As a consequence of oxidative stress the endothelium is activated and various types of adhesion molecules are released, recruiting leukocytes. Initially there is the rolling process in which leukocytes adhere to the endothelium. It is mediated by selectins, expressed by both leukocytes (L-selectin) and endothelial cells (E- and P-selectin). Later, leukocytes more strongly adhere to the endothelium and the process of transendothelial migration begins. This process is mediated by intercellular adhesion molecules (ICAM-1), vascular adhesion molecules (VCAM-1), and platelet endothelial adhesion molecules. Also, inflammatory response in endothelial dysfunction is modulated by platelets. They activate various inflammatory molecules (interleukin-1β, thromboxane A2, CD40L, etc.), which increase endothelial dysfunction and promote leukocyte adhesion by means of stimulation of nuclear factor-kappa B (NF-kB). Metalloproteinases (MMPs), particularly MMP-9, participate in the inflammatory process. Their secretion is related to the oxidative stress that characterizes endothelial dysfunction and causes deterioration of the extracellular matrix, permitting the migration of leukocytes through the endothelium [8, 9].

In this chapter we report the supporting evidence for endothelial dysfunction, oxidative stress, and inflammation in CSVD in humans, considering studies conducted on biohumoral markers, progenitor circulating cells, and genetic associations.

Endothelial dysfunction in sporadic CSVD

There is considerable evidence supporting this issue. Endothelial abnormalities and altered expression of endothelial markers, such as ICAM-1 and P-glycoprotein, have been described in pathologic studies of CSVD [10, 11].

Other data showed possible relations between soluble markers of endothelial function and sporadic CSVD.

Thrombomodulin is produced and expressed on the endothelial cell surface; for example, where it mediates the activation of protein C upon binding thrombin. Activated protein C inhibits, by proteolytic cleavage, the cofactors Va and VIIIa of the coagulation cascade. Loss of endothelial surface thrombomodulin leads to a procoagulant phenotype. Von Willebrand factor is mainly found in endothelial cells (Weibel–Palade bodies), but to some extent also in blood platelets (α-granules). It connects the activated blood platelet to the subendothelial collagen. In blood it circulates in a noncovalent complex with factor VIII. Several different assays are used to determine either the concentration or the function of these molecules. The release of the soluble form of thrombomodulin and von Willebrand factor is regarded as a specific marker of endothelial cell activation. Higher levels of these molecules have been found in patients affected by nonacute lacunar infarcts in comparison with controls not affected by cerebral microangiopathy [12], and in patients with numerous lacunes than in those with only a few [13].

Tissue factor is a protein located at extravascular sites not exposed to the blood, such as adventitial fibroblasts and vascular smooth muscle cells, but it is produced and released into the blood by endothelial cells after different stimuli causing injury or endothelial disruption. Tissue factor is released into the blood when there is injury or endothelial disruption. The contact between tissue factor and factor VIIa initiates the extrinsic coagulation pathway leading to the formation of a complex, which activates factor X and IX. The physiologic inhibitor of tissue factor is the tissue factor pathway inhibitor (TFPI), which binds to activated factor Xa within the tissue factor–VIIa–Xa complex, thus limiting thrombin formation. TFPI is mainly present in endothelial cells. Hassan et al. [12] found an association between elevated levels of soluble tissue factor and the extent of WMLs. Also, they reported elevated levels of TFPI in patients with isolated lacunar infarction compared to either healthy controls or patients with WMLs.

Tissue plasminogen activator (tPA), an endothelial serine protease, converts plasminogen to plasmin, which lyses clots. The activity of tPA is inhibited by binding to plasminogen activator inhibitor type 1 (PAI-1), which is secreted by the endothelium. Elevated levels of tPA and low levels of PAI-1 have been found in patients with extensive WMLs [14]. The imbalance between these components of the fibrinolytic system (i.e., patients with WMLs lack the protective effect of PAI-1 for t-PA-induced tissue damage) could be a possible mechanism of ischemic damage induced by t-PA after crossing the blood–brain barrier.

Selectins are transmembrane glycoproteins expressed on activated vascular endothelium (E- and P-selectin), activated platelets (P-selectin), and leukocytes (L-selectin). These adhesion molecules, elevated in CSVD [15, 16], attract leukocytes from the circulation and promote leukocyte rolling, along the endothelium. Then, leukocytes adhere to the endothelium through the action of ICAM-1 and VCAM-1. ICAM-1 is expressed by both endothelial cells and leukocytes. Soluble isoforms of adhesion molecules are present in the circulation after cellular activation. ICAM-1 levels were found elevated in patients with isolated lacunar infarction and WMLs in comparison with controls not affected by CSVD [12]. In the Austrian Stroke Prevention Study, a prospective population study, ICAM-1 levels correlated with the progression of WMLs after controlling for both conventional risk factors and baseline lesion load, supporting a causal role for endothelial dysfunction in CSVD rather than a secondary one [17].

Asymmetric dimethylarginine (ADMA) is an endogenous inhibitor of eNOS. It competes with L-arginine as substrate of this enzyme. Elevated levels of ADMA have been found in several conditions associated with an increased risk of stroke, including hyperhomocysteinemia. ADMA has also been independently associated with CSVD and correlated with WML severity but not lacunar grade [18].

Circulating endothelial progenitor cells (EPCs) are hematopoietic stem cells with limited pluripotent potential. They are present in peripheral blood of adults and are identified by functional characteristics and expression profiles including $CD133^+$, $VEGFR\text{-}2^+$ (or KDR^+), and $CD34^+$. EPCs are involved in formation of new vessels after ischemia. They play a role also in repairing damaged endothelium and are considered a marker of endothelial function. While in the acute stage after a vascular event, several factors stimulate the release of EPCs and their level rises; in a stable clinical condition, lower EPC numbers reflect a higher consumption of the cells for restoration of endothelial damage. Indeed, lower levels of EPCs have been found to be a strong predictor of cardiovascular events and atherosclerotic disease [19]. Only a few studies have evaluated the association between EPC levels and WMLs in sporadic CSVD. In one study, 172 enrolled patients were divided into three groups according to severity of WMLs on computed tomography (CT) scan. Comparing the levels of EPCs among the groups, the authors found that EPCs were significantly lower in patients with severe WMLs. The association remained significant also after multiple logistic regression analysis [20]. Patients with low levels of EPCs may represent a selected group of subjects more prone to endothelial damage, and thus the development of WMLs. Also, EPC levels have been found to be lower in lacunar stroke compared with cardioembolic ischemic stroke [21].

Recent studies suggest that angiogenic T cells may regulate EPC function. Stimulating the function of EPCs, they promote the formation of new blood vessels and endothelial repair. Rouhl et al. [22] found that 32 hypertensive patients with CSVD had lower levels of both angiogenic T cells and EPCs in comparison with control patients without CSVD and independently of blood pressure levels.

Genetic association studies have demonstrated a correlation between some endothelial candidate genes and CSVD. The angiotensin system has received the most attention. Angiotensin II can promote vasoconstriction, inflammation, thrombosis, and vascular remodeling. An insertion–deletion (I/D) polymorphism in the intron 16 of the angiotensin-converting enzyme (*ACE*) gene is associated with elevated ACE levels. Several studies in whites have been conducted, and an association between this polymorphism and lacunar stroke has been demonstrated in some but not in all the studies [23, 24]. Recently, a meta-analysis of all studies in white populations did not report a significant association, while this was found in Asian populations [25]. Considering the angiotensinogen (*AGT*) gene, several data show its effects on cardiac and vascular function. In the Austrian Stroke Prevention Study the promoter *–20*C polymorphism was associated with WMLs [26]. Other SNPs in the promoter region of the gene have been studied, and haplotype analysis has been performed, but the only significant association remained between the *–20C* polymorphism and WMLs in hypertensive subjects [25].

Variation in the *eNOS* gene also has been studied. In the French GÉNIC study, the 894GG genotype was found to be a risk factor for lacunar stroke but not for other stroke subtypes [27]. A later study did not confirm this association, but the intron 4ab insertion/deletion genotype was found to be protective against CSVD, an effect which was confined to the isolated lacunar infarct (without leukoaraiosis) subtype [28]. Associations were stronger when this was included in a haplotype also comprising the T-786C and G894T polymorphisms [28].

Hyperhomocysteinemia

Several studies have shown a relation between increased homocysteine levels and coronary artery disease, peripheral artery disease, stroke, or venous thrombosis. Moreover, elevated homocysteine levels have been demonstrated in CSVD, particularly in the leukoaraiosis subtype [29]. This association could either be causal or could be secondary to established disease. For example, if CSVD is a systemic arteriopathy and there is also renal microvascular disease, this could lead to impaired clearance of homocysteine and secondary elevation of its levels. Examination of a genetic variant associated with increased homocysteine levels throughout life allows causality to be explored, an approach referred to as "Mendelian randomization." The methylenetetrahydrofolate reductase (MTHFR) C677T polymorphism is associated with elevated homocysteine levels. A number of studies have shown no, or only weak, associations between this common MTHFR polymorphism and stroke as a whole. In contrast, an association was found in a well-phenotyped group of patients affected by CSVD, in particular in patients with an ischemic leukoaraiosis subtype versus patients with isolated lacunar infarction [29]. This supports a causal role for homocysteine in this specific subtype of CSVD. The same authors found that association between hyperhomocysteinemia and CSVD was no longer significant after controlling for the endothelial markers ICAM-1 and thrombomodulin, supporting the hypothesis that homocysteinemia mediates its effect via endothelial damage [29].

Hyperhomocysteine-induced endothelial dysfunction may be explained by several mechanisms such as NO inhibition, prostanoid regulation, endothelium-derived hyperpolarizing factor inhibition, angiotensin II receptor 1 activation, endothelin-1 induction, and oxidative stress. Among these, oxidation has been suggested as a primary biochemical mechanism responsible for hyperhomocysteine-related pathogenesis. Different mechanisms might be involved in the oxidative stress induction mediated by hyperhomocysteine, such as inhibition or disruption of natural antioxidant enzymes (e.g., glutathione peroxidase, superoxide dismutase), homocysteine autooxidation, NOS-dependent generation of superoxide anion via uncoupling of eNOS, and activation of nicotinamide adenine dinucleotide phosphate (NADPH) oxidases [30].

Oxidative stress in sporadic CSVD

Oxidative stress is determined by the action of several vascular risk factors that through different mechanisms lead to an imbalance between formation of ROS (e.g., free oxygen radicals, oxygen ions, and peroxides) and antioxidant defenses against the latter.

Several enzymes and enzyme systems in the vessel wall can potentially produce ROS, the most important being NADPH oxidase, xanthine oxidase, the enzymes of the mitochondrial respiratory chain, and dysfunctional eNOS. Interestingly, the NADPH oxidase-derived superoxide has been implicated in the activation of xanthine oxidase and in eNOS uncoupling (i.e., degradation of NO with formation of peroxynitrite anion). The pathophysiologic mechanisms that link vascular oxidative stress to hypertension are the better understood. These include angiotensin II signaling, through stimulation of angiotensin I receptors, and mechanical stretch-induced NADPH oxidase activation with increase in superoxide production.

Protection against free radicals is provided by a complex interplay of antioxidants. Among these, the superoxide dismutase (SOD) catalyzes the dismutation of superoxide into oxygen and hydrogen peroxide; the glutathione peroxidase reduces lipid hydroperoxides to their corresponding alcohols and free hydrogen peroxide in water; and the paraoxonase circulates in plasma in association with HDL and decreases lipid peroxidation of HDL and LDL. Paraoxonase antioxidative activity has different effects according to the polymorphisms of its coding gene. In particular, two polymorphisms Gln–Arg191 and Met–Leu54, which are in linkage disequilibrium with leucine at position 54, giving rise to arginine at position 191. The presence of LL paraoxonase genotype (position 54) was shown to influence the presence and progression of WMLs in elderly subjects [31].

In addition, there are various small molecular weight redox-active compounds, such as endogenous products of metabolism (i.e., glutathione, uric acid, bilirubin) and ingested substances (vitamins C and E, carotenoids, and polyphenolic compounds). Vitamin C is considered the most efficacious water-soluble antioxidant in human plasma, decreasing ROS and regenerating α-tocopherol. Vitamin E comprises eight different tocopherols and tocotrienols, with α-tocopherol being the most active form, which acts as scavenger of lipid peroxides. Polyphenols (found in fruits, vegetables, cocoa contained in chocolate, red wine, green tea, and grape juice) are mainly mild antioxidants, but some can reduce NADPH oxidase activity, and others can stimulate antioxidative enzymes and eNOS. Antioxidant levels have been found inversely related to CSVD. In particular, in the Austrian Stroke Prevention Study, Schmidt et al. [32] measured the concentrations of 10 antioxidants in 355 clinically normal volunteers (45–75 years of age) and studied possible correlation with the presence of WMLs. They found that the levels of α-tocopherol were significantly lower in subjects with WMLs of moderate and severe degree, while individuals with punctate foci had an antioxidant status similar to those with normal brain MRI scans. Some carotenoids, including β-carotene, inhibit ROS under certain conditions and can block free radical-mediated reactions. An inverse association between carotenoid levels and severe periventricular WMLs has been found in the Rotterdam Scan Study (203 elderly subjects) [33].

Inflammation and sporadic CSVD

Evidence is mounting to suggest that chronic inflammation contributes to the development and consequences of cerebrovascular disease, mainly in relation to large vessel atherosclerosis. Little is known about the relationship between inflammation and CSVD.

C-reactive protein (CRP) has been studied, but conflicting results have been reported. In 1033 participants of the population-based Rotterdam Scan Study, higher CRP levels were associated with the presence and the progression of WMLs, particularly with marked lesion progression [34]. In 3644 patients enrolled in the Cardiovascular Health Study, higher CRP levels were associated with a greater risk of having WMLs [35]. However, in a large community-based group of Japanese elderly (N = 689) the association between CRP levels and CSVD was not confirmed [36]. Moreover, in the Rotterdam Scan Study and in the Memory and Morbidity in Augsburg Elderly (MEMO) study, haplotypes representing common variants in the *CRP* gene in European populations were studied in relation to CSVD. In particular, in the Rotterdam Scan Study, DNA was genotyped for 1184C>T (rs1130864), 2042C>T (rs1205), and 4741C>G (rs3093068) single-nucleotide polymorphisms (SNPs), and in the MEMO study polymorphisms 1184C>T (rs1130864), 2042C>T (rs1205), and 4363C>A (rs3093075) were genotyped. SNPs 4363 C>A and 4741 C>G are in perfect linkage disequilibrium. No differences in WML severity or presence of lacunar infarcts were found among the genotypes of any polymorphism [37]. Similarly, no associations were found between CRP gene polymorphisms and CSVD in the Cardiovascular Health Study [35].

More consistent are data on interleukin-6 (IL-6) in relation with CSVD. Elevated IL-6 levels and common haplotypes of the IL-6 gene, *CC*, were found associated with both silent brain infarcts and WMLs, suggesting a susceptibility of the small cerebral arteries to IL-6-mediated inflammatory damage [35].

Matrix metalloproteinases (MMPs) are a family of metal-dependent proteases, the function of which is the remodeling of the extracellular matrix during tissue injury and repair. They are released from astrocytes, neurons, microglia, leukocytes, and macrophages. They act on collagen, gelatin, fibronectin, laminin, elastin, and proteoglycans. In the central nervous system, MMPs may lead to extracellular matrix destruction, neuronal dysfunction, and death. Common polymorphisms in the genes coding for MMP-1, MMP-2, and MMP-3 have been found associated with vascular dementia (the most common form of which is subcortical vascular dementia due to CSVD) [38].

As a result of leukocyte–endothelial interaction, both leukocytes (e.g., monocytes) and endothelial cells became increasingly activated. Activated monocytes/macrophages produce neopterin, which may itself induce endothelial dysfunction with increased expression of adhesion molecules as a consequence. Higher levels of neopterin where found in patients with asymptomatic lacunar infarcts and WMLs in comparison to patients without these lesions [39].

Levels of Inflammatory Markers in the Treatment of Stroke (LIMITS) is an ongoing prospective, observational study aimed to determine if levels of inflammatory markers, such as high sensitivity CRP, amyloid A, CD40 ligand, and monocyte chemoattractant protein-1 (MCP-1), predict recurrent stroke and other vascular events among people with a history of lacunar infarct [40].

Endothelial dysfunction in CADASIL

Although only a few studies have been conducted in CADASIL evaluating the possible role of endothelial dysfunction as a synergic pathophysiologic factor modulating the clinical–functional phenotype of the disease, available data support this hypothesis.

First, beside the typical alterations of the tunica media in small arteries and arterioles, endothelial changes, including cytoplasmic swelling, disruption of tight junctions, and appearance of bundles of microfilaments, also have been reported in pathologic studies [41]. A recent neuropathologic study conducted on six CADASIL patients showed that endothelial von Willebrand factor accumulates in cerebral penetrating arteries, and in vitro it binds to and inhibits specific ribonucleic acids (RNAs) in smooth muscle cells. These data suggest that von Willebrand factor, likely produced by the endothelium, permeates the vessel wall of CADASIL brains and that the exposure of smooth muscle cells to this molecule could result in impairment of the vascular homeostatic mechanisms [42].

Altered skin microvessel reactivity [43] and endothelial dependent vasodilatation in cerebral and forearm arteries have been observed [44, 45]. Recently, we used a noninvasive plethysmographic method to study peripheral vasoreactivity in 49 CADASIL patients and 25 controls. Endothelium-dependent vasodilatation was assessed by reactive hyperemia (flow-mediated dilation–peripheral arterial tone [FMD-PAT]) and endothelium-independent vasoreactivity by glyceryl trinitrate (GTN) administration (GTN-PAT). Impaired vasoreactivity was found in both FMD-PAT and GTN-PAT in CADASIL patients, supporting the observation that both endothelial and smooth muscle functional alterations may be present in this condition [46].

ADMA levels have been found significantly increased in CADASIL patients with respect to normal controls [47]. The authors hypothesized that one mechanism by which *NOTCH3* mutations could be related to increased ADMA levels in these patients might be the increasing oxidative stress due to abnormal mitochondrial energy metabolism. Several studies suggest concomitant systemic mitochondrial abnormalities in patients with CADASIL including mitochondrial DNA (mtDNA) mutations and complex respiratory chain deficits. Whether these mitochondrial deficits are secondary to oxidative stress due to chronic hypoperfusion and hypoxia or directly associated with *NOTCH3* signaling pathways remains to be elucidated.

In CADASIL patients higher homocysteine levels were demonstrated in comparison with controls, both in the fasting state and after methionine challenge. Also, median differences between homocysteine levels before and after methionine challenge were greater in the CADASIL group than in controls [48]. In a larger sample (127 CADASIL patients), homocysteine levels were higher in migraine sufferers in comparison with nonmigraine-suffering patients, and elevated homocysteine was independently associated with an earlier age of onset of migraine headache [49]. Hyperhomocysteinemia could act by exacerbating the vascular injury, which presumably leads to migraine in CADASIL. Alternatively, hyperhomocysteinemia could increase susceptibility to oxidative injury and excitotoxicity, leading to mitochondrial dysfunction.

Recently, we found that CADASIL patients have a reduced number of EPCs in comparison with controls [50]. Also, we found that CADASIL patients with a more severe clinical picture (i.e., history of stroke and dementia) presented higher circulating progenitor cell (CPC) levels than patients with a milder clinical picture (i.e., no history of stroke or dementia). Moreover, higher CPC levels correlated with worse performances in neuropsychologic, functional, and motor tests. From the biologic viewpoint, EPCs and CPCs likely represent different progenitor cell phenotypes with different biologic properties. The EPC circulating pool represents a population of more mature cells that are just "committed" to differentiate into endothelial cells able to participate mainly in the processes of the re-endothelialization and revascularization. On the other hand, CPCs are a more heterogeneous and undifferentiated cell population that can evolve into different cell types (e.g., neurons, astrocytes, and oligodendrocytes, as well as endothelial cells). These cell lines are known for being involved in sustaining the homeostasis of damaged brains.

References

1. Pantoni L. Cerebral small vessel disease: from pathogenesis and clinical characteristics to therapeutic challenges. *Lancet Neurol* 2010;9:689–701.
2. Charlton RA, Morris RG, Nitkunan A, Markus HS. The cognitive profiles of CADASIL and sporadic small vessel disease. *Neurology* 2006;66: 1523–1526.
3. Chabriat H, Joutel A, Dichgans M, Tournier-Lasserve E, Bousser MG. CADASIL. *Lancet Neurol* 2009;8:643–653.
4. O'Sullivan M, Lythgoe DJ, Pereira AC, et al. Patterns of cerebral blood flow reduction in patients with ischemic leukoaraiosis. *Neurology* 2002;59:321–326.
5. Chabriat H, Pappata S, Ostergaard L, et al. Cerebral hemodynamics in CADASIL before and after acetazolamide challenge assessed with MRI bolus tracking. *Stroke* 2000;31:1904–1912.
6. Gan R, Sacco RL, Kargman DE, et al. Testing the validity of the lacunar hypothesis: the Northern Manhattan Stroke Study experience. *Neurology* 1997;48:1204–1211.
7. Bakker SL, de Leeuw FE, de Groot JC, et al. Cerebral vasomotor reactivity and cerebral white matter lesions in the elderly. *Neurology* 1999;52: 578–583.
8. Szmitko PE, Wang CH, Weisel RD, et al. New markers of inflammation and endothelial cell activation: part I. *Circulation* 2003;108:1917–1923.
9. Blanco M, Rodríguez-Yáñez M, Sobrino T, Leira R, Castillo J. Platelets, inflammation, and atherothrombotic neurovascular disease: the role of endothelial dysfunction. *Cerebrovasc Dis* 2005;20(Suppl 2):32–39.
10. Young VG, Halliday GM, Kril JJ. Neuropathologic correlates of white matter hyperintensities. *Neurology* 2008;71:804–811.
11. Giwa MO, Williams J, Elderfield K, et al. Neuropathologic evidence of endothelial changes in cerebral small vessel disease. *Neurology* 2012;78:167–174.
12. Hassan A, Hunt BJ, O'Sullivan M, et al. Markers of endothelial dysfunction in lacunar infarction and ischaemic leukoaraiosis. *Brain* 2003;126:424–432.
13. Kario K, Matsuo T, Kobayashi H, Asada R, Matsuo M. "Silent" cerebral infarction is associated with hypercoagulability, endothelial cell damage, and high Lp_a levels in elderly Japanese. *Arterioscler Thromb Vasc Biol* 1996;16:734–741.
14. Knottnerus IL, Govers-Riemslag JW, Hamulyak K, et al. Endothelial activation in lacunar stroke subtypes. *Stroke* 2010;41:1617–1622.
15. Fassbender K, Bertsch T, Mielke O, Mühlhauser F, Hennerici M. Adhesion molecules in cerebrovascular diseases. Evidence for an inflammatory endothelial activation in cerebral large- and small-vessel disease. *Stroke* 1999;30:1647–1650.
16. De Leeuw FE, de Kleine M, Frijns CJ, et al. Endothelial cell activation is associated with cerebral white matter lesions in patients with cerebrovascular disease. *Ann NY Acad Sci* 2002;977:306–314.
17. Markus HS, Hunt B, Palmer K, et al. Markers of endothelial and hemostatic activation and progression of cerebral white matter hyperintensities: longitudinal results of the Austrian Stroke Prevention Study. *Stroke* 2005;36:1410–1414.
18. Khan U, Hassan A, Vallance P, Markus HS. Asymmetric dimethylarginine in cerebral small vessel disease. *Stroke* 2007;38: 411–413.
19. Werner N, Kosiol S, Schiegl T, et al. Circulating endothelial progenitor cells and cardiovascular outcomes. *N Engl J Med* 2005;353:999–1007.
20. Jickling G, Salam A, Mohammad A, et al. Circulating endothelial progenitor cells and age-related white matter changes. *Stroke* 2009;40:3191–3196.
21. Chu K, Jung KH, Lee ST, et al. Circulating endothelial progenitor cells as a new marker of endothelial dysfunction or repair in acute stroke. *Stroke* 2008;39:1441–1447.
22. Rouhl RP, Mertens AE, van Oostenbrugge RJ, et al. Angiogenic T-cells and putative endothelial progenitor cells in hypertension-related cerebral small vessel disease. *Stroke* 2012;43:256–258.
23. Ueda S, Weir CJ, Inglis GC, et al. Lack of association between angiotensin converting enzyme gene insertion/deletion polymorphism and stroke. *J Hypertens* 1995;13:1597–1601.
24. Hassan A, Lansbury A, Catto AJ, et al. Angiotensin converting enzyme insertion/deletion genotype is associated with leukoaraiosis in lacunar

syndromes. *J Neurol Neurosurg Psychiatry* 2002;72:343–346.

25. Gormley K, Bevan S, Markus HS. Polymorphisms in genes of the renin–angiotensin system and cerebral small vessel disease. *Cerebrovasc Dis* 2007;232: 148–155.
26. Schmidt H, Fazekas F, Kostner GM, van Duijn CM, Schmidt R. Angiotensinogen gene promoter haplotype and microangiopathy-related cerebral damage: results of the Austrian Stroke Prevention Study. *Stroke* 2001; 32:405–412.
27. Elbaz A, Poirier O, Moulin T, et al. Association between the Glu298Asp polymorphism in the endothelial constitutive nitric oxide synthase gene and brain infarction. The GENIC Investigators. *Stroke* 2000;31:1634–1639.
28. Hassan A, Gormley K, O'Sullivan M, et al. Endothelial nitric oxide gene haplotypes and risk of cerebral small-vessel disease. *Stroke* 2004;35:654–659.
29. Hassan A, Hunt BJ, O'Sullivan M, et al. Homocysteine is a risk factor for cerebral small vessel disease, acting via endothelial dysfunction. *Brain* 2004;127:212–219.
30. Cheng Z, Yang X, Wang H. Hyperhomocysteinemia and endothelial dysfunction. *Curr Hypertens Rev* 2009;5:158–165.
31. Schmidt R, Schmidt H, Fazekas F, et al. MRI cerebral white matter lesions and paraoxonase PON1 polymorphisms: three-year follow-up of the Austrian Stroke Prevention Study. *Arterioscler Thromb Vasc Biol* 2000;20: 1811–1816.
32. Schmidt R, Hayn M, Fazekas F, Kapeller P, Esterbauer H. Magnetic resonance imaging white matter hyperintensities in clinically normal elderly individuals. Correlations with plasma concentrations of naturally occurring antioxidants. *Stroke* 1996;27:2043–2047.
33. den Heijer T, Launer LJ, de Groot JC, et al. Serum carotenoids and cerebral white matter lesions: the Rotterdam Scan Study. *J Am Geriatr Soc* 2001; 49:642–646.
34. Van Dijk EJ, Prins ND, Vermeer SE, et al. C-reactive protein and cerebral small-vessel disease: the Rotterdam Scan Study. *Circulation* 2005;112:900–905.
35. Fornage M, Chiang YA, O'Meara ES, et al. Biomarkers of inflammation and MRI-defined small vessel disease of the brain: the Cardiovascular Health Study. *Stroke* 2008;39:1952–1959.
36. Wada M, Nagasawa H, Kurita K, et al. Cerebral small vessel disease and C-reactive protein: results of a cross-sectional study in community-based Japanese elderly. *J Neurol Sci* 2008;264: 43–49.
37. Reitz C, Berger K, de Maat MP, et al. CRP gene haplotypes, serum CRP, and cerebral small-vessel disease: the Rotterdam Scan Study and the MEMO study. *Stroke* 2007;38:2356–2359.
38. Flex A, Gaetani E, Proia AS, et al. Analysis of functional polymorphisms of metalloproteinase genes in persons with vascular dementia and Alzheimer's disease. *J Gerontol A Biol Sci Med Sci* 2006;61:1065–1069.
39. Rouhl RP, Damoiseaux JG, Lodder J, et al. Vascular inflammation in cerebral small vessel disease. *Neurobiol Aging* 2012;33:1800–1806.
40. Elkind MS, Luna JM, Coffey CS, et al. The Levels of Inflammatory Markers in the Treatment of Stroke Study (LIMITS): inflammatory biomarkers as risk predictors after lacunar stroke. *Int J Stroke* 2010;5:117–125.
41. Ruchoux MM, Maurage CA. Endothelial changes in muscle and skin biopsies in patients with CADASIL. *Neuropathol Appl Neurobiol* 1998;24:60–65.
42. Zhang X, Meng H, Blaivas M, et al. Von Willebrand factor permeates small vessels in CADASIL and inhibits smooth muscle gene expression. *Transl Stroke Res* 2012;3:138–145.
43. Gobron C, Vahedi K, Vicaut E, et al. Characteristic features of in vivo skin microvascular reactivity in CADASIL. *J Cereb Blood Flow Metab* 2007;27:250–257.
44. Peters N, Freilinger T, Opherk C, Pfefferkorn T, Dichgans M. Enhanced L-arginine-induced vasoreactivity suggests endothelial dysfunction in CADASIL. *J Neurol* 2008;255:1203–1208.
45. Stenborg A, Kalimo H, Viitanen M, Terent A, Lind L. Impaired endothelial function of forearm resistance arteries in CADASIL patients. *Stroke* 2007;38:2692–2697.
46. Campolo J, De Maria R, Frontali M, et al. Impaired vasoreactivity in mildly disabled CADASIL patients. *J Neurol Neurosurg Psychiatry* 2012;83:268–274.
47. Rufa A, Blardi P, De Lalla A, et al. Plasma levels of asymmetric dimethylarginine in cerebral autosomal dominant arteriopathy with subcortical infarct and leukoencephalopathy. *Cerebrovasc Dis* 2008;26:636–640.
48. Flemming KD, Nguyen TT, Abu-Lebdeh HS, et al. Hyperhomocysteinemia in patients with cerebral autosomal dominant arteriopathy with subcortical infarcts and leukoencephalopathy (CADASIL). *Mayo Clin Proc* 2001;76: 1213–1218.
49. Singhal S, Bevan S, Barrick T, Rich P, Markus HS. The influence of genetic and cardiovascular risk factors on the CADASIL phenotype. *Brain* 2004;127:2031–2038.
50. Pescini F, Cesari F, Giusti B, et al. Bone marrow-derived progenitor cells in cerebral autosomal dominant arteriopathy with subcortical infarcts and leukoencephalopathy. *Stroke* 2010;41:218–223.

Chapter 17

Cerebral small vessel disease: cerebrospinal fluid aspects

Anders Wallin and Maria Bjerke

Introduction

The most common cerebral small vessel disease is the arteriolosclerotic variant located in the subcortical white and gray matter of the brain [1]. It gives rise to a characteristic phenotype called subcortical vascular dementia (SVD). However, SVD is often underdiagnosed or labeled Alzheimer's disease (AD), although it comprises several features that are not characteristic for AD. The recently published National Institute of Aging/Alzheimer Association criteria [2] are more specific than the very often used, almost 30 years old, diagnostic guidelines for AD [3]. This suggests that now there are improved diagnostic criteria for avoiding error in the identification of SVD and AD.

Another common small vessel disease is cerebral amyloid angiopathy (CAA) situated in meningeal and intracortical arteries. It is a characteristic feature of AD but may also occur without AD pathology [4]. Brains of patients with AD-related CAA often also display subcortical arteriolosclerotic vessel wall lesions [5], whereas those from patients with primary SVD usually lack signs of CAA [6]. The combination of arteriolosclerosis and CAA may underlie what is called "mixed dementia."

Stroke may give rise to cognitive impairment, although it has not been sufficiently clarified that the stoke episode in itself gives rise to progressive cognitive impairment [7]. Principally stroke may manifests itself in two ways: as minor stroke usually as a consequence of arteriolosclerosis but in some cases also as a result of atherosclerosis; and as major stroke which is a consequence of disease of the large arteries.

The driving forces behind small vessel-induced brain tissue dysfunction and the relative contributions of vessel pathology and primary neurodegeneration for the development of SVD, AD, and mixed type dementia i.e., AD and cerebrovascular disease, need to be clarified. One way of doing this is to examine components of the cerebrospinal fluid (CSF) reflecting neurodegenerative and vascular processes of the central nervous system (CNS). Contrary to traditional neuropathology, determination of CSF markers may give information about the pathologic events as they take place. In addition the CSF biomarkers may be useful for diagnostic purposes and surveillance of treatment effects.

Cerebrospinal fluid

CSF surrounds the CNS by occupying the subarachnoid space and further fills the intracerebral space of the ventricular system and the spinal cord. The main part of the CSF is formed by the highly restrictive ependymal cells of the choroid plexus located in the ventricles and by cerebral capillaries [8]. The capillaries of the choroid plexus are fenestrated and leaky; however, the blood–CSF barrier, formed by the modified ependymal cells, is sealed by tight junction proteins [9]. The CSF and the brain interstitial fluid are allowed to mix freely and, thus, share the same composition due to free passage over the ependyma lining the cerebral ventricles and through the cell layers facing the subarachnoid space [10]. In the adult, the total volume of CSF is about 160 ml, and the secretion rate, which is directly proportional to the formation rate, is 0.3–0.6 ml per minute or 500–600 ml per day [11]. About 80% of the total CSF protein content originates from serum, while nearly 20% of the CSF proteins are brain derived; however, less than 1% are brain specific [12].

Cerebral Small Vessel Disease, ed. Leonardo Pantoni and Philip B. Gorelick. Published by Cambridge University Press.

The main exit pathway for CSF is through the cranial arachnoid villi, but a substantial portion is also reabsorbed through spinal nerve arachnoidal pathways. Since the CSF is in continuum with the interstitial fluid surrounding the various CNS cells, it is believed to reflect biochemical changes taking place during remodeling of the extracellular matrix and cellular regeneration as well as degeneration. Furthermore, the CSF provides the brain with mechanical support and delivers nutrients, electrolytes, and signaling molecules to the brain parenchyma, but also functions to clear the brain of metabolic waste and is important in the maintenance of physiologic pH [13].

CSF biomarkers

A biomarker is a substance or feature that can be objectively measured and evaluated as an indicator of normal biological or disease processes. Biomarkers can provide insight into pathophysiologic events, diagnostics, prognostics, and monitoring treatment of diseases. In this chapter, we assume that ischemia-induced breakdown of the blood–brain barrier is the starting event in patients with predominant cerebral small vessel disease followed by glial involvement, inflammation and tissue remodeling, deviations of amyloid metabolism, and, finally, neuronal/axonal degeneration. Similar events may take place in AD and AD plus cerebrovascular disease but presumably in another order. In the text below, first, the substances belonging to the various groups of pathophysiologic events are described and then the clinical biomarker findings of the various patient groups are discussed. The major biomarker findings are summarized in the last part of each section.

Blood–brain barrier breakdown

The endothelial cells of the brain capillaries are, unlike endothelial cells in the periphery, joined together by continuous tight junctions and lack fenestrations. These restrictive features constitute the basis of the blood–brain barrier (BBB). The BBB is an integral part of the neurovascular unit, which consists of brain endothelial cells, astrocytes, pericytes, smooth muscle cells, and neurons. The cells of the neurovascular unit work together to maintain vascular integrity and regulate BBB function through the expression of a wide variety of ion channels, receptors (e.g., for lipoproteins, regulatory peptides and proteins, hormones, and metals such as iron), and transporters (e.g., for glucose, amino acids, vitamins, and nucleosides) and also through biochemical modifiers such as enzymes, all of which allows for effective paracrine interactions in the neurovascular proximity. It not only provides for the regulation of homeostasis of neurotransmitters, but also of water, activity-dependent local regulation of blood flow and angiogenesis, and also elimination of potentially toxic molecules (e.g., waste products from brain interstitial fluid to blood). The interaction is mediated by chemical signals and transducing mechanisms, including those that originate from the remodeling of the basal lamina and extracellular matrix (see below). The numerous mitochondria in the endothelial cells of the brain provide energy for the various transport systems. Metabolic exchange has been found not only in capillaries but also in arterioles, which implies that the latter have BBB features [9, 14–16].

Dysfunction of the BBB is a pathophysiologic feature of a variety of neurologic disorders including traumatic brain injury (TBI), stroke, and vascular cognitive impairment, but it has also been suggested in AD. Mechanisms of BBB disruption are manifested through physical and enzymatic break down of tight junction proteins and altered protein expression. Dysfunction of the neurovascular unit is further reflected by altered function of the astrocytes and degradation of membrane components facilitating extravasation of inflammatory cells into the CNS. Hypoxia is a factor that initially leads to BBB opening through the intrinsic activation of astrocytes, pericytes, and microglia. Hypoxia is further associated with increased expression of hypoxia-inducible factor-1α (HIF-1α), cytokines, matrix metalloproteinases (MMPs), cyclooxygenases (COXs), and free radicals of nitrogen and oxygen [17] (Figure 17.1).

The traditional way of measuring the integrity of the BBB is by determining the CSF : serum ratio for albumin. An increased CSF : serum albumin ratio indicates impaired BBB function. Postmortem studies have found a relation between vascular dementia (VaD) and arteriolosclerosis, lipohyalinosis, and hypertensive angiopathy of the intracerebral capillaries and arterioles of the brain [18]. These changes may lead to dysfunction of the endothelial cells, with increased permeability and extravasation of serum proteins, i.e., BBB damage. An increased CSF : serum albumin ratio in comparison with healthy controls has been found in patients with

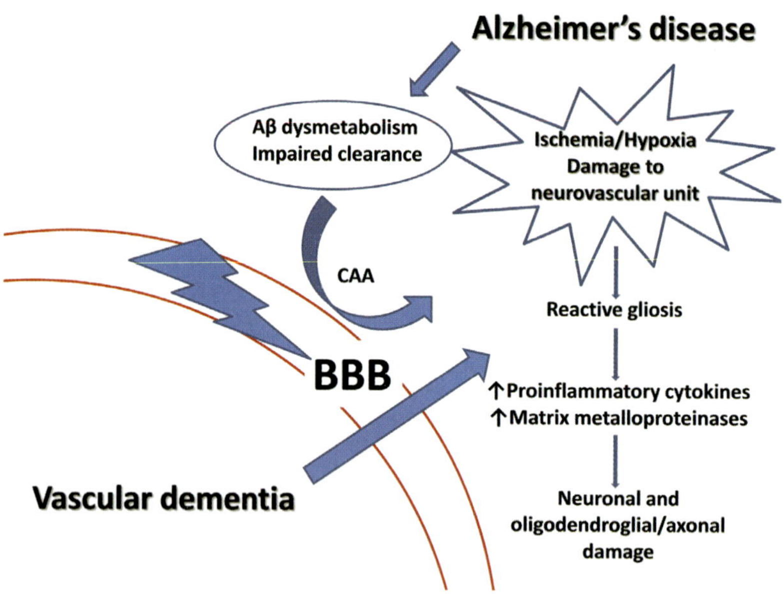

Figure 17.1 A simplified picture of mechanisms related to blood–brain barrier (BBB) disruption and small vessel disease. Evidence indicates that BBB dysfunction, either primary vessel wall damage or secondary to cerebral amyloid angiopathy, is associated with the accumulation of several molecules within the brain parenchyma that are both neurotoxic as well as toxic to the vasculature. Small vessel disease-induced BBB dysfunction is also associated with a reduction in cerebral blood flow with subsequent hypoxia. During ischemia/hypoxia an inflammatory cascade is initiated in order to remove damaged cells and prepare the brain for repair. Enzymes such as matrix metalloproteinases, secreted by various cells including reactive glia, are activated during repair processes such as angiogenesis and neurogenesis to degrade both cellular and extracellular components. However, if the triggering process (BBB/hypoxia) is not attenuated, it might in the long run lead to prolonged BBB, cellular, and tissue damage. Aβ, β-amyloid; CAA, cerebral amyloid angiopathy.

SVD [19] and in patients with increased degrees of white matter change [20, 21].

In a recent study the contrast agent gadolinium diethylene triamine pentaacetic acid (Gd-DTPA) was used to evaluate the BBB through the leakage of the contrast from the plasma into the brain. An overlap between white matter hyperintensities with regions of high contrast permeability was shown in patients with vascular cognitive impairment, indicating a role of vasogenic edema in causing secondary hypoxia and contributing to white matter changes [22]. AD patients with concomitant vascular disorders, e.g., arterial hypertension or white matter changes, have been found to have disturbed BBB function, whereas this function has been found to be normal in patients with pure AD [23]. On the contrary, it also has been shown that a subgroup of AD patients displayed an increased albumin ratio without any obvious relation to vascular factors or magnetic resonance imaging (MRI) changes [24]. The authors speculated about whether the findings could be an effect of amyloid angiopathy.

Thus, BBB dysfunction as measured by albumin ratio does not only emerge as a consequence of acute stroke but also of slowly developing small vessel disease. Leakage of the contrast agent Gd-DTPA in the subcortical regions in patients with white matter changes validates the involvement of the vasculature in this group of patients.

Glial involvement

Reactive astrocytes and microglia/macrophages (i.e., gliosis formation) are associated with white matter changes and fibrohyalinotic vessel wall alterations in patients with SVD. The gliosis is accentuated around infarcted regions in the white matter, and glia are especially prominent around arterioles showing fibrohyalin degeneration [25]. The reactive glia secrete various potentially damaging substances, including proteinases known to degrade extracellular matrix proteins, free radicals, and cytokines.

White matter changes caused by dysfunction of oligodendrocytes could be explained by several etiologies. For instance, hypoxia/ischemia promotes activation of resident astrocytes to protect the brain [26], which may lead to damage of the white matter due to release of various factors. The hypoxia/ischemia is accompanied by an increase in HIF-1α, and this factor has been found in affected white matter at autopsy of patients with vascular cognitive impairment [27]. Furthermore, the fact that hypoxia/ischemia has been associated with extensive damage to cells of the oligodendroglia lines in brain tissue of preterm infants [28], supports a role of hypoxia/ischemia in the process that leads to death of the oligodendrocytes and white matter gliosis. White matter damage could also be exacerbated by the presence of serum proteins, which has been found in the brain of patients with SVD/Binswanger's disease [29].

Myelin basic protein (MBP) is a major component of the myelin, especially in the CNS, where it constitutes approximately 30% of the myelin [30]. The process of demyelination/myelination of the neuronal axon by the oligodendroglial membrane is complex and likely highly influenced by the active/reactive state of astroglial cells and the various promyelinating factors secreted by them [31, 32]. A possible link between white matter changes (i.e., dystrophic oligodendrocytes) and arteriolosclerosis could, thus, be the reactive astroglial cell [33]. Astroglial cells change from their normal quiescent state into a reactive state whenever damage is inflicted on the CNS.

The process of reactive gliosis is characterized by a profound increase of the major intermediate filament (IF) protein in astrocytes, that is the glial fibrillary acidic protein (GFAP) [34]. Increased immunoreactivity of GFAP has been shown in areas of white matter change in patients with SVD [35], and in areas of severe myelin loss visualized by decreased immunoreactivity for MBP. However, these areas also show an increase in remyelinating oligodendrocytes, a process which is likely influenced by the longevity and severity of the demyelinating disease [36]. Elevated levels of MBP and GFAP have previously been found in CSF of patients with VaD and SVD, while GFAP but not MBP has also been shown to be increased in late-onset AD, which is known to display signs of subcortical small vessel disease [37–39]. Increased levels of MBP and GFAP have also been shown in patients with acute ischemic stroke [40, 41], and GFAP was found to correlate with infarct volume, while MBP concentration was significantly higher in subcortical than in cortical infarcts. However, an increase in GFAP has also been found in "pure" AD with predominant cortical symptoms, usually without signs of subcortical engagement [39]. This is explained by the fact that reactive astrocytes seem to be particularly abundant around β-amyloid (Aβ) deposits both in the parenchyma and in the cerebrovasculature [42].

Whether there are differences in the astroglial reactive state that are disease specific is not clear. Even though the reactive astrocytes are localized to different subcortical/cortical departments in small vessel disease as opposed to AD, deviations in CSF GFAP will not provide us with region-specific information.

Sulfatide is the major acidic glycosphingolipid in the oligodendrocytes that constitute the myelin sheath, but it forms only a minor proportion of the membrane lipids in other brain cells. Postmortem findings have indicated significantly reduced levels of the glycolipids in the white matter from the centrum semiovale of patients with VaD [43]. Sulfatide may be detected in CSF, and, thus, it is possible to obtain information about the status of myelin in patients. One study reported CSF concentrations of sulfatide of more than 200% of control values in patients with SVD and normal concentrations in patients with pure AD [44]. In patients with SVD, the CSF levels of sulfatide were significantly higher than in patients with normal pressure hydrocephalus [45]. In contrast, another study with the same design could not replicate the result [46]. The reason might be that the patients in this study were less severely demented than in the other studies.

In cross-sectional studies on normal pressure hydrocephalus/SVD and patients seeking help at a memory clinic, positive correlations between CSF levels of sulfatide and the degree of white matter changes on MRI were found [47, 48]. On the contrary, a longitudinal study found that low sulfatide levels predicted progression of MRI white matter changes [49]. The latter finding in patients with no or only very discrete clinical symptoms suggests the presence of an ongoing remyelination process, whereas the increased sulfatide concentration in those with more pronounced vascular cognitive impairment may reflect insufficient repair mechanism by a degenerative process.

Even though there is an increase in CSF GFAP in both small vessel disease and AD, which points to involvement of astrocytes in both disease processes, it does not necessarily mean that the triggers are the same, or even the response. The increase of MBP in SVD but not in AD speaks in favor of this marker reflecting subcortical alterations. Since GFAP has been shown to be increased in white matter changes in SVD patients, this could be a reflection of an intricate interplay between astrocytes and oligodendrocytes in this disease. Furthermore, as CSF sulfatide seems to vary with regard to the stage of white matter disease, it has a potential as a marker of disease progression. As MRI white matter changes are associated with arteriolosclerotic small vessel disease, it appears reasonable to conclude that this also pertains to CSF sulfatide. However, it cannot be ruled out that CAA, which is a hallmark of AD, also plays a related role in the sulfatide deviations.

Inflammation and tissue remodeling

A crucial function of the inflammatory system is to remove potentially toxic substances and tissue debris from a site of injury and to participate in the subsequent repair processes. To do so, involved cells must release inflammatory regulators such as cytokines and MMPs. Several proteinases, including the MMPs and serine proteases, have been shown to be involved the process of demyelination and BBB opening, and in repair processes such as angiogenesis and neurogenesis [17]. However, the reactive gliosis that initially may be protective to the injured brain might lead to a vicious cycle of inflammation and tissue degeneration rather than repair, unless the initiating process is not arrested. The diverse roles of MMPs might explain the lack of long-term benefit of broad spectrum inhibition, which results in interference with angiogenesis and neurogenesis and, thus, hampers recovery.

Cerebral ischemia has been shown to lead to a biphasic breakdown of the BBB in animal models. The initial opening, which occurs within hours after the ischemia, is associated with activation of the constitutively expressed MMP-2 by membrane-type MMP (MT1-MMP), whereupon MMP-2 acts on the tight junction proteins. The hypoxia induces an increase in HIF-1α that leads to the expression of the protein Furin, which in turn activates MT1–MMP, resulting in the activation of the enzyme MMP-2. The recovery phase is characterized by the induction of vascular endothelial growth factor and transforming growth factor-β, factors important for neurogenesis and angiogenesis, which are also induced by HIF-1α. After the acute phase, HIF-1α reverts to low levels [17]. However, whether HIF-1α remains elevated during chronic low grade hypoxia, and how MMP-2 and other MMPs are affected under these conditions, remains to be investigated.

The second opening of the BBB is mediated by inducible MMPs, such as MMP-3 and MMP-9, which coincide with an elevation of interleukin-1β. The severity of this second opening is more extensive; however, the response is thought to be dependent on the state of the ischemia. Inflammatory cytokines induce both MMPs and COX-2, which is also an important mediator of the damage to the BBB during the second stage. Hypoxia-activated pericytes, microglia, and astrocytes are plausible initiators at this stage of BBB opening. Once the barrier is damaged, neutrophils and monocytes can enter the brain, and the injury is exacerbated by toxic blood products and an amplified source of inflammatory mediators [17].

The intricate relationship between MMPs and cerebrovascular disease has only begun to be elucidated. There are many experimental studies done, but fewer human postmortem studies or studies on human fluids. There is also a question on whether the alterations in CSF arise from inflammation and leakage when there is a damaged BBB. Few studies have combined both plasma and CSF analysis to deal with the issue concerning the origin of the markers. However, autopsy studies have revealed increased expression of MMP-2, MMP-3, and MMP-9 in varying degrees and topology in the human brain after focal ischemia, VaD, and SVD, with higher accumulation around infarcted areas, regions of white matter damage, and around damaged arteries and arterioles [35, 50].

Another study replicated the findings but added MMP-1, MMP-8, MMP-10, and MMP-13 to the list of increased MMPs in the infarcted area after stroke [51]. Some of these findings have been supported by studies in CSF. An increase in the concentration of MMP-9 has been found in patients with VaD and SVD compared to AD patients and controls, while the level of MMP-2 has not been found to be altered [37, 52]. In an attempt to investigate the influence of BBB on the CSF levels, MMP analysis was performed on both CSF and plasma from patients with white matter lesions and mild cognitive impairment (MCI) [53]. The MMP CSF : plasma ratio was compared to the albumin ratio. No correlation between the MMP-9 ratio and the albumin ratio was found, indicating intracerebral production.

Increased CSF levels of MMP-10 have been found in both SVD patients and in patients with AD compared to controls [37], and supposedly contribute to and increase the separation of patients with MCI and cognitively normal controls together with biomarkers known to reflect AD pathology (discussed below)

[54]. Furthermore, reduced CSF levels of MMP-2 and MMP-3 have been found in AD patients with significantly reduced Aβ1–42 levels, possibly reflecting a disturbed clearance mechanism leading to subsequent plaque formation, i.e., a hallmark of AD pathology. Both MMP-2 and MMP-3, as well as MMP-9, have been shown to degrade Aβ in vitro [55, 56], and it has, therefore, been suggested that MMPs are a part of the Aβ clearance system in the brain. MMPs have also been implicated in atherosclerotic plaque pathology of affecting both microvessels and cerebral arteries; however, the exact role has not been established.

Tissue inhibitors of metalloproteinases (TIMP-1 to TIMP-4) regulate the activity of the various MMPs through inhibition. However, TIMP-2 has a unique function since it, in contrast to its name, has been shown to facilitate proMMP-2 activation. In addition, TIMPs have distinct functions independent of those connected to the MMP activity. The proposed functions include regulation of cell fate, such as cell growth promotion and inhibition of mechanisms of cell death, but also growth-inhibitory functions. However, there is still a lot to be learned about the independent effects of TIMPs on cell fate, and there are conflicting reports pointing to the complexity of the TIMP system, including contextual and cell-specific pathways [57].

The expression of MMP-9 and TIMP-1 has been found to be increased after cerebral ischemia in rats, both in cerebral blood vessel smooth muscle cells and in microvessels within the ischemic region [58], and both markers have been associated with white matter changes in human cerebral ischemia [59]. Furthermore, elevated levels of TIMP-1 have been found in patients with subcortical vascular lesions both in overt dementia of mixed Alzheimer/vascular type and in SVD, compared to AD and controls [37], and also in incipient SVD [60]. An upregulation of TIMP-1 has also been found in human brain tissue after stroke [51], and it has been indicated that increased circulating levels of MMP-9 and particularly of TIMP-1 could be related to a higher risk of stroke and cardiovascular mortality [61]. What the consequences are of the increased cerebral levels of these markers in relation to prognosis in patients with cerebrovascular disease remains to be determined.

MMPs and TIMPs are links between the vasculature and the nonvascular extraneuronal tissue areas and deal with a variety of regenerative and degenerative functions. In CSF studies of patients with SVD, it has been found that MMP-9 reflecting BBB abnormalities and TIMP-1, which is a regulator of MMP-9, are affected, whereas those with pure AD lack such findings. As expected the results indicate that in patients with SVD there are more pronounced vessel-related neurochemical deviations than in those with pure AD.

Amyloid precursor protein metabolism

The sporadic forms of VaD and AD are bridged by overlapping pathologies of CAA and lesions induced by arteriolosclerosis of the white matter [62]. CAA can cause hypoperfusion by thickening of the vessel walls with concomitant narrowing of the lumen and impaired response to ischemia due to reduced vascular autoregulation, leading to a higher risk of infarcts and white matter changes [63–65]. Furthermore, CAA has been shown to be associated with cortical infarcts in demented patients with AD pathology [66] and also in VaD [67]. In addition, associations between CAA, white matter changes, and cognitive impairment suggest that advanced CAA causes clinically important vascular dysfunction [68].

Mechanistic knowledge about the deposition of Aβ into parenchymal and vascular plaques is mainly derived from familial forms of AD (FAD) and CAA. The 40–42 amino-acid-long Aβ peptide (Aβ1–40/42) is generated via sequential proteolysis of the transmembrane amyloid precursor protein (APP) by β- and γ-secretases, and the generated peptide has a high tendency to aggregate, leading to the formation of plaques either in the vasculature (Aβ1–40) or in the parenchyma (Aβ1–42).

FAD is mainly associated with mutations in the *APP* gene flanking the Aβ region or mutations within the Presenilin 1 or 2 gene, the protein being a part of the γ-secretase complex. FAD mutations presumably alter the APP metabolism by increasing the production of Aβ1–42 or by increasing the ratio of Aβ1–42 to Aβ1–40. The familial forms of CAA are associated with mutations within the Aβ region, while mutations within the Aβ region might alter the tendency for the produced Aβ peptide to form fibrillar aggregates and shift the aggregation into diffuse plaques in the cerebral vasculature. The vascular Aβ deposit, CAA, is supposedly predominantly composed of Aβ1–40 [69, 70]. However, whether or not the sporadic forms work by the same pathologic mechanisms remains to be elucidated.

One of two well-established neuropathologic hallmarks of sporadic AD is the accumulation of the Aβ1–42 into parenchymal plaques in the brain, but CAA is also a common feature. Whether CAA and parenchymal plaques are reflecting the same pathology or are two pathologies that coincide remains to be clarified.

The importance of vascular disease in the pathology of AD has been brought forward by many groups; however, the role of cause and effect of the diseased vessels remains unclear. CAA in small arteries, arterioles, and capillaries is commonly associated with AD [71]. There are also postmortem studies that indicate that most patients with AD have some form of vascular disease [72–74], at least in the final stage of the disease. Thus, one possible link between AD and cerebral vascular disease could be the accumulation of Aβ in the cerebral vessel wall. Experimental models suggest that CAA may exert a functional effect on cerebral microvasculature, leading to alterations in vessel tone and reactivity [75], and the severity of CAA has also been related to vessel wall destruction [76]. Other clinicopathologic features of CAA are angiitis, intracerebral hemorrhage, and cerebral infarction [64, 77, 78].

The main Aβ clearance pathways are removal from the brain by absorption to the blood, clearance through perivascular lymphatic drainage, or clearance by intracerebral enzymatic cleavage. A dysfunction in any system or an overproduction of Aβ could possibly lead to an accumulation of the peptide in the vicinity of blood vessels causing vascular dysfunction; or, the vascular dysfunction itself gives cause to altered clearance across the BBB and an accumulation of the peptide that further potentiates the impairment of the neurovascular unit. It is also possible that the intracerebral Aβ increase is derived from a peripheral source of the peptide due to damage to the BBB [79, 80].

Several mechanisms account for the transportation of Aβ across the BBB, both determining the entry of the peripheral molecule into the brain as well as the efflux from the brain into the periphery. There are specialized receptors at the BBB that permit the movement of Aβ across the brain endothelium. The main transporter of Aβ into the CNS is the receptor for advanced glycation end products (RAGE) and the low-density lipoprotein receptor-related protein-1 (LRP1) plays a major role in the endothelial transport of Aβ out of the CNS into the bloodstream [14, 15]. However, there is no direct evidence of how, and if, the vascular receptors are actually altered in human challenged brain vessels.

Apolipoprotein E (APOE) ε4 allele is an established genetic risk factor for sporadic AD [81], and it has been related to an increased risk of ischemic cerebrovascular disease [82], and to arteriolosclerosis and microinfarcts in the brains of AD patients [83]. The latter observations suggest that APOE ε4 may play a role in the cerebrovascular changes observed in AD patients. However, the findings regarding the role of the APOE ε4 allele in the development of white matter changes are contradictory [84, 85]. Furthermore, APOE ε4 is associated with increased likelihood and severity of CAA [86], possibly linked to mechanisms such as impaired clearance of Aβ coupled to ApoE along the perivascular interstitial fluid pathways [87, 88].

The role of Aβ as a primary mediator of BBB dysfunction and damage has been supported by experimental studies. In a model of amyloidosis, the increased production of Aβ was shown to be associated with neoangiogenesis and hypervascularity, supposedly triggering the BBB dysfunction by redistribution of tight junction proteins [89]. This study suggests a secondary hypoxic event following the Aβ-induced vascular dysfunction. However, it has been shown that experimental ischemia can lead to CAA by inducing amyloid dysmetabolism and deposition [90, 91]. Nevertheless, a major interest in the intricate relationship between vascular and Alzheimer pathology has arisen, and the question about the interdependence or independence still remains to be clarified.

A decreased CSF concentration of Aβ1–42 in sporadic AD patients as well as in prodromal AD patients with MCI shows high diagnostic accuracy, in combination with tau reflecting neurofibrillary tangles and neurodegeneration as described below, compared to stable patients and controls [92]. Furthermore, extracellular Aβ1–42 seems to be fully decreased in CSF already 5–10 years before conversion to AD, while tau seems to be a later marker in CSF [93]. Decreased levels of Aβ1–42 in CSF also inversely correlate with plaque load, visualized in vivo by Pittsburgh compound B (PiB) positron emission tomography, thus indicating a true biologic relationship between the marker level and the peptide deposition [94]. The deposition of Aβ1–42 along the perivascular pathway, i.e., CAA, has been associated with cognitive dysfunction [68], and the fact that memory performance was associated with low CSF Aβ1–42 in APOE4 positive carriers [95] indicates the clinical importance of the vascular involvement and disturbed clearance. The hypothesis of a disturbed clearance might be further supported by the fact that the early accumulation of both parenchymal and vascular Aβ occur in the cortical region [96], and that a higher burden of the more diffusible Aβ1–40 is prominent in the vascular deposits, possibly due to a subcortical blockage affecting the clearance of extracellular fluid [4]. However, the explanation for the decrease in Aβ1–42 in CSF of SVD patients [97] is somewhat more obscure, due to the fact that CAA is far more common in AD than in VaD [62].

What is even more interesting is that CSF Aβ1–40 has been shown to be decreased in VaD patients but not in AD patients [98], suggesting distinct etiologies. As for the relation between AD and CAA, it could be hypothesized that the decrease in Aβ1–42 is what actually represents the CAA in AD, and that the decrease in CSF of both Aβ1–42 and Aβ1–40 concentrations found in sporadic CAA [99] represents yet another pathologic mechanism. This is supported by findings of a specific subtype of capillary form of CAA that has been associated with AD pathology [100], which seems to involve a more prominent deposition of Aβ1–42 in the pericapillary spaces [101].

Another explanation for differences in CSF findings between patients with AD and cerebrovascular disease is a disturbed trafficking or metabolism of APP. This could explain the decreased levels of the N-terminal soluble APP (sAPPβ) released by cleavage at the β-site seen in patients with cerebrovascular disease [48, 102], which has not been found in patients with AD [103]. It has been shown that ischemia leads to an increased production of the APP isoform containing the Kunitz protease inhibitor (KPI) domain [104]. This could have implications for both intracellular as well as extracellular activity of serine proteases (such as furin, trypsin, and plasmin), which in turn could lead to an altered downstream activation of metalloproteinases such as MMPs [105], membrane-type MMPs (MT-MMP) [106], and A Disintegrin And Metalloproteinases (ADAMs) [107, 108].

It has recently been reported that a metalloproteinase called Meprin β is capable of cleaving APP at the β-secretase site [109]. One could speculate that differences in vascular pathology could, on the one hand, give rise to a local disturbance in clearance with concomitant cerebrovascular deposition of Aβ, as in AD. On the other hand, arteriolosclerosis causing ischemia could lead to an increased expression of the APP-KPI isoform, giving cause to an inhibition of serine proteases and metalloproteases, which in return cause decreased β-secretase activity with a decrease in the release of sAPPβ as well as Aβ1–40 and 1–42 levels.

In summary, CSF amyloid deviations appear in patients with pure AD, AD with signs of cerebrovascular disease ("mixed dementia"), and in those with subcortical brain changes without obvious signs of AD. This implies that low CSF levels of Aβ1–42 are diagnostically nonspecific. However, by using the ratio of Aβ1–42/40 further specificity can be gained, since Aβ1–40 has been found to be altered in patients with VaD with subcortical lesions and lower levels of Aβ1–42, but unaltered Aβ1–40, have been associated with the pure form of AD. Furthermore, a decrease in the soluble extracellular domain of APP, sAPPβ, has been shown to correlate with white matter changes and is not altered in AD patients.

From the pathophysiologic point of view, which is the main focus of the present chapter, it appears that CSF amyloid deviations may arise by different mechanisms. In the group of patients with AD and cerebrovascular disease, clearance obstruction appears to be a strong mechanistic candidate. In those with ischemia, mechanisms associated with BBB alterations and activation/inhibition of different enzymes induced by the ischemia could be the cause of the CSF amyloid deviations.

Axonal degeneration

Neurofilament (NF) belongs to the intermediate filament family, which is one of three types of filaments making up the mammalian cytoskeleton, the other two being microtubules and actin-containing microfilaments. The intermediate filament constitution of a neuronal cell is up to 85% of the total protein [110], which makes this family of proteins very important for the maintenance of cellular structural integrity.

There are three neurofilament chains and they are named according to their molecular sizes: NF-L (light), NF-M (medium), and NF-H (high). The most common of the three chains is the NF-L, with a molar ratio of 4 : 2 : 1 (NF-L : NF-M : NF-H) [111], which forms the backbone of the NF fiber onto which the heavier chains can copolymerize [112–116]. NF-L only constitutes a smaller part of the cytoskeletal components in the neuronal cell body and dendrites relative to axons [117], and thus changes in its concentration in CSF are mainly believed to represent the integrity of the axonal department. Furthermore, the NF seems to regulate the axonal diameter and large caliber myelinated axons outweigh small caliber unmyelinated axons in their NF content. Thus, NF is important for the conduction velocity of nerve impulses since axon caliber is a determinant thereof [118–123].

Increased CSF levels of NF-L have been reported in patients with SVD and AD [37, 124–126], and an increased concentration has been shown already at baseline in prodromal SVD patients at the stage of MCI compared to stable MCI patients and controls [127]. In a meta-analysis of NF-L and NF-H, increased levels were found not only in SVD and AD but also in frontotemporal dementia (FTD) patients [128]. This overlap could be explained by the fact that white matter changes are shown to be more prevalent in all of these groups compared to age-matched controls; however, with a higher incidence and severity in patients with SVD than in AD and FTD patients [129].

Also, NF-L has been found to be increased in normal pressure hydrocephalus, and the degree of MRI white matter changes has been shown to correlate with the CSF concentration [47, 48]. In addition, ventricular CSF NF-L protein levels have been found to decrease in parallel with white matter changes after shunt surgery in normal pressure hydrocephalus [130].

The relationship between NF-L levels in CSF and white matter changes, assessed by semiquantitative MRI, also has been corroborated in patients with SVD and AD [125, 126], indicating a mixed pathology in the latter patient group. One important goal in the future will be to investigate whether the long-term prognosis is correlated to higher levels of NF-L in patients with white matter changes. This has to some extent already been done in patients with aneurysmal subarachnoid hemorrhage where the level of NF-L was found to correlate with stroke severity assessed by the National Institutes of Health Stroke Scale (NIHSS) score on the day of lumbar puncture (10–14 days after acute brain damage) and outcome assessed by Glasgow Outcome Scale (GOS), Mini Mental State Examination (MMSE), and NIHSS after one year [131].

Tau belongs to the microtubule-associated protein (MAP) family, which are proteins essential for the regulation of microtubule stabilization such as assembly and disassembly [132]. Its primary transcript can be alternatively spliced into six different isoforms in the adult brain [133]. The isoforms contain two different domains: a projection domain and a microtubule-binding domain. Some proposed functions of the projection domain are to regulate the spacing between axonal microtubules [134] and to interact with other cytoskeletal proteins [135]. The isoforms differ in the microtubule-binding domain in that they contain three (3R) or four repeats (4R) of a microtubule-binding motif. The 3R and 4R containing isoforms are under normal conditions expressed in a 1 : 1 ratio in the adult brain, and an imbalance in this ratio seems to have implications in some tauopathies [136], since the amount of repeats affects the binding affinity of tau to the microtubules [137].

Furthermore, several post-translational modifications have been described for tau, and the most extensively studied is phosphorylation. The longest tau isoform in the CNS has 79 putative phosphorylation sites. Phosphorylation of tau normally decreases with age but increases under certain pathologic conditions such as AD [138]. The increased phosphorylation of tau leads to a decrease in affinity for microtubules and a subsequent destabilization of the microtubule network [139]. Some findings also indicate that the phosphorylation of tau promotes its self-assembly [140], which could give rise to the AD characteristic neurofibrillary tangles. In addition, phosphorylated tau is more resistant to degradation than nonphosphorylated tau [141].

Increased levels of tau in CSF presumably indicate degeneration of cortical axons as is assumed in both Creutzfeldt–Jakob disease and AD [142]. The total level of tau (T-tau), phosphorylated or not, together with the level of the phosphorylated form (P-tau), has proven useful in identifying AD patients from healthy controls [143]; however, there is a slight overlap with other neurodegenerative diseases such as dementia with Lewy bodies, FTD, and VaD [144], while the T-tau and P-tau levels have been reported to be unchanged in SVD [145]. As mentioned above, by combining the biomarkers T-tau and P-tau with Aβ, reflecting both of the AD pathologic hallmarks of neurofibrillary tangles [138] and amyloid plaques [146], further specificity can be gained [143, 147].

These three biomarkers have also proven useful in identifying patients with MCI who will progress to overt AD [148, 149]. Increased levels of tau in CSF also have been reported in TBI [150, 151] and in CSF from patients with subarachnoid hemorrhage [152], which further implies the nonspecific nature of this axonal injury marker. Even so, the concentration of tau in both AD and subarachnoid hemorrhage correlates with both clinical outcome and injury severity [153]. A previous study of patients with acute ischemic stroke has identified a marked increase of tau in CSF that correlates with infarct volume [154]. Measurements of P-tau, on the other hand, do not seem to be changed in stroke patients, which supports its role as a marker reflecting the neuropathologic alteration in patients with AD [155].

Although not specific for the etiologic SVD diagnostic entity, NF-L is clearly related to changes in the subcortical brain region and to arteriolosclerotic small vessel disease, as identified by MRI white matter changes, whereas T-tau is not. Whether axonal loss of integrity, as measured by NF-L deviations, manifests before or after demyelination as measured by sulfatide and MBP, or vice versa, needs to be further clarified. Nevertheless, the sulfatide findings from the Leukoaraiosis and Disability in the Elderly (LADIS) study suggest demyelinization as being the primary manifestation.

Summary and implications

In patients with subcortical small vessel disease, elevated levels of MBP, NF-L, TIMP-1, and MMP-9 were found, whereas in AD, the levels of P-tau$_{181}$ and T-tau were increased, which reflects cortical involvement. Decreased levels of Aβ1–42 were found in both disorders, which indicates that different pathogenetic pathways may give rise to identical Aβ1–42 deviations.

Thus, the use of a panel of CSF biomarkers in the AD–VaD spectrum reveals variable patterns that support the notion of different mechanisms underlying common dementia disorders, which include involvement of the cerebral small vessels. These results may not only increase our knowledge about the pathophysiologic chain of events that take place in incipient or manifest SVD, AD, and their combinations, but also may be useful for diagnostic and prognostic purposes and for monitoring treatment effects in incipient or manifest SVD.

References

1. Pantoni LG, ed. *Cerebral Small Vessel Disease: Pathological and Pathophysiological Aspects in Relation to Vascular Cognitive Impairment*. London: Dunitz; 2002.
2. McKhann GM, Knopman DS, Chertkow H, et al. The diagnosis of dementia due to Alzheimer's disease: recommendations from the National Institute on Aging – Alzheimer's Association Work Group on diagnostic guidelines for Alzheimer's disease. *Alzheimers Dement* 2011;7: 263–269.
3. McKhann G, Drachman D, Folstein M, et al. Clinical diagnosis of Alzheimer's disease: report of the NINCDS–ADRDA work group under the auspices of Department of Health and Human Services Task Force on Alzheimer's Disease. *Neurology* 1984;34:939–944.
4. Grinberg LT, Thal DR. Vascular pathology in the aged human brain. *Acta Neuropathol* 2010;119:277–290.
5. Thal DR, Grinberg LT, Attems J. Vascular dementia: different forms of vessel disorders contribute to the development of dementia in the elderly brain. *Exp Gerontol* 2012;47:816–824.
6. Brun A. Pathology and pathophysiology of cerebrovascular dementia: pure subgroups of obstructive and hypoperfusive etiology. *Dementia* 1994;5:145–147.
7. Barba R, Martinez-Espinosa S, Rodriguez-Garcia E, et al. Poststroke dementia: clinical features and risk factors. *Stroke* 2000;31:1494–1501.
8. Oreskovic D, Klarica M. The formation of cerebrospinal fluid: nearly a hundred years of interpretations and misinterpretations. *Brain Res Rev* 2010;64:241–262.
9. Abbott NJ, Patabendige AA, Dolman DE, Yusof SR, Begley DJ. Structure and function of the blood–brain barrier. *Neurobiol Dis* 2010;37:13–25.
10. Abbott NJ. Evidence for bulk flow of brain interstitial fluid:

significance for physiology and pathology. *Neurochem Int* 2004;45:545–552.

11. Johanson CE, Duncan JA, 3rd, Klinge PM, et al. Multiplicity of cerebrospinal fluid functions: new challenges in health and disease. *Cerebrospinal Fluid Res* 2008; 5:10.
12. Regeniter A, Kuhle J, Mehling M, et al. A modern approach to CSF analysis: pathophysiology, clinical application, proof of concept and laboratory reporting. *Clin Neurol Neurosurg* 2009;111:313–318.
13. Reiber H. Proteins in cerebrospinal fluid and blood: barriers, CSF flow rate and source-related dynamics. *Restor Neurol Neurosci* 2003;21:79–96.
14. Neuwelt EA, Bauer B, Fahlke C, et al. Engaging neuroscience to advance translational research in brain barrier biology. *Nat Rev Neurosci* 2011;12:169–182.
15. Zlokovic BV. Neurovascular pathways to neurodegeneration in Alzheimer's disease and other disorders. *Nat Rev Neurosci* 2011;12:723–738.
16. Hawkins BT, Davis TP. The blood–brain barrier/ neurovascular unit in health and disease. *Pharmacol Rev* 2005;57:173–185.
17. Rosenberg GA. Neurological diseases in relation to the blood–brain barrier. *J Cereb Blood Flow Metab* 2012;32: 1139–1151.
18. Olsson Y, Brun A, Englund E. Fundamental pathological lesions in vascular dementia. *Acta Neurol Scand Suppl* 1996;168: 31–38.
19. Wallin A, Blennow K, Fredman P, et al. Blood brain barrier function in vascular dementia. *Acta Neurol Scand* 1990;81:318–322.
20. Pantoni L, Inzitari D, Pracucci G, et al. Cerebrospinal fluid proteins in patients with leucoaraiosis: possible abnormalities in blood–brain barrier function. *J Neurol Sci* 1993;115:125–131.
21. Wallin A, Sjogren M, Edman A, Blennow K, Regland B. Symptoms, vascular risk factors and blood–brain barrier function in relation to CT white-matter changes in dementia. *Eur Neurol* 2000;44:229–235.
22. Taheri S, Gasparovic C, Shah NJ, Rosenberg GA. Quantitative measurement of blood–brain barrier permeability in humans using dynamic contrast-enhanced MRI with fast T1 mapping. *Magn Reson Med* 2011;65: 1036–1042.
23. Blennow K, Wallin A, Uhlemann C, Gottfries CG. White-matter lesions on CT in Alzheimer patients: relation to clinical symptomatology and vascular factors. *Acta Neurol Scand* 1991;83:187–193.
24. Bowman GL, Kaye JA, Moore M, et al. Blood–brain barrier impairment in Alzheimer disease: stability and functional significance. *Neurology* 2007;68:1809–1814.
25. Gouw AA, Seewann A, van der Flier WM, et al. Heterogeneity of small vessel disease: a systematic review of MRI and histopathology correlations. *J Neurol Neurosurg Psychiatry* 2011;82:126–135.
26. Pekny M, Nilsson M. Astrocyte activation and reactive gliosis. *Glia* 2005;50:427–434.
27. Fernando MS, Simpson JE, Matthews F, et al. White matter lesions in an unselected cohort of the elderly: molecular pathology suggests origin from chronic hypoperfusion injury. *Stroke* 2006;37:1391–1398.
28. Volpe JJ. Brain injury in premature infants: a complex amalgam of destructive and developmental disturbances. *Lancet Neurol* 2009;8:110–124.
29. Akiguchi I, Tomimoto H, Suenaga T, Wakita H, Budka H. Blood–brain barrier dysfunction in Binswanger's disease; an immunohistochemical study. *Acta Neuropathol* 1998;95: 78–84.
30. Quarles RH, Morell P, eds. *Myelin Formation, Structure, and Biochemistry*. New York, NY: Elsevier Academic Press; 2006.
31. Moore CS, Abdullah SL, Brown A, Arulpragasam A, Crocker SJ. How factors secreted from astrocytes impact myelin repair. *J Neurosci Res* 2011;89:13–21.
32. Nash B, Ioannidou K, Barnett SC. Astrocyte phenotypes and their relationship to myelination. *J Anat* 2011;219:44–52.
33. Iadecola C, Nedergaard M. Glial regulation of the cerebral microvasculature. *Nat Neurosci* 2007;10:1369–1376.
34. Middeldorp J, Hol EM. GFAP in health and disease. *Prog Neurobiol* 2011;3:421–443.
35. Rosenberg GA, Sullivan N, Esiri MM. White matter damage is associated with matrix metalloproteinases in vascular dementia. *Stroke* 2001; 32:1162–1168.
36. Simpson JE, Fernando MS, Clark L, et al. White matter lesions in an unselected cohort of the elderly: astrocytic, microglial and oligodendrocyte precursor cell responses. *Neuropathol Appl Neurobiol* 2007;33:410–419.
37. Bjerke M, Zetterberg H, Edman A, et al. Cerebrospinal fluid matrix metalloproteinases and tissue inhibitor of metalloproteinases in combination with subcortical and cortical biomarkers in vascular dementia and Alzheimer's disease. *J Alzheimers Dis* 2011;27:665–676.
38. Rosen C, Mattsson N, Johansson PM, et al. Discriminatory analysis of biochip-derived protein patterns in CSF and plasma in neurodegenerative diseases. *Front Aging Neurosci* 2011;3:1.

39. Wallin A, Blennow K, Rosengren LE. Glial fibrillary acidic protein in the cerebrospinal fluid of patients with dementia. *Dementia* 1996;7:267–272.
40. Brouns R, De Vil B, Cras P, et al. Neurobiochemical markers of brain damage in cerebrospinal fluid of acute ischemic stroke patients. *Clin Chem* 2010;56: 451–458.
41. Aurell A, Rosengren LE, Karlsson B, et al. Determination of S-100 and glial fibrillary acidic protein concentrations in cerebrospinal fluid after brain infarction. *Stroke* 1991;22:1254–1258.
42. Farfara D, Lifshitz V, Frenkel D. Neuroprotective and neurotoxic properties of glial cells in the pathogenesis of Alzheimer's disease. *J Cell Mol Med* 2008;12:762–780.
43. Wallin A, Gottfries CG, Karlsson I, Svennerholm L. Decreased myelin lipids in Alzheimer's disease and vascular dementia. *Acta Neurol Scand* 1989;80: 319–323.
44. Fredman P, Wallin A, Blennow K, et al. Sulfatide as a biochemical marker in cerebrospinal fluid of patients with vascular dementia. *Acta Neurol Scand* 1992;85: 103–106.
45. Tullberg M, Mansson JE, Fredman P, et al. CSF sulfatide distinguishes between normal pressure hydrocephalus and subcortical arteriosclerotic encephalopathy. *J Neurol Neurosurg Psychiatry* 2000;69: 74–81.
46. Agren-Wilsson A, Lekman A, Sjoberg W, et al. CSF biomarkers in the evaluation of idiopathic normal pressure hydrocephalus. *Acta Neurol Scand* 2007;116: 333–339.
47. Tullberg M, Hultin L, Ekholm S, et al. White matter changes in normal pressure hydrocephalus and Binswanger disease: specificity, predictive value and correlations to axonal degeneration and demyelination. *Acta Neurol Scand* 2002;105: 417–426.
48. Jonsson M, Zetterberg H, van Straaten E, et al. Cerebrospinal fluid biomarkers of white matter lesions – cross-sectional results from the LADIS study. *Eur J Neurol* 2010;17:377–382.
49. Jonsson M, Zetterberg H, Rolstad S, et al. Low cerebrospinal fluid sulfatide predicts progression of white matter lesions: the LADIS study. *Dement Geriatr Cogn Disord* 2012;34:61–67.
50. Clark AW, Krekoski CA, Bou SS, Chapman KR, Edwards DR. Increased gelatinase A (MMP-2) and gelatinase B (MMP-9) activities in human brain after focal ischemia. *Neurosci Lett* 1997;238:53–56.
51. Cuadrado E, Rosell A, Penalba A, et al. Vascular MMP-9/TIMP-2 and neuronal MMP-10 up-regulation in human brain after stroke: a combined laser microdissection and protein array study. *J Proteome Res* 2009;8:3191–3197.
52. Adair JC, Charlie J, Dencoff JE, et al. Measurement of gelatinase B (MMP-9) in the cerebrospinal fluid of patients with vascular dementia and Alzheimer disease. *Stroke* 2004;35:e159–162.
53. Candelario-Jalil E, Thompson J, Taheri S, et al. Matrix metalloproteinases are associated with increased blood–brain barrier opening in vascular cognitive impairment. *Stroke* 2011;42:1345–1350.
54. Craig-Schapiro R, Kuhn M, Xiong C, et al. Multiplexed immunoassay panel identifies novel CSF biomarkers for Alzheimer's disease diagnosis and prognosis. *PLoS One* 2011; 6, e18850.
55. Backstrom JR, Lim GP, Cullen MJ, Tokes ZA. Matrix metalloproteinase-9 (MMP-9) is synthesized in neurons of the human hippocampus and is capable of degrading the amyloid-β peptide (1–40). *J Neurosci* 1996;16:7910–7919.
56. Yan P, Hu X, Song H, et al. Matrix metalloproteinase-9 degrades amyloid-β fibrils in vitro and compact plaques in situ. *J Biol Chem* 2006;281: 24566–24574.
57. Stetler-Stevenson WG. Tissue inhibitors of metalloproteinases in cell signaling: metalloproteinase-independent biological activities. *Sci Signal* 2008;1:e6.
58. Maddahi A, Chen Q, Edvinsson L. Enhanced cerebrovascular expression of matrix metalloproteinase-9 and tissue inhibitor of metalloproteinase-1 via the MEK/ERK pathway during cerebral ischemia in the rat. *BMC Neurosci* 2009;10:56.
59. Romero JR, Vasan RS, Beiser AS, et al. Association of matrix metalloproteinases with MRI indices of brain ischemia and aging. *Neurobiol Aging* 2010;31:2128–2135.
60. Ohrfelt A, Andreasson U, Simon A, et al. Screening for new biomarkers for subcortical vascular dementia and Alzheimer's disease. *Dement Geriatr Cogn Dis Extra* 2011; 1:31–42.
61. Hansson J, Vasan RS, Arnlov J, et al. Biomarkers of extracellular matrix metabolism (MMP-9 and TIMP-1) and risk of stroke, myocardial infarction, and cause-specific mortality: cohort study. *PLoS One* 2011; 6:e16185.
62. Kalaria RN, Ballard C. Overlap between pathology of Alzheimer disease and vascular dementia. *Alzheimer Dis Assoc Disord* 1999;13(Suppl 3):S115–S123.
63. Olichney JM, Hansen LA, Hofstetter CR, et al. Cerebral infarction in Alzheimer's disease is associated with severe amyloid

angiopathy and hypertension. *Arch Neurol* 1995;52:702–708.

64. Cadavid D, Mena H, Koeller K, Frommelt RA. Cerebral β amyloid angiopathy is a risk factor for cerebral ischemic infarction. A case control study in human brain biopsies. *J Neuropathol Exp Neurol* 2000;59:768–773.
65. Zhang F, Eckman C, Younkin S, Hsiao KK, Iadecola C. Increased susceptibility to ischemic brain damage in transgenic mice overexpressing the amyloid precursor protein. *J Neurosci* 1997;17:7655–7661.
66. Soontornniyomkij V, Lynch MD, Mermash S, et al. Cerebral microinfarcts associated with severe cerebral β-amyloid angiopathy. *Brain Pathol* 2010;20:459–467.
67. Haglund M, Passant U, Sjobeck M, Ghebremedhin E, Englund E. Cerebral amyloid angiopathy and cortical microinfarcts as putative substrates of vascular dementia. *Int J Geriatr Psychiatry* 2006;21:681–687.
68. Greenberg SM, Gurol ME, Rosand J, Smith EE. Amyloid angiopathy-related vascular cognitive impairment. *Stroke* 2004;35: 2616–2619.
69. Hardy J, Selkoe DJ. The amyloid hypothesis of Alzheimer's disease: progress and problems on the road to therapeutics. *Science* 2002;297:353–356.
70. Blennow K, de Leon MJ, Zetterberg H. Alzheimer's disease. *Lancet* 2006;368:387–403.
71. Vinters HV, Pardridge WM, Yang J. Immunohistochemical study of cerebral amyloid angiopathy: use of an antiserum to a synthetic 28-amino-acid peptide fragment of the Alzheimer's disease amyloid precursor. *Hum Pathol* 1988;19:214–222.
72. Gold G, Giannakopoulos P, Herrmann FR, Bouras C, Kovari E. Identification of Alzheimer and vascular lesion thresholds for mixed dementia. *Brain* 2007;130:2830–2836.
73. Schneider JA, Boyle PA, Arvanitakis Z, Bienias JL, Bennett DA. Subcortical infarcts, Alzheimer's disease pathology, and memory function in older persons. *Ann Neurol* 2007;62: 59–66.
74. Snowdon DA. Aging and Alzheimer's disease: lessons from the Nun Study. *Gerontologist* 1997;37:150–156.
75. Kimchi EY, Kajdasz S, Bacskai BJ, Hyman BT. Analysis of cerebral amyloid angiopathy in a transgenic mouse model of Alzheimer disease using in vivo multiphoton microscopy. *J Neuropathol Exp Neurol* 2001;60:274–279.
76. Vonsattel JP, Myers RH, Hedley-Whyte ET, et al. Cerebral amyloid angiopathy without and with cerebral hemorrhages: a comparative histological study. *Ann Neurol* 1991;30:637–649.
77. Townsend KP, Obregon D, Quadros A, et al. Proinflammatory and vasoactive effects of Aβ in the cerebrovasculature. *Ann NY Acad Sci* 2002;977:65–76.
78. Scolding NJ, Joseph F, Kirby PA, et al. Aβ-related angiitis: primary angiitis of the central nervous system associated with cerebral amyloid angiopathy. *Brain* 2005;128:500–515.
79. Bjerke M, Portelius E, Minthon L, et al. Confounding factors influencing amyloid β concentration in cerebrospinal fluid. *Int J Alzheimers Dis* 2010; 2010:986310.
80. Catricala S, Torti M, Ricevuti G. Alzheimer disease and platelets: how's that relevant? *Immun Ageing* 2012;9:20.
81. Corder EH, Saunders AM, Strittmatter WJ, et al. Gene dose of apolipoprotein E type 4 allele and the risk of Alzheimer's disease in late onset families. *Science* 1993;261:921–923.
82. McCarron MO, Delong D, Alberts MJ. *APOE* genotype as a risk factor for ischemic cerebrovascular disease: a meta-analysis. *Neurology* 1999;53: 1308–1311.
83. Yip AG, McKee AC, Green RC, et al. *APOE*, vascular pathology, and the AD brain. *Neurology* 2005;65:259–265.
84. Bronge L, Fernaeus SE, Blomberg M, et al. White matter lesions in Alzheimer patients are influenced by apolipoprotein E genotype. *Dement Geriatr Cogn Disord* 1999;10:89–96.
85. Hirono N, Yasuda M, Tanimukai S, Kitagaki H, Mori E. Effect of the apolipoprotein E ε4 allele on white matter hyperintensities in dementia. *Stroke* 2000;31: 1263–1268.
86. Chalmers K, Wilcock GK, Love S. *APOE* ε4 influences the pathological phenotype of Alzheimer's disease by favouring cerebrovascular over parenchymal accumulation of Aβ protein. *Neuropathol Appl Neurobiol* 2003;29:231–238.
87. Thal DR, Larionov S, Abramowski D, et al. Occurrence and co-localization of amyloid β-protein and apolipoprotein E in perivascular drainage channels of wild-type and APP-transgenic mice. *Neurobiol Aging* 2007;28:1221–1230.
88. Greenberg SM, Briggs ME, Hyman BT, et al. Apolipoprotein E ε4 is associated with the presence and earlier onset of hemorrhage in cerebral amyloid angiopathy. *Stroke* 1996;27: 1333–1337.
89. Biron KE, Dickstein DL, Gopaul R, Jefferies WA. Amyloid triggers extensive cerebral angiogenesis causing blood brain barrier permeability and hypervascularity

in Alzheimer's disease. *PLoS One* 2011;6:e23789.

90. Palacios G, Mengod G, Tortosa A, Ferrer I, Palacios JM. Increased β-amyloid precursor protein expression in astrocytes in the gerbil hippocampus following ischaemia: association with proliferation of astrocytes. *Eur J Neurosci* 1995;7: 501–510.

91. Zhang X, Zhou K, Wang R, et al. Hypoxia-inducible factor 1α (HIF-1α)-mediated hypoxia increases BACE1 expression and β-amyloid generation. *J Biol Chem* 2007;282:10873–10880.

92. Blennow K, Zetterberg H, Fagan AM. Fluid biomarkers in Alzheimer disease. *Cold Spring Harb Perspect Med* 2012;2: a006221.

93. Buchhave P, Minthon L, Zetterberg H, et al. Cerebrospinal fluid levels of β-amyloid 1–42, but not of tau, are fully changed already 5 to 10 years before the onset of Alzheimer dementia. *Arch Gen Psychiatry* 2012;69: 98–106.

94. Fagan AM, Mintun MA, Mach RH, et al. Inverse relation between in vivo amyloid imaging load and cerebrospinal fluid Aβ42 in humans. *Ann Neurol* 2006;59:512–519.

95. Thorvaldsson V, Nordlund A, Reinvang I, et al. Memory in individuals with mild cognitive impairment in relation to APOE and CSF Aβ42. *Int Psychogeriatr* 2010;22:598–606.

96. Thal DR, Rub U, Orantes M, Braak H. Phases of Aβ-deposition in the human brain and its relevance for the development of AD. *Neurology* 2002;58: 1791–1800.

97. Sjogren M, Davidsson P, Gottfries J, et al. The cerebrospinal fluid levels of tau, growth-associated protein-43 and soluble amyloid precursor protein correlate in Alzheimer's disease, reflecting a common pathophysiological process. *Dement Geriatr Cogn Disord* 2001;12:257–264.

98. Goos JD, Teunissen CE, Veerhuis R, et al. Microbleeds relate to altered amyloid-β metabolism in Alzheimer's disease. *Neurobiol Aging* 2012;33:e1011–1019.

99. Verbeek MM, Kremer BP, Rikkert MO, et al. Cerebrospinal fluid amyloid β40 is decreased in cerebral amyloid angiopathy. *Ann Neurol* 2009;66:245–249.

100. Attems J, Jellinger KA. Only cerebral capillary amyloid angiopathy correlates with Alzheimer pathology – a pilot study. *Acta Neuropathol* 2004;107:83–90.

101. Attems J, Lintner F, Jellinger KA. Amyloid β peptide 1–42 highly correlates with capillary cerebral amyloid angiopathy and Alzheimer disease pathology. *Acta Neuropathol* 2004;107: 283–291.

102. Selnes P, Blennow K, Zetterberg H, et al. Effects of cerebrovascular disease on amyloid precursor protein metabolites in cerebrospinal fluid. *Cerebrospinal Fluid Res* 2010;7:10.

103. Zetterberg H, Andreasson U, Hansson O, et al. Elevated cerebrospinal fluid BACE1 activity in incipient Alzheimer disease. *Arch Neurol* 2008;65:1102–1107.

104. Kim HS, Lee SH, Kim SS, et al. Post-ischemic changes in the expression of Alzheimer's APP isoforms in rat cerebral cortex. *Neuroreport* 1998;9:533–537.

105. Gasche Y, Soccal PM, Kanemitsu M, Copin JC. Matrix metalloproteinases and diseases of the central nervous system with a special emphasis on ischemic brain. *Front Biosci* 2006;11: 1289–1301.

106. Thomas G. Furin at the cutting edge: from protein traffic to embryogenesis and disease. *Nat Rev Mol Cell Biol* 2002;3: 753–766.

107. Srour N, Lebel A, McMahon S, et al. TACE/ADAM-17 maturation and activation of sheddase activity require proprotein convertase activity. *FEBS Lett* 2003;554:275–283.

108. Anders A, Gilbert S, Garten W, Postina R, Fahrenholz F. Regulation of the alpha-secretase ADAM10 by its prodomain and proprotein convertases. *FASEB J* 2001;15:1837–1839.

109. Bien J, Jefferson T, Causevic M, et al. The metalloprotease meprin β generates amino terminal-truncated amyloid β peptide species. *J Biol Chem* 2012;287:33304–33313.

110. Fuchs E, Cleveland DW. A structural scaffolding of intermediate filaments in health and disease. *Science* 1998;279:514–519.

111. Scott D, Smith KE, O'Brien BJ, Angelides KJ. Characterization of mammalian neurofilament triplet proteins. Subunit stoichiometry and morphology of native and reconstituted filaments. *J Biol Chem* 1985;260:10736–10747.

112. Weber K, Shaw G, Osborn M, Debus E, Geisler N. Neurofilaments, a subclass of intermediate filaments: structure and expression. *Cold Spring Harb Symp Quant Biol* 1983;48: 717–729.

113. Geisler N, Weber K. Self-assembly in vitro of the 68 000 molecular weight component of the mammalian neurofilament triplet proteins into intermediate-sized filaments. *J Mol Biol* 1981;151:565–571.

114. Hoffman PN, Cleveland DW, Griffin JW, et al. Neurofilament gene expression: a major determinant of axonal caliber. *Proc Natl Acad Sci USA* 1987;84:3472–3476.

115. Lee MK, Xu Z, Wong PC, Cleveland DW. Neurofilaments

are obligate heteropolymers in vivo. *J Cell Biol* 1993;122: 1337–1350.

116. Cohlberg JA, Hajarian H, Tran T, Alipourjeddi P, Noveen A. Neurofilament protein heterotetramers as assembly intermediates. *J Biol Chem* 1995;270:9334–9339.

117. Lasek RJ. *Studying the Intrinsic Determinants of Neuronal Form and Function*. New York, NY: Alan R. Liss; 1988.

118. Friede RL, Samorajski T. Axon caliber related to neurofilaments and microtubules in sciatic nerve fibers of rats and mice. *Anat Rec* 1970;167: 379–387.

119. Kriz J, Zhu Q, Julien JP, Padjen AL. Electrophysiological properties of axons in mice lacking neurofilament subunit genes: disparity between conduction velocity and axon diameter in absence of NF-H. *Brain Res* 2000;885: 32–44.

120. Xu Z, Marszalek JR, Lee MK, et al. Subunit composition of neurofilaments specifies axonal diameter. *J Cell Biol* 1996;133:1061–1069.

121. Lawson SN, Waddell PJ. Soma neurofilament immunoreactivity is related to cell size and fibre conduction velocity in rat primary sensory neurons. *J Physiol* 1991;435:41–63.

122. Kong J, Tung VW, Aghajanian J, Xu Z. Antagonistic roles of neurofilament subunits NF-H and NF-M against NF-L in shaping dendritic arborization in spinal motor neurons. *J Cell Biol* 1998;140:1167–1176.

123. Zhu Q, Couillard-Despres S, Julien JP. Delayed maturation of regenerating myelinated axons in mice lacking neurofilaments. *Exp Neurol* 1997;148:299–316.

124. Rosengren LE, Karlsson JE, Sjogren M, Blennow K, Wallin A. Neurofilament protein levels in CSF are increased in dementia. *Neurology* 1999;52: 1090–1093.

125. Sjogren M, Blomberg M, Jonsson M, et al. Neurofilament protein in cerebrospinal fluid: a marker of white matter changes. *J Neurosci Res* 2001;66:510–516.

126. Wallin A, Sjogren M. Cerebrospinal fluid cytoskeleton proteins in patients with subcortical white-matter dementia. *Mech Ageing Dev* 2001;122:1937–1949.

127. Bjerke M, Andreasson U, Rolstad S, et al. Subcortical vascular dementia biomarker pattern in mild cognitive impairment. *Dement Geriatr Cogn Disord* 2009;28:348–356.

128. Petzold A, Keir G, Warren J, Fox N, Rossor MN. A systematic review and meta-analysis of CSF neurofilament protein levels as biomarkers in dementia. *Neurodegener Dis* 2007;4:185–194.

129. Varma AR, Laitt R, Lloyd JJ, et al. Diagnostic value of high signal abnormalities on T2 weighted MRI in the differentiation of Alzheimer's, frontotemporal and vascular dementias. *Acta Neurol Scand* 2002;105:355–364.

130. Tullberg M, Blennow K, Mansson JE, et al. Ventricular cerebrospinal fluid neurofilament protein levels decrease in parallel with white matter pathology after shunt surgery in normal pressure hydrocephalus. *Eur J Neurol* 2007;14:248–254.

131. Nylen K, Csajbok LZ, Ost M, et al. CSF–neurofilament correlates with outcome after aneurysmal subarachnoid hemorrhage. *Neurosci Lett* 2006;404:132–136.

132. Weingarten MD, Lockwood AH, Hwo SY, Kirschner MW. A protein factor essential for microtubule assembly. *Proc Natl Acad Sci USA* 1975;72: 1858–1862.

133. Goedert M, Spillantini MG, Jakes R, Rutherford D, Crowther RA. Multiple isoforms of human microtubule-associated protein tau: sequences and localization in neurofibrillary tangles of Alzheimer's disease. *Neuron* 1989;3:519–526.

134. Chen J, Kanai Y, Cowan NJ, Hirokawa N. Projection domains of MAP2 and tau determine spacings between microtubules in dendrites and axons. *Nature* 1992;360: 674–677.

135. Hirokawa N, Shiomura Y, Okabe S. Tau proteins: the molecular structure and mode of binding on microtubules. *J Cell Biol* 1988;107:1449–1459.

136. Cairns NJ, Bigio EH, Mackenzie IR, et al. Neuropathologic diagnostic and nosologic criteria for frontotemporal lobar degeneration: consensus of the Consortium for Frontotemporal Lobar Degeneration. *Acta Neuropathol* 2007;114:5–22.

137. Lu M, Kosik KS. Competition for microtubule-binding with dual expression of tau missense and splice isoforms. *Mol Biol Cell* 2001;12:171–184.

138. Grundke-Iqbal I, Iqbal K, Tung YC, et al. Abnormal phosphorylation of the microtubule-associated protein tau (tau) in Alzheimer cytoskeletal pathology. *Proc Natl Acad Sci USA* 1986;83:4913–4917.

139. Yamamoto A, Lucas JJ, Hen R. Reversal of neuropathology and motor dysfunction in a conditional model of Huntington's disease. *Cell* 2000;101:57–66.

140. Alonso A, Zaidi T, Novak M, Grundke-Iqbal I, Iqbal K. Hyperphosphorylation induces self-assembly of tau into tangles of paired helical filaments/ straight filaments. *Proc Natl Acad Sci USA* 2001;98: 6923–6928.

141. Wang JZ, Gong CX, Zaidi T, Grundke-Iqbal I, Iqbal K. Dephosphorylation of Alzheimer paired helical filaments by protein phosphatase-2A and -2B. *J Biol Chem* 1995;270:4854–4860.

142. Hampel H, Blennow K, Shaw LM, et al. Total and phosphorylated tau protein as biological markers of Alzheimer's disease. *Exp Gerontol* 2010;45:30–40.

143. Blennow K, Zetterberg H. Cerebrospinal fluid biomarkers for Alzheimer's disease. *J Alzheimers Dis* 2009;18: 413–417.

144. Van Harten AC, Kester MI, Visser PJ, et al. Tau and p-tau as CSF biomarkers in dementia: a meta-analysis. *Clin Chem Lab Med* 2011;49:353–366.

145. Sjogren M, Davidsson P, Tullberg M, et al. Both total and phosphorylated tau are increased in Alzheimer's disease. *J Neurol Neurosurg Psychiatry* 2001;70:624–630.

146. Masters CL, Simms G, Weinman NA, et al. Amyloid plaque core protein in Alzheimer disease and Down syndrome. *Proc Natl Acad Sci USA* 1985;82: 4245–4249.

147. Blennow K, Hampel H, Weiner M, Zetterberg H. Cerebrospinal fluid and plasma biomarkers in Alzheimer disease. *Nat Rev Neurol* 2010;6:131–144.

148. Hansson O, Zetterberg H, Buchhave P, et al. Association between CSF biomarkers and incipient Alzheimer's disease in patients with mild cognitive impairment: a follow-up study. *Lancet Neurol* 2006; 5:228–234.

149. Blennow K, Hampel H. CSF markers for incipient Alzheimer's disease. *Lancet Neurol* 2003;2:605–613.

150. Franz G, Beer R, Kampfl A, et al. Amyloid β1–42 and tau in cerebrospinal fluid after severe traumatic brain injury. *Neurology* 2003;60:1457–1461.

151. Kay AD, Petzold A, Kerr M, et al. Alterations in cerebrospinal fluid apolipoprotein E and amyloid β-protein after traumatic brain injury. *J Neurotrauma* 2003;20:943–952.

152. Zemlan FP, Jauch EC, Mulchahey JJ, et al. C-tau biomarker of neuronal damage in severe brain injured patients: association with elevated intracranial pressure and clinical outcome. *Brain Res* 2002;947:131–139.

153. Kay A, Petzold A, Kerr M, et al. Temporal alterations in cerebrospinal fluid amyloid β-protein and apolipoprotein E after subarachnoid hemorrhage. *Stroke* 2003;34:e240–243.

154. Hesse C, Rosengren L, Vanmechelen E, et al. Cerebrospinal fluid markers for Alzheimer's disease evaluated after acute ischemic stroke. *J Alzheimers Dis* 2000; 2:199–206.

155. Hesse C, Rosengren L, Andreasen N, et al. Transient increase in total tau but not phospho-tau in human cerebrospinal fluid after acute stroke. *Neurosci Lett* 2001;297:187–190.

Chapter 18

Acute stroke syndromes caused by small vessel disease

Mark I. Boulos, Ranjith K. Menon, Richard I. Aviv, Sandra E. Black, and Richard H. Swartz

Introduction

The term small vessel disease (SVD) refers to all pathologic processes that affect the small arteries and veins of the brain. SVD in the brain parenchyma typically gives rise to lesions located in the subcortical structures and brainstem, and includes small subcortical infarcts (i.e., lacunar strokes), white matter lesions, perivascular spaces, some large hemorrhages, microbleeds, and can lead to brain atrophy [1]. In the present work, we will focus on acute presentations of cerebral SVD. As lacunar syndromes have been the most studied subtype in the acute setting, this will be our area of focus.

Overview of lacunar infarcts

Lacunar infarcts are small subcortical infarcts typically located in the basal ganglia, thalamus, internal capsule, corona radiata, or brainstem, which result from occlusion of a single perforating artery [2]. The precise definition, including site and size, of these infarcts has varied across studies [3]. This subtype of stroke is so named because lacunar infarctions are thought to evolve into lacunar cavities ("lacunes") over time; however, the actual proportion of lacunar strokes that have been demonstrated to cavitate has varied across imaging studies [4, 5].

Epidemiology of lacunar infarctions

Percentage of acute strokes

Lacunar infarcts account for approximately 25% of all acute ischemic stroke presentations [6]. In comparison, using the TOAST (Trial of ORG 10172 in Acute Stroke Treatment) classification for stroke subtype [7], 30% of strokes are estimated to be due to cardioembolism, 15% secondary to large artery atherosclerosis, and the remaining 30% are thought to be caused by less common or undetermined etiologies [6].

Demographics and risk factors

The Secondary Prevention of Small Subcortical Strokes (SPS3) study [8], the largest trial to date investigating symptomatic small subcortical (i.e., lacunar) stroke, provided valuable insights into the demographic and clinical characteristics of patients with lacunar stroke. In the 3020 randomized patients who were recruited within 6 months of having sustained a lacunar stroke, the mean age was 63 years and 63% of the patients were male; other large population-based studies have also demonstrated a mean age in the 60s and a slight male predominance for patients with lacunar stroke [9]. The most prevalent vascular risk factors were hypertension (75%), hyperlipidemia (49%), diabetes (37%), and 60% of patients were current or former smokers [10]. These findings were consistent with earlier reports which also demonstrated that age, hypertension, diabetes, and smoking were associated with an increased the risk of lacunar infarction [11–13]. Lacunar infarction is also the most common stroke subtype in patients with type 2 diabetes [14].

Ethnicity

In the SPS3 trial, 51% of the patients were white, 30% Hispanic, and 16% black. Important differences in clinical characteristics emerged among the different ethnicities. For example, the average age of black patients at the time of enrollment (58 years) was significantly lower than that for both Hispanics and white patients (64 years; $P<0.001$). Hispanic and black patients were more likely than white patients to have had a prior history of hypertension and

Cerebral Small Vessel Disease, ed. Leonardo Pantoni and Philip B. Gorelick. Published by Cambridge University Press.

diabetes (P <0.001) [10]. Previous work has also demonstrated that blacks and Hispanics with stroke have a higher prevalence of hypertension and diabetes compared to whites [15, 16]. Finally, despite having a higher likelihood of a prior lacunar stroke compared to whites (13% vs. 9%; P <0.01), blacks were still less likely to have been using aspirin during the seven days leading to the qualifying event (21% vs. 33%; P <0.001). Hispanics were also less likely than whites to report regular aspirin use (21% vs. 33%; P <0.001) [10], also consistent with prior reports [17].

Within six months of a lacunar stroke, most patients made a good recovery, with 67% of patients reporting a modified Rankin Scale (mRS) score of 0 or 1 (indicating no symptoms or no significant disability despite some symptoms). Seventy-one percent of whites had an mRS of 0–1; however, only 65% of Hispanics and 55% of blacks had achieved a similar degree of recovery [10].

Complexity of SVD

Heterogeneity in stroke mechanism

Arterial stroke syndromes arising as a result of SVD are usually attributed to various pathologic processes affecting small intracranial perforating arteries [18]. Since these small perforating arteries are branches of larger cerebral arteries, proximal causes (such as large artery thromboembolic and cardioembolic disease) also need to be considered since these can also occlude small intracranial arteries, and several large studies have supported this. For example, in the three-city – Dijon (3C-Dijon) study (N = 1800 participants), markers of large vessel disease (i.e., carotid lumen diameter and carotid stiffness) were associated with increased prevalence of lacunar infarcts and white matter hyperintensities on multivariable regression analyses [19]. Multiple patient series case reports have also demonstrated large artery disease giving rise to lacunar syndromes [20, 21]. Similarly, in the Warfarin Aspirin Symptomatic Intracranial Disease (WASID) trial, which enrolled 347 stroke patients with cerebrovascular events attributable to angiographically verified severe (i.e., 50–99%) stenosis of a major intracranial artery, more than 10% (38/347) of the strokes were lacunar in nature [22]. Cardioembolism has also been demonstrated to give rise to lacunar infarcts, although this is a less common mechanism (about 2.6–10.0% of all lacunar strokes) [23, 24]. Overall, 75–83% of lacunar syndromes are thought to be due to intrinsic SVD, with 17–25% of lacunar syndromes associated with other etiologic mechanisms (such as large artery or cardioembolic sources: see Figure 18.1) [25, 26]. Pure sensory strokes seem to be the most predictive, and pure motor hemiparesis least predictive of lacunar infarction on imaging [25]. In addition, lacunar infarcts that arise from non-SVD mechanisms carry a poorer prognosis than lacunar strokes that are associated with SVD [27]. These findings emphasize the need for noninvasive neurovascular imaging and cardiac evaluations in patients with lacunar stroke.

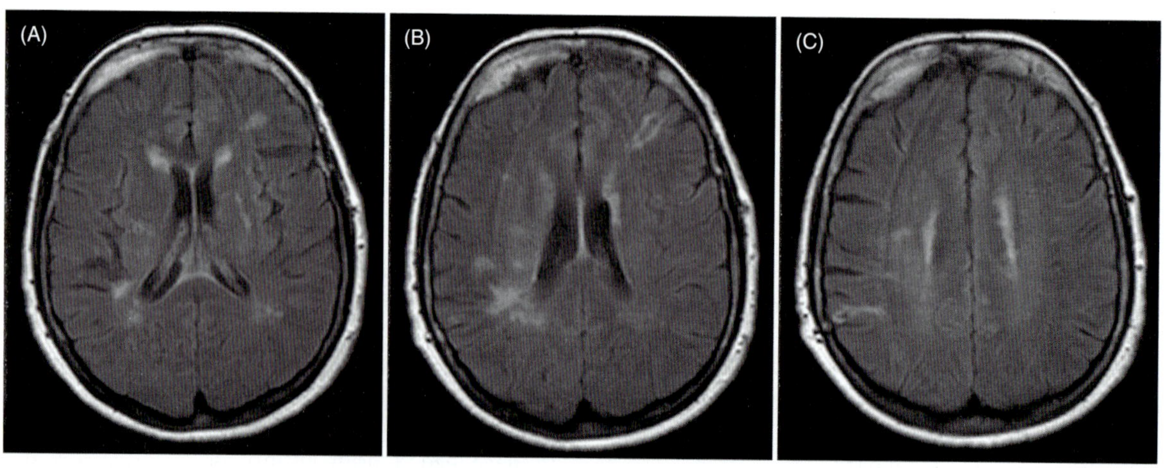

Figure 18.1 Heterogeneity in underlying mechanism when evaluating acute stroke syndromes caused by small vessel disease. In this 70-year-old woman with an initial clinical evaluation suggestive of a pure motor lacunar syndrome, the presence of both deep and cortical infarcts in multiple vascular territories on magnetic resonance fluid-attenuated inversion recovery (FLAIR) images (A–C) prompted the search for an underlying cardioembolic source.

Not all authors agree with screening for nonlacunar mechanisms in patients with confirmed lacunar stroke. Atherosclerosis of medium-sized intracranial vessels shares many of the same risk factors as SVD, so people may have both. Thus, the identification of severe stenosis in a large vessel (e.g., internal carotid artery or middle cerebral artery) in a patient with lacunar stroke does not necessarily prove that large artery disease was the culprit. For example, in a study of 259 patients with lacunar stroke, there was no difference in the prevalence of severe contralateral or ipsilateral stenosis of the internal carotid artery or middle cerebral artery [28]; coexisting large artery disease may or may not be coincidental, as severe stenosis can cause subtle brain changes [29]. However, in another series carotid disease was less common in lacunar infarcts compared with nonlacunar infarcts [30]. Such findings have led some authors to argue that investigating for carotid disease in patients with noncortical lacunar stroke is unnecessary [30]. Since severe ipsilateral carotid stenosis or cardioembolic source of stroke have different management implications, and since patients with lacunar syndromes were included in the seminal trials of these treatments, on balance the evidence still favors noninvasive screening for these alternative causes of lacunar syndromes (Figure 18.1).

Heterogeneity in lesion localization

As discussed in further detail below, multiple lacunar syndromes have been reported. These are usually attributed to SVD involving the subcortical structures or brainstem. However, a patient who presents clinically with a typical lacunar syndrome may not always have a stroke syndrome that localizes to the subcortical region or brainstem. For example, the pure sensory syndrome – a typical lacunar syndrome – can infrequently localize to the parietal cortex without direct involvement of the thalamus [31].

To complicate matters further, multiple lacunar syndromes can also result from a lesion in the same region of the brain. For example, a lesion in the posterior limb of the internal capsule can give rise to four lacunar syndromes, namely: (1) pure motor hemiparesis; (2) sensorimotor stroke; (3) ataxic hemiparesis; and (4) dysarthria–clumsy hand syndrome [32]. This highlights the complexity of brain–behavior relationships in lacunar syndromes: one lacunar syndrome can be caused by lesions in a variety of locations (including those not associated with SVD), and lesions in a specific location can cause a variety of lacunar syndromes [33].

Acute stroke syndromes

Brief vascular anatomy of the arteries that give rise to lacunar stroke

Small arteries in the brain, which are usually perforators branching off larger blood vessels, irrigate broad neuroanatomical substrates such as subcortical nuclei, white matter, and the brainstem. The anatomy of these small blood vessels and the regions they supply are briefly reviewed below.

Branches of the middle cerebral artery

The *lateral lenticulostriate arteries* arise from the proximal portion of the middle cerebral artery (MCA) (M1 segment), prior to the entry of the MCA into the Sylvian fissure. These arteries irrigate much of the basal ganglia and internal capsule. As a result of pathologic changes that result from hypertension and other vascular risk factors, the lateral lenticulostriate arteries become particularly prone to constriction or rupture, giving rise to lacunar stroke or intracerebral hemorrhage, respectively. The lateral lenticulostriate arteries are the most common vessels involved in lacunar stroke syndromes (Figure 18.2).

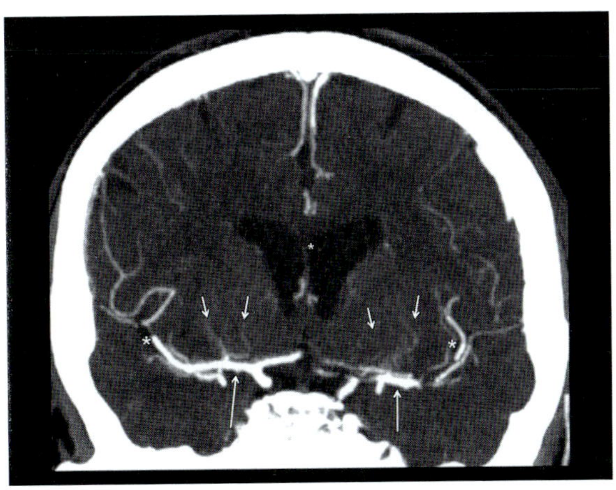

Figure 18.2 Origins of the lenticulostriate arteries. Coronal maximum intensity projection, multiplanar reformatted computed tomography (CT) angiogram illustrating the lenticulostriates arteries (white short arrows) as they arise from the proximal and mid portions of the middle cerebral artery (MCA) (long arrows) prior to entry of the MCA into the Sylvian fissure (*).

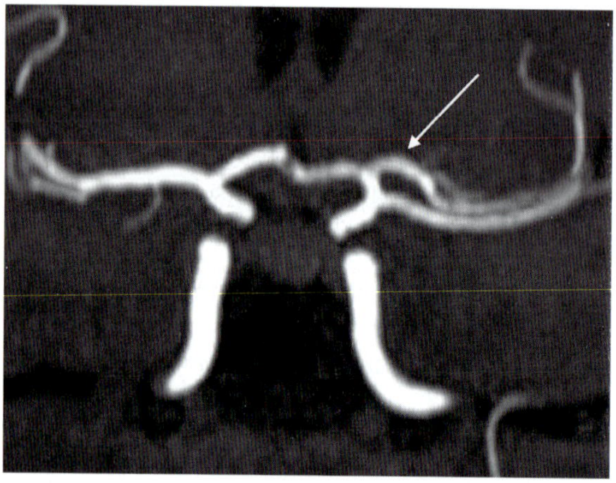

Figure 18.3 Heubner's artery. Coronal maximum intensity projection, multiplanar reformatted computed tomography (CT) angiogram illustrating a so-called "duplicated" left middle cerebral artery. Heubner's artery (also known as the recurrent artery of Heubner [arrow]) arises from the A1 segment of the anterior cerebral artery. In this case, a persistent cortical supply of Heubner's artery gives the appearance of a second (hence "duplicated") middle cerebral artery.

Branches of the internal carotid artery

The internal carotid artery (ICA) gives rise to several arterial branches including the *anterior choroidal artery*, which irrigates deep cerebral structures, such as the posterior limb of internal capsule, globus pallidus, putamen, and the thalamus (sometimes involving the lateral geniculate body).

Branches of the anterior cerebral artery

The *medial lenticulostriate arteries* and *Heubner's artery* (a.k.a. the recurrent artery of Heubner) arise from the initial portion (A1 segment) of the anterior cerebral artery (ACA). These supply the head of the caudate, anterior putamen, globus pallidus, and internal capsule (Figure 18.3).

Branches of the posterior cerebral artery

The *thalamoperforator, thalamogeniculate*, and *posterior choroidal arteries* arise from the proximal portion (P1 segment) of the posterior cerebral artery (PCA). These supply the thalamus and sometimes a portion of the posterior limb of the internal capsule.

Branches of the vertebrobasilar system

- The *posterior inferior cerebellar artery* arises from the vertebral artery at the level of the medulla and irrigates the lateral medulla and the inferior cerebellum.
- The *anterior inferior cerebellar artery* arises from the *basilar artery* at the level of the caudal pons and supplies the lateral caudal pons and part of the cerebellum.
- The *superior cerebellar artery* comes off the top of the basilar artery at the level of the rostral pons, and supplies the superior aspects of the pons and cerebellum.
- Several smaller blood vessels arise from these main arteries and irrigate various portions of the brainstem:
  - *Paramedian branches* supply midline brainstem structures.
  - *Short and long circumferential arteries* supply more lateral brainstem structures.

Stroke syndromes

Multiply localized clinical syndromes: Miller–Fisher's lacunar syndromes

More than 20 lacunar syndromes have been described in the literature [34], but five are most commonly recognized: (1) pure motor hemiparesis; (2) pure sensory stroke; (3) sensorimotor stroke; (4) dysarthria–clumsy hand syndrome; and (5) ataxic hemiparesis. The syndromes are characterized by the absence of cortical signs, such as visual field defects and cognitive deficits (e.g., hemispatial neglect, apraxia, and aphasia). Face, arm, and leg involvement is present in the first three syndromes [2].

Pure motor hemiparesis

This is the most common lacunar syndrome, and represents 33–50% of all lacunar strokes [10, 35] and approximately 10% of all strokes [35]. Patients present with contralateral weakness of the face, arm, and leg in the absence of additional clinical symptoms or signs. While this syndrome is typically associated with lacunar infarction from SVD [36], as discussed above, approximately one out of every seven patients with a pure motor stroke will have a nonlacunar mechanism such as cardioembolism, large artery atherosclerosis, or a hemorrhagic event [35]. Brain regions most typically associated with this syndrome are the posterior limb of the internal capsule (most common), ventral pons, corona radiata, medial medulla, and the cerebral peduncle [33, 35]. In-hospital mortality is low (0.5%) and about 20% of patients are symptom-free upon discharge from hospital [35].

Pure sensory stroke

Seven to ten percent of lacunar infarcts are pure sensory strokes [10, 25]. Patients present with contralateral sensory loss involving the face, arm, and leg, which can be incomplete, and is without additional clinical symptoms or signs. In a series of 99 patients with pure sensory stroke, 81% of participants (80/99) presented with a complete hemisensory syndrome, while 19% (19/99) had an incomplete hemisensory syndrome, involving only one or two of the face, arm, hand, or leg.

While pure sensory strokes are traditionally attributed to an infarction in the ventral posterior lateral nucleus of the thalamus [37], other localizations have been reported, such as the internal capsule, corona radiata, pontine tegmentum, and parietal cortex [31, 38]. This lacunar syndrome is thought to be highly predictive of a lacunar infarction, with imaging confirming the presence of a lacunar stroke in 89–100% of cases [25, 38]. The syndrome carries a good prognosis, with 0% in-hospital mortality and 41.5% absence of neurologic disability at discharge [38].

A unique thalamic pain syndrome (also known as Dejerine–Roussy syndrome) most commonly occurs in patients with right-sided thalamic lesions, particularly after involvement of the inferolateral artery. Onset occurs within one week post-stroke in 36% of patients, between one week and one month post-stroke in an additional 20%, and after one month in the majority of the remainder of patients; only 11% are noted to develop the syndrome one year after stroke onset. Patients complain of painful paraesthesias, allodynia, and hyperalgesia [39]. Few large studies have examined the management of post-stroke central pain such as that seen in the Dejerine–Roussy syndrome. Amitriptyline and lamotrigine have been recommended as first-line therapies, and mexiletine, fluvoxamine, and gabapentin as second-line drugs. In pharmacoresistant patients, repetitive transcranial magnetic stimulation and deep brain stimulation have been noted to be beneficial [40].

Sensorimotor stroke

In the SPS3 trial, 31% of lacunar strokes were sensorimotor in nature [10]; other studies have reported a lower frequency of 20% [25]. Patients present with both contralateral weakness and sensory loss involving the face, arm, and leg in the absence of additional clinical symptoms or signs. Associated lesions tend to occur in the posterior limb of the internal capsule, thalamocapsular region [41], and the lateral medulla [33]. SVD is the most commonly reported mechanism for this lacunar syndrome, with large artery disease and cardioembolism being less frequently implicated [42].

Ataxic hemiparesis

Ataxic hemiparesis syndrome accounted for 9% of lacunar strokes in the SPS3 trial [10]; other work has shown both higher (18%) [25] and lower (3–4%) [43, 44] prevalence among patients with lacunar stroke. Patients manifest with a combination of weakness and incoordination (out of proportion to the weakness) on the same side of the body. This syndrome localizes to the internal capsule, pons, corona radiata, and frontal–subcortical region, as well as to cortical regions such as the insula, or precentral gyrus with or without involvement of the post-central gyrus [33, 43–45]; thalamic involvement has also been rarely reported [46]. The clinical features of ataxic hemiparesis with different lesion locations is almost identical [47]. In a series of 29 patients, hemiparesis with predominantly leg weakness was seen in 28% (eight patients) and predominantly arm weakness in 14% (four patients) [45]. Mechanistically, ataxic hemiparesis has been reported to be caused by SVD in 47–87%, artery to artery embolism in 7–9%, and cardioembolism in 4–11% [44, 48]. The prognosis is generally good, with 39% of patients discharged without neurologic disability [44].

It has been hypothesized that this syndrome arises from disruption of the corticopontocerebellar pathway at the level of the frontal cortex or subcortical structures [45]. Crossed cerebellar diaschisis, i.e., deafferentation of the affected cerebellar hemisphere because of contralateral interruption of corticopontocerebellar fibers, has also been proposed as another mechanism for this lacunar stroke subtype [49].

Dysarthria–clumsy hand syndrome

Dysarthria–clumsy hand syndrome is the least common of the lacunar syndromes. In series of patients with lacunar stroke, only 2–6% manifest with the dysarthria–clumsy hand syndrome [10, 43, 50]. Patients present with simultaneous dysarthria and poor dexterity of the hand contralateral to the brain lesion. SVD is the underlying mechanism in 94% of patients, with artery to artery embolism and cardioembolism being much less common [50]. Implicated brain regions include the posterior limb of the internal capsule, pons, corona radiata, caudate nucleus, and thalamus [33, 50]. Like the other lacunar syndromes, prognosis is generally good, with approximately 46% of patients leaving the hospital free of neurologic disability [50].

Uniquely localized clinical syndromes: brainstem syndromes

Compared to lacunar syndromes typically associated with infarcts in subcortical regions of the brain, brainstem stroke syndromes are far less common. As eponyms for vascular syndromes have varied across authors, we will discuss both the eponymous name and possible lesion localizations.

Midbrain syndromes

In patients with symptomatic vertebrobasilar ischemic lesions, midbrain involvement occurs in about 9% of patients [51]; isolated midbrain involvement is quite rare [52]. In a series of 39 patients with midbrain stroke, cardioembolism (28%) was the most common mechanism, with large artery thrombosis (23%), large artery to artery embolism (18%), and SVD (13%) being less common mechanisms [51].

Medial midbrain syndrome (Weber's syndrome) Weber's syndrome occurs as a result of a midbrain lesion involving the ipsilateral third nerve nucleus and cerebral peduncle. The syndrome is characterized by ipsilateral oculomotor palsy (which can be pupil-sparing [53]) with contralateral hemiparesis. Only a few reports are available in the present literature. Although originally described in the context of midbrain hemorrhage [54], the most common etiology is cerebrovascular occlusion; less commonly reported are intracranial aneurysms, demyelination, neoplastic lesions [55], and infections [56].

Midbrain tegmentum syndrome (Claude's syndrome) This syndrome was first described by the French neurologist Henri Claude. Patients typically manifest with a partial ipsilateral oculomotor palsy (nuclear lesion of the third nerve) and contralateral ataxia; in addition, patients can also occasionally present with a fourth nerve palsy [57]. Several studies have shown that Claude syndrome is localized to a lesion of the ventromedial midbrain [57, 58]; whether the red nucleus needs to be specifically involved remains controversial [59, 60]. In addition to SVD, large artery stenosis of the PCA [61] and cardioembolism [62] have been reported as stroke mechanisms. The few cases in the literature suggest that the prognosis for this syndrome is good; however, patients may be left with persisting neurologic deficits such as the presenting ataxia and oculomotor difficulties [57]. Aside from stroke, Claude syndrome has also been reported in association with neurocysticercosis [63].

Midbrain tegmentum syndrome (Benedikt's syndrome) Benedikt's syndrome is a rare syndrome characterized by a unilateral third nerve palsy, as well as hemiparesis and tremor in the contralateral limbs [64]. This syndrome has been attributed to lesions in the ipsilateral red nucleus, substantia nigra, oculomotor fibers, and the cerebral peduncle [65]. The syndrome has been reported in the context of stroke, stereotactic surgery [64], trauma [66], neoplastic lesions [67], and vascular malformations [68].

Pontine syndromes

Pontine infarcts account for 25% of lacunar strokes [69]. In a series of patients with isolated pontine infarcts, the etiology was basilar artery branch disease in 59 patients (39%); SVD in 31 (21%); large-artery disease of the vertebrobasilar arteries in 27 patients (18%); cardioembolism in 12 (8%); and in 16 patients (11%) no cause for stroke was found [70]. Pure motor hemiparesis is the most common pontine syndrome, followed by sensorimotor stroke and ataxic hemiparesis. Eye movement abnormalities and neuropsychological deficits are also commonly seen. Short-term functional prognosis is usually good with lacunar presentations [69]. Four classical pontine syndromes are outlined below; very few reports in the literature describe these syndromes.

Lateral pontine syndrome (Marie–Foix syndrome) This syndrome consists of ataxia in the ipsilateral arm and leg, contralateral weakness in the upper and lower extremities, and contralateral hemisensory loss (pain and temperature). The long circumferential branches of the basilar artery or the anterior inferior cerebellar artery are involved.

Inferior medial pontine syndrome (Foville's syndrome) Patients manifest with contralateral weakness in the upper and lower extremities, ipsilateral facial weakness, and an ipsilateral lateral gaze deficit. The short circumferential arteries or paramedian branches of the basilar artery are implicated.

Ventral pontine syndrome (Raymond's syndrome) Patients manifest with contralateral weakness in the upper and lower extremities and an ipsilateral lateral gaze deficit; contralateral facial weakness has rarely been reported [71, 72]. The paramedian branches of the basilar artery are implicated. The most common etiology is ischemic or hemorrhagic stroke [73].

Ventral pontine syndrome (Millard–Gubler syndrome) Patients manifest with contralateral weakness in the upper and lower extremities, ipsilateral lower motor neuron facial weakness, and an ipsilateral lateral gaze deficit. The short circumferential arteries or paramedian branches of the basilar artery are implicated. Millard–Gubler syndrome has been reported in the context of stroke [74], traumatic subarachnoid hematoma [75], vascular malformation [76, 77], and neurocysticercosis [78].

Medullary syndromes

SVD accounts for about 20% of all acute medullary infarctions; large artery disease (LAD) and dissection are other common mechanisms for both the lateral and medial medullary syndromes [79].

Lateral medullary syndrome (Wallenberg's syndrome) This syndrome accounts for about 3% of all ischemic strokes [80]. LAD is implicated in 42–50% of cases, SVD in 13–17%, dissection in 15–31%, cardioembolism in 5–9%, and the remainder of cases are attributed to undetermined etiologies [79–81]. The vertebral artery is involved in 67% of patients, with the posterior inferior cerebellar artery the culprit in 10% of cases [81].

Patients present with ataxia, nystagmus, facial sensory disturbance, Horner's syndrome, and paralysis of the soft palate and pharynx on the side ipsilateral to the lesion, as well as reduced pain and temperature sensation in the upper and lower extremities contralateral to the infarct. Sneezing and hiccups have also been reported at the onset of lateral medullary syndrome [82]. All these clinical symptoms are unlikely to manifest simultaneously, with most patients presenting with several but not all symptoms [80]. Ataxia, sensory symptoms, and Horner's syndrome are the most common manifestations [81, 83].

At times, differentiating the vestibular symptoms of the lateral medullary syndrome from acute peripheral vestibulopathy on clinical grounds alone can pose a challenge. A negative horizontal head impulse test (i.e., normal vestibulo-ocular reflex) strongly suggests a central lesion, while a positive test is in keeping with a peripheral vestibulopathy; however, in one series, 9% of patients presenting with stroke also had a positive horizontal head impulse test [84]. Adding additional oculomotor tests can increase the yield of the clinical evaluation; for example, the presence of a negative horizontal head impulse test, direction-changing nystagmus in eccentric gaze, or skew deviation can be 100% sensitive and 96% specific for stroke [85]. These three oculomotor tests (together called the "HINTS" assessment, for Head Impulse, Nystagmus, and Test of Skew) have been reported to be more sensitive for stroke than early magnetic resonance imaging (MRI) [85].

Lesion location may predict the most prominent clinical features, with more rostral lesions associated with severe dysphagia, dysarthria, and facial paralysis [81], and caudal lesions correlating with marked gait ataxia [86]. Patients with large rostral lesions tend to have severe dysphagia, aspiration pneumonia, and prolonged admission [81]. Respiratory and cardiovascular events are the major threats to life in the acute phase; however, the risk of recurrent stroke in the long term is thought to be low [87]. Depending on the series, in-hospital mortality ranges from 0.8 to 11.6% (Figure 18.4) [81].

Medial medullary syndrome (Dejerine's syndrome) This syndrome is thought to account for about 1% of all ischemic strokes [80]. LAD causes about 55–62% of cases, SVD is implicated in 28–32% of patients, dissection in 9–13%, and the remainder have undetermined etiologies [79, 80, 88]. Diabetes is frequently associated with medial medullary syndrome [89].

Patients manifest with tongue weakness and atrophy ipsilateral to the side of the stroke; hemiplegia and reduced vibration and joint position sensation occur in the upper and lower extremities contralateral to the lesion. As in the lateral medullary syndrome, all these symptoms rarely occur simultaneously [80]. Motor dysfunction is the most common manifestation and is associated with more ventral lesions, while sensory dysfunction is correlated with lesions in the middle portion of the medial medulla [88]. Occasionally hemiparesis can be the first and even remain the sole manifestation of medial medullary syndrome, in which case clinical differentiation from

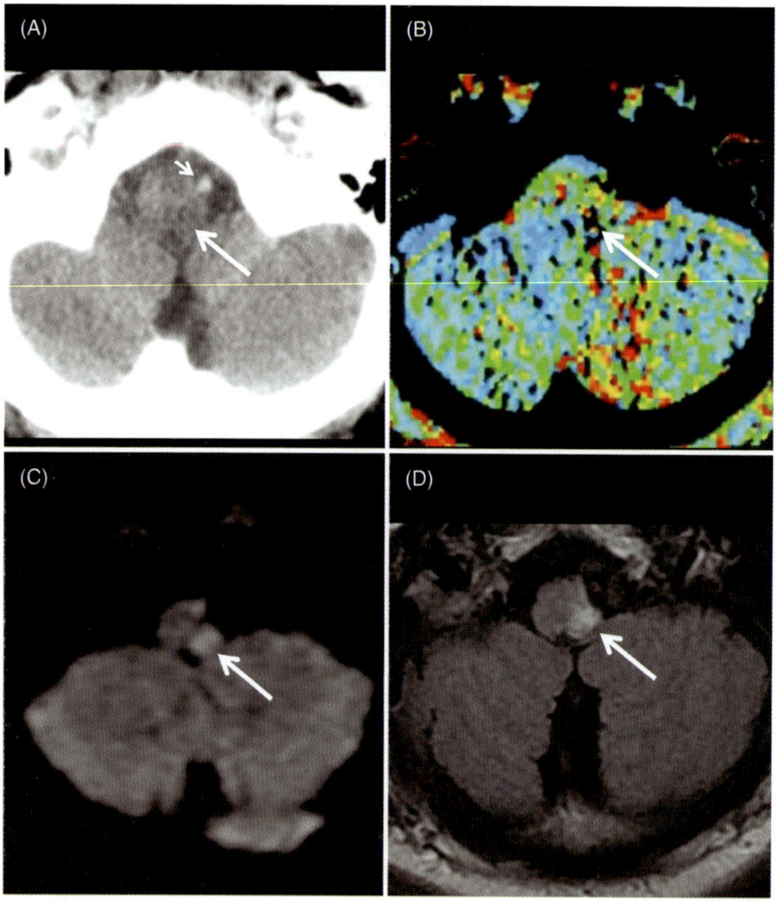

Figure 18.4 Left lateral medullary syndrome. Noncontrast computed tomography (CT) scan of the brain illustrating a hyperdense left vertebral artery (small arrow) and hypodensity of the left lateral medulla and inferior cerebellar peduncle (longer arrow) (A). Mean transit time CT perfusion demonstrates prolongation in the territory of the posterior inferior cerebellar artery including both the lateral medulla (arrow) and the medial cerebellum (B). Left lateral medulla appears hyperintense on both the magnetic resonance diffusion-weighted imaging (MR DWI) (C), and fluid-attenuated inversion recovery (FLAIR) sequences consistent with infarct (D). The cerebellar distribution of the posterior inferior cerebellar artery, although initially ischemic (see increased mean transit time in B), did not progress to infarction.

a subcortical or pontine lacunar infarction giving rise to a pure motor syndrome can be challenging [90].

Patients with medial medullary infarcts have higher baseline National Institutes of Health Stroke Scale (NIHSS) scores compared to those with involvement of the lateral medulla [79]. In the largest series to date of 86 patients with medial medullary syndrome, 13% (11/86 patients) died during the mean 71-month follow-up period; older age and severe motor dysfunction at admission were factors predictive of poor prognosis. Central post-stroke pain occurred in 24% (21/86 patients) and was also associated with a poor clinical outcome [88]. However, earlier series demonstrated more favorable outcomes [90, 91].

Uniquely localized clinical syndromes: thalamic syndromes

Anatomically, the thalamus is one of the most complicated structures in the brain and boasts an intricate array of nuclei and connections [92–94]. This explains the wide range of behavioral manifestations seen after thalamic stroke; virtually all "cortical" syndromes may be mimicked by thalamic infarction, with aphasia, agnosia, amnesia, and neglect commonly reported. Vascular syndromes arising after thalamic stroke have been reported in detail elsewhere [95, 96]. Below, we briefly describe the thalamic syndromes that arise after infarction of the four main vascular territories of the thalamus.

Anterior territory infarction

The anterior territory (also known as the tuberothalamic or polar territory) is supplied by the tuberothalamic or polar artery, which usually originates from the posterior communicating artery [96]. Infarcts in the anterior thalamic territory account for about 12% of all thalamic infarctions [97]. Acutely, patients display a fluctuating level of consciousness and appear withdrawn. Personality changes include apathy, abulia, lack of insight, and disorientation to time

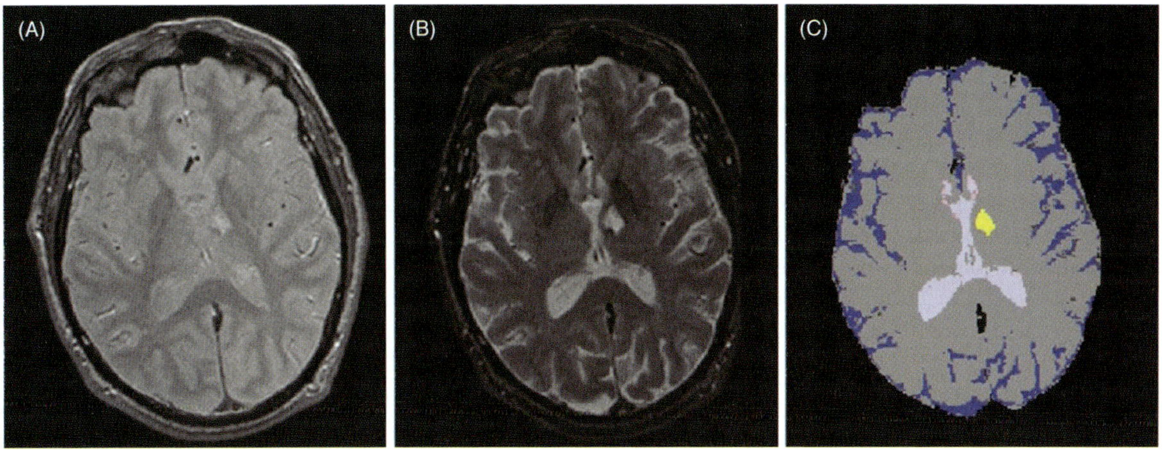

Figure 18.5 Strategic lacunar infarcts can cause sudden changes in cognitive status. Images from a patient with vascular dementia after a left-sided anterior-medial thalamic infarct. (A) Proton density-weighted and (B) T2-weighted images of a single slice are shown, along with (C) the corresponding slice from the segmented image. Adapted from Swartz and Black [98].

and place [95]. Patients also experience impairment of recent memory and anterograde amnesia. Visuospatial impairment, such as hemispatial neglect and visual memory deficits, may occur after right-sided lesions. Verbal impairment characterized by a reduction in speech output and fluency, impaired comprehension, paraphasias, hypophonic speech, and occasional neologisms are associated with left-sided lesions. Anterior-medial thalamic lesions greater than 55 mm [3] are associated with a stepwise decline in cognitive function [98] There may also be hemispheric specialization with thalamic lesions. Left thalamic lesions are more likely to result in language impairment and a clinical diagnosis of vascular dementia, while right hemisphere thalamic lesions are associated with cognitive impairment not meeting the criteria for dementia (Figure 18.5) [98].

A characteristic finding after anterior territory infarction of the thalamus is "palipsychism," where patients exhibit superimposition of temporally unrelated information, yielding parallel expression of mental activities; for example, a patient may correctly solve a mathematical question and talk about his garden simultaneously. Palipsychism is frequently associated with perseverations in thought and speech output [95, 96].

Paramedian territory infarction

The paramedian territory is supplied by the thalamoperforating arteries, which originate from the P1 segment of the PCA [96]. Infarcts in the paramedian thalamic territory account for about 35% of all thalamic infarctions [97]. The characteristic features of acute paramedian infarction include decreased level of consciousness, vertical gaze paresis, and cognitive impairment. Behavioral changes, such as disinhibition with apathy and amnesia, become apparent when the decreased level of consciousness resolves [96].

After paramedian infarction, thalamofrontal disconnection can give rise to disinhibition syndromes such as cyclical psychosis and manic delirium. In addition, frontal syndromes are also seen, such as utilization behavior, where patients impulsively manipulate objects that are within their reach or inappropriately respond to cues in their environment [96].

In addition, after bilateral paramedian infarctions, patients may become severely apathetic and lose their motor and affective drives; full recovery after bilateral paramedian infarction is rare [96]. Some authors also report transient global amnesia after left paramedian infarction [99].

Inferolateral territory infarction

The inferolateral territory (also known as the thalamogeniculate territory) is supplied by the thalamogeniculate arteries, which arise from the P2 segment of the PCA [96]. Infarcts in the inferolateral thalamic territory account for about 45% of all thalamic infarctions [97]. A common clinical manifestation is ataxia and reduced sensitivity to sensory stimuli [100]. In addition, executive function can be impaired and cause difficulties with planning and initiation, and regulation of goal-directed behavior; these deficits can lead to significant long-term disability [96].

As mentioned above, patients with inferolateral artery infarction also present with the thalamic pain syndrome of Dejerine–Roussy, particularly after right-sided lesions [39]. This syndrome is characterized by variable sensory loss, impaired extremity movement, and sometimes post-lesional pain, which can emerge weeks to months following the infarct. Ataxia with hemiparesis can also coexist [95].

Posterior territory infarction

The posterior territory is supplied by the medial and lateral branches of the posterior choroidal artery, which originates from the P2 segment of the PCA; the pulvinar is the main thalamic nucleus in this territory [96]. Infarcts in the posterior thalamic territory account for about 8% of all thalamic infarctions [97]. The most common symptoms are contralateral hemibody sensory loss and homonymous horizontal sectoranopsia (from involvement of the lateral geniculate body) [95, 96]. Hemispatial neglect may be seen in association with right pulvinar lesions [101]. In addition, other neuropsychological dysfunction may also be observed, such as transcortical aphasia and memory disturbances [102]. Finally, some authors report a delayed complex hyperkinetic motor syndrome, including ataxia, rubral tremor, dystonia, myoclonus, and chorea after infarcts restricted to the pulvinar [103].

Capsular warning syndrome

Capsular warning syndrome is characterized by multiple stereotyped motor, sensory or sensorimotor transitory ischemic attacks (TIAs) involving the face, arm, and/or leg [104]. This syndrome is uncommon, and represents only 1.5–4.5% of all TIAs [104, 105]. The prognosis for capsular warning syndrome is generally poor, with a 60% seven-day risk of stroke. Indeed, capsular warning syndrome may be the main contributor to the increased stroke risk seen early after recurrent TIAs, with other mechanisms such as atrial fibrillation and large artery disease conferring comparatively lower early stroke risk [105].

The underlying mechanism for capsular warning is thought to be hemodynamic compromise or thrombosis within a small, single penetrating artery or stenosis of the proximal portion of the MCA, which ultimately results in fluctuating arterial blood flow to the internal capsule [105–107]. Case reports describe other mechanisms, such as spontaneous MCA dissection [108], microscopic polyangiitis [109], and even dural sinus thrombosis [110] as being associated with a clinical picture consistent with the capsular warning syndrome.

Although capsular warning syndrome is traditionally associated with ischemia involving the internal capsule, an identical clinical scenario can also result from involvement of the anterior or paramedian pons, with small vessel perforators branching off the basilar artery being implicated; this has been coined the "pontine warning syndrome" [111–113], and is thought to primarily involve the fibers of the corticospinal tract as they travel through the brainstem. Consistent with this, imaging studies of patients presenting clinically with capsular warning symptoms demonstrate diffusion-weighted MRI abnormalities involving the basal ganglia or pons, close to the central motor pathways [114].

Treatment of acute stroke syndromes caused by SVD

Acute stroke care

Thrombolytic therapy

Acute thrombus in a small penetrating artery is a recognized mechanism for lacunar infarction, which implies that thrombolytic therapy may be potentially beneficial in some cases of acute lacunar stroke [115]. A management challenge, however, is that acute arterial occlusion of a small blood vessel is not readily visualized using current imaging techniques; this has dissuaded some from offering acute thrombolysis in this clinical setting. However, perfusion imaging may assist in this regard. For example, in a study of perfusion and diffusion MRI, a patient with lacunar stroke was initially shown to have a perfusion deficit and a matching diffusion abnormality; following thrombolytic therapy, a reversal of the perfusion and diffusion deficits, as well as clinical recovery, were observed [116].

Accumulating evidence suggests that thrombolytic therapy is effective in lacunar stroke. In the National Institute of Neurological Disorders and Stroke (NINDS) study, those with lacunar stroke who were randomized to receive intravenous tissue plasminogen activator (tPA) had more favorable outcomes than those who received placebo (mRS ≤1 in 63 vs. 40%) [117]. In a review of 11 503 ischemic stroke patients from the Registry of the Canadian Stroke Network, patients with lacunar strokes, partial anterior circulation syndromes, and total anterior circulation syndromes all benefitted equally from thrombolysis [118]. Furthermore, in a retrospective study of 957 patients with ischemic stroke receiving thrombolysis, those with SVD had a better clinical outcome (mRS ≤2 at three months) than patients with strokes caused by other etiologies [119]. Thrombolytic therapy is also associated with significantly lower hemorrhagic complications after acute cerebral ischemia attributable to a single penetrator artery compared to ischemia caused by large artery disease; in one series, no patients with single penetrator artery infarcts experienced any hemorrhagic transformation, whereas radiologic hemorrhagic transformation occurred in 29.3% of large artery infarcts ($P = 0.03$) [120].

Limited evidence also supports a role for thrombolytic therapy in capsular warning syndrome. For example, in four patients who received intravenous thrombolytic therapy for capsular warning syndrome, three patients made a complete recovery without subsequent neurologic episodes; these patients had a NIHSS score of zero at the time of discharge [121]. A single case report also demonstrates a full neurologic recovery after administration of intravenous thrombolysis in a patient with recurrent lacunar stroke [122]. Of note, stroke centers that had unfavorable outcomes after thrombolyzing patients with capsular warning may have not published their results, so interpretation of the small studies reported here may be limited by a publication bias. Nonetheless, since a postulated mechanism for the clinical fluctuations seen in capsular warning syndrome is unstable thrombus within a small branching artery of the proximal portion of the MCA, thrombolysis in this clinical situation may be biologically justified.

Blood pressure management

Systolic blood pressure levels below 140 mmHg after acute stroke occurs may be associated with higher rates of death and disability [123], but the optimal blood pressure target for hyperacute stroke has not been determined. In lacunar stroke, particularly in the setting of fluctuating neurologic symptoms seen in capsular warning syndrome, a temporal relationship has been observed between decreases in blood pressure and clinical worsening [124]. It has been proposed that blood pressure elevation in the acute stroke setting may be beneficial by increasing perfusion to the peri-infarct penumbra. To investigate this possibility, Lim et al. [125] studied 82 patients with lacunar infarction who experienced motor progression; hypertension was induced using phenylephrine in 52 patients. Compared to patients in the conventional treatment group, patients receiving phenylephrine had lower NIHSS motor scores and shorter hospitalizations; however, these results were not significantly different compared to the baseline clinical findings.

At this time, good theoretical arguments exist for inducing blood pressure elevation in acute ischemic stroke to increase blood flow to the ischemic penumbra. Unfortunately, few trials are available to support routine clinical use of this practice. Future studies are needed to establish the safety and potential benefits of pressor therapy in various acute stroke subtypes [123].

In the absence of clinical trial evidence, most experts do not induce hypertension but favor permissive hypertension. Canadian Best Practice Recommendations recommend treatment of high blood pressure (>185/110 mmHg) in ischemic stroke patients eligible for thrombolytic therapy in order to reduce the risk of secondary intracranial hemorrhage. In ischemic stroke patients not eligible for thrombolytic therapy, treatment of hypertension in the setting of acute ischemic stroke is not routinely recommended; extreme blood pressure elevations (e.g., systolic >220 or diastolic >120 mmHg) may be treated to reduce the blood pressure by about 15%, and not more than 25%, over the first 24 hours with gradual reduction thereafter [126].

Antiplatelet therapy

In large randomized controlled trials, the use of aspirin in acute stroke has been shown to be effective in reducing future vascular events and mortality. In the International Stroke Trial (IST), which randomized 19 435 patients in a 2 × 2 factorial design to heparin, aspirin, neither medication, or both medications, aspirin-allocated patients had significantly fewer recurrent ischemic strokes within 14 days (2.8 vs. 3.9%) with no significant excess of hemorrhagic strokes (0.9 vs. 0.8%); in addition, after adjustment for baseline prognosis, the use of aspirin was associated with lower rates of death or dependency at six months. In the IST study, 24% of patients presented with lacunar stroke [127]. In the Chinese Acute Stroke Trial (CAST), in which 21 106 patients were randomized to aspirin versus placebo within 48 hours of acute stroke, aspirin-allocated patients experienced a 14% reduction in total mortality at four weeks (3.3 vs. 3.9%; $P = 0.04$). In this study, 30% of patients presented with lacunar stroke [128]. Taken together, the IST and CAST trials demonstrated that aspirin therapy in acute ischemic stroke led to a reduction of approximately nine nonfatal strokes or deaths for every 1000 patients treated early [129].

Only preliminary evidence is available concerning the use of antiplatelet agents other than aspirin immediately after acute ischemic stroke. In the FASTER trial, 392 patients were randomized within 24 hours of symptom onset to aspirin plus clopidogrel (300 mg loading dose, then 75 mg daily) or aspirin alone. The trial ended prematurely due to failure to recruit patients at the prespecified minimum enrolment rate. At 90 days, there was no significant difference between treatment groups (aspirin plus clopidogrel vs. aspirin alone) for the primary outcome measure of combined ischemic and hemorrhagic stroke (7.1 vs. 10.8%; $P = 0.19$). Twenty-nine percent of patients in the FASTER trial had presented with lacunar stroke [130]. In the EARLY trial, 539 patients were randomly assigned within 24 hours of symptom onset to treatment with either the combination of aspirin–extended-release dipyridamole (aspirin 25 mg and extended-release dipyridamole 200 mg twice daily) or aspirin (100 mg daily) alone. After seven days, all patients received open-label aspirin and extended-release dipyridamole. At 90 days, there was no significant difference between the aspirin and extended-release dipyridamole group and the aspirin group in the primary endpoint of good neurologic outcome, defined as an mRS score of 0–1 assessed by telephone (56 vs. 52%; $P = 0.45$) [131]. The EARLY trial did not report the number of patients who had presented with lacunar stroke [131]. Evidence from future larger randomized controlled trials is required to ascertain whether other antiplatelet regimens are equivalent or superior to aspirin for the early treatment of acute ischemic stroke, including lacunar stroke.

As discussed above with regards to capsular warning syndrome, unstable thrombus in small penetrating arteries may be implicated in the pathogenesis of this syndrome; antiplatelet therapy may stabilize unstable thrombus, as well as mitigate inflammation and excitotoxicity at the site of ischemia during the acute phase [115]. Combination therapy with loading doses of clopidogrel with aspirin has been demonstrated in small case series to provide an excellent clinical outcome [132, 133]. In addition, two glycoprotein IIb/IIIa inhibitors, tirofiban and eptifibatide, have shown promising results in improving outcomes in patients with progressive lacunar or subcortical stroke [134, 135].

Anticoagulation

There is no evidence at this time to support the role of anticoagulation in acute lacunar stroke. The IST was the largest trial to compare heparin to antiplatelet therapy in the acute stroke setting. In this study, treatment with heparin did not confer any clinical advantage at six months; subgroup analyses were not reported, however nearly 25% of the patients had manifested with a lacunar stroke [127]. Smaller studies that specifically examined the efficacy of heparin in lacunar stroke have also failed to find a beneficial effect [136, 137].

Intra-arterial stenting

Small arteries are not readily amendable to stenting with presently available devices, and it is unlikely that trials in the near future will examine the role of stenting small subcortical or brainstem arteries. However, a few trials have examined the role of stenting large arteries in patients with recent cerebrovascular events attributable to severe intracranial stenosis – a recognized mechanism for lacunar stroke. The largest of these studies was the Stenting and Aggressive Medical Management for Preventing Recurrent Stroke in Intracranial Stenosis (SAMMPRIS) trial. This trial demonstrated that aggressive medical management was superior to stenting with the Wingspan stent system, a result likely seen because both the post-stenting risk of stroke was high (14.7%) and the risk of stroke with aggressive medical therapy alone was lower than expected (5.3%) [138]. While the study did not specifically examine lacunar stroke or subcortical/brainstem TIA, it is likely that many patients had presented with lacunar syndromes given the fact that nearly 80% of the patients presented with a significant stenosis in either the middle cerebral, vertebral, or basilar artery, which are arteries known to directly irrigate small blood vessels in the subcortex and brainstem. On the basis of the SAMMPRIS trial, lacunar strokes thought to originate from significant

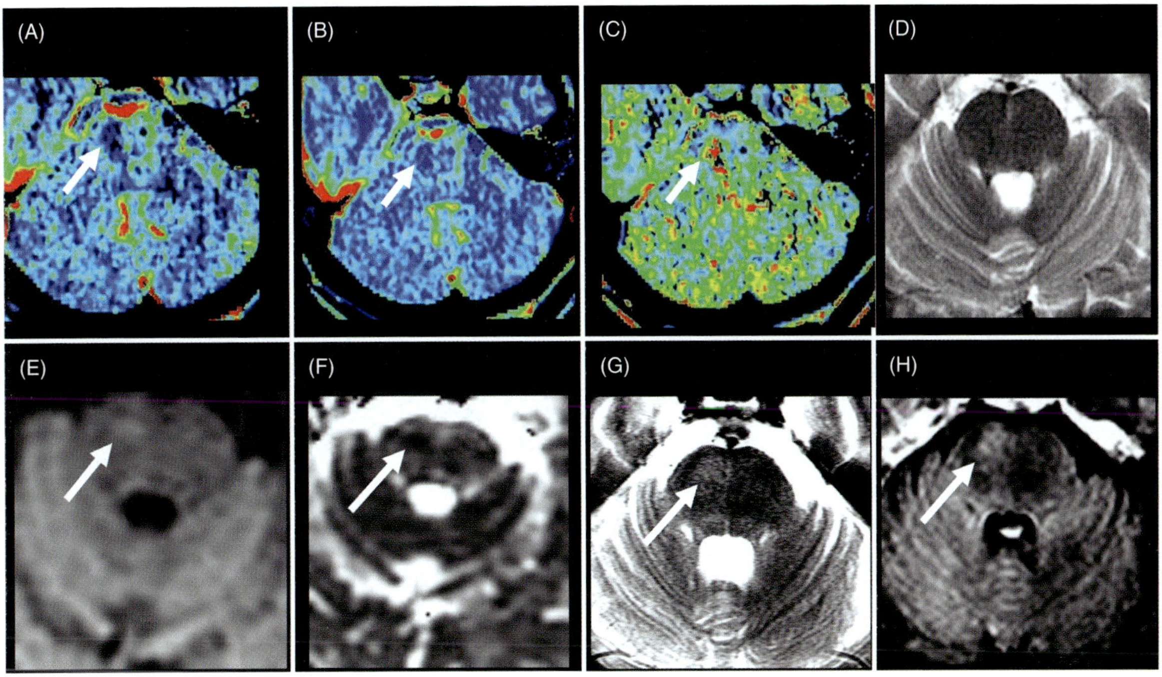

Figure 18.6 Use of computed tomography (CT) perfusion in the acute detection of lacunar infarctions (arrows) of the brainstem. Acute noncontrast CT and CT angiogram were unremarkable (not shown). CT perfusion sequences (A, blood flow; B, blood volume; C, mean transit time) demonstrated a matched perfusion deficit in the right paramedian pons consistent with a perforator territory infarct. Initial magnetic resonance imaging (MRI) T2 sequence was unrevealing (D); however, the diffusion-weighted (E) and apparent diffusion–coefficient sequences (F) confirm subtle changes consistent with acute infarct. An MRI conducted four days later confirmed infarction with interval development of signal change on both the T2 (G) and fluid-attenuated inversion recovery (FLAIR) (H) sequences.

intracranial stenosis should be managed with aggressive, multimodal medical therapies, including dual antiplatelets, statins, and antihypertensives to time-defined targets, smoking cessation, and lifestyle counseling.

Stroke unit care

A stroke unit is defined as "A multidisciplinary team consisting of physicians, nurses, occupational therapists, speech language pathologists, physiotherapists, and social workers provided at any geographical area in a hospital where stroke patients are admitted, and where care is provided" [139]. Multiple studies have demonstrated that all stroke subtypes benefit from admission to a stroke unit. For example, reductions in 30-day mortality are seen with stroke unit admissions: for lacunar stroke, to prevent one patient death at 30 days, there is a number needed to treat of nine [140]. Canadian Best Practice Guidelines recommend that all acute stroke patients, including those with SVD, be treated on an interprofessional stroke unit [126].

Acute imaging in lacunar stroke

Diffusion-weighted MRI

Diffusion-weighted MRI plays an important role in the diagnosis of acute stroke, and is more sensitive than computed tomography (CT) [141] or conventional MRI in this setting [142]. As discussed above, lacunar syndromes are not always attributable to SVD, as some patients are found to have large artery disease or cardioembolism as the underlying mechanism for their lacunar syndrome. Diffusion-weighted MRI improves the accuracy of the subtype diagnosis of stroke; inaccuracy has to be expected in about one third of cases if a diagnosis of lacunar syndrome is based on clinical and CT findings alone [143]. Although lacunar syndromes are typically attributed to subcortical lesions less than 15 mm in size on diffusion-weighted MRI, a larger size criteria may more accurately capture these events [144].

Multimodal CT

Conventional noncontrast CT (NCCT) is insensitive to cerebral infarction in the first three hours. CT perfusion (CTP) significantly improves sensitivity

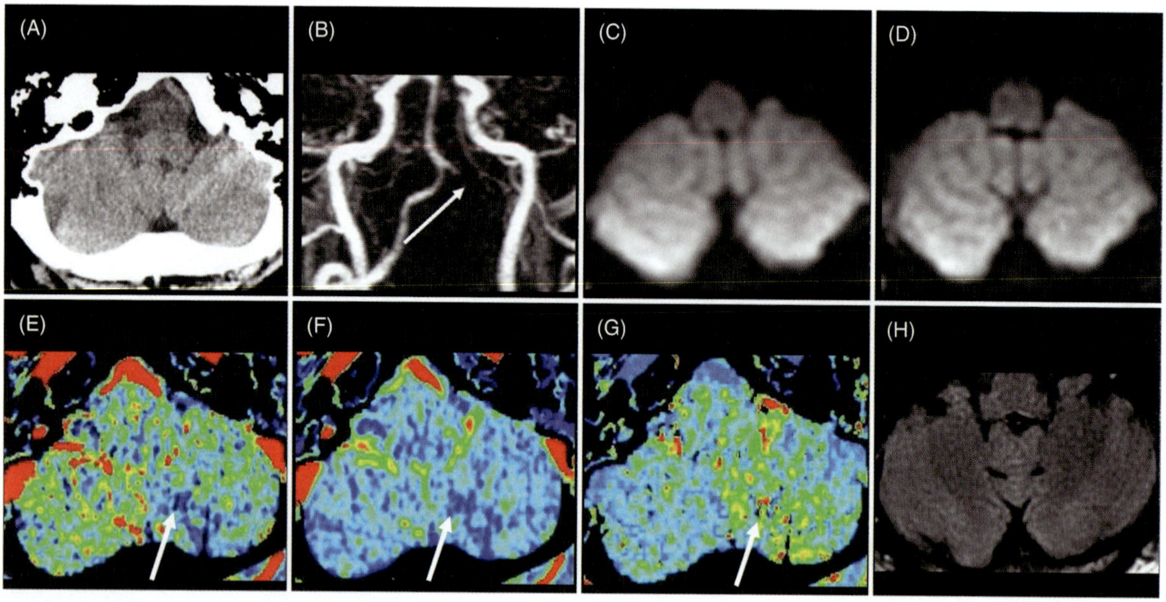

Figure 18.7 Computed tomography (CT) perfusion in the acute detection of small vessel disease in the absence of any magentic resonance imaging (MRI) abnormality. A 51-year-old man presented with an acute onset of left hemisensory loss, dysmetria, and difficulties with gait. Non-contrast CT was unremarkable (A). CT angiography demonstrated a left vertebral artery occlusion (arrow) (B). Magnetic resonance diffusion-weighted imaging (MR DWI) performed minutes after the CT study (C), and approximately 24 hours later (D) were both negative for acute stroke. No imaging support for an underlying cerebrovascular lesion was present until CT perfusion was performed. CT perfusion demonstrated low-level ischemia in the territory of the left posterior inferior cerebellar artery (arrows) (E, blood flow; F, blood volume; G, mean transit time). The patient's symptoms persisted despite absence of infarction on MRI brain T2 fluid-attenuated inversion recovery (FLAIR) sequence eight days later (H).

and accuracy in the detection of hyperacute stroke compared to NCCT (Figure 18.6); for example, CTP has been shown to be more frequently diagnostic than NCCT (80 vs. 50%, $P<0.001$) [145]. In addition, CTP is not associated with any clinically significant contrast nephropathy when patients with low estimated glomerular filtration rate (eGFR <50 ml/min) or diabetes with unknown eGFR are excluded; the median time for processing and interpreting a non-contrast CT, CT perfusion, from aortic arch to vertex (NCCT/CTP/arch-vertex) CT angiogram can be as low as 12 minutes [145]. In some cases, CTP can miss lacunar type infarcts (≤15 mm in size) when diffusion-weighted MRI is also used to confirm acute infarction [146]; in other situations, CT perfusion may demonstrate an ischemic insult even in the absence of findings on MRI (Figure 18.7).

References

1. Pantoni L. Cerebral small vessel disease: from pathogenesis and clinical characteristics to therapeutic challenges. *Lancet Neurol* 2010;9:689–701.
2. Norrving B. Long-term prognosis after lacunar infarction. *Lancet Neurol* 2003;2:238–245.
3. Potter GM, Marlborough FJ, Wardlaw JM. Wide variation in definition, detection, and description of lacunar lesions on imaging. *Stroke* 2011;42:359–366.
4. Potter GM, Doubal FN, Jackson CA, et al. Counting cavitating lacunes underestimates the burden of lacunar infarction. *Stroke* 2010;41:267–272.
5. Moreau F, Patel S, Lauzon ML, et al. Cavitation after acute symptomatic lacunar stroke depends on time, location, and MRI sequence. *Stroke* 2012;43:1837–1842.
6. Kolominsky-Rabas PL, Weber M, Gefeller O, et al. Epidemiology of ischemic stroke subtypes according to TOAST criteria: incidence, recurrence, and long-term survival in ischemic stroke subtypes: a population-based study. *Stroke* 2001;32:2735–2740.
7. Adams HP, Jr., Bendixen BH, Kappelle LJ, et al. Classification of subtype of acute ischemic stroke. Definitions for use in a multicenter clinical trial. TOAST. Trial of Org 10172 in Acute Stroke Treatment. *Stroke* 1993;24:35–41.
8. Benavente OR, White CL, Pearce L, et al. The Secondary Prevention of Small Subcortical Strokes

(SPS3) study. *Int J Stroke* 2011;6:164–175.

9. Fang XH, Wang WH, Zhang XQ, et al. Incidence and survival of symptomatic lacunar infarction in a Beijing population: a six-year prospective study. *Eur J Neurol* 2012;19:1114–1120.

10. White CL, Szychowski JM, Roldan A, et al. Clinical features and racial/ethnic differences among the 3020 participants in the Secondary Prevention of Small Subcortical Strokes (SPS3) trial. *J Stroke Cerebrovasc Dis* 2012.

11. You R, McNeil JJ, O'Malley HM, Davis SM, Donnan GA. Risk factors for lacunar infarction syndromes. *Neurology* 1995;45:1483–1487.

12. Tanizaki Y, Kiyohara Y, Kato I, et al. Incidence and risk factors for subtypes of cerebral infarction in a general population: the Hisayama study. *Stroke* 2000;31:2616–2622.

13. Ohira T, Shahar E, Chambless LE, et al. Risk factors for ischemic stroke subtypes: the atherosclerosis risk in communities study. *Stroke* 2006;37:2493–2498.

14. Shah IM, Ghosh SK, Collier A. Stroke presentation in type 2 diabetes and the metabolic syndrome. *Diabetes Res Clin Pract* 2008;79:e1–4.

15. Sacco RL, Boden-Albala B, Abel G, et al. Race–ethnic disparities in the impact of stroke risk factors: the Northern Manhattan Stroke Study. *Stroke* 2001;32:1725–1731.

16. Bravata DM, Wells CK, Gulanski B, et al. Racial disparities in stroke risk factors: the impact of socioeconomic status. *Stroke* 2005;36:1507–1511.

17. Morgenstern LB, Smith MA, Lisabeth LD, et al. Excess stroke in Mexican Americans compared with non-Hispanic whites: the brain attack surveillance in the Corpus Christi project. *Am J Epidemiol* 2004;160:376–383.

18. Bailey EL, Smith C, Sudlow CL, Wardlaw JM. Pathology of lacunar ischemic stroke in humans – a systematic review. *Brain Pathol* 2012;22:583–591.

19. Brisset M, Boutouyrie P, Pico F, et al. Large-vessel correlates of cerebral small-vessel disease. *Neurology* 2013;80:662–669.

20. Cho KH, Kang DW, Kwon SU, Kim JS. Location of single subcortical infarction due to middle cerebral artery atherosclerosis: proximal versus distal arterial stenosis. *J Neurol Neurosurg Psychiatry* 2009; 80:48–52.

21. Chan DK, Silver FL. Basilar artery stenosis mimicking the lacunar syndrome of pure motor hemiparesis. *Can J Neurol Sci* 2003;30:159–162.

22. Khan A, Kasner SE, Lynn MJ, Chimowitz MI, Warfarin Aspirin Symptomatic Intracranial Disease Trial I. Risk factors and outcome of patients with symptomatic intracranial stenosis presenting with lacunar stroke. *Stroke* 2012;43:1230–1233.

23. Arboix A, Alio J. Cardioembolic stroke: clinical features, specific cardiac disorders and prognosis. *Curr Cardiol Rev* 2010;6:150–161.

24. Chowdhury D, Wardlaw JM, Dennis MS. Are multiple acute small subcortical infarctions caused by embolic mechanisms? *J Neurol Neurosurg Psychiatry* 2004;75:1416–1420.

25. Gan R, Sacco RL, Kargman DE, et al. Testing the validity of the lacunar hypothesis: the Northern Manhattan Stroke Study experience. *Neurology* 1997;48:1204–1211.

26. Arboix A, Massons J, Garcia-Eroles L, et al. Clinical predictors of lacunar syndrome not due to lacunar infarction. *BMC Neurol* 2010;10:31.

27. Baumgartner RW, Sidler C, Mosso M, Georgiadis D. Ischemic lacunar stroke in patients with and without potential mechanism other than small-artery disease. *Stroke* 2003;34:653–659.

28. Mead GE, Lewis SC, Wardlaw JM, Dennis MS, Warlow CP. Severe ipsilateral carotid stenosis and middle cerebral artery disease in lacunar ischaemic stroke: innocent bystanders? *J Neurol* 2002;249:266–271.

29. Hougaku H, Matsumoto M, Handa N, et al. Asymptomatic carotid lesions and silent cerebral infarction. *Stroke* 1994;25:566–570.

30. Rajapakse A, Rajapakse S, Sharma JC. Is investigating for carotid artery disease warranted in non-cortical lacunar infarction? *Stroke* 2011;42:217–220.

31. Kim JS. Pure sensory stroke. Clinical–radiological correlates of 21 cases. *Stroke* 1992;23:983–987.

32. Tei H, Uchiyama S, Maruyama S. Capsular infarcts: location, size and etiology of pure motor hemiparesis, sensorimotor stroke and ataxic hemiparesis. *Acta Neurol Scand* 1993;88:264–268.

33. Schonewille WJ, Tuhrim S, Singer MB, Atlas SW. Diffusion-weighted MRI in acute lacunar syndromes. A clinical–radiological correlation study. *Stroke* 1999;30:2066–2069.

34. Fisher CM. Lacunes: small, deep cerebral infarcts. *Neurology* 1965;15:774–784.

35. Arboix A, Padilla I, Massons J, et al. Clinical study of 222 patients with pure motor stroke. *J Neurol Neurosurg Psychiatry* 2001;71:239–242.

36. Fisher CM, Curry HB. Pure motor hemiplegia of vascular origin. *Arch Neurol* 1965;13:30–44.

37. Fisher CM. Thalamic pure sensory stroke: a pathologic study. *Neurology* 1978;28:1141–1144.

38. Arboix A, Garcia-Plata C, Garcia-Eroles L, et al. Clinical study of 99 patients with

pure sensory stroke. *J Neurol* 2005;252:156–162.

39. Nasreddine ZS, Saver JL. Pain after thalamic stroke: right diencephalic predominance and clinical features in 180 patients. *Neurology* 1997;48:1196–1199.
40. Kumar B, Kalita J, Kumar G, Misra UK. Central poststroke pain: a review of pathophysiology and treatment. *Anesth Analg* 2009;108:1645–1657.
41. Mohr JP, Kase CS, Meckler RJ, Fisher CM. Sensorimotor stroke due to thalamocapsular ischemia. *Arch Neurol* 1977; 34:739–741.
42. Staaf G, Samuelsson M, Lindgren A, Norrving B. Sensorimotor stroke; clinical features, MRI findings, and cardiac and vascular concomitants in 32 patients. *Acta Neurol Scand* 1998;97:93–98.
43. Arboix A, Marti-Vilalta JL, Garcia JH. Clinical study of 227 patients with lacunar infarcts. *Stroke* 1990;21:842–847.
44. Arboix A. [Clinical study of 23 patients with ataxic hemiparesis.] *Med Clin (Barc)* 2004;122:342–344 [in Spanish].
45. Hiraga A, Uzawa A, Kamitsukasa I. Diffusion weighted imaging in ataxic hemiparesis. *J Neurol Neurosurg Psychiatry* 2007;78:1260–1262.
46. Emori T, Kuriyama Y, Imakita S, Sawada T. Ataxic hemiparesis following thalamic lacunar infarction. *Intern Med* 1992;31:889–892.
47. Moulin T, Bogousslavsky J, Chopard JL, et al. Vascular ataxic hemiparesis: a re-evaluation. *J Neurol Neurosurg Psychiatry* 1995;58:422–427.
48. Gorman MJ, Dafer R, Levine SR. Ataxic hemiparesis: critical appraisal of a lacunar syndrome. *Stroke* 1998;29:2549–2555.
49. Flint AC, Naley MC, Wright CB. Ataxic hemiparesis from strategic frontal white matter infarction with crossed cerebellar diaschisis. *Stroke* 2006;37:e1–2.
50. Arboix A, Bell Y, Garcia-Eroles L, et al. Clinical study of 35 patients with dysarthria–clumsy hand syndrome. *J Neurol Neurosurg Psychiatry* 2004;75:231–234.
51. Martin PJ, Chang HM, Wityk R, Caplan LR. Midbrain infarction: associations and aetiologies in the New England medical center posterior circulation registry. *J Neurol Neurosurg Psychiatry* 1998;64:392–395.
52. Bogousslavsky J, Maeder P, Regli F, Meuli R. Pure midbrain infarction: clinical syndromes, MRI, and etiologic patterns. *Neurology* 1994;44:2032–2040.
53. Umasankar U, Huwez FU. A patient with reversible pupil-sparing Weber's syndrome. *Neurol India* 2003;51:388–389.
54. Silverman IE, Liu GT, Volpe NJ, Galetta SL. The crossed paralyses. The original brain-stem syndromes of Millard-Gubler, Foville, Weber, and Raymond–Cestan. *Arch Neurol* 1995;52:635–638.
55. Sitthinamsuwan B, Nunta-Aree S, Sitthinamsuwan P, Suwanawiboon B, Chiewvit P. Two patients with rare causes of Weber's syndrome. *J Clin Neurosci* 2011;18:578–579.
56. Patel R, Jha S, Yadav RK. Pleomorphism of the clinical manifestations of neurocysticercosis. *Trans R Soc Trop Med Hyg* 2006;100: 134–141.
57. Broadley SA, Taylor J, Waddy HM, Thompson PD. The clinical and MRI correlate of ischaemia in the ventromedial midbrain: Claude's syndrome. *J Neurol* 2001;248:1087–1089.
58. Asakawa H, Yanaka K, Nose T. MRI of Claude's syndrome. *Neurology* 2003;61:575.
59. Seo SW, Heo JH, Lee KY, et al. Localization of Claude's syndrome. *Neurology* 2001;57:2304–2307.
60. Coppola RJ. Localization of Claude's syndrome. *Neurology* 2002;58:1707; author reply 1707–1708.
61. Dhanjal T, Walters M, MacMillan N. Claude's syndrome in association with posterior cerebral artery stenosis. *Scott Med J* 2003;48:91–92.
62. Serrano-Pozo A, Montes-Latorre E, Gonzalez-Marcos JR, Gil-Peralta A. Cardiac embolism in a Claude's syndrome without involvement of the red nucleus. *Eur J Neurol* 2007;14:e1–2.
63. Song TJ, Suh SH, Cho H, Lee KY. Claude's syndrome associated with neurocysticercosis. *Yonsei Med J* 2010;51:978–979.
64. Borras JM, Salazar FG, Grandas F. Oculomotor palsy and contralateral tremor (Benedikt's syndrome) following a stereotactic procedure. *J Neurol* 1997;244:272–274.
65. Liu GT, Crenner CW, Logigian EL, Charness ME, Samuels MA. Midbrain syndromes of Benedikt, Claude, and Nothnagel: setting the record straight. *Neurology* 1992;42:1820–1822.
66. Paidakakos NA, Rokas E, Theodoropoulos S, Dimogerontas G, Konstantinidis E. Posttraumatic Benedikt's syndrome: a rare entity with unclear anatomopathological correlations. *World Neurosurg* 2012;78:e713–715.
67. Loseke N, Retif J, Noterman J, Flament-Durand J. Inferior red nucleus syndrome (Benedikt's syndrome) due to a single intramesencephalic metastasis from a prostatic carcinoma. Case report. *Acta Neurochir (Wien)* 1981;56:59–64.
68. Maduri R, Barbagallo G, Iofrida G, Signorelli M, Signorelli F. Regression of Benedikt's syndrome after single-stage

removal of mesencephalic cavernoma and temporal meningioma: a case report. *Clin Neurol Neurosurg*, in press.

69. Field TS, Benavente OR. Penetrating artery territory pontine infarction. *Rev Neurol Dis* 2011;8:30–38.

70. Kumral E, Bayulkem G, Evyapan D. Clinical spectrum of pontine infarction. Clinical–MRI correlations. *J Neurol* 2002;249:1659–1670.

71. Zaorsky NG, Luo JJ. A case of classic Raymond syndrome. *Case Rep Neurol Med* 2012;2012:583123.

72. Ogawa K, Suzuki Y, Kamei S. Two patients with abducens nerve palsy and crossed hemiplegia (Raymond syndrome). *Acta Neurol Belg* 2010;110:270–271.

73. Satake M, Kira J, Yamada T, Kobayashi T. Raymond syndrome (alternating abducent hemiplegia) caused by a small haematoma at the medial pontomedullary junction. *J Neurol Neurosurg Psychiatry* 1995;58:261.

74. Onbas O, Kantarci M, Alper F, Karaca L, Okur A. Millard–Gubler syndrome: MR findings. *Neuroradiology* 2005;47:35–37.

75. Matsuyama T, Masuda A. [A rare case of delayed traumatic Millard–Gubler syndrome.] *No Shinkei Geka* 1992;20:697–699.

76. Gardela G, Kusmiderski J, Slowik S. [Millard–Gubler syndrome in a young man after hemorrhage from arteriovenous hemangioma to the brainstem.] *Neurol Neurochir Pol* 1989;23:149–152 [in Polish].

77. Kesikburun S, Safaz I, Alaca R. Pontine cavernoma hemorrhage leading to Millard-Gubler syndrome. *Am J Phys Med Rehabil* 2011;90:263.

78. Prasad R, Kapoor K, Srivastava A, Mishra O. Neurocysticercosis presenting as Millard–Gubler syndrome. *J Neurosci Rural Pract* 2012;3:375–377.

79. Lee MJ, Park YG, Kim SJ, et al. Characteristics of stroke mechanisms in patients with medullary infarction. *Eur J Neurol* 2012;19:1433–1439.

80. Fukuoka T, Takeda H, Dembo T, et al. Clinical review of 37 patients with medullary infarction. *J Stroke Cerebrovasc Dis* 2012;21:594–599.

81. Kim JS. Pure lateral medullary infarction: clinical–radiological correlation of 130 acute, consecutive patients. *Brain* 2003;126:1864–1872.

82. Swenson AJ, Leira EC. Paroxysmal sneezing at the onset of lateral medullary syndrome: cause or consequence? *Eur J Neurol* 2007;14:461–463.

83. Sacco RL, Freddo L, Bello JA, et al. Wallenberg's lateral medullary syndrome. Clinical-magnetic resonance imaging correlations. *Arch Neurol* 1993;50:609–614.

84. Newman-Toker DE, Kattah JC, Alvernia JE, Wang DZ. Normal head impulse test differentiates acute cerebellar strokes from vestibular neuritis. *Neurology* 2008;70:2378–2385.

85. Kattah JC, Talkad AV, Wang DZ, Hsieh YH, Newman-Toker DE. Hints to diagnose stroke in the acute vestibular syndrome: three-step bedside oculomotor examination more sensitive than early MRI diffusion-weighted imaging. *Stroke* 2009;40:3504–3510.

86. Kim JS, Lee JH, Suh DC, Lee MC. Spectrum of lateral medullary syndrome. Correlation between clinical findings and magnetic resonance imaging in 33 subjects. *Stroke* 1994;25:1405–1410.

87. Norrving B, Cronqvist S. Lateral medullary infarction: prognosis in an unselected series. *Neurology* 1991;41:244–248.

88. Kim JS, Han YS. Medial medullary infarction: clinical, imaging, and outcome study in 86 consecutive patients. *Stroke* 2009;40:3221–3225.

89. Kameda W, Kawanami T, Kurita K, et al. Lateral and medial medullary infarction: a comparative analysis of 214 patients. *Stroke* 2004;35:694–699.

90. Bassetti C, Bogousslavsky J, Mattle H, Bernasconi A. Medial medullary stroke: report of seven patients and review of the literature. *Neurology* 1997;48:882–890.

91. Toyoda K, Imamura T, Saku Y, et al. Medial medullary infarction: analyses of 11 patients. *Neurology* 1996;47:1141–1147.

92. Percheron G. [Arteries of the human thalamus. II. Arteries and paramedian thalamic territory of the communicating basilar artery.] *Rev Neurol (Paris)* 1976;132:309–324 [in French].

93. Percheron G. [Arteries of the human thalamus. I. Artery and polar thalamic territory of the posterior communicating artery.] *Rev Neurol (Paris)* 1976;132:297–307 [in French].

94. Percheron G. [Arteries of the thalamus in man. Choroidal arteries. III. Absence of the constituted thalamic territory of the anterior choroidal artery. IV. Arteries and thalamic territories of the choroidal and postero-median thalamic arterial system. V. Arteries and thalamic territories of the choroidal and postero-lateral thalamic arterial system.] *Rev Neurol (Paris)* 1977;133:547–558 [in French].

95. Schmahmann JD. Vascular syndromes of the thalamus. *Stroke* 2003;34:2264–2278.

96. Carrera E, Bogousslavsky J. The thalamus and behavior: effects of anatomically distinct strokes. *Neurology* 2006;66:1817–1823.

97. Bogousslavsky J, Regli F, Uske A. Thalamic infarcts: clinical syndromes, etiology, and prognosis. *Neurology* 1988;38:837–848.

98. Swartz RH, Black SE. Anterior-medial thalamic lesions in

dementia: frequent and volume-dependently associated with sudden cognitive decline. *J Neurol Neurosurg Psychiatry* 2006;77:1307–1312.

99. Gorelick PB, Amico LL, Ganellen R, Benevento LA. Transient global amnesia and thalamic infarction. *Neurology* 1988;38:496–499.

100. Melo TP, Bogousslavsky J. Hemiataxia-enhypesthesia: a thalamic stroke syndrome. *J Neurol Neurosurg Psychiatry* 1992;55:581–584.

101. Karnath HO, Himmelbach M, Rorden C. The subcortical anatomy of human spatial neglect: putamen, caudate nucleus and pulvinar. *Brain* 2002;125:350–360.

102. Neau JP, Bogousslavsky J. The syndrome of posterior choroidal artery territory infarction. *Ann Neurol* 1996;39:779–788.

103. Ghika J, Bogousslavsky J, Henderson J, Maeder P, Regli F. The "jerky dystonic unsteady hand": a delayed motor syndrome in posterior thalamic infarctions. *J Neurol* 1994;241:537–542.

104. Donnan GA, O'Malley HM, Quang L, Hurley S, Bladin PF. The capsular warning syndrome: pathogenesis and clinical features. *Neurology* 1993;43:957–962.

105. Paul NL, Simoni M, Chandratheva A, Rothwell PM. Population-based study of capsular warning syndrome and prognosis after early recurrent TIA. *Neurology* 2012;79:1356–1362.

106. Abetz L, Allen R, Follet A, et al. Evaluating the quality of life of patients with restless legs syndrome. *Clin Ther* 2004;26:925–935.

107. Lee J, Albers GW, Marks MP, Lansberg MG. Capsular warning syndrome caused by middle cerebral artery stenosis. *J Neurol Sci* 2010;296:115–120.

108. Chen ZC, Sun JZ, Shi ZH, Lou M. Capsular warning syndrome caused by spontaneous middle cerebral artery dissection. *CNS Neurosci Ther* 2012;18:702–704.

109. Tang CW, Wang PN, Lin KP, et al. Microscopic polyangiitis presenting with capsular warning syndrome and subsequent stroke. *J Neurol Sci* 2009;277:174–175.

110. Ferro JM, Falcao F, Melo TP, Campos JG. Dural sinus thrombosis mimicking "capsular warning syndrome." *J Neurol* 2000;247:802–803.

111. Farrar J, Donnan GA. Capsular warning syndrome preceding pontine infarction. *Stroke* 1993;24:762.

112. Saposnik G, Noel de Tilly L, Caplan LR. Pontine warning syndrome. *Arch Neurol* 2008;65:1375–1377.

113. Muengtaweepongsa S, Singh NN, Cruz-Flores S. Pontine warning syndrome: case series and review of literature. *J Stroke Cerebrovasc Dis* 2010;19:353–356.

114. Staaf G, Geijer B, Lindgren A, Norrving B. Diffusion-weighted MRI findings in patients with capsular warning syndrome. *Cerebrovasc Dis* 2004;17:1–8.

115. Del Bene A, Palumbo V, Lamassa M, et al. Progressive lacunar stroke: review of mechanisms, prognostic features, and putative treatments. *Int J Stroke* 2012;7:321–329.

116. Chalela JA, Ezzeddine M, Latour L, Warach S. Reversal of perfusion and diffusion abnormalities after intravenous thrombolysis for a lacunar infarction. *J Neuroimaging* 2003;13:152–154.

117. National Institute of Neurological Disorders and Stroke rt-PA Stroke Study Group. Tissue plasminogen activator for acute ischemic stroke. *N Engl J Med* 1995;333:1581–1587.

118. Shobha N, Fang J, Hill MD. Do lacunar strokes benefit from thrombolysis? Evidence from the Registry of the Canadian Stroke Network. *Int J Stroke* 2013; 8 (Suppl A100):45–9.

119. Mustanoja S, Meretoja A, Putaala J, et al. Outcome by stroke etiology in patients receiving thrombolytic treatment: descriptive subtype analysis. *Stroke* 2011;42:102–106.

120. Lee SJ, Saver JL, Liebeskind DS, et al. Safety of intravenous fibrinolysis in imaging-confirmed single penetrator artery infarcts. *Stroke* 2010;41:2587–2591.

121. Vivanco-Hidalgo RM, Rodriguez-Campello A, Ois A, et al. Thrombolysis in capsular warning syndrome. *Cerebrovasc Dis* 2008;25:508–510.

122. Nguyen TH, Vo D, Ngo MB, et al. Thrombolysis in recurrent lacunar stroke: a case example. *Eur J Neurol* 2008;15:1409–1411.

123. Mistri AK, Robinson TG, Potter JF. Pressor therapy in acute ischemic stroke: systematic review. *Stroke* 2006;37:1565–1571.

124. Lalive PH, Mayor I, Sztajzel R. The role of blood pressure in lacunar strokes preceded by TIAs. *Cerebrovasc Dis* 2003;16:88–90.

125. Lim TS, Hong JM, Lee JS, et al. Induced-hypertension in progressing lacunar infarction. *J Neurol Sci* 2011;308:72–76.

126. Canadian Stroke Strategy. *Canadian Best Practice Recommendations for Stroke Care: update 2010.* http://www.strokebestpractices.ca/wp-content/uploads/2011/04/2010BPR_ENG.pdf (accessed May 5, 2013).

127. The International Stroke Trial (IST). A randomised trial of aspirin, subcutaneous heparin, both, or neither among 19 435 patients with acute ischaemic stroke. International Stroke Trial Collaborative Group. *Lancet* 1997;349:1569–1581.

128. Chinese Acute Stroke Trial (CAST) Collaborative Group. Randomised placebo-controlled

trial of early aspirin use in 20 000 patients with acute ischaemic stroke. *Lancet* 1997;349:1641–1649.

129. Chen ZM, Sandercock P, Pan HC, et al. Indications for early aspirin use in acute ischemic stroke: a combined analysis of 40 000 randomized patients from the Chinese Acute Stroke Trial and the International Stroke Trial. On behalf of the CAST and IST Collaborative Groups. *Stroke* 2000;31:1240 1249.

130. Kennedy J, Hill MD, Ryckborst KJ, et al. Fast Assessment of Stroke and Transient Ischaemic Attack to Prevent Early Recurrence (FASTER): a randomised controlled pilot trial. *Lancet Neurol* 2007;6:961–969.

131. Dengler R, Diener HC, Schwartz A, et al. Early treatment with aspirin plus extended-release dipyridamole for transient ischaemic attack or ischaemic stroke within 24 h of symptom onset (EARLY trial): a randomised, open-label, blinded-endpoint trial. *Lancet Neurol* 2010;9:159–166.

132. Fahey CD, Alberts MJ, Bernstein RA. Oral clopidogrel load in aspirin-resistant capsular warning syndrome. *Neurocrit Care* 2005;2:183–184.

133. Asil T, Ir N, Karaduman F, Cagli B, Tuncel S. Combined antithrombotic treatment with aspirin and clopidogrel for patients with capsular warning syndrome: a case report. *Neurologist* 2012;18:68–69.

134. Philipps J, Thomalla G, Glahn J, Schwarze M, Rother J. Treatment of progressive stroke with tirofiban – experience in 35 patients. *Cerebrovasc Dis* 2009;28:435–438.

135. Martin-Schild S, Shaltoni H, Abraham AT, et al. Safety of eptifibatide for subcortical stroke progression. *Cerebrovasc Dis* 2009;28:595–600.

136. Dobkin BH. Heparin for lacunar stroke in progression. *Stroke* 1983;14:421–423.

137. Haley EC, Jr., Kassell NF, Torner JC. Failure of heparin to prevent progression in progressing ischemic infarction. *Stroke* 1988;19:10–14.

138. Chimowitz MI, Lynn MJ, Derdeyn CP, et al. Stenting versus aggressive medical therapy for intracranial arterial stenosis. *N Engl J Med* 2011;365: 993–1003.

139. Saposnik G, Hassan KA, Selchen D, et al. Stroke unit care: does ischemic stroke subtype matter? *Int J Stroke* 2011;6:244–250.

140. Smith EE, Hassan KA, Fang J, et al. Do all ischemic stroke subtypes benefit from organized inpatient stroke care? *Neurology* 2010;75:456–462.

141. Lansberg MG, Albers GW, Beaulieu C, Marks MP. Comparison of diffusion-weighted MRI and CT in acute stroke. *Neurology* 2000;54:1557–1561.

142. Albers GW, Lansberg MG, Norbash AM, et al. Yield of diffusion-weighted MRI for detection of potentially relevant findings in stroke patients. *Neurology* 2000;54:1562–1567.

143. Wessels T, Rottger C, Jauss M, et al. Identification of embolic stroke patterns by diffusion-weighted MRI in clinically defined lacunar stroke syndromes. *Stroke* 2005;36:757–761.

144. Kang DW, Chalela JA, Ezzeddine MA, Warach S. Association of ischemic lesion patterns on early diffusion-weighted imaging with TOAST stroke subtypes. *Arch Neurol* 2003;60:1730–1734.

145. Campbell BC, Weir L, Desmond PM, et al. CT perfusion improves diagnostic accuracy and confidence in acute ischaemic stroke. *J Neurol Neurosurg Psychiatry* 2013;84:613–618.

146. Lin K, Do KG, Ong P, et al. Perfusion CT improves diagnostic accuracy for hyperacute ischemic stroke in the three-hour window: study of 100 patients with diffusion MRI confirmation. *Cerebrovasc Dis* 2009;28: 72–79.

Chapter 19

Cognitive consequences of cerebral small vessel disease

José M. Ferro, Ana Verdelho, and Sofia Madureira

Cognitive implications of small vessel disease

White matter changes, lacunes, and microbleeds are all visible expressions of small vessel disease (SVD). The cognitive impact of SVD has gained interest in the last decades. In this section, we review: (1) the cognitive impact of the different types of SVD; (2) the influence of other clinical variables on cognition of subjects with SVD; and (3) the neuropsychological approach.

Cognitive implications of white matter changes

Age-related white matter changes (WMCs) are frequent findings in magnetic resonance imaging (MRI) of elderly individuals in population-based studies [1–3]. In the Rotterdam Scan Study only 5% of the 1077 subjects aged between 60 and 90 years, randomly sampled from the general population, were free of any WMCs [1]. Among the 3301 subjects aged over 65 years from the community included in the Cardiovascular Health Study, only 4.4% were free of any abnormal signal in the white matter [2]. Even in younger ages (under 55 years), mild WMCs are frequently described in asymptomatic subjects [4], and prevalence is increased in symptomatic subjects in population studies. A clear increase with age has been reported over the different studies [1–4].

The frequency and severity of WMCs in different degenerative dementias remains a controversial issue. In demented older patients, periventricular WMCs have been reported in almost all patients, irrespective of dementia type [4], and subcortical lesions were described in 96% of vascular dementia patients, 89% of Alzheimer's disease (AD) patients, and in 85% of patients with dementia with Lewy bodies [5]. However, some authors found WMCs more frequent in dementia with Lewy bodies and dementia associated with Parkinson disease [5, 6], mainly associated with periventricular hyperintensities [7], compared with AD. Others found WMCs more frequent in both pathologies without differences in the severity of WMC [8, 9].

Among nondemented independent elderly subjects, cerebral age-related WMCs (ARWMCs) are associated with cognitive deficits, mainly in executive functions, attention, speed, and motor control [10–12], but also in global measures of cognition [2, 10, 12–14], visuoconstructional [10, 12, 13], naming [12], and memory tasks [15, 16]. Despite controversy in extant publications [17–20], WMC severity is also implicated in decline in specific neuropsychological domains, mainly attention, executive functions, and processing speed in longitudinal studies [16, 21–26]. Moreover, progression of WMCs is associated with deterioration in global cognitive function [27, 28] in specific cognitive domains, such as executive functions and processing speed [17, 23, 27, 28], memory and visuospatial abilities [29], and with the progression towards cognitive impairment and dementia [14, 26, 30, 31].

WMCs are associated with a significant risk of all types of dementia in population-based studies [32–34]. Consistent associations were described between WMCs and risk of vascular dementia [25, 35, 36]. Among nondemented stroke survivors, WMCs were related with worse performance in speed and attention cognitive domains [37]. Among mild cognitive impairment (MCI) patients, severe WMCs were associated with risk of vascular or mixed dementia [8, 35].

Cerebral Small Vessel Disease, ed. Leonardo Pantoni and Philip B. Gorelick. Published by Cambridge University Press.

WMC severity predicted progression towards cognitive impairment and dementia of independent elderly subjects with evidence of SVD, even when controlling for demographic variables, vascular risk factors, lacunes, and mesial temporal lobe atrophy [38]. Recent meta-analysis and reviews yielded a significant association between WMCs and risk of AD [25, 33, 35, 39].

Recent neuropathologic data suggested that vascular disease could affect cognition, not only through the effects on subcortical connections and WMC, but also through exacerbating cortical atrophy [40], suggesting a synergistic effect. Capizzano et al. [41] found WMCs significantly associated with cortical atrophy in AD patients and compromising independently neuropsychological performance. In vivo, diffusion tensor imaging techniques provide evidence of white matter tract degeneration in early AD [42]. These findings support the idea that degeneration of structures in the interconnected limbic–diencephalic network appear in association with very early stages of AD.

Increasing loads of WMC volume were recently correlated with atrophy of the corpus callosum (rostrum and splenium, but also corpus callosum global atrophy), suggesting that WMCs may lead to a gradual loss of corpus callosum tissue [43]. Corpus callosum atrophy has been found associated with cognitive deficits [44, 45], mainly in mental speed and executive functions, and with AD and vascular dementia [46, 47]. Very recently, Frederiksen et al. [48] showed that subjects who converted to dementia had a higher rate of tissue loss in the splenium, compared to nonconverters, independently of the effect of medial temporal atrophy.

Cognitive implications of lacunes

Silent lacunes are prevalent in elderly subjects [49, 50], but their clinical significance has been difficult to establish. Among cognitively normal elderly subjects, the total number of subcortical lacunes was an independent predictor of executive functioning [51], speed, and motor control [52]. Lacunes are implicated in higher risk of incident dementia [53], mainly among those with WMC [54], cortical atrophy, and recurrent stroke [53]. Specific locations, such as thalamic and basal ganglia lacunes, were independent predictors of cognitive decline in elderly subjects [55]. Progression of lacunes was associated with cognitive function, particularly in processing speed [28, 56] and executive functions [56], along with WMC progression.

In cerebral autosomal dominant arteriopathy with subcortical infarcts and leukoencephalopathy (CADASIL) patients – a pathology that represents a model of brain SVD – lacunar lesion load was the most important neuroimaging parameter associated with cognitive impairment [57, 58], in contrast with WMCs and microbleeds, which were not [58]. Among individuals with AD, cognitive function was markedly influenced by thalamic, basal ganglia, and deep white matter lacunes identified in neuropathologic study [59]. However, in a large neuropathologic series, lacunes were present in approximately one quarter of elderly cases without psychiatric or neurologic disease [60]. Van de Pol et al. [61] found that lacunes no longer predicted any of the cognitive test outcomes when adjusting for age and medial temporal atrophy, and evidence of the independent influence of lacunes for the progression to other dementias, taking into consideration other confounders, is still lacking.

Cognitive implications of cerebral microbleeds

Cerebral microbleeds (CMBs) – small hemorrhages seen in susceptible MRI sequences as isolated circular hypointense lesions – have been recently recognized as one of the manifestations of SVD. They have been progressively identified in specific and sensitive MRI sequences (T2* gradient-recalled echo [GRE] or susceptibility-weighted imaging [SWI]), accompanying white matter lesions and lacunes [62].

CMBs increase with age, but prevalence values are quite variable depending upon the MRI technique used. In a community setting, 15% had one or more CMBs, ranging from 7% in younger ages (45–55 years old) to 36% in those older than 80 [63].

Among AD patients, a pooled prevalence of 23% of CMBs was yielded by a recent meta-analysis [64]. Prevalence can be as high as 50% in multiple lacunar stroke patients [62] and can reach 85% of subjects with criteria for subcortical vascular dementia [65].

The impact of CMBs on cognition has been approached in recent years: CMBs were associated with impairment in frontal executive functions [66–68], information processing [68, 69] and motor speed [69], attention [70], immediate and delayed visual memory [71], and with a lower global measure of cognition [70, 72, 73]. Among survivors of stroke, those without CMBs were more prone to recover from neuropsychological deficits in the language domain and in the visuospeed domain [74]. However, the study designs were quite variable, and those findings were yielded by very few longitudinal studies [66, 75], and some cross-sectional [67, 70, 72, 73, 75] and retrospective studies [65, 67, 76]. Besides, controlling for other confounders was not systematic [66, 67, 72, 75].

Few and controversial data exist concerning CMB location and implications in cognitive functions. Most studies distinguished between cortical and deep or infratentorial CMBs. Lobar CMBs were associated with information processing and motor speed [69], but also with global cognitive performance and attention [70]. Deep CMBs were associated with motor speed [69], processing speed and executive functions [68], global cognitive performance [70, 77], and attention [70]. Infratentorial CMBs were associated with motor speed, attention [68], and visual memory [71].

Some studies found that cognitive implications were stronger with multiple CMBs [68], and an increasing number of CMBs was found associated with increasing cognitive deterioration [75].

CMBs are highly frequent among patients with a diagnosis of vascular dementia [65, 68, 78] and in patients with other SVD. In vascular dementia patients, the number of CMBs is associated with cognitive function mainly in attention and executive functions, but also with global measure of cognition, memory, language, and visuospatial function [65].

Among subjects with subcortical vascular dementia, CMBs are associated with worse performance in orientation and attention/calculation items of the Mini Mental State Examination (MMSE), an effect that was proposed to be mediated through a decrease in the cholinergic function [79]. In CADASIL patients, CMBs were associated with worse executive functions [80].

Among MCI patients and in subjects with AD, available data are still scarce and controversial. In one study with MCI patients, CMBs were associated with higher risk of progression to dementia [81], but, in another study, multidomain MCI subjects did not differ in the number of CMBs when compared with cognitive normal controls [75].

Within subjects with AD, patients with multiple CMBs performed worse on MMSE, semantic fluency, naming and digit span, compared to patients with AD and no CMBs [76], but others were not able to find differences in cognitive performance, according to the presence or absence of CMBs [82]. One of the possible reasons associated with the differences reported among AD patients is that, in this particular setting, CMBs can be a result of cerebral amyloid angiopathy rather then lipohyalinolysis and hyaline degeneration. Another explanation is that the number of subjects included in these studies is not sufficiently large to identify statistical effects.

Other clinical correlates that influence cognition in subjects with SVD

Increasing age is the most frequent factor associated with dementia [83] among subjects with SVD [84], and education has been consistently found a protective factor for dementia [84, 85]. There are, however, subjects with severe WMCs who appear cognitively and physically intact, and it is probable that protective factors, for instance cognitive reserve, could partially explain this phenomenon.

Epidemiologic studies indicate that vascular risk factors, which are known risk factors for SVD, play a role in the development of cognitive impairment and dementia, including degenerative dementia, and, among vascular risk factors, the main risks were hypertension, stroke, and diabetes [86–88].

Hypertension in mid life has been consistently associated with later development of cognitive decline and dementia, not only of vascular dementia, but also of degenerative dementia such as AD [89–92]. The relationship between late-onset hypertension and cognitive decline and dementia is less clear: some studies were negative for this association [93–95] or sustain that a very low systolic and/or diastolic value was associated with higher risk of cognitive decline [90, 91]. In cross-sectional studies, hypertension in late life was associated with worse performance in several cognitive tests mainly related with executive functions and attention, digit–symbol test, and word fluency [96], and also with difficulties in some global cognitive functioning [97–99]. One possible explanation for these discrepancies is that the relationship between hypertension and cognitive decline changes with time [92]: hypertension in mid life probably is associated with chronic vascular damage that later originates cognitive impairment, while late-life hypertension does not have this impact. Trials focusing on the prevention of dementia using antihypertensive medication have failed to show a consistent protective effect [100–103]. From the six main randomized placebo-controlled studies, four were negative for a protective effect [104–107], one found a small effect on the prevention of dementia [108], and the other [109] found a protective effect only for post-stroke dementia. Those studies were probably performed in older ages than what was desirable to prevent dementia (subjects older than 60 years), and the follow-up was short, not long enough to have sufficient patients converting into dementia.

An association between diabetes and higher risk of cognitive impairment and dementia has been described [38, 86, 110–115]. A recent meta-analysis showed that diabetes was a risk factor not only for AD but also MCI and all dementias, including vascular dementia [115]. Observational studies suggest that diabetic subjects have a twofold increase in risk of MCI and dementia comparing to nondiabetics [98, 116]. Nondemented diabetic patients performed worse on several cognitive tasks (global tests, attention, executive functions, processing speed and motor control, memory, praxis, and language) compared with healthy controls, even taking into account SVD [12, 117].

Diabetes was initially implicated in the progression of dementia due to the higher risk of vascular disease, but this higher frequency has been also mediated through metabolic changes due to the insulin and glycemia pathways that are implicated in the metabolic production of β-amyloid protein and tau protein [111], and so directly implicated in pathogenesis of AD [116, 118], or even suggesting that diabetes and AD share common metabolic pathways [119] and could be an expression of the same disease.

Stroke (irrespective of being large territorial or lacunar stroke) has been associated with progression to cognitive impairment [87, 120, 121] and dementia [120–122], not only to vascular dementia and vascular cognitive impairment [38], but also to degenerative dementias such as AD [122]. In nondemented subjects with WMCs, previous stroke is associated with worse performance on mental flexibility, attention, and memory recognition tests, independently of the severity of ARWMC [12]. Stroke could be a mediator between cerebral SVD and cognitive decline [22].

Acute lacunar infarction was associated with mild neuropsychological disturbances, especially among those with atypical lacunar syndrome and pure motor hemiparesis [123]. Controversial data exist about cognitive long-term evolution after lacunar stroke, with some authors reporting a high prevalence of cognitive impairment in the first three to four years after stroke, with a stepwise progression, and decreasing slightly after [121]. Impaired processing speed, attention, working memory, and executive function are the most frequent deficits associated with lacunar strokes, and verbal episodic memory was also described in a large cohort; however, cognitive impairment prior to stroke could not be ruled out [124].

One of the most interesting findings is that the risk for developing dementia provided by the association of multiple vascular risk factors is much higher when compared to the risk provided from each vascular risk factor [125]. A recent systematic review stressed that the risk of dementia in diabetes is increased when associated with other vascular risk factors [126]. Even among subjects free of stroke, with vascular risk factors, risk of cognitive impairment is increased [114, 127]. These results suggest an additive effect between several vascular risk factors and the progression towards dementia. To sustain this hypothesis, in several reports, treatment of several risk factors simultaneously was more effective than the treatment of a single vascular risk factor [128, 129].

Neuropsychological assessment of SVD patients

The cognitive dysfunction features related with SVD are distinctive from the ones present in AD patients, or even in patients with post-stroke vascular dementia, and neuropsychological assessment should be directed to the specific deficits due to SVD.

SVD and global cognitive measures

Since SVD is an insidious disease, early subtle cognitive changes are difficult to detect, especially in the absence of other clinical complaints. Some recent longitudinal studies, performed within the general population and reporting data from cognitively intact participants, have demonstrated that increasing volume and extension of WMCs are related to lower global cognitive measures, such as MMSE [130], and to conversion to MCI [26, 131]. Nevertheless, in both studies, MMSE mean scores at baseline were over the cut-off point for cognitive impairment (total baseline score 29 and 28, respectively). Global cognitive decline associated with progression of WMCs was also found in the Rotterdam Scan Study [22]. Using both MMSE and a composed cognitive score (cognitive index) based on the performance in information processing speed, executive functions, and verbal memory tests, the authors found a significant decline with increasing periventricular WMC. Decline on global functioning was mainly caused by impairment in speed (Stroop naming colors) and efficiency of processing (letter–digit substitution test) [22].

Decrease in global cognitive functioning associated with SVD has been more clearly observed in studies reporting the evolution of cognitive status in persons with other complaints or vascular risk factors. In a population identified with memory complaints and diagnosed with MCI, WMC volume was associated with an annual change in the Cambridge Cognitive Examination (CAMCOG) global score [132]. Additionally, in the Leukoaraiosis And DISability Study (LADIS) [133] – a three-year follow-up project that evaluated the transition into a dependent functional status of nondisabled independent elderly people with WMC – a steeper decline in MMSE associated with small ischemic vascular disease (SIVD) was also reported [30]. However, changes in MMSE are usually seen with the progression and/or severity of the disease, when a global compromise is already installed. In patients with very subtle cognitive changes, the sensitivity and specificity of the MMSE tend to decrease. For instance, in a cohort of patients with acute lacunar infarcts, the MMSE failed to identify 30% of the patients diagnosed with cognitive deficits with another neuropsychological battery [134].

The same occurs with other global cognitive scales or batteries such as CAMCOG [135] or the Alzheimer's Disease Assessment Scale–cognitive subscale (ADAS-cog) [136]. This might be explained by the lack of sensitivity of these instruments in identifying subtle changes or deficits in other cognitive domains other than orientation, memory, language, or visual constructional praxis. For instance, memory functioning seems to be less vulnerable to the presence of WMCs, unless the increasing WMCs represents a significant loss of brain volume [17].

To decrease the risk of underdiagnosing cognitive impairment in the initial phases of the disease, it is generally recommended to add more specific tests to well-studied and known batteries in order to improve their sensitivity to executive, attentional, and speed processing deficits. An example of such a combination is the Vascular Dementia Assessment Scale–cognitive subscale (VADAS-cog) battery [137], which resulted from the addition of five tests to assess working memory, psychomotor speed, attention, and executive functions (namely, digit span backwards, maze simple task, digit–symbol, digit cancellation, and verbal fluency) to the ADAS-cog battery. In the LADIS study, VADAS-cog proved to be not only more sensitive than ADAS-cog on significantly differentiating groups of mild, moderate, and severe WMC [138] at baseline, but also to be a neuropsychological predictor of dementia in a three-year period of follow-up [139].

The Montreal Cognitive Assessment (MoCA) scale [140] is another global cognitive measure that has been recently developed and used as a more sensitive instrument than MMSE in detecting vascular cognitive impairment. However, except for one study reporting that MoCA was a useful instrument differentiating a small group of SVD patients from controls [141], there is still a lack of data regarding its sensitivity and specificity to detect subtle cognitive changes in SVD patients.

SVD and executive functions

The effect of SVD on the decline of global cognitive measures is mainly due to the compromise and decrease of specific cognitive functions and not, at least in the initial and intermediate stages of the disease, to a diffuse cognitive impairment pattern. Executive dysfunction – mainly characterized by deficits in set shifting, verbal fluency, abstract problem solving, and attention – and decrease on speed of information processing might be detectable even in the initial stages of the disease. Multiple lacunes located in the subcortical structures and confluent and extensive WMCs can result in a disconnection of frontal–subcortical circuits (in particular, the dorsolateral prefrontal circuit) interrupting the central cholinergic pathway [142], and causing this pattern of frontal-lobe dysfunction.

For this reason, tailored instruments should be used in the clinical assessment of patients with SVD. The National Institute of Neurological Disorders and Stroke–Canadian Stroke Network (NINDS–CSN) Group [143] recently proposed the use of standard neuropsychological protocols to assess vascular cognitive impairment. The importance given to measures of executive, attention, and speed processing functioning is well established, even in the short-form protocols [143].

Executive and activation functions are frequently assessed using timed tests with a variety of set shifting, mental flexibility, and response inhibition tasks. Both executive functions and speed of processing are frequently impaired in patients with SVD. Lower scores on verbal fluency (both semantic and phonemic), Stroop reading and color naming tasks [144], and Trail Making tests [145] have been repeatedly associated with SVD [22, 146–148]. On other nontimed instruments used to assess mental flexibility and conceptualization, such as the Wisconsin Card Sorting Test [149], changes on scores were also associated with progression of WMCs in healthy community-dwelling elderly volunteers [17].

On a brief assessment battery used to differentiate patients with ischemic leukoaraiosis from normal controls, Trail Making and digit–symbol substitution tasks were the best individual tests identifying cognitive impairment [25]. Also on other studies, a decline in the digit–symbol substitution test performance was associated with worsening and progression of WMCs [26]. Tests sensitive to reductions in psychomotor speed, mental flexibility, working memory, and attention, such as the digit–symbol, or Trail Making are useful instruments for detecting early subtle changes in SVD patients.

Attention, slowing, and motor skills

Decrease in attention and speed of mental processing has been frequently associated with the presence and progression of WMCs, either in healthy elderly populations [22, 28, 150] or in elderly populations with high risk for vascular disease [29, 30, 151]. Changes in attention and processing speed due to SVD are explained by a disruption in brain structures involving the frontal–subcortical pathway circuits causing a frontal lobe-related cognitive impairment pattern.

In studies reporting an association between cognitive functions and WMC localization, impairment in speed of mental processing is usually related to WMCs located in periventricular regions rather than in subcortical deep areas [22, 28, 29].

A recent study performed by Duering et al. [152], in a cohort of 215 patients with CADASIL, tried to explore the role of strategic lesions detected for both lacunar and white matter changes on different patterns of cognitive decline, including mental processing speed. Using a voxel-based approach, the authors were able to report an association between a decrease in processing speed and the volume of WMCs and lacunar lesions located on the anterior thalamic radiation and forceps minor. These findings are in accordance with the previously described involvement of these structures in executive functions [153–155], as they are composed of white matter tracts that project between the thalamus, prefrontal cortex, and striatum, which play an important role in the prefrontal–subcortical circuits.

However, results are still controversial concerning the strategic locations for cognitive symptoms related with SVD. Different results might be explained by differences in imaging techniques, in cohorts of participants, and also in the different instruments used in the neuropsychological evaluation. In the majority of the studies, tests used to assess processing speed are usually complex since they require multiple cognitive capacities to perform the task. Instruments such as Trail Making and symbol–digit modalities are dependent on attention, memory, and motor skills, and require the involvement of different cerebral structures. The role of corpus callosum in processing speed and executive functions was also addressed in previous studies [156]. In a study performed in a nondemented elderly population, Jokinen et al. [44, 157] reported an association between atrophy of the total corpus callosum and decrease of processing speed, measured by the Trail Making, Part A, reading words, and colored dots of Stroop. In the same study, atrophy of the anterior corpus callosum was mainly associated with poorer performance on attention and executive functions, assessed by symbol–digit modalities, digit cancellation tests, Trail Making, Part B, and Stroop naming noncorresponding colored dots.

On the other hand, it is still difficult to identify if slowing is an effect of compromised executive functioning or an impairment in sensory motor ability. Wright et al. [158], using the Grooved pegboard test, confirmed the association between the volume of WMCs and poorer performance on sensorimotor tasks. The authors emphasized the use of the Grooved pegboard test as a robust marker of white matter damage, since it is sensitive to slow neural transmission or conduction of integrative rostral–caudal pathways. Still, the majority of the studies do not use such specific tests to assess sensorimotor skills. However, the inclusion of Pegboard tests in the evaluation of patients with SVD, as recommended for the assessment of vascular cognitive impairment [159], would help in differentiating measures of psychomotor speed from those more dependent on executive/activation abilities.

SVD and memory performance

Memory deficits observed in SVD are distinctive from those observed in other pathologies such as MCI and AD. Studies comparing patients with MCI, with and without SVD, tried to identify different cognitive profiles [148, 160, 161]. Zhou et al. [148] reported a nonspecific profile in MCI–SVD patients, since they found extensive cognitive deficits in these patients. Comparatively, patients with MCI–AD had a more specific pattern, characterized by a significantly worse performance on verbal and visual delay recall and recognition measures, with a relatively preserved performance on processing speed tasks.

MCI patients with severe WMCs were compared with MCI patients with severe hippocampal atrophy using a comprehensive neuropsychological battery [162]. The authors found that patients with hippocampal atrophy exhibited specific episodic memory impairment, while patients with WMCs exhibited deficits on episodic memory (assessed by a 36-item object color-association task), working memory (patients were tested on two verbal working memory tasks and a spatial working memory task), and attention–control tasks (continuous performance test), suggesting that the episodic memory deficit was secondary to a more general impairment of executive control. In fact, working memory performance requires an ability to hold, manipulate, and quickly access information that is dependent on mental flexibility and speed. The mediation effect of executive functions on verbal and visual memory performance of SVD patients is already described [146].

Distinctive patterns can be observed in relation to memory impairment. Ability to store information is mainly dependent on the limbic and hippocampal structures, while retrieval and short-term memory capacities are more related with the integrity of frontal–subcortical structures and temporoparietal lesions, respectively. In SVD patients, episodic memory impairment is usually absent or mild in the initial phases, being the most frequent deficit characterized by difficulty in recalling information that improves in the presence of cues. However, these findings are frequently associated with other variables, such as medial temporal lobe atrophy [163] and corpus callosum atrophy [44]. Poorer episodic memory has been associated with age-related differences in central white matter regions [164]. Recent studies with SVD patients have explored the relationship of microstructural integrity of the hippocampus – not detected with conventional MRI – and verbal memory impairment [165, 166]. These authors found that deficits in verbal memory (immediate, delayed recall, and delayed recognition), but not in psychomotor speed, were related to changes in the hippocampus microstructure and, consequently, in the cingulum. These results might lead us into a new perspective in the understanding of memory impairment related to SVD.

Language

Impairment in language functions is not frequent in SVD. Comparing patients with initial dementia, Kertesz et al. [167] found that patients with periventricular hyperintensities performed worse on comprehension and attention tasks compared to those with no hyperintensities, who showed worse performances on memory and conceptualization tasks. However, other studies performed within the general population and with high-risk nondemented patients with WMCs did not find a relationship between the presence of WMCs or lacunes and language deficits (see [33] for a review). Nevertheless, lexical and semantic fluency measures should be included in the assessment of SVD patients. Impairment in lexical tasks is more frequent and prominent that semantic difficulties, showing a different pattern of MCI or AD patients [168]. As occurs in other cognitive functional deficits observed in patients with SVD, the type of impairment found in verbal functions seems to be related to the decrease in speed of processing and access to information that affect word-generation tasks.

Visuospatial construction and visuopractical functions

Previous studies with healthy elderly or community-dwelling populations did not find any relationship between visuoconstructional impairment and the presence of WMCs [150, 169–171].

Similar results were also reported in patients with vascular risk factors [151] or initial dementia [167]. On the contrary, in a cohort with more severe dementia, impairment in visuospatial abilities measured by the Wechsler Adult Intelligence Scale – Revised (WAIS-R) object assembly subtest was associated with the volume of WMCs located on the posterior periventricular regions [172]. The WAIS-R Picture Arrangement and Mattis Dementia Rating Scale (MDRS) motor performance subtests were also found to be important contributors to discriminating between groups with severe vascular dementia and AD [173]. Nevertheless, both WAIS-R subtests used in the two studies are sensitive to constructional abilities and visuospatial organization skills, while they are also time-dependent and highly sensitive to frontal-lobe dysfunction.

Results from the Austrian Stroke Prevention Study [17] also show an association between visuopractical skill decline assessed by the Pordue pegboard [174] and the progression of WMCs and related loss of brain volume. Again, the performance on this test is highly dependent on the speed of motor response.

More recently, decline in spatial organization and visuoconstructional skills, measured by the Benton Visual Retention Test (BVRT) and the Consortium to Establish a Registry in Alzheimer's Diseases (CERAD) geometric design copying test, was found to be uniquely associated with progression of posterior WMCs [175].

Another recent study [176] investigated the impact of WMCs on cognitive impairment and motor dysfunction in a cohort of neurologically intact elderly subjects. Measuring the percentage of WMCs in well-defined cerebral regions (frontal, temporal, parietal, occipital, periventricular, and subcortical) and the performance in memory, language, executive functions, and visuospatial–reasoning domains, the authors found only a trend toward worse performance in visuospatial abilities (measured by the WAIS-R picture completion and block design subtests) with a greater percentage of WMC. Interestingly, in this study, a higher percentage of WMCs in all regions except occipital lobe was associated with worse performance in executive tasks (measured by Trail Making, Part B and digit–symbol tests). No significant relationship was found between WMCs and memory or language standard scores. These findings support the importance of the integrity of white matter fibers in anterior brain regions for global cognitive functioning, and might reflect the contribution of executive functions to visual reasoning, as both tests – picture completion and block design – depend also on subjects' abilities of reasoning and judgment about practical and conceptual relevancies and problem-solving techniques.

Although some variability depending on the type (multiple lacunes vs. widespread WMCs) and location of the lacunes and WMCs (thalamus vs. other locations, posterior vs. anterior, deep vs. periventricular) and severity of the lesions (punctuate vs. confluent WMCs), the pattern of cognitive impairment in SVD is mainly characterized by a predominance of deficits in executive functions, slowed processing speed, attention, and related working-memory deficits.

Executive functions, defined as the abilities of set shifting, abstract reasoning, and problem solving, as well as the ability to plan, initiate, sequence, and monitor complex behaviors, are the most vulnerable cognitive domains to SVD. The use of sensitive neuropsychological tools to assess these patients is important to detect subtle changes and to understand the initial mechanisms that contribute to decline in cognitive functions, functional impairment, and dementia.

Conclusion

SVD is implicated in cognitive decline and dementia. The knowledge of the specific contribution of each form of SVD is essential to understanding and diagnosing this type of cognitive impairment. Additionally several concomitant clinical factors contribute to decline in cognitive abilities in patients with SVD.

In this setting, the use of specific neuropsychological instruments is crucial for the identification and follow-up of cognitive changes.

References

1. De Leeuw FE, de Groot JC, Achten E, et al. Prevalence of cerebral white matter lesions in elderly people: a population based magnetic resonance imaging study. The Rotterdam Scan Study. *J Neurol Neurosurg Psychiatry* 2001;70:9–14.
2. Longstreth WT, Manolio TA, Arnold A. Clinical correlates of white matter findings on cranial magnetic resonance imaging of 3301 elderly people: the Cardiovascular Health Study. *Stroke* 1996;27: 1274–1282.

3. Ylikoski A, Erkinjuntti T, Raininko R, et al. White matter hyperintensities on MRI in the neurologically nondiseased elderly. Analysis of cohorts of consecutive subjects aged 55 to 85 years living at home. *Stroke* 1995;26:1171–1177.
4. Schmidt R, Schmidt H, Haybaeck J, et al. Heterogeneity in age-related white matter changes. *Acta Neuropathol* 2011;122:171–185.
5. Barber R, Scheltens P, Gholkar A, et al. White matter lesions on magnetic resonance imaging in dementia with Lewy bodies, Alzheimer's disease, vascular dementia, and normal aging. *J Neurol Neurosurg Psychiatry* 1999;67:66–72.
6. Silbert LC, Kaye J. Neuroimaging and cognition in Parkinson's disease dementia. *Brain Pathol* 2010;20:646–653.
7. Barber R, Gholkar A, Scheltens P, et al. MRI volumetric correlates of white matter lesions in dementia with Lewy bodies and Alzheimer's disease. *Int J Geriatr Psychiatry* 2000;15:911–916.
8. Meyer JS, Huang J, Chowdhury MH. MRI confirms mild cognitive impairments prodromal for Alzheimer's, vascular and Parkinson–Lewy body dementias. *J Neurol Sci* 2007;257:97–104.
9. Burton EJ, McKeith IG, Burn DJ, Firbank MJ, O'Brien JT. Progression of white matter hyperintensities in Alzheimer's disease, dementia with Lewy bodies, and Parkinson disease dementia: a comparison with normal aging. *Am J Geriatr Psychiatry* 2006;14:842–849.
10. Skoog IBS, Johansson B, Palmertz B, Andreasson LA. The influence of white matter lesions on neuropsychological functioning in demented and non-demented 85-year-olds. *Acta Neurol Scand* 1996;93:142–148.
11. De Leeuw FE, de Groot JC, Oudkerk M, et al. Hypertension and cerebral white matter lesions in a prospective cohort study. *Brain* 2002;125:765–772.
12. Verdelho A, Madureira S, Ferro JM, et al. Differential impact of cerebral white matter changes, diabetes, hypertension and stroke on cognitive performance among non-disabled elderly. The LADIS study. *J Neurol Neurosurg Psychiatry* 2007;78:1325–1330.
13. Ylikoski R, Ylikoski A, Raininko R, et al. Cardiovascular diseases, health status, brain imaging findings and neuropsychological functioning in neurologically healthy elderly individuals. *Arch Gerontol Geriatr* 2000;30:115–130.
14. Inaba M, White L, Bell C, et al. White matter lesions on brain magnetic resonance imaging scan and five-year cognitive decline: the Honolulu–Asia Aging Study. *J Am Geriatr Soc* 2011;59:1484–1489.
15. Breteler MM, Swieten JCV, Bots ML. Cerebral white matter lesions, vascular risk factors and cognitive function in a population-based study: the Rotterdam Study. *Neurology* 1994;44:1246–1253.
16. Garde E, Mortensen EL, Krabbe K, Rostrup E, Larsson HB. Relation between age-related decline in intelligence and cerebral white-matter hyperintensities in healthy octogenarians: a longitudinal study. *Lancet* 2000;356:628–634.
17. Schmidt R, Ropele S, Enzinger C, et al. White matter lesion progression, brain atrophy, and cognitive decline: the Austrian Stroke Prevention Study. *Ann Neurol* 2005;58:610–616.
18. Hirono N, Kitagaki H, Kazui H, Hashimoto M, Mori E. Impact of white matter changes on clinical manifestation of Alzheimer's disease – a quantitative study *Stroke* 2000;31:2182–2188.
19. Mungas D, Harvey D, Reed BR, et al. Longitudinal volumetric MRI change and rate of cognitive decline. *Neurology* 2005;65:565–571.
20. DeCarli C, Mungas D, Harvey D, et al. Memory impairment, but not cerebrovascular disease, predicts progression of MCI to dementia. *Neurology* 2004;63: 220–227.
21. Tzourio C, Dufouil C, Ducimetiere P, Alperovitch A. Cognitive decline in individuals with high blood pressure: a longitudinal study in the elderly. EVA Study Group. Epidemiology of vascular aging. *Neurology* 1999;53:1948–1952.
22. Prins ND, van Dijk EJ, den Heijer T, et al. Cerebral small-vessel disease and decline in information processing speed, executive function and memory. *Brain* 2005;128:2034–2041.
23. Kramer JH, Mungas D, Reed BR, et al. Longitudinal MRI and cognitive change in healthy elderly. *Neuropsychology* 2007;21:412–418.
24. Tullberg M, Fletcher E, DeCarli C, et al. White matter lesions impair frontal lobe function regardless of their location. *Neurology* 2004;63:246–253.
25. Kuller LH, Lopez OL, Newman A, et al. Risk factors for dementia in the Cardiovascular Health Cognition Study. *Neuroepidemiology* 2003;22:13–22.
26. Silbert LC, Howieson DB, Dodge H, Kaye JA. Cognitive impairment risk: white matter hyperintensity progression matters. *Neurology* 2009;73:120–125.
27. Longstreth WT, Jr., Arnold AM, Beauchamp NJ, Jr., et al. Incidence, manifestations, and predictors of worsening white matter on serial cranial magnetic resonance imaging in the elderly: the Cardiovascular Health Study. *Stroke* 2005;36:56–61.
28. Van Dijk EJ, Prins ND, Vrooman HA, et al. Progression of cerebral small vessel disease in relation to

risk factors and cognitive consequences: Rotterdam Scan Study. *Stroke* 2008;39: 2712–2719.

29. Van den Heuvel DM, ten Dam VH, de Craen AJ, et al. Increase in periventricular white matter hyperintensities parallels decline in mental processing speed in a non-demented elderly population. *J Neurol Neurosurg Psychiatry* 2006;77:149–153.
30. Jokinen H, Kalska H, Ylikoski R, et al. Longitudinal cognitive decline in subcortical ischemic vascular disease – the LADIS study. *Cerebrovasc Dis* 2009;27:384–391.
31. Steffens DC, Potter GG, McQuoid DR, et al. Longitudinal magnetic resonance imaging vascular changes, apolipoprotein E genotype, and development of dementia in the neurocognitive outcomes of depression in the elderly study. *Am J Geriatr Psychiatry* 2007;15:839–849.
32. Debette S, Beiser A, DeCarli C, et al. Association of MRI markers of vascular brain injury with incident stroke, mild cognitive impairment, dementia, and mortality: the Framingham Offspring Study. *Stroke* 2010;41:600–606.
33. Debette S, Markus HS. The clinical importance of white matter hyperintensities on brain magnetic resonance imaging: systematic review and meta-analysis. *BMJ* 2010;341:3666.
34. Prins ND, van Dijk EJ, den Heijer T, et al. Cerebral white matter lesions and the risk of dementia. *Arch Neurol* 2004;61:1531–1534.
35. Bombois S, Debette S, Bruandet A, et al. Vascular subcortical hyperintensities predict conversion to vascular and mixed dementia in mci patients. *Stroke* 2008;39:2046–2051.
36. Meguro K, Ishii H, Kasuya M, et al. Incidence of dementia and associated risk factors in Japan: the Osaki–Tajiri project. *J Neurol Sci* 2007;260:175–182.
37. Burton EJ, Kenny RA, O'Brien J, et al. White matter hyperintensities are associated with impairment of memory, attention, and global cognitive performance in older stroke patients. *Stroke* 2004;35:1270–1275.
38. Verdelho A, Madureira S, Moleiro C, et al. White matter changes and diabetes predict cognitive decline in the elderly: the LADIS study. *Neurology* 2010;75:160–167.
39. Staekenborg SS, Koedam EL, Henneman WJ, et al. Progression of mild cognitive impairment to dementia: contribution of cerebrovascular disease compared with medial temporal lobe atrophy. *Stroke* 2009;40:1269–1274.
40. Jagust WJ, Zheng L, Harvey DJ, et al. Neuropathological basis of magnetic resonance images in aging and dementia. *Ann Neurol* 2008;63:72–80.
41. Capizzano AA, Acion L, Bekinschtein T, et al. White matter hyperintensities are significantly associated with cortical atrophy in Alzheimer's disease. *J Neurol Neurosurg Psychiatry* 2004;75:822–827.
42. Acosta-Cabronero J, Williams GB, Pengas G, Nestor PJ. Absolute diffusivities define the landscape of white matter degeneration in Alzheimer's disease. *Brain* 2010;133:529–539.
43. Ryberg C, Rostrup E, Paulson OB, et al. Corpus callosum atrophy as a predictor of age-related cognitive and motor impairment: a three-year follow-up of the LADIS study cohort. *J Neurol Sci* 2011;307:100–105.
44. Jokinen H, Ryberg C, Kalska H, et al. Corpus callosum atrophy is associated with mental slowing and executive deficits in subjects with age-related white matter hyperintensities: the LADIS study. *J Neurol Neurosurg Psychiatry* 2007;78:491–496.
45. Ryberg C, Rostrup E, Stegmann MB, et al. Clinical significance of corpus callosum atrophy in a mixed elderly population. *Neurobiol Aging* 2007;28:955–963.
46. Di Paola M, Luders E, Di Iulio F, et al. Callosal atrophy in mild cognitive impairment and Alzheimer's disease: different effects in different stages. *Neuroimage* 2010;49:141–149.
47. Teipel SJ, Bayer W, Alexander GE, et al. Progression of corpus callosum atrophy in Alzheimer disease. *Arch Neurol* 2002;59:243–248.
48. Frederiksen KS, Garde E, Skimminge A, et al. Corpus callosum tissue loss and development of motor and global cognitive impairment: the LADIS study. *Dement Geriatr Cogn Disord* 2011;32:279–286.
49. Roman GC, Erkinjuntti T, Wallin A, Pantoni L, Chui HC. Subcortical ischaemic vascular dementia. *Lancet Neurol* 2002;1:426–436.
50. Vermeer SE, Den Heijer T, Koudstaal PJ, et al. Incidence and risk factors of silent brain infarcts in the population-based Rotterdam Scan Study. *Stroke* 2003;34:392–396.
51. Carey CL, Kramer JH, Josephson SA, et al. Subcortical lacunes are associated with executive dysfunction in cognitively normal elderly. *Stroke* 2008;39:397–402.
52. Benisty S, Gouw AA, Porcher R, et al. Location of lacunar infarcts correlates with cognition in a sample of non-disabled subjects with age-related white-matter changes: the LADIS study. *J Neurol Neurosurg Psychiatry* 2009;80:478–483.
53. Loeb C, Gandolfo C, Crose R, Conti M. Dementia associated with lacunar infarction. *Stroke* 1992;23:1225–1229.

54. Miyao S, Takano A, Teramoto J, Takahashi A. Leukoaraiosis in relation to prognosis for patients with lacunar infarction. *Stroke* 1992;23:1434–1438.

55. Gold G, Kovari E, Herrmann FR, et al. Cognitive consequences of thalamic, basal ganglia, and deep white matter lacunes in brain aging and dementia. *Stroke* 2005;36:1184–1188.

56. Jokinen H, Gouw AA, Madureira S, et al. Incident lacunes influence cognitive decline: the LADIS study. *Neurology* 2011;76:1872–1878.

57. Viswanathan A, Gschwendtner A, Guichard JP, et al. Lacunar lesions are independently associated with disability and cognitive impairment in CADASIL. *Neurology* 2007;69:172–179.

58. Liem MK, van der Grond J, Haan J, et al. Lacunar infarcts are the main correlate with cognitive dysfunction in CADASIL. *Stroke* 2007;38:923–928.

59. Snowdon D, Greiner L, Mortimer J, et al. Brain infarction and the clinical expression of Alzheimer disease. *JAMA* 1997;277:813–817.

60. Jellinger KA, Attems J. Incidence of cerebrovascular lesions in Alzheimer's disease: a postmortem study. *Acta Neuropathol* 2003;105:14–17.

61. Van de Pol LA, Korf ES, van der Flier WM, et al. Magnetic resonance imaging predictors of cognition in mild cognitive impairment. *Arch Neurol* 2007;64:1023–1028.

62. Hanyu H, Tanaka Y, Shimizu S, et al. Cerebral microbleeds in Binswanger's disease: a gradient-echo T2*-weighted magnetic resonance imaging study. *Neurosci Lett* 2003;340:213–216.

63. Poels MM, Vernooij MW, Ikram MA, et al. Prevalence and risk factors of cerebral microbleeds: an update of the Rotterdam Scan Study. *Stroke* 2010;41:S103–S106.

64. Cordonnier C, van der Flier WM. Brain microbleeds and Alzheimer's disease: innocent observation or key player? *Brain* 2011;134:335–344.

65. Seo SW, Hwa Lee B, Kim EJ, et al. Clinical significance of microbleeds in subcortical vascular dementia. *Stroke* 2007;38:1949–1951.

66. Gregoire SM, Smith K, Jager HR, et al. Cerebral microbleeds and long-term cognitive outcome: longitudinal cohort study of stroke clinic patients. *Cerebrovasc Dis* 2012;33:430–435.

67. Werring DJ, Frazer DW, Coward LJ, et al. Cognitive dysfunction in patients with cerebral microbleeds on T2*-weighted gradient-echo MRI. *Brain* 2004;127:2265–2275.

68. Qiu C, Cotch MF, Sigurdsson S, et al. Cerebral microbleeds, retinopathy, and dementia: the Ages–Reykjavik study. *Neurology* 2010;75:2221–2228.

69. Poels MM, Ikram MA, van der Lugt A, et al. Cerebral microbleeds are associated with worse cognitive function: the Rotterdam Scan Study. *Neurology* 2012;78:326–333.

70. Van Norden AG, van den Berg HA, de Laat KF, et al. Frontal and temporal microbleeds are related to cognitive function: the Radboud University Nijmegen Diffusion Tensor and Magnetic Resonance Cohort (RUN DMC) study. *Stroke* 2011;42:3382–3386.

71. Van Es AC, van der Grond J, de Craen AJ, et al. Cerebral microbleeds and cognitive functioning in the PROSPER study. *Neurology* 2011;77:1446–1452.

72. Takashima Y, Mori T, Hashimoto M, et al. Clinical correlating factors and cognitive function in community-dwelling healthy subjects with cerebral microbleeds. *J Stroke Cerebrovasc Dis* 2011;20:105–110.

73. Yakushiji Y, Nishiyama M, Yakushiji S, et al. Brain microbleeds and global cognitive function in adults without neurological disorder. *Stroke* 2008;39:3323–3328.

74. Tang WK, Chen YK, Lu JY, et al. Absence of cerebral microbleeds predicts reversion of vascular "cognitive impairment no dementia" in stroke. *Int J Stroke* 2011;6:498–505.

75. Ayaz M, Boikov AS, Haacke EM, Kido DK, Kirsch WM. Imaging cerebral microbleeds using susceptibility weighted imaging: one step toward detecting vascular dementia. *J Magn Reson Imaging* 2010;31:142–148.

76. Goos JD, Kester MI, Barkhof F, et al. Patients with Alzheimer disease with multiple microbleeds: relation with cerebrospinal fluid biomarkers and cognition. *Stroke* 2009;40:3455–3460.

77. Yakushiji Y, Noguchi T, Hara M, et al. Distributional impact of brain microbleeds on global cognitive function in adults without neurological disorder. *Stroke* 2012;43:1800–1805.

78. Cordonnier C, van der Flier WM, Sluimer JD, et al. Prevalence and severity of microbleeds in a memory clinic setting. *Neurology* 2006;66:1356–1360.

79. Nardone R, De Blasi P, Seidl M, et al. Cognitive function and cholinergic transmission in patients with subcortical vascular dementia and microbleeds: a TMS study. *J Neural Transm* 2011;118:1349–1358.

80. Liem MK, Lesnik Oberstein SA, Haan J, et al. MRI correlates of cognitive decline in CADASIL: a seven-year follow-up study. *Neurology* 2009;72:143–148.

81. Kirsch W, McAuley G, Holshouser B, et al. Serial susceptibility weighted MRI measures brain iron and microbleeds in dementia. *J Alzheimers Dis* 2009;17:599–609.

82. Pettersen JA, Sathiyamoorthy G, Gao FQ, et al. Microbleed topography, leukoaraiosis, and cognition in probable Alzheimer disease from the Sunnybrook Dementia Study. *Arch Neurol* 2008;65:790–795.

83. Tyas SL, Salazar JC, Snowdon DA, et al. Transitions to mild cognitive impairments, dementia, and death: findings from the Nun Study. *Am J Epidemiol* 2007;165:1231–1238.

84. Madureira S, Verdelho A, Ferro J, et al. Development of a neuropsychological battery for the Leukoaraiosis And DISability in the elderly (LADIS) study: experience and baseline data. *Neuroepidemiology* 2006;27:101–116.

85. Dufouil C, Alperovitch A, Tzourio C. Influence of education on the relationship between white matter lesions and cognition. *Neurology* 2003;60:831–836.

86. Biessels GJ, Staekenborg S, Brunner E, Brayne C, Scheltens P. Risk of dementia in diabetes mellitus: a systematic review. *Lancet Neurol* 2006;5:64–74.

87. Henon H, Pasquier F, Leys D. Poststroke dementia. *Cerebrovasc Dis* 2006;22:61–70.

88. Kivipelto M, Helkala EL, Laakso MP, et al. Midlife vascular risk factors and Alzheimer's disease in later life: longitudinal, population based study. *BMJ* 2001;322:1447–1451.

89. Launer LJ, Ross GW, Petrovitch H, et al. Midlife blood pressure and dementia: the Honolulu–Asia Aging Study. *Neurobiol Aging* 2000;21:49–55.

90. Qiu C, Winblad B, Fratiglioni L. Low diastolic pressure and risk of dementia in very old people: a longitudinal study. *Dement Geriatr Cogn Disord* 2009;28:213–219.

91. Razay G, Williams J, King E, Smith AD, Wilcock G. Blood pressure, dementia and Alzheimer's disease: the OPTIMA longitudinal study. *Dement Geriatr Cogn Disord* 2009;28:70–74.

92. Stewart R, Xue QL, Masaki K, et al. Change in blood pressure and incident dementia: a 32-year prospective study. *Hypertension* 2009;54:233–240.

93. Hebert LE, Scherr PA, Bennett DA, et al. Blood pressure and late-life cognitive function change: a biracial longitudinal population study. *Neurology* 2004;62:2021–2024.

94. Shah RC, Wilson RS, Bienias JL, et al. Relation of blood pressure to risk of incident Alzheimer's disease and change in global cognitive function in older persons. *Neuroepidemiology* 2006;26:30–36.

95. Di Carlo A, Baldereschi M, Amaducci L, et al. Cognitive impairment without dementia in older people: prevalence, vascular risk factors, impact on disability. The Italian Longitudinal Study on Aging. *J Am Geriatr Soc* 2000;48:775–782.

96. Cerhan JR, Folsom AR, Mortimer JA, et al. Correlates of cognitive function in middle-aged adults. Atherosclerosis Risk in Communities (ARIC) study investigators. *Gerontology* 1998;44:95–105.

97. Budge MM, de Jager C, Hogervorst E, Smith AD. Total plasma homocysteine, age, systolic blood pressure, and cognitive performance in older people. *J Am Geriatr Soc* 2002;50:2014–2018.

98. Kilander L, Nyman H, Boberg M, Hansson L, Lithell H. Hypertension is related to cognitive impairment: a 20-year follow-up of 999 men. *Hypertension* 1998;31:780–786.

99. Cacciatore F, Abete P, Ferrara N, et al. The role of blood pressure in cognitive impairment in an elderly population. Osservatorio Geriatrico Campano Group. *J Hypertens* 1997;15:135–142.

100. Gorelick PB, Scuteri A, Black SE, et al. Vascular contributions to cognitive impairment and dementia: a statement for healthcare professionals from the American Heart Association/ American Stroke Association. *Stroke* 2011;42:2672–2713.

101. McGuinness B, Todd S, Passmore P, Bullock R. Blood pressure lowering in patients without prior cerebrovascular disease for prevention of cognitive impairment and dementia. *Cochrane Database Syst Rev* 2009;4:CD004034.

102. Guan JW, Huang CQ, Li YH, et al. No association between hypertension and risk for Alzheimer's disease: a meta-analysis of longitudinal studies. *J Alzheimers Dis* 2011;27:799–807.

103. Chang-Quan H, Hui W, Chao-Min W, et al. The association of antihypertensive medication use with risk of cognitive decline and dementia: a meta-analysis of longitudinal studies. *Int J Clin Pract* 2011;65:1295–1305.

104. SHEP Cooperative Research Group. Prevention of stroke by antihypertensive drug treatment in older persons with isolated systolic hypertension. Final results of the Systolic Hypertension in the Elderly Program (SHEP). *JAMA* 1991;265:3255–3264.

105. Lithell H, Hansson L, Skoog I, et al. The Study on Cognition and Prognosis in the Elderly (SCOPE): principal results of a randomized double-blind intervention trial. *J Hypertens* 2003;21:875–886.

106. Peters R, Beckett N, Forette F, et al. Incident dementia and blood pressure lowering in the Hypertension in the Very Elderly Trial cognitive function assessment (HYVET-cog): a double-blind, placebo controlled trial. *Lancet Neurol* 2008;7:683–689.

107. Yusuf S, Diener HC, Sacco RL, et al. Telmisartan to prevent

recurrent stroke and cardiovascular events. *N Engl J Med* 2008;359:1225–1237.

108. Forette F, Seux ML, Staessen JA, et al. Prevention of dementia in randomised double-blind placebo-controlled systolic hypertension in Europe (SYST-Eur) trial. *Lancet* 1998;352:1347–1351.

109. Tzourio C, Anderson C, Chapman N, et al. Effects of blood pressure lowering with perindopril and indapamide therapy on dementia and cognitive decline in patients with cerebrovascular disease. *Arch Intern Med* 2003;163: 1069–1075.

110. Cukierman T, Gerstein HC, Williamson JD. Cognitive decline and dementia in diabetes – systematic overview of prospective observational studies. *Diabetologia* 2005;48:2460–2469.

111. Luchsinger JA. Adiposity, hyperinsulinemia, diabetes and Alzheimer's disease: an epidemiological perspective. *Eur J Pharmacol* 2008;585:119–129.

112. Yaffe K, Falvey C, Hamilton N, et al. Diabetes, glucose control, and nine-year cognitive decline among older adults without dementia. *Arch Neurol* 2012;69:1170–1175.

113. Wang KC, Woung LC, Tsai MT, et al. Risk of Alzheimer's disease in relation to diabetes: a population-based cohort study. *Neuroepidemiology* 2012;38:237–244.

114. Kaffashian S, Dugravot A, Brunner EJ, et al. Midlife stroke risk and cognitive decline: a 10-year follow-up of the Whitehall II Cohort Study. *Alzheimers Dement* 2013;9:572-579.

115. Cheng G, Huang C, Deng H, Wang H. Diabetes as a risk factor for dementia and mild cognitive impairment: a meta-analysis of longitudinal studies. *Intern Med J* 2012;42:484–491.

116. Arvanitakis Z, Wilson RS, Bienias JL, Evans DA, Bennett DA. Diabetes mellitus and risk of Alzheimer disease and decline in cognitive function. *Arch Neurol* 2004;61:661–666.

117. Manschot SM, Brands AM, van der Grond J, et al. Brain magnetic resonance imaging correlates of impaired cognition in patients with type 2 diabetes. *Diabetes* 2006;55:1106–1113.

118. Liu F, Shi J, Tanimukai H, et al. Reduced O-glcNacylation links lower brain glucose metabolism and tau pathology in Alzheimer's disease. *Brain* 2009;132:1820–1832.

119. De la Monte SM. Brain insulin resistance and deficiency as therapeutic targets in Alzheimer's disease. *Curr Alzheimer Res* 2012;9:35–66.

120. Reitz C, Bos MJ, Hofman A, Koudstaal PJ, Breteler MM. Prestroke cognitive performance, incident stroke, and risk of dementia: the Rotterdam Study. *Stroke* 2008;39:36–41.

121. Douiri A, Rudd AG, Wolfe CD. Prevalence of poststroke cognitive impairment: South London Stroke Register 1995–2010. *Stroke* 2013;44:138–145.

122. Savva GM, Stephan BC. Epidemiological studies of the effect of stroke on incident dementia: a systematic review. *Stroke* 2010;41:e41–46.

123. Grau-Olivares M, Arboix A, Bartres-Faz D, Junque C. Neuropsychological abnormalities associated with lacunar infarction. *J Neurol Sci* 2007;257:160–165.

124. Jacova C, Pearce LA, Costello R, et al. Cognitive impairment in lacunar strokes: the SPS3 trial. *Ann Neurol* 2012;72:351–362.

125. Kivipelto M, Ngandu T, Fratiglioni L, et al. Obesity and vascular risk factors at midlife and the risk of dementia and Alzheimer disease. *Arch Neurol* 2005;62:1556–1560.

126. Purnell C, Gao S, Callahan CM, Hendrie HC. Cardiovascular risk factors and incident Alzheimer disease: a systematic review of the literature. *Alzheimer Dis Assoc Disord* 2009;23:1–10.

127. Unverzagt FW, McClure LA, Wadley VG, et al. Vascular risk factors and cognitive impairment in a stroke-free cohort. *Neurology* 2011;77:1729–1736.

128. Li L, Wang Y, Yan J, et al. Clinical predictors of cognitive decline in patients with mild cognitive impairment: the Chongqing Aging Study. *J Neurol* 2012;259:1303–1311.

129. Deschaintre Y, Richard F, Leys D, Pasquier F. Treatment of vascular risk factors is associated with slower decline in Alzheimer disease. *Neurology* 2009;73:674–680.

130. Folstein M, Folstein S, McHugh PJ. Mini-Mental State: a practical method for grading the cognitive state of patients for clinicians. *J Psychiatr Res* 1975;12:189–198.

131. Smith EE, Egorova S, Blacker D, et al. Magnetic resonance imaging white matter hyperintensities and brain volume in the prediction of mild cognitive impairment and dementia. *Arch Neurol* 2008;65:94–100.

132. Van der Flier WM, van der Vlies AE, Weverling-Rijnsburger AW, et al. MRI measures and progression of cognitive decline in nondemented elderly attending a memory clinic. *Int J Geriatr Psychiatry* 2005;20:1060–1066.

133. Pantoni L, Basile AM, Pracucci G, et al. Impact of age-related cerebral white matter changes on the transition to disability – the LADIS study: rationale, design and methodology. *Neuroepidemiology* 2005;24:51–62.

134. Fure B, Bruun Wyller T, Engedal K, Thommessen B. Cognitive impairments in acute lacunar stroke. *Acta Neurol Scand* 2006;114:17–22.

135. Roth M, Tym E, Mountjoy CQ, et al. CAMDEX. A standardised instrument for the diagnosis of mental disorder in the elderly with special reference to the early detection of dementia. *Br J Psychiatry* 1986;149:698–709.

136. Rosen W, Mohs R, Davis K. A new rating scale for Alzheimer's disease. *Am J Psychiatry* 1984;141:1356–1364.

137. Ferris S. General measures of cognition. *Int Psychogeriatr* 2003;15:215–217.

138. Ylikoski R, Jokinen H, Andersen P, et al. Comparison of the Alzheimer's Disease Assessment Scale cognitive subscale and the Vascular Dementia Assessment Scale in differentiating elderly individuals with different degrees of white matter changes. The LADIS study. *Dement Geriatr Cogn Disord* 2007;24:73–81.

139. Madureira S, Verdelho A, Moleiro C, et al. Neuropsychological predictors of dementia in a three-year follow-up period: data from the LADIS study. *Dement Geriatr Cogn Disord* 2010;29:325–334.

140. Nasreddine ZS, Phillips NA, Bedirian V, et al. The Montreal Cognitive Assessment, MoCA: a brief screening tool for mild cognitive impairment. *J Am Geriatr Soc* 2005;53:695–699.

141. Wong A, Xiong YY, Kwan PW, et al. The validity, reliability and clinical utility of the Hong Kong Montreal Cognitive Assessment (HK-MoCA) in patients with cerebral small vessel disease. *Dement Geriatr Cogn Disord* 2009;28:81–87.

142. Ishikawa H, Meguro K, Ishii H, Tanaka N, Yamaguchi S. Silent infarction or white matter hyperintensity and impaired attention task scores in a nondemented population: the Osaki–Tajiri Project. *J Stroke Cerebrovasc Dis* 2012;21:275–282.

143. Hachinski V, Iadecola C, Petersen RC, et al. National Institute of Neurological Disorders and Stroke–Canadian Stroke Network vascular cognitive impairment harmonization standards. *Stroke* 2006;37:2220–2241.

144. Stroop JR. Studies of interference in serial verbal reactions. *J Exp Psychol* 1935;18:643–662.

145. Reitan R. Validity of the Trail Making test as an indicator of organic brain damage. *Percept Mot Skills* 1958;8:271–276.

146. Jokinen H, Kalska H, Mantyla R, et al. White matter hyperintensities as a predictor of neuropsychological deficits post-stroke. *J Neurol Neurosurg Psychiatry* 2005;76:1229–1233.

147. Jokinen H, Kalska H, Mantyla R, et al. Cognitive profile of subcortical ischaemic vascular disease. *J Neurol Neurosurg Psychiatry* 2006;77:28–33.

148. Zhou A, Jia J. Different cognitive profiles between mild cognitive impairment due to cerebral small vessel disease and mild cognitive impairment of Alzheimer's disease origin. *J Int Neuropsychol Soc* 2009;15:898–905.

149. Heaton R, Chelune G, Talley JL, Kay G, Curtiss G. *Wisconsin Card Sorting Test Manual: Revised and Expanded.* Odessa, FL: Psychological Assessment Resources; 1993.

150. Ylikoski R, Ylikoski A, Erkinjuntti T, et al. White matter changes in healthy elderly persons correlate with attention and speed of mental processing. *Arch Neurol* 1993;50:818–824.

151. Junque C, Pujol J, Vendrell P, et al. Leuko-araiosis on magnetic resonance imaging and speed of mental processing. *Arch Neurol* 1990;47:151–156.

152. Duering M, Zieren N, Herve D, et al. Strategic role of frontal white matter tracts in vascular cognitive impairment: a voxel-based lesion-symptom mapping study in CADASIL. *Brain* 2011; 134:2366–2375.

153. Cummings JL. Frontal–subcortical circuits and human behavior. *J Psychosom Res* 1998;44:627–628.

154. Tekin S, Cummings JL. Frontal–subcortical neuronal circuits and clinical neuropsychiatry: an update. *J Psychosom Res* 2002;53:647–654.

155. Behrens TE, Johansen-Berg H, Woolrich MW, et al. Non-invasive mapping of connections between human thalamus and cortex using diffusion imaging. *Nat Neurosci* 2003;6:750–757.

156. Meguro K, Constans JM, Shimada M, et al. Corpus callosum atrophy, white matter lesions, and frontal executive dysfunction in normal aging and Alzheimer's disease. A community-based study: the Tajiri Project. *Int Psychogeriatr* 2003;15:9–25.

157. Jokinen H, Frederiksen KS, Garde E, et al. Callosal tissue loss parallels subtle decline in psychomotor speed. A longitudinal quantitative MRI study. The LADIS study. *Neuropsychologia* 2012;50:1650–1655.

158. Wright CB, Festa JR, Paik MC, et al. White matter hyperintensities and subclinical infarction: associations with psychomotor speed and cognitive flexibility. *Stroke* 2008;39:800–805.

159. Paul R, Lane E, Jefferson A. Vascular cognitive impairment. In Ravdin LD, Katzen HL, eds. *Handbook on the Neuropsychology of Aging and Dementia.* New York, NY: Springer; 2012: pp. 281–294.

160. De Mendonca A, Ribeiro F, Guerreiro M, Palma T, Garcia C. Clinical significance of subcortical vascular disease in patients with mild cognitive impairment. *Eur J Neurol* 2005;12:125–130.

161. Loewenstein DA, Acevedo A, Agron J, et al. Cognitive profiles in Alzheimer's disease and in mild cognitive impairment of different

etiologies. *Dement Geriatr Cogn Disord* 2006;21:309–315.

162. Nordahl CW, Ranganath C, Yonelinas AP, et al. Different mechanisms of episodic memory failure in mild cognitive impairment. *Neuropsychologia* 2005;43:1688–1697.

163. Jokinen H, Lipsanen J, Schmidt R, et al. Brain atrophy accelerates cognitive decline in cerebral small vessel disease: the LADIS study. *Neurology* 2012;78:1785–1792.

164. Kennedy KM, Raz N. Aging white matter and cognition: differential effects of regional variations in diffusion properties on memory, executive functions, and speed. *Neuropsychologia* 2009;47:916–927.

165. Van der Holst HM, Tuladhar AM, van Norden AG, et al. Microstructural integrity of the cingulum is related to verbal memory performance in elderly with cerebral small vessel disease: the RUN DMC study. *Neuroimage* 2012;65C:416–423.

166. Van Norden AG, de Laat KF, Fick I, et al. Diffusion tensor imaging of the hippocampus and verbal memory performance: the RUN DMC study. *Hum Brain Mapp* 2012;33:542–551.

167. Kertesz A, Polk M, Carr T. Cognition and white matter changes on magnetic resonance imaging in dementia. *Arch Neurol* 1990;47:387–391.

168. Canning SJ, Leach L, Stuss D, Ngo L, Black SE. Diagnostic utility of abbreviated fluency measures in Alzheimer disease and vascular dementia. *Neurology* 2004;62:556–562.

169. Rao SM, Mittenberg W, Bernardin L. Neuropsychological test findings in subject with leukoaraiosis. *Arch Neurol* 1989;46:40–44.

170. Hunt AL, Orrison WW, Yeo RA. Clinical significance of MRI white matter lesions in the elderly. *Neurology* 1989;39:1470–1474.

171. Breteler M, van Amerongen N, van Swieten J, et al. Cognitive correlates of ventricular enlargement and cerebral white matter lesions on magnetic resonance imaging. The Rotterdam Study. *Stroke* 1994;25:1109–1115.

172. Almkvist O, Wahlund LO, Andersson-Lundman G, Basun H, Backman L. White-matter hyperintensity and neuropsychological functions in dementia and healthy aging. *Arch Neurol* 1992;49:626–632.

173. Kertesz A, Clydesdale S. Neuropsychological deficits in vascular dementia versus Alzheimer's disease. Frontal lobe deficits prominent in vascular dementia. *Arch Neurol* 1994;51:1226–1231.

174. Tiffin J, Asher EJ. The Purdue Pegboard: norms and studies of reliability and validity. *J Appl Psychol* 1948;32:234.

175. Marquine MJ, Attix DK, Goldstein LB, et al. Differential patterns of cognitive decline in anterior and posterior white matter hyperintensity progression. *Stroke* 2010;41:1946–1950.

176. Murray ME, Senjem ML, Petersen RC, et al. Functional impact of white matter hyperintensities in cognitively normal elderly subjects. *Arch Neurol* 2010;67:1379–1385.

Chapter 20

Motor, stance, and balance consequences of cerebral small vessel disease

Hansjoerg Baezner, Christian Blahak, and Michael G. Hennerici

Introduction

Gait and balance disturbances and falls are major symptoms of patients with cerebral small vessel disease (CSVD), and an important cause of morbidity and mortality in the elderly. Nevertheless, gait disorders and their impact on the burden of disability in the growing elderly population are under-represented in medical scientific literature. The absence of a clear framework for the diagnosis and classification of gait disorders caused by CSVD has multiple reasons: (1) neither movement disorder specialists nor stroke specialists are truly familiar with this topic and feel responsible for its treatment; (2) the existing terminology lacks a clear concept and a consistent classification; and (3) only in recent years have large prospective trials started to address the natural course of this condition.

Clearly, increasing age is not sufficient to explain the majority of cases. A promising theory to explain the progressive decline in motor abilities refers to the complex motor network that guarantees the integrity of central coordination of stance and gait. This network may be challenged through a critical amount of lesions in subcortical regions [1]. Motor deficits associated with CSVD present in different ways, such as unsteadiness of gait, impaired balance on walking, and increased risk of falls. Furthermore, gait abnormalities have been shown to predict non-Alzheimer's dementia, i.e., mainly vascular dementia [2].

The systematic analysis of a possible association of gait and balance disorders in CSVD started in the 1990s, when heterogeneous results were reported from different study populations, including population-based groups of healthy elderly but also cohorts of severely disabled patients [3, 4]. Moreover, only a few studies provided prospective data [5, 6]. In the recent decade, larger systematic studies confirmed an association of the severity of CSVD with the severity of gait problems and falls both in cross-sectional and in longitudinal studies [7–10]. Hence, recognition and early diagnosis of this disabling condition will be feasible by early detection of gait abnormalities. As a future step, there is an urgent need to aim at preventive medical treatment.

Historical and modern classification of gait and balance disorders in patients with CSVD

Unfortunately, diagnosis of gait and postural problems is incapacitated by the lack of a clear framework for classification [1]. This is rather amazing, because extensively detailed descriptions have existed for more than 100 years. The terminology, however, is quite confusing, due to the existence of more than a dozen terms for the same type of gait disturbance.

Recent efforts to classify gait disturbances yielded rather unsuitable solutions for this important problem, because they consist of a mixture of presumed anatomic location and of clinical phenomenology, or use the much debated notion of apraxia [11].

Therefore, we propose to avoid anatomic and disease references (such as frontal gait or hydrocephalic gait) and to stay with the clinically relevant elements of stance and gait. Proposals like the "higher level gait disorders" are unsuitable because they do not provide clear-cut definitions and mix presumed anatomic location and clinical phenomenology.

We suggest classifying gait disorders in CSVD and other "higher level" gait disorders as follows:

1. Locomotion failure (LF)
2. Postural control failure (PCF)
3. Gait ignition failure and freezing (GIF).

Cerebral Small Vessel Disease, ed. Leonardo Pantoni and Philip B. Gorelick. Published by Cambridge University Press.

Table 20.1 Grading of gait disturbance in small vessel disease

Gait disturbance	Grade 1	Grade 2	Grade 3
Locomotion failure	Mild unsteadiness, walks slowly, small steps, broadened base, regular rhythm	Severe unsteadiness, breakdown of gait rhythm with irregular step length and timing	Unable to walk
Postural control failure	Difficulties with turns and on stairs without handrail, occasional falls	Stands with minor support, falls if unsupported when turning or raising from chair	Unable to stand unsupported
Gait ignition failure and freezing	Mild start hesitation, occasional freezing	Severe start hesitation, frequent freezing	Unable to initiate walking

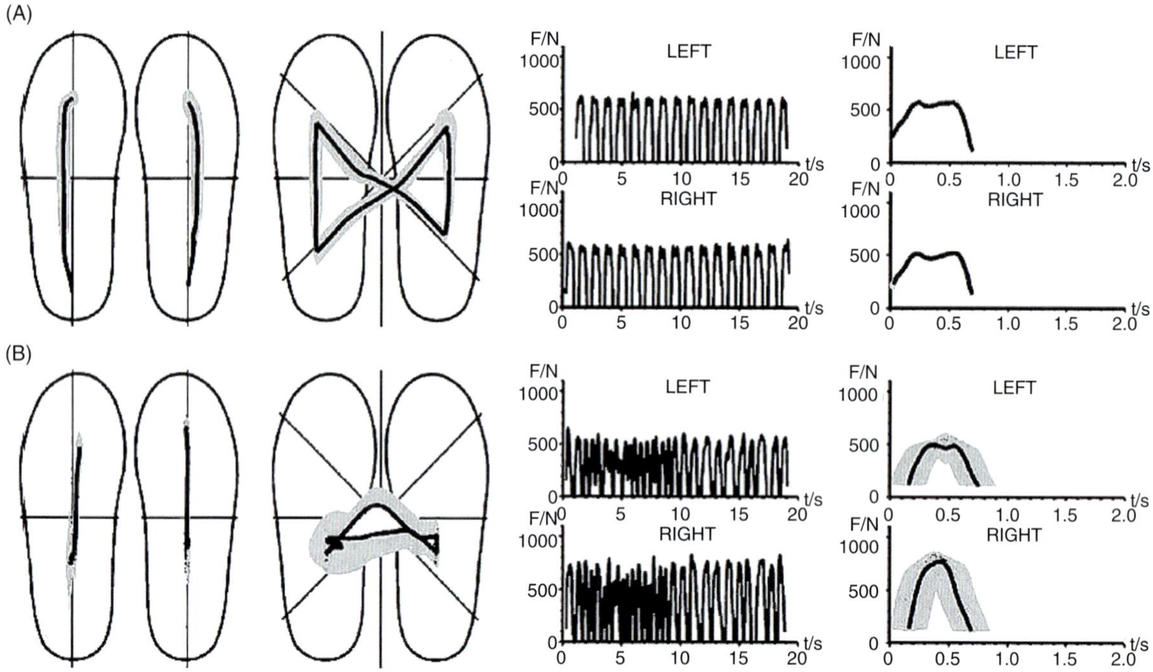

Figure 20.1 Gait pattern in a healthy person (A) and gait disturbances in a patient with small vessel disease (B), measured with the Computer Dyno Graphy gait analysis system.

According to symptom severity, we suggest classifying the patients into three categories indicating mild, moderate, or severe disturbances (Table 20.1).

Certainly, many patients show overlaps of two or three of the above mentioned categories and will have to be classified into "mixed" categories. On the other hand, previous categories will easily be placed in either category, or overlaps of two categories, or the full picture of all three components, which reflects the often progressive course of the syndrome starting with mild PCF and progressing to additional gait ignition and LF.

In our clinical experience, most patients present with slowing of gait, small shuffling steps, and a broad base in gait and stance. A further early feature is a mild disturbance of postural control. Later in the course, patients may show gait initiation failure, magnetic feet, and dysrhythmic steps (Figure 20.1).

Clinical tests to measure these syndromes quantitatively include walking speed and rhythmicity for LF, as well as chair stands, tandem stand, and single leg stand for PCF. GIF are clinically easy to diagnose. However, to rely exclusively on clinical observations leads to uncertainty in long-term follow-up. Therefore, the application of instrumental gait analysis has been shown to be useful to measure gait abnormalities in CSVD, because results are reproducible and can be compared independently of the rater over the course of many years [5]. If instrumental computerized analysis is not available, clinical scales using rater-independent simple clinical tests will be sufficient to control for progressive versus stable conditions.

The LADIS study

One of the main goals of the Leukoaraiosis And DISability (LADIS) study was to analyze the strength of association of gait and balance disturbances with the degree of CSVD reflected in the severity of age-related white matter changes (ARWMCs) [12]. In order to quantify motor performance, several clinical measures, including the Short Physical Performance Battery, single leg stance time, and walking speed, have been used in a large study sample consisting of a clinically well-defined group and originating from a prospective, prestandardized study. The results of this study are now available both in cross-section and in longitudinal-section analysis.

LADIS: cross-sectional results

In the LADIS study, 11 European centers evaluated the role of ARWMCs as an independent determinant of the transition to disability in the elderly (65–84 years). Since previous smaller studies had reported conflicting results as to the impact of ARWMCs on gait and motor abilities in cross-sectional analysis, the aim was to determine their influence on different objective measures of gait and balance.

Six hundred and thirty-nine nondisabled individuals were prospectively enrolled and followed-up for three years. At baseline and during follow-up, subjects were graded in three standardized categories of ARWMCs (mild, moderate, and severe) according to central magnetic resonance imaging (MRI) readings.

In order to assess the occurrence and severity of gait and motor disturbances, a test battery was chosen, including the Short Physical Performance Battery (SPPB) [13, 14]. This test battery comprises three simple tests of gait and balance (Figure 20.2). Balance was tested by scoring stand, semitandem stand, tandem stand, and repetitive chair stands. In addition, walking speed was measured. A composite score with a maximum of 12 points and a minimum of 0 points was calculated by adding stands score (0–4 points), walk score (0–4 points), and chair stands (0–4 points). Two additional simple measures of gait and balance (gait velocity, single leg stance time) were performed. Gait velocity was calculated after individuals walked at their usual pace on an 8 m course. Single Leg Stance Time was measured by asking individuals, with hands on hips, to balance as long as possible on one leg with an upper limit of 30 seconds.

In cross-sectional analysis, deficiencies in motor performance were correlated with the severity of

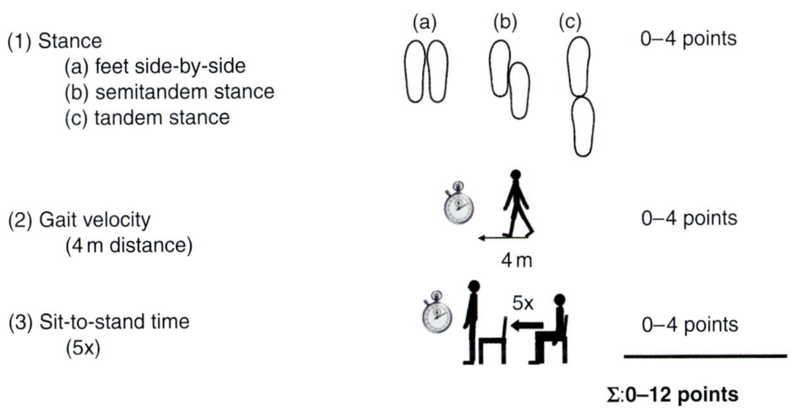

Figure 20.2 The Short Physical Performance Battery: a simple test to assess gait and balance function [13, 14].

ARWMCs reflected in SPPB scores of 10.2 ± 2.1 in the mild, 9.9 ± 2.0 in the moderate, and significantly worse with a score of 8.9 ± 2.6 in the severe group ($P<0.001$). Walking speed was reduced depending on the severity of ARWMCs (1.24 ± 0.28 m/s in the mild, 1.18 ± 0.32 m/s in the moderate, and 1.09 ± 0.31 m/s in the severe group, $P<0.001$). Balance as reflected in single leg stance time was worst in individuals with severe ARWMCs (13.6 ± 11.2s) compared to moderate and mild ARWMCs (16.4 ± 10.8 s and 18.9 ± 10.8 s, $P<0.001$). These results remained stable after correction for several sociodemographic factors and for various prespeçified factors interfering with gait and balance. Physically inactive individuals had a significantly higher risk of a pathologic SPPB score (moderate vs. mild ARWMC: odds ratio [OR] 1.60, 95% confidence interval [CI] 1.02–2.52; severe vs. mild ARWMC: OR 1.75, 95% CI 1.09–2.80) [10].

These cross-sectional results of the LADIS study had shown a clear-cut relationship between the severity of ARWMCs and the severity of gait and motor compromise. Physical activity was associated with a reduced risk of limitations in mobility [10].

LADIS: longitudinal results

For the longitudinal data analysis we focused on the potential change of SPPB scores over time versus the severity of ARWMC.

Overall, LADIS participants' lower body motor function deteriorated as measured by a decline in the SPPB score of 2.6% per year. However, after adjustment for baseline motor impairment and potential confounders, only subjects with moderate (0.22 points/year on the SPPB [= 2.3%]; 95% CI 0.09–0.35, $P<0.01$) or severe (0.46 points/year [= 4.7%]; 95% CI 0.28–0.63, $P<0.001$) degrees of ARWMCs showed a decline in balance and gait ability. Interestingly, age showed a differential effect: relatively younger subjects across all degrees of ARWMC severity had comparable temporal dynamics of SPPB change; subjects with severe ARWMCs but older than 75.9 years deteriorated significantly more rapidly than their counterparts with only mild or moderate white matter pathology [15].

In conclusion, the LADIS study has shown that only moderate and severe CSVD are independently associated with a deterioration of lower body motor function.

Evidence of an association between CSVD and gait disturbances originating from large-scale prospective studies

Few large population-based studies of community-dwelling disability-free elderly have provided data supporting the clinical observation that a greater burden of white matter pathology is associated with a more pronounced increase in gait impairment over time.

In the Cardiovascular Health Study, Rosano et al. [7] studied brain MRI abnormalities, such as ventricular enlargement, white matter hyperintensities (WMHs), subcortical and basal ganglia small brain infarcts. They asked participants for physical impairment (difficulty walking half a mile or with one or more Activities of Daily Living), and studied motor performance (gait speed, timed chair stand) for an average follow-up of four years.

These authors found a 35% greater risk of incident self-reported physical impairment for those participants with severe ventricular enlargement than for those with minimal ventricular enlargement, a 22% greater risk for those with moderate white matter lesions (WMLs) than for those with minimal WMLs, and a 26% greater risk for participants with at least one brain infarct than for those with no infarcts. Interestingly, participants with moderate to severe brain abnormalities experienced faster gait speed decline than those with no MRI abnormalities.

Soumaré et al. [9] postulated a threshold effect of WML load: a pathologic change in the white matter will be compensated up to a certain degree without leading to functional decline. Once this threshold is surpassed, subjects will show impairment.

WMLs as independent predictors of physical decline have been shown in a recent longitudinal study comprising 287 community-dwelling people aged 70–90 years [16]. In multivariate logistic regression analyses, people with WML volumes in the fourth quartile showed greater physical decline (OR 3.02, 95% CI 1.02–8.95) while controlling for age, baseline physical function, general health, physical activity, and cognitive function. The strongest associations with physical decline could be shown for WMHs in the deep frontoparietal and periventricular parieto-occipital regions.

In a series of publications originating from the same study population of 431 independently living, nondemented elderly aged between 50 and 85 years with CSVD, de Laat et al. [8, 17, 18] found that in cross-sectional analysis WMLs and lacunar infarcts were associated with a series of quantitatively assessed gait parameters, the most sensitive of which was stride length. Furthermore, they were able to show using MR diffusion tensor imaging (DTI) of white matter integrity that WMLs in the centrum semiovale and frontal periventricular regions were associated with deterioration in several gait parameters. Interestingly, the same was true for a reduction of integrity in areas of normal-appearing white matter. The authors conclude that particularly the loss of fibers interconnecting bilateral cortical regions, especially in the prefrontal cortex, may be an important determinant of gait disorders in the elderly. Importantly, areas especially relevant to cognitive control of motor processing, such as callosal fibers of the genu projecting to prefrontal areas, were shown to be affected. Finally, the same group has recently shown that cortical atrophy is part of the disease process and a further finding associated with gait impairment in patients with CSVD [19].

Summarizing these data and citing a recent meta-analysis [20], CSVD is commonly associated with disturbances of balance and gait, although in most studies, they are only evident in patients with the most severe degree of CSVD.

Role of falls and balance disturbances in impaired mobility in the elderly

Other important factors contributing to impaired mobility in elderly people are falls and balance disturbances. Over one third of older people have one or more falls per year, with approximately half of these resulting in injuries [21]. Among older people, falls account for >10% of emergency admissions and are the leading cause of injury-related deaths [21–23]. Recurrent falls are associated with physical decline and disability, resulting in psychosocial problems and a significant reduction in quality of life [24]. Thus, falls and related injuries result in substantial medical and socioeconomic burdens [24, 25].

Various risk factors for falls have been proposed, among them visual impairment, functional limitations in daily living, an abnormal postural sway, and an increased gait and stride variability [24, 26, 27]. Several neurodegenerative disorders, such as Parkinson's disease [28], Alzheimer's disease, and various conditions associated with cerebellar ataxia [29], and also psychiatric diseases, such as depression, are correlated with an increased risk of falls. In recent years, there is growing evidence that CSVD is also associated with impaired balance and an increased rate of falls in elderly people.

Association of balance disturbances with WMLs and CSVD

Several cross-sectional and longitudinal studies assessed the relationship between CSVD and impaired balance control in elderly people [30–35]. The first notable results on an association came from the Cardiovascular Health Study: in a substudy of more than 700 community-dwelling elderly people, WMLs were found to be correlated with poorer performance in balance tests using both clinical measures and dynamic posturography [31, 35].

As already mentioned above, in the LADIS study we could demonstrate a significant correlation between the global severity of CSVD and balance disturbances, as assessed by simple clinical tests like the single leg stance time and the stance subscore of the SPPB [32]. Impaired balance was found to be associated with deep frontal and periventricular WMLs, but not with parietal and periventricular WML regions despite a considerable prevalence of WMLs in all of these regions. In another community-based study, brainstem lesions also appeared to be associated with reduced balance control [33]. A single study suggested that the association between WMLs and balance might be influenced by gender, and reported a significant association between WMLs and single leg stance performance in men only [35].

The integration of complex interactions among sensory, motor, and central processes is an important aspect of balance control during quiet standing and, in the first instance, in dynamic circumstances like turning during gait. By using the diagnostic tool of a dynamic posturography with a force platform, Novak et al. [30] demonstrated a significant association of periventricular and focal WMLs with changes in certain balance measures in elderly community-living subjects without history of falls, in particular an increased sway in the mediolateral direction with more random fluctuations.

The first longitudinal data were collected by Whitman et al. [36], who compared the progression of WMLs in otherwise healthy people with impaired postural control. Subjects whose scores dropped more than four points on the Tinetti Performance Oriented Mobility score over four years had a greater increase in WML volume than those with unchanged scores. In another 10-year longitudinal study, Baloh et al. [6] also reported a correlation between yearly changes in the Tinetti Balance score and the WML severity.

Association of falls with WMLs and CSVD

A number of studies have investigated the association between WMLs and falls, and most of them reported that fallers have greater WML volumes compared with nonfallers [3, 6, 20, 32, 36–38]. The methodology to assess the fall rate, however, varied widely in these studies, in particular with regard to definition of falls, retrospective or prospective recording, quantification of WMLs, statistical analysis, and also study population, making it difficult to review and interpret the findings.

The strongest evidence for an association between WMLs and falls comes from three large prospective studies. In a population-based study of 294 elderly people over a 12-month observation period, the risk of falls was twice as high as in people with WML volumes in the highest quintile of distribution compared with those in the lowest quintile [37]. In another prospective study of 820 community-dwelling older people, in a nine-year follow-up a significant association between WMLs and fall-related hip fractures was reported in participants <80 years [38]. Finally, in a recently published study in 287 community-dwelling people aged between 70 and 90 years, subjects with severe WMLs had a 55% greater risk of suffering multiple or injurious falls when compared with subjects with mild WML burden during the 12-month follow-up period [16].

Within the LADIS study we also analyzed the location of WMLs in relation to falls: in a multivariate analysis of the cross-sectional results of the semiquantitative Scheltens scale on the baseline MRI, periventricular and deep frontal WMLs were found to be independently associated with falls [32]. The key link between WMLs and fall risk therefore is the impairment of balance control: compared with subjects without a history of falls, the mean single leg stance time was significantly reduced both in individuals with a history of a single or multiple falls.

Pathophysiologic mechanisms and implications

Neurologic symptoms are traditionally analyzed with regard to lesion localization. The classical strategy is based on the endeavor to find a close causal relationship between a lesion in pathologic brain section or brain imaging and a functional deficit. More recently, however, based on the steadily increasing quality of brain imaging, the concept of an immediate relationship of clinical signs and expected anatomic lesion sites is often challenged in patients with multiple or diffuse lesions. Hence, the hypothesis was promoted that new lesions may generate symptoms unrelated to the specific anatomic or functional area affected through the breakdown of neuronal networks. Several anatomic–functional networks have been proposed and models such as (pre)frontal–subcortical circuits have been established [39]. Consequently, we suggest the disturbance of a widespread subcortical motor network through pathologically and neuroradiologically proven focal or diffuse white matter and basal ganglia lesions as the reason for gait and postural control disturbances in CSVD. In addition, neuronal dysfunction in the normal-appearing white matter may already cause relevant clinical problems.

The few studies that considered not only the global severity but also the topography of WMLs demonstrated that, in particular, balance disturbances and falls are associated with deep frontal, periventricular, and also infratentorial WMLs. It is a well-known fact that different frontal lesions such as bilateral subdural hematomas, tumors, or hydrocephalus are associated with gait and balance disturbances [40]. In normal pressure hydrocephalus, characterized by a "frontal" gait disorder similar to that in CSVD, gait dysfunction and balance disturbances have been attributed to interruptions of cortico-cortical fibers projecting to the frontal cortex or lesions of the frontocerebellar pathways [40], as well as frontal cortical–subcortical circuits for motor control [39]. Lesions in the frontal deep white matter and lateral to the frontal horns of the ventricles may also affect the fronto-occipital fasciculus and the more laterally located superior longitudinal fasciculus [41], which are likewise involved in postural control and sensorimotor integration.

As outlined above, in patients with CSVD rather than an interruption of a single tract or circuit, an increasing impairment of the functional integrity of widespread subcortical neural networks necessary for processing sensorimotor input from vision, proprioception, and peripheral sensation, and, therefore, for maintaining balance control, might be the reason for balance disturbances and falls [1, 5, 6, 20, 36, 42]. This network failure affects in particular certain parameters of dynamic balance control, specifically those associated with long-term control of postural sway that require engagement of central and peripheral feedback mechanisms [30]. In healthy persons, spontaneous body sway in one direction is compensated by movement in the opposite direction through engagement of compensatory feedback mechanisms. WMLs impair these mechanisms and sway fluctuations become more random, finally affecting postural control even during quiet standing and contributing to mobility decline in the elderly [30].

In addition, impaired frontal executive function with disturbed planning, control, and execution of movements is likely to increase the rate of falls [43, 44]. Reduced executive functions may increase the fall risk in different ways: (1) reduced attentional capacity, impaired central processing and integration, and impaired execution of postural responses leads to balance and gait dysfunction and falls; (2) reduced executive functions may also increase falls risk by decreased judgment and diminished self-regulation; and (3) disruptions in executive function-related behavior, such as a loss in motivation and initiation, indirectly results in an increased fall risk by a decrease in physical activity and, thus, impaired physical function [45].

The exact pathophysiology and biology of how WMLs affect frontal and subcortical networks is unclear. In a combined MRI and positron emission tomography (PET) study, Tullberg et al. [46] demonstrated that WMLs were associated with frontal hypometabolism, irrespective of their location. Given that the frontal and periventricular areas are the predominant locations for WMLs, it could simply be that WMLs in these regions are good estimates of global WML magnitude [46]. Some studies, however, revealed that only frontal and periventricular WMLs are associated with balance disturbances and falls despite considerable WML scores even in other brain areas, such as the parietal white matter or the basal ganglia [32], clearly pointing to a prominent role of WMLs in these regions in the occurrence of balance disturbances and falls. In addition, regional brain metabolism may be exposed to fluctuations in perfusion pressure, compromising especially the periventricular watershed areas and regions with high metabolic demands [30].

Another traditional hypothesis for the cause of a "frontal" gait disorder and falls, at least in hydrocephalus, is the interference with descending motor tracts related to lower extremity control, arising from medial cortical areas and passing close to the lateral ventricle before entering the internal capsule [47]. A significant association of WMLs located in the internal capsule with balance disturbances and falls, however, could not be proven [32], and the rate of upper motor neuron signs in patients with WMLs is only about 15% [48]. Thus a direct effect of WMLs on descending motor fibers seems to be of minor importance for balance disturbances and the risk of falls. On the other hand, besides supratentorial WMLs also infratentorial WMLs located in the brainstem have been shown to be associated with reduced balance control [33]. These brainstem lesions may affect not primarily corticospinal tracts but vestibulospinal, vestibulocerebellar, and numerous cerebellovestibular connections, all of which pass through the brainstem [49]. Because vestibular fibers and vestibular nuclei are recognized to communicate between regions thought to be associated with balance and mobility [49], it has been hypothesized that also brainstem WMLs might affect balance and hence mobility [30].

Therapy

Following the hypothesis that the effect of extensive WMLs does not translate into manifest disability until compensatory mechanisms falter or the body can no longer be held upright as the brain ages, our focus should therefore be on how we can prevent further aggravation of the underlying pathophysiologic processes in order to maintain lower body motor function and, as a consequence, general health in the elderly. This may be reached by a thorough control of cardiovascular risk factors, such as arterial hypertension, diabetes, and hyperlipidemia.

In the LADIS study, a clear association with better scores in SPPB was noted in individuals who regularly did physical exercise. This effect remained significant after correction for demographic variables and was even independent of a history of gait disturbance or falls [10]. This finding may point to possible therapeutic interventions. A putative independent intrinsic effect of physical exercise may be explained by a stabilization of the labile neuronal motor network. This is a rather new message because, so far, several small studies have shown a positive effect of physical exercise on selected aspects of mobility in the elderly, but there still is contradictory evidence regarding its influence on gait, balance, and Activities of Daily Living. Just recently, we were able to demonstrate that physical activity reduces the risk of cognitive impairment in the LADIS study population [50].

Two of the most important determinants of gait impairment and disability are falls and the fear of falls; therefore, in clinical practice an early identification of patients with CSVD at risk of falls using simple clinical tests to assess balance ability, such as the single leg stance time, is of particular relevance. In general populations of community-dwelling elderly persons, some exercise and strength-training programs have been shown to be effective in preventing falls. In a meta-analysis on controlled studies, the mean reduction of falls, averaged over 44 studies with a total of 9600 patients, was 22% [51]. Controlled trials on the effect of exercise programs on balance and fall risk in patients with CSVD are not yet available. In the LADIS study, however, our group could show that physical activity was clearly associated not only with the results of the SPPB but also with a reduced rate of falls [10, 32]. These results support published data indicating that exercise, in particular when combined with balance training, can reduce the risk of falls [52, 53] and mobility impairment [54]. Nevertheless, the causal direction of an association between physical activity and improvement of balance and reduced fall risk remains unclear, as on the other hand fear of falls as well as balance and motor disturbances might restrain patients from partaking in physical activity.

References

1. Baezner H, Hennerici M. From trepidant abasia to motor network failure – gait disorders as a consequence of subcortical vascular encephalopathy (SVE): review of historical and contemporary concepts. *J Neurol Sci* 2005;229:81–88.
2. Verghese J, Lipton RB, Hall CB, et al. Abnormality of gait as a predictor of non-Alzheimer's dementia. *N Engl J Med* 2002;347:1761–1768.
3. Masdeu JC, Wolfson L, Lantos G, et al. Brain white-matter changes in the elderly prone to falling. *Arch Neurol* 1989;46:1292–1296.
4. Kerber KA, Enrietto JA, Jacobson KM, Baloh RW. Disequilibrium in older people: a prospective study. *Neurology* 1998;51:574–580.
5. Baezner H, Oster M, Daffertshofer M, Hennerici M. Assessment of gait in subcortical vascular encephalopathy by computerized analysis: a cross-sectional and longitudinal study. *J Neurol* 2000;247:841–849.
6. Baloh RW, Ying SH, Jacobson KM. A longitudinal study of gait and balance dysfunction in normal older people. *Arch Neurol* 2003;60:835–839.
7. Rosano C, Kuller LH, Chung H, et al. Subclinical brain magnetic resonance imaging abnormalities predict physical functional decline in high-functioning older adults. *J Am Geriatr Soc* 2005;53:649–654.
8. De Laat KF, van Norden AG, Gons RA, et al. Gait in elderly with cerebral small vessel disease. *Stroke* 2010;41:1652–1658.
9. Soumaré A, Elbaz A, Zhu Y, et al. White matter lesions volume and motor performances in the elderly. *Ann Neurol* 2009;65:706–715.
10. Baezner H, Blahak C, Poggesi A, et al. Association of gait and balance disorders with age-related white matter changes: the LADIS study. *Neurology* 2008;70:935–942.
11. Nutt JG, Marsden CD, Thompson PD. Human walking and higher-level gait disorders, particularly in the elderly. *Neurology* 1993;43:268–279.
12. Pantoni L, Basile AM, Pracucci G, et al. Impact of age-related cerebral white matter changes on the transition to disability – the LADIS study: rationale, design and methodology. *Neuroepidemiology* 2005; 24:51–62.
13. Guralnik JM, Simonsick EM, Ferrucci L, et al. A Short Physical Performance Battery assessing lower extremity function: association with self-reported disability and prediction of mortality and nursing home admission. *J Gerontol* 1994; 49:85–94.
14. Guralnik JM, Ferrucci L, Simonsick EM, Salive ME, Wallace RB. Lower-extremity function in persons over the age of 70 years as a predictor of subsequent disability. *N Engl J Med* 1995;332:556–561.
15. Kreisel SH, Blahak C, Baezner H, et al. Deterioration of gait and balance over time: the effects of age-related white matter change. *Cerebrovasc Dis* 2013; 35:544–553.
16. Zheng JJ, Delbaere K, Close JC, et al. White matter hyperintensities are an independent predictor of physical decline in community-dwelling older people. *Gerontology* 2012;58:398–406.

17. de Laat KF, Tuladhar AM, van Norden AG, et al. Loss of white matter integrity is associated with gait disorders in cerebral small vessel disease. *Brain* 2011; 134:73–83.
18. de Laat KF, van Norden AG, Gons RA, et al. Diffusion tensor imaging and gait in elderly persons with cerebral small vessel disease. *Stroke* 2011;42:373–379.
19. de Laat KF, Reid AT, Grim DC, et al. Cortical thickness is associated with gait disturbances in cerebral small vessel disease. *Neuroimage* 2012;59:1478–1484.
20. Zheng JJ, Delbaere K, Close JC, Sachdev PS, Lord SR. Impact of white matter lesions on physical functioning and fall risk in older people: a systematic review. *Stroke* 2011;42:2086–2090.
21. Whiting P, Rutjes AW, Reitsma JB, Bossuyt PM, Kleijnen J. The development of quadas: a tool for the quality assessment of studies of diagnostic accuracy included in systematic reviews. *BMC Med Res Methodol* 2003;3:25.
22. Rubenstein LZ, Powers CM, MacLean CH. Quality indicators for the management and prevention of falls and mobility problems in vulnerable elders. *Ann Intern Med* 2001; 135:686–693.
23. Murray ME, Senjem ML, Petersen RC, et al. Functional impact of white matter hyperintensities in cognitively normal elderly subjects. *Arch Neurol* 2010;67:1379–1385.
24. Bloem BR, Steijns JAG, Smits-Engelsman BC. An update on falls. *Curr Opin Neurol* 2003;16:15–26.
25. Alexander BH, Rivara FP, Wolf ME. The cost and frequency of hospitalisation for fall related injuries in older adults. *Am J Public Health* 1992; 82:1020–1023.
26. Tinetti ME, Speechley M, Ginter SF. Risk factors for falls among elderly persons living in the community. *N Engl J Med* 1988;319:1701–1707.
27. Maki BE. Gait changes in older adults: predictors of falls or indicators of fear. *J Am Geriatr Soc* 1997;45:313–320.
28. Bloem BR, Grimbergen YAM, Cramer M, et al. Prospective assessment of falls in Parkinson's disease. *J Neurol* 2001;248:950–958.
29. Ebersbach G, Sojer M, Valldeoriola F, et al. Comparative analysis of gait in Parkinson's disease, cerebellar ataxia and subcortical arteriosclerotic encephalopathy. *Brain.* 1999;122:1349–1355.
30. Novak V, Haertle M, Zhao P, et al. White matter hyperintensities and dynamics of postural control. *Magn Reson Imaging* 2009;27:752–759.
31. Longstreth WT Jr, Manolio TA, Arnold A, et al. Clinical correlates of white matter findings on cranial magnetic resonance imaging of 3301 elderly people. The Cardiovascular Health Study. *Stroke* 1996;27:1274–1282.
32. Blahak C, Baezner H, Pantoni L, et al. Deep frontal and periventricular age-related white matter changes but not basal ganglia and infratentorial hyperintensities are associated with falls: cross-sectional results from the LADIS study. *J Neurol Neurosurg Psychiatry* 2009;80:608–613.
33. Starr JM, Leaper SA, Murray AD, et al. Brain white matter lesions detected by magnetic resonance imaging are associated with balance and gait speed. *J Neurol Neurosurg Psychiatry* 2003; 74:94–98.
34. Camicioli R, Moore MM, Sexton G, Howieson DB, Kaye JA. Age-related brain changes associated with motor function in healthy older people. *J Am Geriatr Soc* 1999;47:330–334.
35. Tell GS, Lefkowitz DS, Diehr P, Elster AD. Relationship between balance and abnormalities in cerebral magnetic resonance imaging in older adults. *Arch Neurol* 1998;55:73–79.
36. Whitman GT, Tang T. A prospective study of cerebral white matter abnormalities in older people with gait dysfunction. *Neurology* 2001;57:990–994.
37. Srikanth V, Beare R, Blizzard L, et al. Cerebral white matter lesions, gait, and the risk of incident falls: a prospective population-based study. *Stroke* 2009;40:175–180.
38. Corti MC, Baggio G, Sartori L, et al. White matter lesions and the risk of incident hip fracture in older persons: results from the Progetto Veneto Anziani Study. *Arch Intern Med* 2007;167:1745–1751.
39. Alexander GE, DeLong MR, Strick PL. Parallel organization of functionally segregated circuits linking basal ganglia and cortex. *Annu Rev Neurosci* 1986;9: 357–381.
40. Stolze H, Kuhtz-Buschbeck JP, Drücke H, et al. Comparative analysis of the gait disorder of normal pressure hydrocephalus and Parkinson's disease. *J Neurol Neurosurg Psychiatry* 2001;70:289–297.
41. Curnes JT, Burger PC, Djang WT, Boyko OB. MR imaging of compact white matter pathways. *AJNR Am J Neuroradiol* 1988;9:1061–1068.
42. Guttmann CR, Benson R, Warfield SK, et al. White matter abnormalities in mobility impaired older persons. *Neurology* 2000;54:1277–1283.
43. Kerber KA, Enrietto JA, Jacobson KM, Baloh RW. Disequilibrium in older people: a prospective study. *Neurology* 1998;51:574–580.
44. Sparto PJ, Aizenstein HJ, Vanswearingen JM, et al. Delays

in auditory-cued step initiation are related to increased volume of white matter hyperintensities in older adults. *Exp Brain Res* 2008;188:633–640.

45. Liu-Ambrose T, Nagamatsu LS, Hsu CL, Bolandzadeh N. Emerging concept: "central benefit model" of exercise in falls prevention. *Br J Sports Med* 2013;47:115–117.
46. Tullberg M, Fletcher E, DeCarli C, et al. White matter lesions impair frontal lobe function regardless of their location. *Neurology* 2004;63:246–253.
47. Yakovlev PI. Paraplegias of hydrocephalics. *Am J Ment Defic* 1947;51:561–576.
48. Poggesi A, Gouw A, van der Flier W, et al. Cerebral white matter changes are associated with abnormalities on neurological examination in non-disabled elderly: the LADIS study. *J Neurol* 2013;260:1014–1021.
49. Afifi AK, Bergman RA. *Functional Neuroanatomy*. New York, NY: McGraw-Hill; 1998: pp. 105–179.
50. Verdelho A, Madureira S, Ferro JM, et al. Physical activity prevents progression for cognitive impairment and vascular dementia: results from the LADIS (Leukoaraiosis And DISability) study. *Stroke* 2012;43:3331–3335.
51. Sherrington C, Whitney JC, Lord SR, et al. Effective exercise for the prevention of falls: a systematic review and meta-analysis. *J Am Geriatr Soc* 2008;56:2234–2243.
52. Province MA, Hadley EC, Hornbrook MC, et al. The effects of exercise on falls in elderly patients. A preplanned meta-analysis of the FICSIT trials. Frailty and injuries: cooperative studies of intervention techniques. *JAMA* 1995;273:1341–1347.
53. Day L, Fildes B, Gordon I, et al. Randomised factorial trial of falls prevention among older people living in their own homes. *BMJ* 2002;325: 128–134.
54. Lang IA, Guralnik JM, Melzer D. Physical activity in middle-aged adults reduces risks of functional impairment independent of its effect on weight. *J Am Geriatr Soc* 2007;55:1836–1841.

Chapter 21

Psychiatric consequences of small vessel disease

Perminder S. Sachdev and Sharon Reutens

Introduction

Not only is small vessel disease (SVD) common, especially in older individuals, it often occurs silently and manifests insidiously, with the result that the scope of the problem is under-recognized. The manifestations of SVD are widespread, with an impact on psychiatric status, quality of life, and functional ability through the development of symptoms of depression, cognitive impairment, and amotivational syndromes, as well as noncognitive manifestations, such as poorer physical health, urinary incontinence, and gait disturbance.

For the purposes of this chapter, the presence of cerebral SVD is identified by neuroimaging, particularly findings on magnetic resonance imaging (MRI), rather than neuropathology. While neuropathologic studies of dementia as well as cognitively unimpaired individuals reveal the common occurrence of SVD manifesting as lacunar infarcts, microbleeds, and noninfarct white matter ischemic changes [1–3], determining the relationship between these and premortem psychiatric disorder is methodologically constrained. Earlier work relating psychiatric symptoms and disorders to SVD was based on computerized tomography (CT). With the evidence that modern MRI is more sensitive in detecting SVD [4], and the large number of studies that have related psychiatric symptomatology to MRI findings, this is indeed the appropriate basis for any current analysis.

Technological advances in MRI have repeatedly posed challenges to this field of investigation. The introduction of T2-weighted imaging using fluid-attenuated inversion recovery (FLAIR) sequences showed that white matter hyperintensities (WMHs) were present in the vast majority of older individuals [5] and nearly one half of otherwise healthy people in their late 40s [6], even though the extent of these lesions was small in most cases. These lesions have been referred to as "leukoaraiosis" (literally, thinning of the white matter) [7], because they are seen as hypodense or reduced signal abnormalities on CT scan and T1-weighted MRI. The frequency of such "incidental" findings has posed a problem for the determination of their clinical significance, both in relation to cognitive function and in psychiatric disorder. The issue is further confounded by the fact that WMHs are nonspecific in terms of etiology with a large number of causes, which include inflammation, demyelination, degeneration, developmental abnormality, and edema in addition to ischemia [8]. Persuasive arguments have been presented to support the view that the WMHs seen incidentally in older individuals are most likely ischemic in nature and, therefore, markers of damage due to SVD [9]. FLAIR imaging has been useful in characterizing lacunar infarcts, and distinguishing dilated perivascular or Virchow–Robin spaces from WMHs.

The recent use of diffusion tensor imaging (DTI) to investigate white matter tract integrity in neuropsychiatric conditions has revealed more subtle perturbations not seen on other imaging modalities. DTI measures the diffusivity of water molecules in multiple planes, and damage to white matter leads to increase in diffusivity and reduction of fractional anisotropy, a measure of the directionality of diffusion [10]. Therefore, DTI can detect abnormalities in white matter that is normal-appearing on T2-weighted imaging. This added sensitivity is both an advantage as well as a challenge, as it is not always possible to relate abnormalities on DTI to psychiatric symptoms or cognitive function.

Another recent imaging modality is T2*-weighted MRI, which uses gradient-echo sequences, and its

Cerebral Small Vessel Disease, ed. Leonardo Pantoni and Philip B. Gorelick. Published by Cambridge University Press.

special application is susceptibility-weighted imaging (SWI), which is very sensitive for cerebral microbleeds [11]. This modality has highlighted the common occurrence of microbleeds in the brain and opened up the area of hemorrhagic SVD and its neuropsychiatric consequences. Other techniques such as magnetic resonance spectroscopy (MRS), blood oxygen level dependent (BOLD) functional MRI (fMRI), and perfusion MRI (pMRI) have been less influential in this field.

Establishing a relationship between SVD and neuropsychiatric symptoms and disorders

The high prevalence of SVD, which is usually insidious in onset and may be widespread in the brain, makes it difficult to relate it etiologically to psychiatric disorders, which themselves are common and, therefore, incidental co-occurrence is not unlikely. A simple association between markers of SVD and psychiatric disorders is, therefore, not sufficient to establish causality. A number of strategies have been used in the literature to establish an etiologic relationship, with varying degrees of success:

1. *Prevalence estimates.* Much of the research has attempted to demonstrate that psychiatric symptoms and disorders are more common in individuals with SVD, and vice versa. As an example, WMHs have been reported to be more common in patients with late-life depression [12], late-onset schizophrenia [13], and bipolar disorder [14]. Psychiatric disorders, in particular depression, are common in cerebral autosomal dominant arteriopathy with subcortical infarcts and leukoencephalopathy (CADASIL), an inherited cerebrovascular disease with extensive SVD [15]. While this association is a useful first step, it by no means establishes that these lesions cause the psychiatric syndromes. It is possible that a common etiologic factor may account for both increased WMHs and the psychiatric syndrome. For example, in one population-based study, poor physical health could explain both increased occurrence of WMHs and depression, and the relationship between WMHs and depression was no longer significant once physical health status had been accounted for [16]. Risk factors for SVD, such as hypertension, diabetes, high homocysteine, etc. [17], have been independently associated with neuropsychiatric disorders, including depression, and cognitive impairment, and must be accounted for in any study. The importance of matching for confounding factors in any case – control study is very important, as statistical correction for differences fails to achieve an optimal result [12].
2. *Temporal association.* If it can be clearly established that the occurrence of the psychiatric syndrome is temporally related to that of SVD, it increases the likelihood of an etiologic relationship. Considerable literature has examined the occurrence of psychiatric disorders, in particular depression and apathy, after stroke [18, 19]. This is more difficult to examine in relation to SVD, except in patients with symptomatic lacunar infarction. A factor to consider is that patients with stroke or transient ischemic attacks (TIAs) usually have additional evidence of SVD that precedes the event, which confounds the interpretation of the findings.
3. *Longitudinal course.* Longitudinal studies may be better able to establish etiologic relationships if SVD and psychiatric disorders can be demonstrated to co-vary over time. For WMHs, this has been examined in relation to cognitive dysfunction [20] and depression [21, 22].
4. *Prognostic implications.* If the presence of SVD in someone with a psychiatric disorder affects treatment response and/or long-term outcome, it is likely that the SVD has an etiologic role, although this may be a partial or contributory one only. This issue has been studied in relation to late-life depression to some extent [23, 24].
5. *Anatomic specificity.* Another approach taken to examine etiologic significance is to demonstrate a tight relationship between the anatomic location of the vascular lesion and the psychiatric syndrome. The finding that left frontal and left basal ganglia strokes were more likely to be followed by depression [25] has, however, been hotly contested [26], and, moreover, does not relate to SVD. There is some literature linking cognitive function with location of lacunar infarcts [27] and even WMHs [28]. The literature examining the anatomical location of SVD and psychiatric syndromes is small [29–31] and inconclusive, partly because SVD is rarely

restricted to one brain region. The other reason is that the neuroanatomical basis of most psychiatric disorders is only partially understood, and even though there is recognition of neuronal circuits being dysfunctional, the precise constituents of these circuits are still not known.

Because of the above reasons, the relationship between SVD and psychiatric disorders continues to attract much controversy. We will discuss some of these issues in the following pages.

Specific disorders

Depression

Major depression is common in the elderly, with a reported prevalence of between 1 and 16% [32]. The prevalence of minor depression is 4–13% [33], indicating that depressive symptoms are common in the elderly population. Cerebrovascular disease is also common in asymptomatic elderly people and increases with age [34, 35], thereby suggesting the possibility that the two are inter-related. There are some challenges to this deduction, however. It must be stated at this point that many mental health surveys have shown that rates of mood and anxiety disorders are lower in the elderly than in middle-aged individuals [36, 37], contrary to the popularly held view of increasing mental illness with age. Moreover, the relationship between SVD and depression does not necessarily have to be one-sided. While SVD could arguably lead to depression, the reverse may also be true as depression has been seen as a risk factor for vascular disease [38]. Additionally, apathy is often mistaken for depression in the elderly, and rates of apathy increase with age and cerebrovascular disease [39]. Attempts are necessary to distinguish the two syndromes.

There is considerable literature on depression following stroke, or post-stroke depression (PSD). Estimates vary, depending upon the setting of the study and the ascertainment methods use. In community settings, the lowest estimates were 14% for major and 9% for minor depression, and in clinical settings, 21.6% for major and 21% for minor depression [18]. There have been many attempts to understand this association, which have bearing on our discussion of the role of SVD in depression. The most consistent association of PSD has been with the severity of impairment in Activities of Daily Living (ADL), with 15 out of 18 studies showing this association [40]. Whether it is the severity of the functional impairment that leads to depression, or depression compounds the impairment, remains debatable. PSD has been shown to delay recovery following stroke, and increase mortality [41]. The relationship to the site of the stroke has been contentious. Depression occurring soon after a stroke, generally within three months, has been noted to occur more often with left anterior hemispheric strokes [18]. Studies of depression between 3 and 12 months after stroke have failed to show a laterality bias [42]. A number of controlled investigations have shown that PSD can be effectively treated with antidepressants, and one study showed that it could be prevented by prophylactic medication [18].

There is considerable literature on depression in association with SVD, but the conclusions are more tentative than those for PSD. The main arguments suggesting that subcortical ischemic lesions are associated with depression are as follows:

(a) Older individuals with depression are more likely to have subcortical lesions than nondepressed control subjects [29].
(b) Subcortical lesions are more common in late-onset depression when compared to early-onset depression, even after controlling for age of the patients, with a reported difference in rate of WMHs being as high as fivefold [43, 44].
(c) Community-based studies have also shown an association between subcortical ischemic disease and depression, which is not necessarily major depression [16, 45].
(d) There is some evidence to suggest that depressed individuals with WMHs have poorer response to antidepressant drugs and electroconvulsive (ECT) treatment [29, 30, 46], and that the depression may persist and even worsen over time [45]. The increased potential for the development of delirium in depression with subcortical lesions has also been suggested [47]. It has also been shown by at least one group of investigators that treatment of vascular risk factors with the calcium channel antagonist nimodipine augmented the response to antidepressants [48, 49].
(e) Taylor et al. [21] followed subjects diagnosed with DSM-IV Major Depressive Disorder over two years and determined that subjects who sustained

remission of depression had a lower WMH volume that those that did not sustain remission, even when controlled for baseline depression severity. They calculated a 7% increased risk of poor outcome with every 1% increase of WMH volume [21]. In a four-year longitudinal study of elderly subjects, Godin et al. [50] found a relationship between lifetime major depression and WMH volume, WMH progression and lifetime major depression, and for the development of depression in subjects with higher WMH volumes.

(f) Some studies have found lower rates of familial mood disorders and psychiatric illness in those with SVD-associated depression [29, 51].

(g) Several studies have found evidence for the placement of strategic lesions resulting in the development of depression [52–54], with most studies implicating frontal lobe lesions. Taylor et al. [29] demonstrated that older depressed subjects were more likely to show WMHs in bilateral frontal and left parietotemporal regions, compared with control subjects who were more likely to demonstrate WMHs in parietotemporal areas only. Lesion placement has been found to influence prognosis with reported poorer prognosis in subjects with lesions located in the basal ganglia, pons, and frontal lobes [29, 45, 52, 55]. Similarly, Alexopoulos et al. [55] found that elderly subjects with depression had a poorer response if they demonstrated DTI evidence of disruption of frontal white matter tracts.

The above arguments supported the concept of a *vascular depression* proposed in the 1990s [43, 56], as a depressive disorder with a late age of onset, or a change in course of an early-onset illness coupled with vascular risk factors and significant diffuse or multiple localized cerebrovascular lesions [43]. The proposed mechanism was the disruption of subcortical pathways underlying mood regulation. Neuroimaging studies of depression implicate limbic, subcortical gray nuclei, and prefrontal areas of the brain. Alexopoulos et al. [56] suggested that depression might result from the accumulation of lesions sufficient to reach a threshold level from which nonbiologic factors could lead to the development of depression, or the direct disruption of circuits critical for mood regulation.

A number of arguments can, however, be presented against the concept of Vascular Depression as a specific condition:

(a) There is no good evidence that a specific phenomenological entity of Vascular Depression can be delineated. A number of studies, as reviewed recently [57], show that Vascular Depression is more commonly associated with lassitude, poor motivation, anhedonia, and psychomotor retardation, but the findings are inconsistent. Other authors have also argued that it is difficult to symptomatically characterize a syndrome of Vascular Depression [58].

(b) The evidence for the influence of WMH load on depression is conflicting, with some studies [59, 60] not finding a relationship between progression of WMHs and depression. In their seven-year population-based study, Ikram et al. [61] were unable to find any relationship between neuroimaging markers and incident depression. The authors suggested several potential explanations, including the possibility that cerebrovascular disease is related to persistence of depression rather than its incidence.

(c) The mechanism by which SVD results in depression has not been elucidated, particularly noting the high prevalence of WMHs with increasing age in normal elderly people. While direct damage to the brain parenchyma occurs as a result of ischemia and inflammation, this may be a vulnerability factor that results in depression as a result of other triggers, biologic or nonbiologic [56]. Nonbiologic factors such as adversity, bereavement, and disability are common in older populations and may be the determining factors.

(d) The possibility that medical disease may be a common factor underlying both depression and SVD must be considered, as one study showed that the relationship between depression and WMHs was no longer significant if physical health was added as a covariate in the analysis [16].

(e) The reverse relationship, i.e., depression increasing the risk of SVD, should not be dismissed.

Does the concept of Vascular Depression have any treatment implications? Greater treatment resistance and chronicity of illness have indeed been noted in subjects with WMHs [23, 29, 51], and one study demonstrated poor response to treatment in depression with progression of WMHs [21]. Some studies have related the location of white matter abnormalities to treatment response, implicating the basal ganglia [55] or the frontal white matter [21]. ECT has been used in depressed patients with SVD, with good effect [47, 62]. However, two studies reported a poorer response to ECT in patients with vascular-related depression [63], with one study noting a correlation between severity of subcortical gray matter hyperintensities and poorer response [62].

In view of putative vascular etiology, strategies addressing SVD have been used in secondary prevention. Drugs such as vasodilators, calcium antagonists, and antioxidants that have been tried, albeit unsuccessfully, in vascular dementia (VaD) have not been tried for depression with SVD. An exception is a trial of nimodipine, a calcium channel antagonist, as an augmenting agent for antidepressant medications that found a higher rate of remission and lower rate of recurrence in treatment responders [49].

It is suggested that the focus of pharmacologic treatment may need to change from modulating neurotransmitters in the damaged tracts to one of neuroprotection. Decreasing neuroinflammatory processes, improving cerebral perfusion, and the optimal treatment of hypertension are potential targets for limiting SVD and reducing the psychiatric consequences. Primary prevention should be focused on reducing risk factors for the development of SVD, and this must begin in mid life or earlier. Reduction of hypertension, smoking cessation, blood glucose and lipid control, and increased physical, mental, and social activities are paramount. The role of folic acid supplementation and reduction in homocysteine levels has been debated but not proven.

In summary, the proposal of a Vascular Depression has limited appeal and warrants further study to best elucidate the relationship between SVD and depression. With the current state of knowledge, it might be best to refer to "Depression with SVD" instead of Vascular Depression, as the former is agnostic in its etiologic implications. At the same time, one is best advised not to ignore the SVD as it has treatment, preventative, and prognostic implications.

Bipolar disorder

The relationship between bipolar disorder (BD) and cerebrovascular disease has been examined from a number of perspectives. The early interest related to the occurrence of secondary mania following stroke, which has been generally considered to be rare [64]. The majority of reports of post-stroke mania are single case reports or small series of cases, although a few cohort studies have examined this as well, as reviewed recently [65]. One study found only three cases in 700 stroke patients [66], attesting to its rarity. The recent review found post-stroke mania to be more common in men who had no family or personal history of psychiatric disorder and who had at least one vascular risk factor, although selection bias in case reports can make these findings somewhat tentative. Some studies, on the other hand, have suggested a role for genetic predisposition [66, 67], and the inconsistent literature partly relates to the fact that some studies excluded those with a past or family history of BD and others did not. Mania was related more often to a right cerebral infarct [65] and there is inconsistent literature relating it to subcortical atrophy [67]. BD patients are also at increased risk of stroke [68], and this may be related to increased rates of hypertension, metabolic syndrome, and obesity in these individuals [69].

The relationship between BD or mania and SVD has also been examined in a number of studies. In addition to higher rates of stroke, silent brain infarction is not uncommon in BD patients. In one study of older people with BD with a mean age 65.3 years [70], silent infarcts, most commonly in the corona radiata and the basal ganglia, were present in nearly 60%, with rates somewhat higher in those with onset after 50 years, and a rate of 47% in those with onset before age 50. A rate of 65% of silent infarcts in late-onset mania has been previously reported [71]. However, this high rate, even in those with an earlier onset, suggests that the infarction cannot be implicated in etiology and must be regarded as being a consequence of the increased vascular risk factors in these patients.

BD patients are also likely to have higher rates of WMHs. A recent meta-analysis of 27 studies found a 2.5-fold increase relative to controls, although there was much heterogeneity [72]. Surprisingly, WMHs were much more likely to be present in children and adolescents with BD (odds ratio = 5.7). This review also found that the deep WMHs and subcortical gray matter, but not periventricular hyperintensities, were increased in BD. However, the studies do not suggest that this finding is specific for BD, and the differences from unipolar depression and schizophrenia were not significant. The relationship between age or age of onset of BD and rates of WMHs is inconsistent in the literature. While WMHs have a definite relationship with age, not all studies have shown a clear distinction between early- and late-onset cases. The high prevalence of WMHs in children with BD suggests that these may not be related to SVD, at least those that are secondary to vascular risk factors, and genetic factors may be important. Studies of white matter integrity using DTI have produced inconsistent results. While the majority demonstrate decreased frontal and prefrontal fractional anisotropy and higher diffusivity, several studies have reported increased fractional anisotropy, as summarized recently [73, 74].

The relationship between BD and SVD, therefore, remains uncertain. Some investigators have focused on individuals who develop mania for the first time after age 50 years, who comprise about 10% of all BD patients [75]. While it is true that they have more stigmata of cerebrovascular disease than a nondisease control group, it is likely that this is due to increased vascular risk factors and any causative role cannot be attributed to the SVD. The concept of "vascular mania," defined as mania with onset after 50 years and with clinical, neuropsychological, or neuroimaging evidence of cerebrovascular disease [76], does not, therefore, have empirical support.

Psychosis

The prevalence of schizophrenia in community-dwelling people aged over 65 ranges from 0.1 to 0.5% [77]. A study of the very old found the prevalence of psychotic symptoms in nondemented 85 year olds to be 10.1%, with delusions in 5.5%, hallucinations in 6.9%, and paranoid ideation in 6.9% [78]. A number of investigators have attempted to relate this to neurodegenerative and cerebrovascular disorders.

Only a few studies have systematically examined the association between stroke and psychosis. In a study of 390 consecutive stroke in-patients, 4.2% were reported to develop delusions within three months [79]. In another study of 1008 incident strokes, 3.5% developed a delusional or schizophreniform disorder within two years, giving an incidence rate of post-stroke psychosis of 1.1 per 1000 person-years [80]. Since these are hospital-based studies, the community incidence of post-stroke psychosis is likely to be lower than 1 per 1000 person–years. Hallucinations appear to be particularly characteristic of psychosis occurring after stroke [81], which may be related to sensory deficits.

Psychosis has been well described in VaD. Ballard et al. [81] estimated that 37% of subjects experienced psychosis, deriving their figure from combined data. Of these, 19–50% experienced delusions, 14–60% visual hallucinations, and 19–30% delusional misidentification. In their own study [81], they determined that 22% of VaD subjects had visual hallucinations, 8% auditory hallucinations, 36% delusions, and 23% delusional misidentification. The one-month prevalence of psychosis was 46%. Whether psychotic symptoms relate to severity of dementia is not clear. There is some suggestion that delusional ideation is more likely to arise in moderate dementia and hallucinations in severe dementia [81, 82]. Whether psychosis is related to SVD or large infarctions, or simply has a nonspecific association with dementia, is not known.

There are few studies of psychosis related to cerebrovascular SVD. Some studies have reported an increased prevalence of WMHs in late-onset schizophrenia [83–86], but other studies have not supported this finding [87–90]. A recent DTI study did not find a difference in frontal white matter tracts in subjects with onset of psychosis after 60 years [13]. However, another recent study examining subjects with Alzheimer's disease noted that subjects with concomitant SVD, as evidenced by WMHs or lacunes, were more likely to have delusions and depression [91]. These findings suggest that SVD is generally not a major factor in the development of psychosis in late life. However, it is possible that white matter perturbations caused by SVD may be a contributing factor.

Anxiety

Anxiety is common after stroke, often in conjunction with depression. One study reported that the three-year prevalence of Generalized Anxiety Disorder (GAD) was 28% [92]. Poor prognosis for recovery was also noted, with only 23% of patients' symptoms remitting in the first year, and no significant further decrease for the remainder of follow-up. Another study found similar results, with 27% of subjects meeting DSM-III criteria for GAD, most with comorbid depressive disorders [93]. There is a paucity of neuroimaging studies of late-life anxiety disorders. Most studies have only examined anxiety using scores on combined anxiety and depression scales [94], or are case reports, such as one reporting post-traumatic stress disorder following a thalamic infarct [95]. The evidence linking SVD with anxiety disorder is, therefore, weak.

Obsessive Compulsive Disorder (OCD) is the subject of a large number of neuroimaging and neuropsychological studies. WMHs have been described in early-onset OCD [96]. Late-onset OCD is, however, uncommon, with only 15% presenting after the age of 35 [97], and neuroimaging data on these are not available. Late-onset OCD has been associated with more frequent brain lesions, including silent strokes, with lesions largely being in the cerebral cortex or the basal ganglia [98]. In one case series, four of five subjects with late-onset OCD had lesions (tumor, stroke) in the frontal lobes or caudate nucleus [99].

Neuroimaging findings in OCD have suggested an orbital–frontal–striatal circuit underlying the disorder, and microstructural abnormalities of white matter demonstrated on DTI have added weight to the underlying disruption of a circuit comprising of frontal, striatal, and thalamic connectivity [100]. However, the contribution of SVD to this disruption has not received strong empirical support.

Apathy

Apathy is conceptualized as a diminution of motivation, but is variously described as a symptom as well as a syndrome, leading to a lack of clarity as to its definition. Marin [101] described the syndrome as combining emotional, behavioral, and cognitive components. Levy and Dubois [102] emphasized the observable behavioral components arising from disruptions in the basal ganglia and prefrontal cortex, and Starkstein and Leentjens [103] proposed a definition of reduced goal-orientated behaviors and cognitions. Stuss et al. [104] have gone so far as to suggest several subtypes of apathy based on the involvement of various frontal–subcortical circuits. Despite the varying definitions of apathy, most authors note the characteristics of lack of initiation and motivation manifesting as limited self-generated behaviors. Apathy is often mistaken for depression, although the correlation between apathy and depression ratings is often low [39], and the neuropsychological profiles differ [104]. Notwithstanding the lack of conceptual clarity, it is generally agreed that apathy has major adverse outcomes in relation to function, caregiver distress, treatment response, and cognitive decline [102–104].

Apathy is very common in brain disorders, with one review suggesting that the prevalence in disorders with substantial cortical dysfunction, such as Alzheimer's disease, is about 60%, and that in subcortical disorders it is about 40%. The point prevalence in VaD was calculated to be 33.8%, while the prevalence of apathy in patients with stroke ranges from 22.5 to 56.7% [105]. Patients with frontal lesions are particularly prone to developing apathy, with an average point prevalence of 60.3%. Since stroke and SVD are quite likely to affect the frontal lobes and basal ganglia, structures often associated with apathy, their relationship to vascular disease is not surprising. Even in Alzheimer's disease, neuroimaging studies have associated apathy with WMHs in the frontal lobe [106]. Apathy is common in people with CADASIL [107], with one study reporting a prevalence of 41%, using the Neuropsychiatric Inventory [108].

The association of apathy with SVD has been supported by a number of neuroimaging studies. In the SMART-Medea study [109], 650 patients with SVD were examined, and an association was found between lacunar infarcts in the deep white matter and depression. Interestingly, the relationship was driven largely by motivational symptoms, raising the question whether the syndrome being examined was in reality apathy. The authors concluded that disruption of the cortical–subcortical circuits with SVD led to an amotivational syndrome, and the exclusion of subjects with major depression did not affect the findings [109, 110]. Frontal WMHs have been associated with apathy in Alzheimer's disease [103, 111]. Brodaty et al. [31] examined 205 people admitted to a stroke unit and found that apathy was five times more common in stroke patients than controls, even three to six months after the stroke, but interestingly not correlated with stroke severity. Stroke patients had greater WMHs in the right hemisphere, as reported in another study [112]. Stroke patients with apathy were older, had lower cognitive function, and were less independent in their functioning.

In summary, apathy is an important syndrome associated with SVD, and attempts should be made to distinguish it from depression. Not only are its consequences different from those of depression, the treatment strategies also differ. The drugs used to treat apathy include stimulants, dopamine agonists, neuroleptics, and cholinesterase inhibitors, often depending upon the setting in which it occurs. The evidence for the efficacy of these drugs is, however, limited.

Conclusion

SVD is common and, considering its wide anatomical distribution, it can have diverse psychiatric consequences. A number of psychiatric syndromes associated with SVD have been described. These must be examined in the context of physical and cognitive dysfunction related to SVD. Any study of SVD must, therefore, include its neuropsychiatric manifestations. An important corollary is that this association is a pointer to considerations for the prevention of neuropsychiatric disorders, especially in the elderly in whom this association is more likely to manifest. It is, therefore, an extremely important area of clinical interest and future research.

References

1. Neuropathology Group of the Medical Research Council Cognitive Function and Ageing Study (MRC CFAS). Pathological correlates of late-onset dementia in a multicentre, community-based population in England and Wales. *Lancet* 2001;357:169–175.
2. White L. Brain lesions at autopsy in older Japanese-American men as related to cognitive impairment and dementia in the final years of life: a summary report from the Honolulu–Asia Aging Study. *J Alzheimers Dis* 2009;18:713–725.
3. Fisher CM. Lacunar strokes and infarcts: a review. *Neurology* 1982;32:871–876.
4. Black S, Gao F, Bilbao J. Understanding white matter disease: imaging–pathological correlations in vascular cognitive impairment. *Stroke* 2009;40:S48–S52.
5. Wen W, Sachdev PS. The topography of white matter hyperintensities on brain MRI in healthy 60- to 64-year-old individuals. *Neuroimage* 2004;22:144–154.
6. Wen W, Sachdev PS, Li JJ, Chen X, Anstey KJ. White matter hyperintensities in the forties: their prevalence and topography in an epidemiological sample aged 44–48. *Hum Brain Mapp* 2009;30:1155–1167.
7. Hachinski VC, Potter P, Merskey H. Leukoaraiosis. *Arch Neurol* 1987;44:21–23.
8. Ovbiagele B, Saver JL. Cerebral white matter hyperintensities on MRI: current concepts and therapeutic implications. *Cerebrovasc Dis* 2006;22:83–90.
9. Pantoni L, Garcia JH. Pathogenesis of leukoaraiosis: a review. *Stroke* 1997;28:652–659.
10. Nucifora PG, Verma R, Lee SK, Melhem ER. Diffusion-tensor MR imaging and tractography: exploring brain microstructure and connectivity. *Radiology* 2007;245:367–384.
11. Chavhan GB, Babyn PS, Thomas B, Shroff MM, Haacke EM. Principles, techniques, and applications of T2*-based MR imaging and its special applications. *Radiographics* 2009;29:1433–1449.
12. Sheline YI, Price JL, Vaishnavi SN, et al. Regional white matter hyperintensity burden in automated segmentation distinguishes late-life depressed subjects from comparison subjects matched for vascular risk factors. *Am J Psychiatry* 2008:524–532.
13. Sachdev P, Brodaty H, Rose N, Cathcart S. Schizophrenia with onset after age 50 years. 2: Neurological, neuropsychological and MRI investigation. *Br J Psychiatry* 1999;175:416–421.
14. McDonald W, Krishnan K, Doaiswamy P, Blazer D. Occurance of subcortical hyperintensities in elderly subjects with mania. *Psychiatry Res* 1991;40:211–220.
15. Valenti R, Poggesi A, Pescini F, Inzitari D, Pantoni L. Psychiatric disturbances in CADASIL: a brief review. *Acta Neurol Scand* 2008;118:291–295.
16. Jorm AF, Anstey KJ, Christensen H, et al. MRI hyperintensities and depressive symptoms in a community sample of individuals 60–64 years old. *Am J Psychiatry* 2005;162:699–705.
17. Khan U, Porteous L, Hassan A, Markus HS. Risk factor profile of cerebral small vessel disease and its subtypes. *J Neurol Neurosurg Psychiatry* 2007;78:702–706.
18. Robinson RG, Spalletta G. Poststroke depression: a review. *Can J Psychiatry* 2010;55:341–349.
19. Jorge RE, Starkstein SE, Raobinson RG. Apathy following stroke. *Can J Psychiatry* 2010;55:350–354.
20. Van Dijk EJ, Prins ND, Vrooman HA, et al. Progression of cerebral small vessel disease in relation to risk factors and cognitive consequences: Rotterdam Scan Study. *Stroke* 2008;39:2712–2719.
21. Taylor WD, Steffens DC, MacFall JR, et al. White matter hyperintesity progression and late life depression outcomes. *Arch Gen Psychiatry* 2003;60:1090–1096.
22. Versluis CE, van der Mast RC, van Buchem MA, et al. Progression of cerebral white matter lesions is not associated with development of depressive symptoms in elderly subjects at risk of cardiovascular

disease: the PROSPER study. *Int J Geriatr Psychiatry* 2006;21:375–381.

23. Hickie I, Scott E, Mitchell P, et al. Subcortical hyperintensities on magnetic resonance imaging: clinical correlates and prognostic significance in patients with severe depression. *Biol Psychiatry* 1995;37:151–160.
24. O'Brien J, Ames D, Chiu E, et al. Severe deep white matter lesions and in elderly patients with major depressive disorder: follow up study. *BMJ* 1998;317:982–984.
25. Robinson RG. Poststroke depression: prevalence, diagnosis, treatment, and disease progression. *Biol Psychiatry* 2003;54:376–587.
26. Goodwin GM. Neuropsychological and neuroimaging evidence for the involvement of the frontal lobes in depression. *J Psychopharmacol* 1997;11:971–975.
27. Benisty S, Gouw AA, Porcher R, et al. Location of lacunar infarcts correlates with cognition in a sample of non-disabled subjects with age-related white-matter changes: the LADIS study. *J Neurol Neurosurg Psychiatry* 2009;80:478–483.
28. Bunce D, Anstey KJ, Cherbuin N, et al. Cognitive deficits are associated with frontal and temporal lobe white matter lesions in middle-aged adults living in the community. *PLoS One* 2010;5: e13567.
29. Taylor WD, MacFall JR, Steffens DC, et al. Localization of age-associated white matter hyperintensities in late-life depression. *Prog Neuropsychopharmacol Biol Psychiatry* 2003;27:539–544.
30. Steffens DC, Helms MJ, Krishnan KR, Burke GL. Cerebrovascular disease and depression symptoms in the Cardiovascular Health Study. *Stroke* 1999;30:2159–2166.
31. Brodaty H, Sachdev PS, Withall A, et al. Frequency and clinical, neuropsychological and neuroimaging correlates of apathy following stroke – the Sydney Stroke Study. *Psychol Med* 2005;35:1707–1716.
32. Djernes JK. Prevalence and predictors of depression in populations of elderly: a review. *Acta Psychiatr Scand* 2006;113:372–387.
33. Blazer DG. Depression in late life: review and commentary. *J Gerontol Med Sci* 2003; 56A:249–265.
34. Bryan RN, Cai J, Burke G, et al. Prevalence and anatomic characteristics of infarct-like lesions on MR images of middle-aged adults: the Atherosclerosis Risk In Communities Study. *AJNR Am J Neuroradiol* 1999;20:1273–1280.
35. De Leeuw FE, de Groot JC, Achten E, et al. Prevalence of cerebral white matter lesions in elderly people: a population based magnetic resonance imaging study. The Rotterdam Scan Study. *J Neurol Neurosurg Psychiatry* 2001;70:9–14.
36. Regier DA, Boyd JH, Burke JDJ, et al. One-month prevalence of mental disorders in the United States: based on five epidemiologic catchment area sites. *Arch Gen Psychiatry* 1988;45:977–986.
37. Trollor JN, Anderson TM, Sachdev PS, Brodaty H, Andrews G. Age shall not weary them: mental health in the middle-aged and the elderly. *Aust N Z J Psychiatry* 2007; 41:581–589.
38. Taylor CB, Conrad A, Wilhelm FH, et al. Psychophysiological and cortisol responses to psychological stress in depressed and nondepressed older men and women with elevated cardiovascular disease risk. *Psychosom Med* 2006;68:538–546.
39. Withall A, Brodaty H, Altendorf A, Sachdev PS. A longitudinal study examining the independence of apathy and depression after stroke: the Sydney Stroke Study. *Int Psychogeriatr* 2011;23:264–273.
40. Robinson RG. *The Clinical Neuropsychiatry of Stroke.* Cambridge, MA: Cambridge University Press; 2006.
41. Sinyor D, Amato P, Kaloupek P. Post-stroke depression: relationship to functional impairment, coping strategies, and rehabilitation outcome. *Stroke* 1986;17:112–117.
42. Carson AJ, MacHale S, Allen K, et al. Depression after stroke and lesion location: a systematic review. *Lancet* 2000;356:122–126.
43. Krishnan KR, Hays JC, Blazer DG. MRI-defined vascular depression. *Am J Psychiatry* 1997;154:497–501.
44. Lavretsky H, Lesser IM, Wohl M, Miller BL. Relationship of age, age at onset, and sex to depression in older adults. *Am J Geriatr Psychiatry* 1998;6:248–256.
45. Steffens DC, Krishnan KRR, Crump C, Burke GL. Cerebrovascular disease and evolution of depressive symptoms in the Cardiovascular Health Study. *Stroke* 2002;33:1636–1644.
46. O'Brien J, Ames D, Chiu E, et al. Severe deep white matter lesions in elderly patients with major depressive disorder: follow up study. *BMJ* 1998;317.
47. Figiel GS, Krishnan KR, Doraiswamy PM. Subcortical structural changes in ECT-induced delirium. *J Geriatr Psychiatry Neurol* 1990;3:172–176.
48. Taragano FE, Allegri R, Vicario A, Bagnatti P, Lyketsos CG. A double blind, randomized clinical trial assessing the efficacy and safety of augmenting standard antidepressant therapy with nimodipine in the treatment of

vascular depression. *Int J Geriatr Psychiatry* 2001;16:254–260.

49. Taragano FE, Bagnatti P, Allegri R. A double-blind, randomized clinical trial to assess the augmentation with nimodipine of antidepressant therapy in the treatment of vascular depression. *Int Psychogeriatr* 2005;17:487–498.
50. Godin O, Dufouil C, Maillard P, et al. White matter lesions as a predictor of depression in the elderly: the 3C-Dijon study. *Biol Psychiatry* 2008;63:663–669.
51. Simpson SW, Jackson A, Baldwin RC, Burns A. Subcortical hyperintensities in late-life depression: acute response to treatment and neuropsychological impairment. *Int Psychogeriatr* 1997;9:257–275.
52. MacFall JR, Taylor WD, Rex DE, et al. Lobar distribution of lesion volumes in late-life depression: the Biomedical Information Research Network (BIRN). *Neuropsychopharmacology* 2006;31:1500–1507.
53. Greenwald BS, Kramer-Ginsberg E, Krishnan KRR, et al. Neuroanatomic localization of magnetic resonance imaging signal hyperintensities in geriatric depression. *Stroke* 1998;29:613–617.
54. MacFall JR, Payne ME, Provenzale JM, Krishnan KRR. Medial orbital frontal lesions in late-onset depression. *Biol Psychiatry* 2001;49:803–806.
55. Alexopoulos GS, Kiosses DN, Choi SJ, Murphy CF, Lim KO. Frontal white matter microstructure and treatment response of late-life depression: a preliminary study. *Am J Psychiatry* 2002;159:1929–1923.
56. Alexopoulos GS, Meyers BS, Young RC, et al. "Vascular depression" hypothesis. *Arch Gen Psychiatry* 1997;54:915–922.
57. McDougall F, Brayne C. Systematic review of the depressive symptoms associated with vascular conditions. *J Affect Disord* 2007;104:25–35.
58. Baldwin RC. Is vascular depression a distinct sub-type of depressive disorder? A review of causal evidence. *Int J Geriatr Psychiatry* 2005;20:1–11.
59. Chen PS, McQuoid DR, Payne ME, Steffens DC. White matter and subcortical gray matter lesion volume changes and late-life depression outcome: a four-year magnetic resonance imaging study. *Int Psychogeriatr* 2006;18:445–456.
60. Sanders ML, Lyness JM, Eberly S, King DA, Caine ED. Cerebrovascular risk factors, executive dysfunction, and depression in older primary care patients. *Am J Geriatr Psychiatry* 2006;14:145–152.
61. Ikram MA, Luijendijk HJ, Vernooij MW, et al. Vascular brain disease and depression in the elderly. *Epidemiology* 2010;21:78–81.
62. Steffens DC, Conway CR, Dombeck CB, et al. Severity of subcortical gray matter hyperintensity predicts ECT response in geriatric depression. *J ECT* 2001;17:45–49.
63. Coffey CE, Figiel GS, Djang WT, et al. Effects of ECT on brain structure: a pilot prospective magnetic resonance imaging study. *Am J Psychiatry* 1988;145:701–706.
64. Krauthammer C, Klerman G. Secondary mania. Manic syndromes associated with antecedent physical illness or drugs. *Arch Gen Psychiatry* 1978;35:1333–1339.
65. Santos CO, Caeiro L, Ferro JM, Figueira ML. Mania and stroke: a systematic review. *Cerebrovasc Dis* 2011;32:11–21.
66. Robinson RG, Boston JD, Starkstein SE, Price TR. Comparison of mania and depression after brain injury: causal factors. *Am J Psychiatry* 1988;145:172–178.
67. Starkstein SE, Pearlson GD, Boston JD, Robinson RG. Mania after brain injury. A controlled study of causative factors. *Arch Neurol* 1987;44:1069–1073.
68. Lin HC, Tsai SY, Lee HC. Increased risk of developing stroke among patients with bipolar disorder after an acute mood episode: a six-year follow-up study. *J Affect Disord* 2007;100:49–54.
69. Newcomer JW. Medical risk in patients with bipolar disorder and schizophrenia. *J Clin Psychiatry* 2006;67:25–30.
70. Huang SH, Chung KH, Hsu JL, et al. The risk factors for elderly patients with bipolar disorder having cerebral infarction. *J Geriatr Psychiatry Neurol* 2012;25:15–19.
71. Fujikawa T, Yamawaki S, Touhouda Y. Silent cerebral infarctions in patients with late-onset mania. *Stroke* 1995;26:946–949.
72. Beyer JL, Young R, Kuchibhatla M, Krishnan KR. Hyperintense MRI lesions in bipolar disorder: a meta-analysis and review. *Int Rev Psychiatry* 2009;21:394–409.
73. Vederine FE, Wessa M, Leboyer M, Houenou J. A meta-analysis of whole-brain diffusion tensor imaging studies in bipolar disorder. *Prog Neuropsychopharmacol Biol Psychiatry* 2011;35:1820–1826.
74. Bellani M, Brambilla P. Diffusion imaging studies of white matter integrity in bipolar disorder. *Epidemiol Psychiatr Sci* 2011;20:137–140.
75. Kennedy N, Everitt B, Boydell J, et al. Incidence and distribution of first-episode mania by age: results from a 35-year study. *Psychol Med* 2005;35:855–863.
76. Steffens DC, Krishnan KR. Structural neuroimaging and

mood disorders: recent findings, implications for classification, and future directions. *Biol Psychiatry* 1998;43:705–712.

77. Howard R, Rabins PV, Seeman MV, Jeste DV. Late-onset schizophrenia and very late-onset schizophrenia-like psychosis: an international consensus. *Am J Psychiatry* 2000;157:172–178.
78. Östling S, Skoog I. Psychotic symptoms and paranoid ideation in a nondemented population-based sample of the very old. *Arch Gen Psychiatry* 2002; 59:53–59.
79. Kumral E, Öztürk Ö. Delusional state following acute stroke. *Neurology* 2004;62:110–113.
80. Almeida OP, Xiao J. Mortality associated with incident mental health disorders after stroke. *Aust N Z J Psychiatry* 2007;41:274–281.
81. Ballard C, Neill D, O'Brien J, et al. Anxiety, depression and psychosis in vascular dementia: prevalence and associations. *J Affective Disord* 2000;59:97–106.
82. Hope T, Keene J, Gedling K, et al. Behaviour changes in dementia 1: Point of entry data of a prospective study. *Int J Geriatr Psychiatry* 1997;12:1062–1073.
83. Breitner JCS, Husain MM, Figiel GS, Krishnan KR, Boyko OB. Cerebral white matter disease in late-onset paranoid psychosis. *Biol Psychiatry* 1990;28:266–274.
84. Sachdev P, Brodaty H. Quantitative study of signal hyperintensities on T2-weighted magnetic resonance imaging in late-onset schizophrenia. *Am J Psychiatry* 1999;156:1958–1967.
85. Keshavan MS, Mulsant BH, Sweet RA, et al. MRI changes in schizophrenia in late life: a preliminary controlled study. *Psychiatry Res* 1996;60:117–123.
86. Lesser IM, Jeste DV, Boone KB, et al. Late-onset psychotic disorder, not otherwise specified: clinical and neuroimaging findings. *Biol Psychiatry* 1992;31:419–423.
87. Corey-Bloom J, Jernigan T, Archibald S, Harris MJ, Jeste DV. Quantitative magnetic resonance imaging of the brain in late-life schizophrenia. *Am J Psychiatry* 1995;152:447–449.
88. Howard R, Cox T, Almeida O, et al. White matter signal hyperintensities in the brains of patients with late paraphrenia and the normal community-living elderly. *Biol Psychiatry* 1995;38:86–91.
89. Rivkin P, Kraut M, Barta P, et al. White matter hyperintensity volume in late-onset and early-onset schizophrenia. *Int J Geriatr Psychiatry* 2000;15:1085–1089.
90. Symonds LL, Olichney JM, Jernigan TL, et al. Lack of clinically significant gross structural abnormalities in MRIs of older patients with schizophrenia and related psychoses. *J Neuropsychiatry Clin Neurosci* 1997;9:251–258.
91. Ogawa Y, Hashimoto M, Yatabe Y, et al. Association of cerebral small vessel disease with delusions in patients with Alzheimer's disease. *Int J Geriatr Psychiatry* 2013;28:18–25.
92. Aström M. Generalized anxiety disorder in stroke patients: a three-year longitudinal study. *Stroke* 1996;27:270–275.
93. Castillo CS, Schultz SK, Robinson RG. Clinical correlates of early-onset and late-onset post-stroke generalized anxiety. *Am J Psychiatry* 1995;152:1174–1179.
94. Sultzer DL, Mahler ME, Cummings JL, et al. Cortical abnormalities associated with subcortical lesions in vascular dementia: clinical and positron emission tomographic findings. *Arch Neurol* 1995;52:773–780.
95. Duggal HS. New-onset PTSD after thalamic infarct. *Am J Psychiatry* 2002;159:2113–2114.
96. Fan Q, Yan X, Wang J, et al. Abnormalities of white matter microstructure in unmedicated obsessive-compulsive disorder and changes after medication. *PLoS One* 2012;7:e35889.
97. Nestadt G, Bienvenu OJ, Cai G, Samuels J, Eaton WW. Incidence of obsessive-compulsive disorder in adults. *J Nerv Ment Dis* 1998:401–406.
98. Berthier ML, Kulisevsky J, Gironell A, Heras JA. Obsessive-compulsive disorder associated with brain lesions: clinical phenomenology, cognitive function, and anatomic correlates. *Neurology* 1996;47:353–361.
99. Weiss AP, Jenike MA. Late-onset obsessive-compulsive disorder: a case series. *J Neuropsychiatry Clin Neurosci* 2000;12:265–268.
100. Menzies L, Chamberlain SR, Laird AR, et al. Integrating evidence from neuroimaging and neuropsychological studies of obsessive-compulsive disorder: the orbitofronto-striatal model revisited. *Neurosci Biobehav Rev* 2008;32:525–549.
101. Marin RS. Apathy: a neuropsychiatric syndrome. *J Neuropsychiatry Clin Neurosci* 1991;3:243–254.
102. Levy R, Dubois B. Apathy and the functional anatomy of the prefrontal cortex-basal ganglia circuits. *Cereb Cortex* 2006;16:916–928.
103. Starkstein SE, Leentjens AF. The nosological position of apathy in clinical practice. *J Neurol Neurosurg Psychiatry* 2008;79:1088–1092.
104. Stuss DT, van Reekum R, Murphy KJ. Differentiation of states and causes of apathy. In Borod J, ed. *The Neuropsychology of Emotion*. New York, NY: Oxford University Press; 2000: pp. 340–363.
105. Van Reekum R, Stuss DT, Ostrander L. Apathy: why care? *J Neuropsychiatry Clin Neurosci* 2005;17:7–19.

106. Starkstein SE, Mizrahi R, Capizzano AA, et al. Neuroimaging correlates of apathy and depression in Alzheimer's disease. *J Neuropsychiatry Clin Neurosci* 2009;21:259–265.

107. Jouvent E, Reyes S, Mangin JF, et al. Apathy is related to cortex morphology in CADASIL: a sulcal-based morphometry study. *Neurology* 2011;76:1472–1477.

108. Reyes S, Viswanathan A, Godin O, et al. Apathy: a major symptom in CADASIL. *Neurology* 2009;72:905–910.

109. Grool AM, Gerritsen L, Zuithoff NP, et al. Lacunar infarcts in deep white matter are associated with higher and more fluctuating depressive symptoms during three years follow-up. *Biol Psychiatry* 2013;73:169–176.

110. Grool AM, van der Graaf Y, Mali WP, et al. Location and progression of cerebral small-vessel disease and atrophy, and depressive symptom profiles: the Second Manifestations of Arterial Disease (SMART)-Medea study. *Psychol Med* 2011;42:359–370.

111. Jonsson M, Edman A, Lind K, et al. Apathy is a prominent neuropsychiatric feature of radiological white-matter changes in patients with dementia. *Int J Geriatr Psychiatry* 2010;25:588–595.

112. Andersson S, Krogstad JM, Finset A. Apathy and depressed mood in acquired brain damage: relationship to lesion localization and psychophysiological reactivity. *Psychol Med* 1999;29:447–456.

Chapter 22

Consequences of cerebral small vessel disease: disability, mortality, and prognosis

Anna Poggesi, Leonardo Pantoni, and Domenico Inzitari

Introduction

Brain small vessel disease (SVD) causes selective lesions, including lacunar infarcts, white matter lesions, microbleeds, and intracerebral hemorrhage, all located in the subcortical structures of the brain. Over the last decade, evidence has accumulated about the prevalence, clinical significance, and prognostic value of each of these lesions. SVD has been shown to play an important role related to stroke, cognitive decline, and psychiatric and motor disorders, as outlined in other chapters of this book. Also, changes induced by SVD have been considered major determinants of disability, mortality, and, overall, as a marker of poor prognosis. Death and disability are of importance from ethical, personal, family, society, and economic viewpoints.

This chapter deals with the available evidence of the association of white matter changes, lacunar infarcts, and microbleeds with disability and mortality. We begin with a brief introduction to the definition of disability.

In 1980 the World Health Organization developed a first model of health, which was the International Classification of Impairments, Disabilities and Handicaps [1]. In the model, health was divided into three domains: (1) impairments of body functions and structures; (2) disability or an inability to undertake tasks; and (3) handicap or the loss of role that accompanies impairment and disability. This framework provoked much debate as the cause of disability and handicap was assumed solely to be due to disease, while environmental and societal factors were not taken into account. In 2001, a revised framework was validated responding to such criticisms. In the International Classification of Functioning, Disability and Health (ICF), health is defined by the interaction between body functions and structures and their impairments, activities and their activity limitations ("disability" in the previous definition), participation and restriction in participation ("handicap" in the previous definition), and also contextual or environmental factors and personal factors [2]. Thus, functioning and disability are viewed as a complex interaction between health condition of the individual and the contextual factors of the environment as well as personal factors. The picture produced by this combination of factors and dimensions is that of "the person in his or her world."

In geriatric medicine, functional status refers to the ability to perform activities necessary or desirable in daily life. Functional status is directly influenced by health conditions, particularly in the context of an elder's environment and social support network. Changes in functional status should prompt further diagnostic evaluation and intervention.

Table 22.1 summarizes some of the different instruments adopted in neurology and geriatric medicine for assessing global functioning, which will be cited in the following paragraphs [3–7]. In the same table, the evidenced effect of each of the subcortical vascular lesions is highlighted.

White matter changes: prognostic effects in terms of death and disability

White matter changes (WMCs), appearing as bilateral, patchy, or diffuse areas of hypodensity on computed tomography (CT) or hyperintensities on T2-weighted magnetic resonance imaging (MRI) scans, are frequently observed in the brains of elderly subjects, particularly those with history of arterial hypertension often combined with other vascular

Cerebral Small Vessel Disease, ed. Leonardo Pantoni and Philip B. Gorelick. Published by Cambridge University Press.

Table 22.1 Main clinical instruments adopted in neurologic and geriatric clinical fields for the assessment of global functioning

Instrument	Brief description	Small vessel disease		
		White matter changes	Lacunes	Microbleeds
BADL [3] *Basic Activities of Daily Living*	Consists of self-care tasks (personal hygiene and grooming, dressing, feeding, functional transfers, bowel and bladder management, and ambulation)	X		
IADL [4] *Instrumental Activities of Daily Living*	Not necessary for fundamental functioning but they let the individual live independently in the community (ability to use the telephone, shopping, food preparation, housekeeping, laundry, mode of transportation, responsibilities for own medications, and ability to handle finances)	X		
DAD [5] *Disability Assessment for Dementia scale*	Forty-item questionnaire including: (1) Basic Activities of Daily Living; (2) Instrumental Activities of Daily Living; (3) leisure activities (recreational activities). Each item is considered by the cognitive processing involved as being: (a) an initiation; (b) planning and organization; or (c) an effective performance item	X		
mRS [6] *Modified Rankin Scale*	Measures the degree of disability of people after a stroke or other causes of neurologic disability. The scale runs from 0 to 6, from perfect health without symptoms to death		X	X
Barthel Index [7]	Ordinal scale measuring functional performance in 10 variables describing Activities of Daily Living and mobility in people after stroke or hospital discharge		X	X

risk factors. WMCs may be seated in the periventricular white matter, corona radiata, and centrum semiovale, may be more or less extensive, usually have irregular margins, and do not follow specific vascular territories. Figure 22.1 shows the MRI appearance of WMCs of different degrees of severity according to the Fazekas visual rating scale [8]. Nowadays, WMCs are fully recognized as one of the most typical neuroimaging expressions of cerebral SVD [9]. The clinicopathologic significance of WMCs has been the object of several studies over the last 30 years. In the 1990s there was no full consensus on the clinical significance of WMCs, although some data existed (reviewed in 1995, see [10]) supporting a possible association with cognitive, motor, mood, and micturition disorders. Moreover, an increased risk of cardiovascular events and death was reported in patients showing extensive WMCs [11–14]. Currently, evidence consistently indicates that, particularly when severe, WMCs are associated with a number of significant clinical and functional outcomes [15–17].

To reach an agreement on the pathologic and clinical significance of WMCs, and to harmonize and promote research in this field, a European collaboration was started in 1996, the European Task Force on Age-Related White Matter Changes [18]. This collaboration was an ideal setting for planning the Leukoaraiosis And DISability (LADIS) study. In 2001, this project succeeded in obtaining both endorsement and financial support from the European Union, after applying for funding to the Fifth European Framework Program "Quality of life and management of living resources." The main aim of the project was to assess the role of WMCs as a determinant of the transition from functional autonomy to dependency in the elderly [19]. This definition was based on the Instrumental Activities of Daily Living (IADL) scale. At study entry, patients had to perform without help on all the activities of the IADL

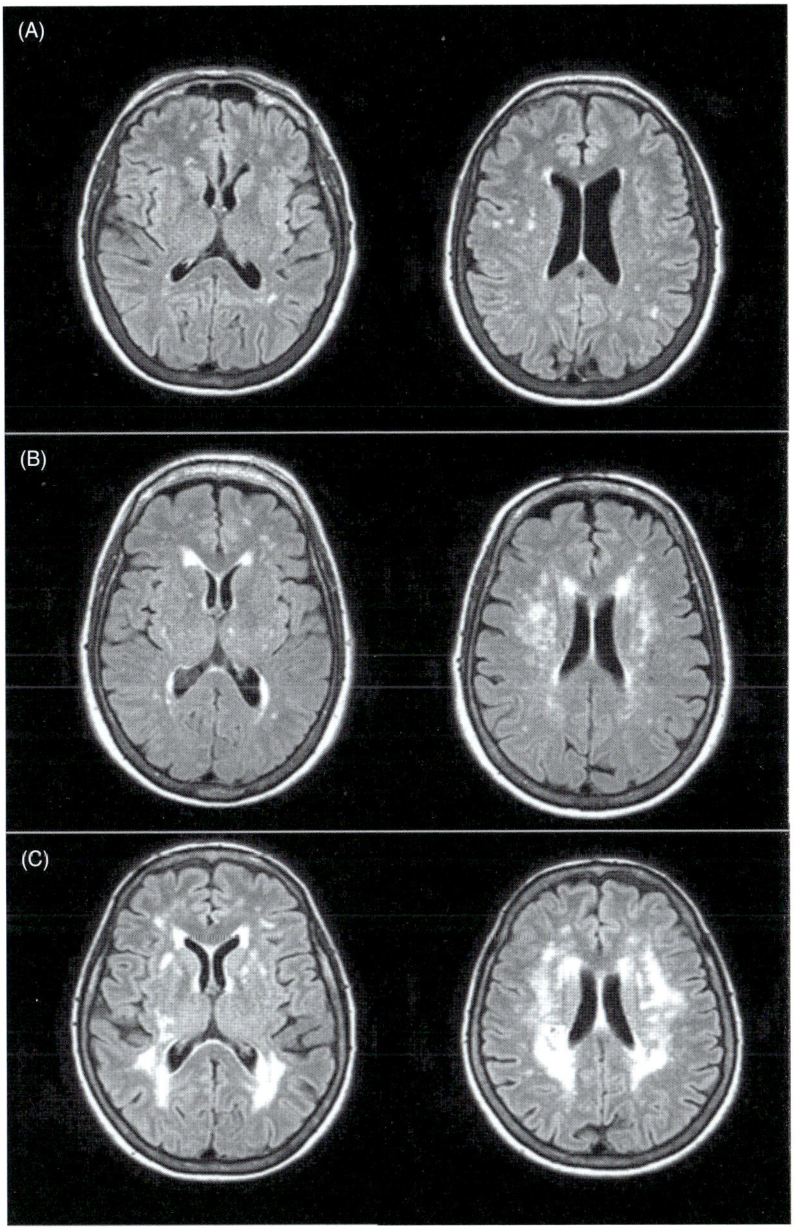

Figure 22.1 Magnetic resonance imaging (MRI) appearance of white matter changes (WMCs) of different severity. There are different ways of assessing severity of WMCs. For the visual assessment of WMCs on fluid-attenuated inversion recovery (FLAIR) images there is one simple scoring system which is the modified version of the Fazekas scale [8], as adopted in the Leukoaraiosis And DISability (LADIS) study. The modified Fazekas scale scores range from mild to severe. In these examples: (A) Mild WMCs: punctuate lesions in the deep white matter with a maximum diameter of a single lesion of 9 mm and of grouped lesions of 20 mm. (B) Moderate WMCs: early confluent lesions, with single lesions between 10 and 20 mm, grouped lesions more than 20 mm in any diameter, and no more than connecting bridges between individual lesions. (C) Severe WMCs: single lesions or confluent areas of hyperintensity of 20 mm or more in any diameter.

scale, or to be impaired on just one activity. The endpoint was the progression to impairment in more than one activity. Figure 22.2 illustrates the design and main methodological issues of LADIS. Results achieved from LADIS have been summarized in a recently published review paper [20].

A cross-sectional analysis of the baseline LADIS cohort showed that patients with the highest severity of WMCs, even if independent in IADL at entry, already had a small but measurable degree of functional impairment as measured by the 40-item Disability Assessment for Dementia (DAD) scale [21]. A trend towards declining performance on the DAD scale was apparent with increasing WMC score severity. The independent effect of WMCs on global functioning was maintained after a multiple regression analysis, controlling for numerous other determinants of disability in the elderly. Possible links between WMC degree of severity and global functional performance was a selective impairment in

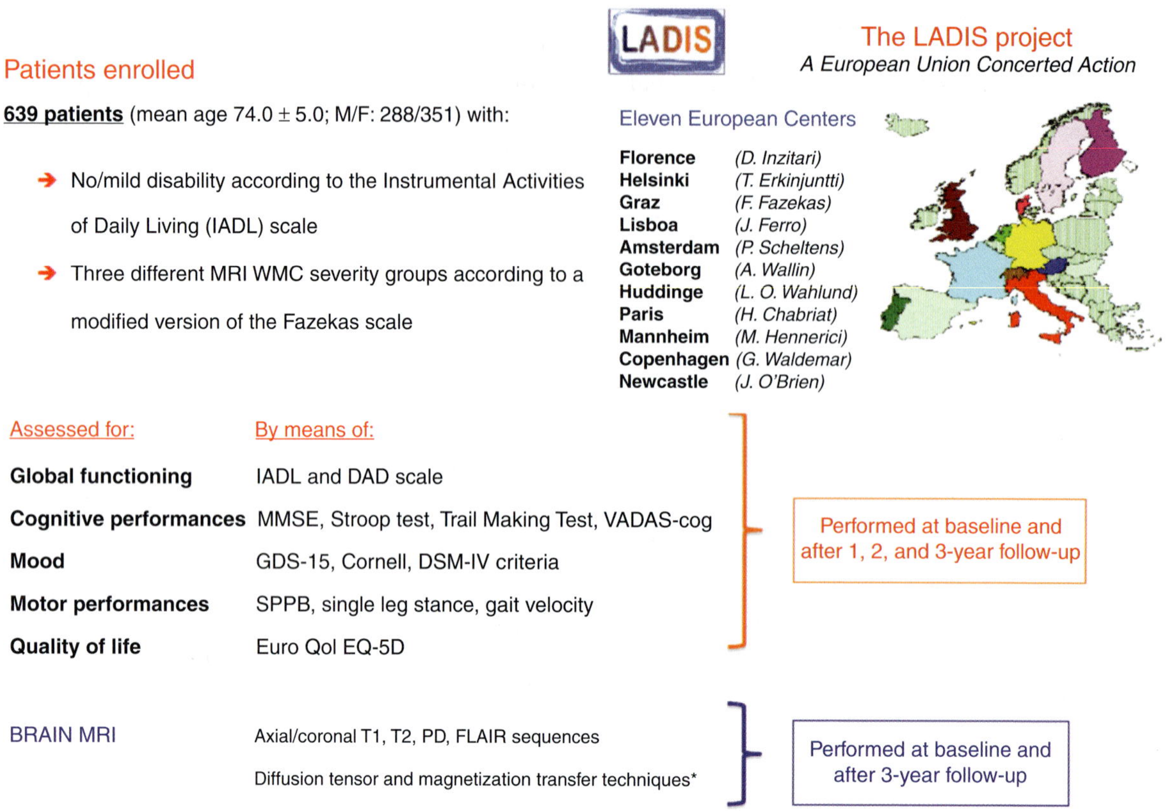

Figure 22.2 Design and main methodological aspects of the Leukoaraiosis And DISability (LADIS) study. DAD, Disability Assessment for Dementia scale; FLAIR, fluid-attenuated inversion recovery; GDS-15, Geriatric Depression Scale 15 items; IADL, Instrumental Activities of Daily Living scale; MMSE, Mini Mental State Examination; PD, proton density; SPPB, Short Physical Performance Battery; WMC, white matter change. *Available only in selected centers.

the executive domain, which worsened along with increasing WMC severity and was significantly correlated with the DAD total score [21].

Considering the prospective phase of LADIS, an interim analysis, performed after just one year from enrolment, showed that the rate of transition from functional autonomy to disability was 9%, 15%, and 26% respectively in the mild, moderate, and severe groups of WMCs. Subjects with severe degrees of WMCs had a risk of transition more than twofold higher compared to the mild group, independent of a large number of other predictors of disability [22].

The analysis of the three-year follow-up data offered the conclusive proof of the original hypothesis of the study [23]. After a median follow-up period of 2.9 years, information on the main outcome was available from over 90% of the enrolled patients. The annual rate of transition or death was 10.5%, 15.1%, and 29.5% respectively for patients with mild, moderate, and severe WMCs (Kaplan–Meier log-rank test $P<0.001$). Comparing severe with mild WMCs, and adjusting by a Cox model for other factors of functional decline, the risk of transition to disability or death was more than twofold higher (hazard ratio [HR] 2.43; 95% confidence interval [CI]: 1.70–3.47). The effect of severe WMCs on disability was also independent of baseline degree of cerebral atrophy and number of infarcts, while incident stroke and dementia only slightly modified that effect [23].

A systematic review and meta-analysis of 46 prospective studies has recently provided strong evidence that the presence of WMCs is associated with a poor prognosis in terms of death, stroke, and dementia [17]. Studies were included in the meta-analyses if they provided longitudinal data on the association of WMCs (detected by MRI) with risk of stroke, dementia, cognitive decline, and death. Only studies using a categorical measure of WMCs were included, and when more than two categories were present, HRs for the highest category compared with the lowest category were used. Focusing on mortality data, four population-based and six hospital-based studies (these last had included only high-risk patients, i.e., those presenting with a history of stroke, depression, or minor neurologic symptoms), consistently provided proof of evidence that WMCs predict an increased risk of death. From pooled data, the adjusted HR for death among subjects with WMCs, compared to those without, was doubled (HR 2.0, 95% CI 1.6–2.7) [17].

Lacunar infarcts: prognostic effects in terms of death and disability

Lacunar stroke, one of the main stroke types, is a widely accepted consequence of SVD. Lacunar infarcts are mainly located in the basal ganglia, internal capsule, thalamus, corona radiata, and brainstem. On MRI they appear as hypointense foci on T1-weighted sequences with a maximum diameter conventionally fixed at 15 mm (Figure 22.3). Lacunar infarcts may be symptomatic, causing a clinically evident stroke, or asymptomatic, also referred to as "silent," depending on whether they are located in clinically eloquent or ineloquent areas of the brain. Importantly, both types of lacunar infarcts, silent and symptomatic, share the same risk factor profile and impact [24]. Thus, the term "silent" has a misleading connotation.

When symptomatic, lacunar infarcts are associated typically with the "classical" Fisher lacunar syndromes: pure motor hemiparesis, sensorimotor stroke, pure sensory stroke, dysarthria–clumsy hand, and ataxic hemiparesis [25]. Lacunar strokes account for about one fourth of the total cases of ischemic stroke. Incidence rates reported in previous studies range from 13/100 000 per year up to 59/100 000 per year [26]. Data from a French prospective population-based registry (1989–2006) showed a significant increase in the incidence of lacunar stroke, especially in patients under 65 years of age [27].

Among all ischemic stroke subtypes, lacunar strokes were once considered the most benign, with good prognosis given the frequently good recovery and a relatively small risk of recurrence. This view has been modified during the last decade [24]. The fact that prognosis is more favorable in terms of survival and disability in the short term, compared to other stroke subtypes, probably depends on the smaller size of the brain lesion. However, in the long term, an excess risk of death, disability, stroke recurrence, and cognitive impairment has been consistently documented.

In 2003, Norrving [24] analyzed 24 studies reporting data on survival and stroke recurrence among patients with lacunar infarcts. Most of these studies found a low risk of death immediately after stroke onset that may be explained, at least in part, by the limited size of the primary lesion, the typical rapid rate of recovery, and the fact that cardiac

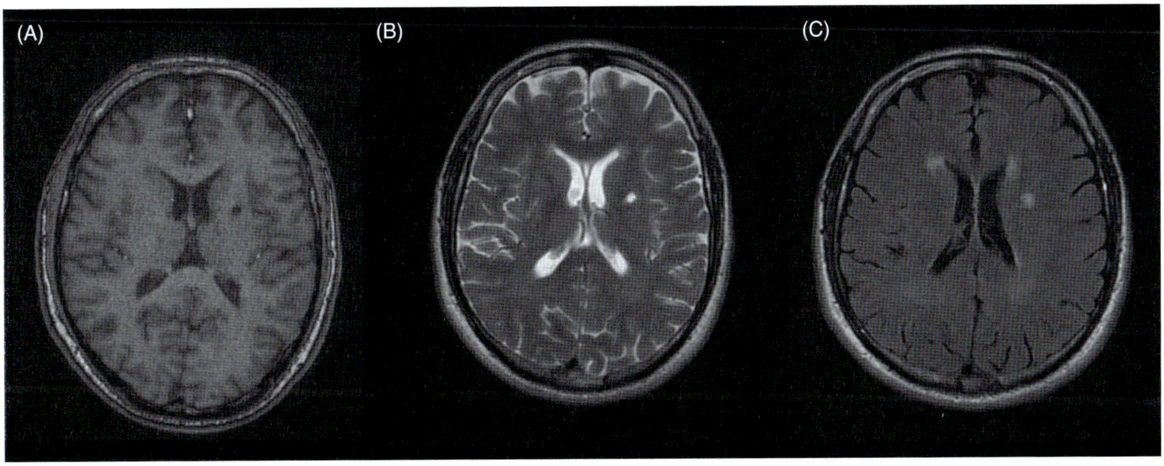

Figure 22.3 Magnetic resonance imaging (MRI) appearance of lacunar infarcts. Different aspects of lacunar infarcts according to MRI sequences: T1-weighted sequence (A), T2-weighted sequence (B), and fluid-attenuated inversion recovery (FLAIR) sequence (C). The combination of the three-scan sequences is useful to distinguish lacunes from Virchow–Robin spaces and microbleeds. In the above case, one lacunar infarct is seated in the left globus pallidus.

comorbidities are less common in these patients compared to other stroke types. The mean case fatality rate was 2.5% (range 0–10%) at 30 days, and 2.8% (range 2–15%) at 1 year. This scenario changed after reports of studies with longer follow-up. In a 10-year follow-up study, the risk of death in lacunar stroke patients was similar to that in the general population for the first 5 years, but increased by 10–15% between 5 and 10 years, and after 10 years 60% of the patients had died [28]. In another study with 14 years of follow-up, death rates in patients with lacunar stroke were significantly lower compared with the general population after 6 years, while after 14 years almost 75% of the patients had died [29]. In a population-based study, the five-year survival was longer in patients with lacunar stroke compared to nonlacunar strokes but, when comparing average annual mortality rates, the longer survival mostly depended on low early mortality, while from the third year onward rates were similar between the two groups or slightly higher in patients with lacunar stroke [26].

Long-term global functioning as an outcome after lacunar infarction has received less attention than survival and stroke recurrence. Bamford et al. [30] compared lacunar stroke patients with patients with other stroke types: the former had more favorable functional outcomes shortly after the index stroke. However, the proportion of patients with lacunar infarct strokes that were dependent in daily activities was as high as 18–33% at 1 year, 36% at 2 years, and 42% at 3 years [24]. Moreover about 10% of the patients who were independent in daily living had measurable impairments in other domains; for example, those connected with restricted customary social relations or reduced recreational activities [31].

In Norrving's review [24], among factors predicting disability in lacunar stroke patients, besides age, diabetes, and initial stroke severity, imaging markers such as asymptomatic lacunar lesions and WMCs proved to be the most important contributors, suggesting that the more advanced are imaging signs of cerebral small artery disease, the more limited is the possibility of functional recovery of the brain after an, albeit small, focal lesion. The same applies when death is taken as the outcome, as lacunar stroke patients with silent infarcts and WMCs show higher mortality rates [32]. These data reinforce the concept that in patients presenting with lacunar stroke the coexistence of silent infarcts and WMCs seems to have additive or synergistic effects with stroke on disability or death. In the last decade it has become clear that small infarcts that do not cause acute stroke symptoms are more common than symptomatic ones [33].

In summary, lacunar infarcts cannot be considered an innocent vascular bystander lesion. Although the prognosis associated with these lesions is more favorable in the short term, in the long term they are associated with an excess risk of death, increased recurrence rate of stroke, and increased risk of disability. Moreover in the long term, patients with a lacunar stroke show a higher risk of developing cognitive decline and dementia [31, 34, 35]. Factors that are associated with cognitive decline with lacunar infarcts are the presence of multiple lacunes and their location [36, 37]. Recently, data from the Secondary Prevention of Small Subcortical Strokes (SPS3) study have shown that mild cognitive impairment was present in nearly half of this cohort of lacunar stroke patients [38].

Microbleeds: prognostic effects in terms of death and disability

Microbleeds are small dot-like lesions appearing as hyposignals on gradient echo T2*-weighted MR sequences or on susceptibility-weighted MR images. As WMCs and lacunes are accepted signs of ischemic cerebral SVD, microbleeds, together with larger cerebral bleeding (i.e., intracerebral hemorrhage or macrohemorrhages), are considered as the MRI expression of hemorrhagic SVD [39]. Based on available evidence, the etiology of cerebral microbleeds may differ according to their location. Cortical–subcortical, also defined as lobar, microbleeds are more closely associated with underlying cerebral amyloid angiopathy, thus, also relevant in the context of Alzheimer's disease pathology; whereas deep and infratentorial microbleeds are presumed to result from hypertensive SVD [40]. These latter are in fact found more frequently in hypertensive persons, both in the general population and in patients with cerebrovascular disorders [41]. Figure 22.4 shows MRI examples of predominantly subcortical microbleeds.

Prevalence of cerebral microbleeds is variably reported from different study populations, ranging from 5% in the general population, to 35% in patients with ischemic stroke, and up to 60% in patients with hemorrhagic stroke [41]. Their true prevalence in the different settings is presumed to be even higher, and figures are expected to increase in the future, mostly

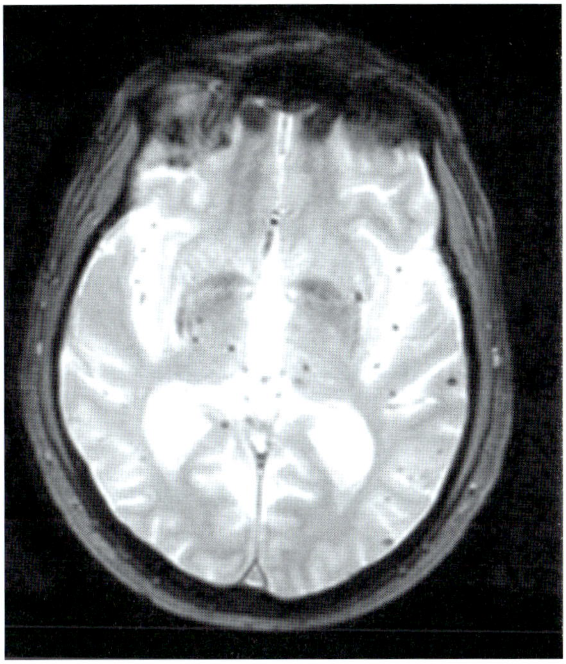

Figure 22.4 Magnetic resonance imaging (MRI) appearance of predominantly subcortical microbleeds. MRI, axial plane, T2* gradient-echo sequence showing multiple brain microbleeds predominantly in the basal ganglia.

due to the development of new and more sensitive scanning techniques, including susceptibility-weighted MRI and ultra-high field strength techniques [42, 43].

Cerebral microbleeds have been considered for a long time to be incidental lesions, but evidence is rapidly increasing documenting their association with cognitive impairment, dementia, bleeding risk, and stroke. Studies focusing on the relationship between microbleeds and disability or death are scarce. Data sustaining such relations have been recently reviewed (see [39]). A first demonstration of this possible association derives from studies of patients affected by cerebral autosomal dominant arteriopathy with subcortical infarcts and leukoencephalopathy (CADASIL) [44–46], a disease where WMCs, lacunar infarcts, and microbleeds occur in association with the typical CADASIL angiopathy, similarly to other forms of small vessel angiopathy. In a cohort of 147 patients, microbleeds were observed in 35%, mostly occurring in deep regions such as the thalamus, basal ganglia, and brainstem [45]. Both the presence and the number of microbleeds turned out to be associated with handicap or disability, assessed by the modified Rankin Scale or the Barthel Index, independent of other clinical determinants of disability and of other MRI lesions [45, 46].

In a memory clinic setting, Henneman et al. [47] assessed the predictive value of cerebral microbleeds, together with other MRI markers, with respect to death risk. The study cohort was composed of 1138 patients with diagnosis of subjective memory complaints, mild cognitive impairment, Alzheimer's disease, vascular dementia, or other dementia types. During a mean follow-up of about 2.5 years both microbleeds and, to a lesser extent, WMCs proved to be independent determinants of death, adjusting for confounders, (HR [95% CI] 1.5 [1.1–2.0] for microbleeds and HR [95% CI] 1.2 [1.0–1.4] for WMCs) [47].

Data from the PROspective Study of Pravastatin in the Elderly at Risk (PROSPER) trial have recently confirmed the predictive value of microbleeds in relation to a few adverse outcomes [48]. Among 435 patients at increased risk of vascular disease followed up for an average of seven years, nonlobar microbleeds were independently associated with cardiovascular mortality, while lobar ones predicted stroke-related mortality [48].

Conclusion

We have reviewed the available evidence concerning the prognostic effects of three forms of SVD – WMCs, lacunar infarcts, and microbleeds – on disability and death. WMCs, particularly when of severe degree, are recognized as an important determinant of functional loss in elderly persons. In LADIS, it has clearly been shown that an older person with extensive MRI-based WMCs has a risk of rapid decline in global functioning. Also for lacunar infarcts, the available evidence shows that both clinically manifest and so-called "silent" (i.e., asymptomatic) lesions are regarded as important markers of unfavorable functional outcome. Finally, preliminary data suggest that cerebral microbleeds may be considered an independent marker of the risk of deterioration in global functioning.

Furthermore, there is adequate evidence that SVD has an important role in cerebrovascular disease and is a leading cause of functional, as well as cognitive, decline in the elderly. Given the frequent coexistence of different forms of SVD (i.e., WMCs, lacunar infarcts, and cerebral microbleeds), all relevant lesion types need to be taken into account. We are in need of specific preventive and therapeutic measures to reduce the burden of functional loss caused by SVD. In this regard, neuroimaging could be a major tool to help assess efficacy of these measures. As an example, some studies have considered WMC progression as a surrogate marker in therapeutic trials of cerebral SVD. In the Perindopril Protection aGainst Recurrent Stroke Study (PROGRESS) trial, MRI was used to demonstrate that a regimen of active blood pressure lowering was associated with reduction of progression of WMCS [49]. Two other trials have investigated the effect of statins on WMC progression, showing conflicting results [50, 51]. Preliminary experience suggests that more sophisticated MRI techniques, such as diffusion imaging and spectroscopy, should be utilized in future studies.

References

1. World Health Organization. *International Classification of Impairments, Disabilities and Handicaps*. Geneva: World Health Organization; 1980.
2. World Health Organization. *International Classification of Functioning, Disability and Health*. Geneva: World Health Organization; 2001. Available from: http://www3.who.int/icf/intros/ICF-Eng-Intro.pdf (accessed January 3, 2014).
3. Katz S. Assessing self-maintenance: Activities of Daily Living, mobility, and Instrumental Activities of Daily Living. *J Am Geriatr Soc* 1983;31:721–727.
4. Lawton MP, Brody EM. Assessment of older people: self-maintaining and Instrumental Activities of Daily Living. *Gerontologist* 1969;9:179–186.
5. Gelinàs I, Gauthier L, McIntyre M, et al. Development of a functional measure for persons with Alzheimer's disease: the Disability Assessment for Dementia. *Am J Occup Ther* 1999;53:471–481.
6. Van Swieten J, Koudstaal P, Visser M, et al. Interobserver agreement for the assessment of handicap in stroke patients. *Stroke* 1988;19:604–607.
7. Mahoney FI, Barthel DW. Functional evaluation: the Barthel Index. *MD State Med J* 1965;14:61–65.
8. Fazekas F, Chawluk JB, Alavi A, Hurtig HI, Zimmerman RA. MR signal abnormalities at 1.5 T in Alzheimer's dementia and normal aging. *AJR Am J Roentgenol* 1987;149:351–356.
9. Pantoni L. Cerebral small vessel disease: from pathogenesis and clinical characteristics to therapeutic challenges. *Lancet Neurol* 2010;9:689–701.
10. Pantoni L, Garcia JH. The significance of cerebral white matter abnormalities 100 years after Binswanger's report. A review. *Stroke* 1995;26:1293–1301.
11. Tarvonen-Schröder S, Kurki T, Räihä I, Sourander L. Leukoaraiosis and cause of death: a five year follow up. *J Neurol Neurosurg Psychiatry* 1995;58:586–589.
12. Inzitari D, Di Carlo A, Mascalchi M, Pracucci G, Amaducci L. The cardiovascular outcome of patients with motor impairment and extensive leukoaraiosis. *Arch Neurol* 1995;52:687–691.
13. Inzitari D, Cadelo M, Marranci ML, Pracucci G, Pantoni L. Vascular deaths in elderly neurological patients with leukoaraiosis. *J Neurol Neurosurg Psychiatry* 1997;62:177–181.
14. Briley DP, Haroon S, Sergent SM, Thomas S. Does leukoaraiosis predict morbidity and mortality? *Neurology* 2000;54:90–94.
15. Inzitari D. Leukoaraiosis: an independent risk factor for stroke? *Stroke* 2003;34:2067–2071.
16. Pantoni L. Leukoaraiosis: from an ancient term to an actual marker of poor prognosis. *Stroke* 2008;39:1401–1403.
17. Debette S, Markus HS. The clinical importance of white matter hyperintensities on brain magnetic resonance imaging: systematic review and meta-analysis. *BMJ* 2010;341:3666.
18. Erkinjuntti T, Pantoni L, Scheltens P. Cooperation and networking on white matter disorders: the European Task Force on Age-Related White Matter Changes. *Dement Geriatr Cogn Disord* 1998;9(Suppl 1): 44–45.
19. Pantoni L, Basile AM, Pracucci G, et al. Impact of age-related cerebral white matter changes on the transition to disability – the LADIS study: rationale, design and methodology. *Neuroepidemiology* 2005; 24:51–62.
20. The LADIS Study Group. 2001–2011: a decade of the LADIS (Leukoaraiosis And DISability) study: what have we learned about white matter changes and small-vessel disease? *Cerebrovasc Dis* 2011;32:577–588.
21. Pantoni L, Poggesi A, Basile AM, et al. LADIS Study Group. Leukoaraiosis predicts hidden global functioning impairment in nondisabled older people: the LADIS (Leukoaraiosis And DISability in the elderly) study. *J Am Geriatr Soc* 2006;54:1095–2101.
22. Inzitari D, Simoni M, Pracucci G, et al. LADIS Study Group. Risk of rapid global functional decline in

elderly patients with severe cerebral age-related white matter changes: the LADIS study. *Arch Intern Med* 2007; 167:81–88.

23. Inzitari D, Pracucci G, Poggesi A, et al. LADIS Study Group. Changes in white matter as determinant of global functional decline in older independent outpatients: three year follow-up of LADIS (Leukoaraiosis And DISability) study cohort. *BMJ* 2009;339:2477.
24. Norrving B. Long-term prognosis after lacunar infarction. *Lancet Neurol* 2003;2:238–245.
25. Fisher CM. Lacunar stroke and infarcts: a review. *Neurology* 1982;32:871–876.
26. Sacco S, Marini C, Totaro R, et al. A population-based study of the incidence and prognosis of lacunar stroke. *Neurology* 2006;66:1335–1338.
27. Bejot Y, Catteau A, Caillier M, et al. Trends in incidence, risk factors, and survival in symptomatic lacunar stroke in Dijon, France, from 1989 to 2006: a population-based study. *Stroke* 2008;39:1945–1951.
28. Staaf G, Lindgren A, Norrving B. Pure motor stroke from presumed lacunar infarct: long-term prognosis for survival and risk of recurrent stroke. *Stroke* 2001;32:2592–2596.
29. Eriksson S-E, Olsson JE. Survival and recurrent strokes in patients with different subtypes of stroke: a 14-year follow-up study. *Cerebrovasc Dis* 2001;12: 171–180.
30. Bamford J, Sandercock P, Dennis M, Burn J, Warlow C. Classification and natural history of clinically identifiable subtypes of cerebral infarction. *Lancet* 1991;337:1521–1526.
31. Samuelsson M, Söderfelt B, Olsson GB. Functional outcome in patients with lacunar infarction. *Stroke* 1996;27:842–846.
32. De Jong G, Kessels F, Lodder J. Two types of lacunar infarcts. Further arguments from a study on prognosis. *Stroke* 2002;33:2072–2076.
33. Vermeer S, Longstreth WT Jr, Koudstaal PJ. Silent brain infarcts: a systematic review. *Lancet Neurology* 2007;6:611–619.
34. Miyao S, Takano A, Teramoto J, Takahashi A. Leukoaraiosis in relation to prognosis for patients with lacunar infarction. *Stroke* 1992;23:1434–1438.
35. Yamamoto Y, Akiguchi I, Oiwa K, et al. Twenty-four-hour blood pressure and MRI as predictive factors for different outcomes in patients with lacunar infarct. *Stroke* 2002;33:297–305.
36. Koga H, Takashima Y, Murakawa R, et al. Cognitive consequences of multiple lacunes and leukoaraiosis as vascular cognitive impairment in community-dwelling elderly individuals. *J Stroke Cerebrovasc Dis* 2009;18:32–37.
37. Benisty S, Gouw AA, Porcher R, et al. Location of lacunar infarcts correlates with cognition in a sample of non disabled subjects with age-related white matter changes: the LADIS study. *J Neurol Neurosurg Psychiatry* 2009;80:478–483.
38. Jacova C, Pearce LA, Costello R, et al. Cognitive impairment in lacunar strokes: the SPS3 trial. *Ann Neurol* 2012;72:351–362.
39. Van der Flier WM, Cordonnier C. Microbleeds in vascular dementia: clinical aspects. *Exp Gerontol* 2012;47:853–857.
40. Cordonnier C, van der Flier WM. Brain microbleeds and Alzheimer's disease: innocent observation or key player? *Brain* 2011;134:335–344.
41. Cordonnier C, Al-Shahi SR, Wardlaw J. Spontaneous brain microbleeds: systematic review, subgroup analyses and standards for study design and reporting. *Brain* 2007;130: 1988–2003.
42. Biessels GJ, Zwanenburg JJ, Visser F, Frijns CJ, Luijten PR. Hypertensive cerebral hemorrhage: imaging the leak with 7-T MRI. *Neurology* 2010;75:572–573.
43. Theysohn JM, Kraff O, Maderwald S, et al. Seven Tesla MRI of microbleeds and white matter lesions as seen in vascular dementia. *J Magn Reson Imaging* 2011;33:782–791.
44. Lesnik Oberstein SA, van den Boom R, van Buchem MA, et al. Cerebral microbleeds in CADASIL. *Neurology* 2001; 57:1066–1070.
45. Viswanathan A, Guichard JP, Gschwendtner A, et al. Blood pressure and haemoglobin A1c are associated with microhaemorrhage in CADASIL: a two-centre cohort study. *Brain* 2006;129:2375–2383.
46. Viswanathan A, Gschwendtner A, Guichard JP, et al. Lacunar lesions are independently associated with disability and cognitive impairment in CADASIL. *Neurology* 2007; 69:172–179.
47. Henneman WJ, Sluimer JD, Cordonnier C, et al. MRI biomarkers of vascular damage and atrophy predicting mortality in a memory clinic population. *Stroke* 2009;40:492–498.
48. Altmann-Schneider I, Trompet S, de Craen AJ, et al. Cerebral microbleeds are predictive of mortality in the elderly. *Stroke* 2011;42:638–644.
49. Dufouil C, Chalmers J, Coskun O, et al. Effects of blood pressure lowering on cerebral white matter hyperintensities in patients with stroke: the PROGRESS (Perindopril Protection aGainst Recurrent Stroke Study)

Magnetic Resonance Imaging Substudy. *Circulation* 2005;112:1644–1650.

50. Mok VC, Lam WW, Fan YH, et al. Effects of statins on the progression of cerebral white matter lesion: post hoc analysis of the ROCAS (Regression of Cerebral Artery Stenosis) study. *J Neurol* 2009;256:750–757.

51. Ten Dam VH, van den Heuvel DM, van Buchem MA, et al. for the PROSPER Study Group. Effect of pravastatin on cerebral infarcts and white matter lesions. *Neurology* 2005;64:1807–1809.

Chapter 23

Clinical aspects of genetic forms of small vessel disease

Maria Teresa Dotti and Antonio Federico

Introduction

Thanks to recent advances in molecular genetics, several rare disorders due to mutations in single genes involved in the regulation of small vessel development and function have been identified. They mainly affect brain white matter and share features with age-related leukoaraiosis and/or so-called Binswanger's disease. The most frequent are cerebral autosomal dominant arteriopathy with subcortical infarcts and leukoencephalopathy (CADASIL) and Fabry's disease (FD). Only a few families with other forms (cerebral autosomal recessive arteriopathy with subcortical infarcts and leukoencephalopathy [CARASIL], COL4A1-related disorders, and retinal vasculopathy with cerebral leukodystrophy [RVCL]) have been published. Here we describe in detail the clinical aspects of all these disorders, mainly focusing on CADASIL and FD. In all of them, abnormal cerebral small vessel blood flow leads to similar clinical and neuroimaging phenotypes. However, different age at onset, type of inheritance, and certain associated symptoms can help in the differential diagnosis.

Cerebral autosomal dominant arteriopathy with subcortical infarcts and leukoencephalopathy

Cerebral autosomal dominant arteriopathy with subcortical infarcts and leukoencephalopathy (CADASIL) is the most common form of hereditary small vessel disease (SVD). It is caused by highly stereotyped mutations in exons 2–24 of the *NOTCH3* gene, leading to an odd number of cysteine residues in epidermal growth factor-like repeats (EGFR) of the heterodimeric Notch3 receptor. Since its clinical and genetic definition in the early 1990s [1], hundreds of families in different ethnic groups have been reported worldwide. The largest series of patients are described in European countries, including Germany, United Kingdom, France, Scandinavia, and Italy [1–5]. More recently, increasing numbers of CADASIL patients have been reported in Asian countries [6, 7]. The prevalence of the disease is unknown. The few population studies, limited to circumscribed areas of west Scotland and northeast England, have estimated a similar minimum prevalence of defined CADASIL cases (1.98 and 1.32/100 000 adults, respectively) and individuals at risk (>4/100 000) [8]. A higher prevalence of defined cases (~4/100 000) has been estimated in Finland [9] and in central Italy (personal data). This variability may be due to a different population-related frequency of the disease or to other factors, including partial mutational screening of the *NOTCH3* gene, often limited to the exons known to be the most common mutation sites. However, it is widely held that CADASIL is underestimated because it is still largely unknown and frequently misdiagnosed due to overlap with other common neurologic disorders. The limited availability of genetic testing in some countries should also be taken into account.

Arteriolar pathology, mostly affecting the penetrating and leptomeningeal arteries, but also extending to extracranial vessels, is dominated by progressive loss of vascular smooth muscle cells from the media, wall thickening, narrowing of the lumen, and extracellular deposition of granular osmiophilic material (GOM). Only the latter is pathognomonic of the disease and therefore of diagnostic value. In addition to GOM, CADASIL mutations also cause accumulation of the Notch3 ectodomain leading to a

Cerebral Small Vessel Disease, ed. Leonardo Pantoni and Philip B. Gorelick. Published by Cambridge University Press.

characteristic immunostaining pattern, absent in normal controls [10]. Morphological and functional endothelial changes in vessel walls have also been reported, suggesting that endothelial dysfunction may be a causal factor. The functional consequences of these vascular wall modifications, still incompletely elucidated, are presumably responsible for altered cerebral vasoreactivity leading to chronic subcortical hypoperfusion and ischemic lacunar lesions. Cerebral hypoperfusion has been documented in CADASIL in different studies using blood flow imaging. In spite of generalized small vessel involvement with similar pathologic changes in cerebral and systemic microcirculation, the CADASIL phenotype is virtually restricted to cerebral manifestations, which are highly heterogeneous in their clinical expression between and within families. The reasons for this great, commonly observed clinical variability are still substantially unknown and the subject of much basic and clinical research.

Magnetic resonance imaging (MRI) is an essential tool in CADASIL diagnosis and follow-up monitoring. Typical neuroimaging findings include multifocal or extensive abnormalities in the cerebral white matter (leukoaraiosis), often involving the anterior temporal pole and external capsule, multiple lacunar lesions, and cerebral microbleeds (CMBs). Clinical manifestations result from diffuse cerebral white matter damage and lacunar infarcts (LIs) in both white and deep gray matter. The main clinical characteristic is young-adult presentation of a variable combination of one or more of the following symptoms: migraine often with aura, transient ischemic attacks and/or strokes, cognitive impairment progressively leading to dementia, and mood disorders. Apart from these "core symptoms," few other neurologic and, occasionally, extraneurologic manifestations have been reported. The course of CADASIL is usually progressive and disabling, eventually evolving into a pseudobulbar syndrome with reduced lifespan [11]. Some patients, however, have few symptoms and a milder course, even in old age.

Clinical features

Ischemic events

Cerebral microvascular pathology in CADASIL leads to chronic white matter hypoperfusion and repeated infarcts in the subcortical white matter of the cerebral hemispheres, brainstem, and deep gray matter of the basal ganglia. The cortex is usually spared. Clinical signs of classical lacunar syndromes manifesting as transient ischemic attacks (TIAs) or stroke are observed with pure motor or pure sensory stroke, mixed sensory–motor stroke, ataxic hemiparesis, or dysarthria–clumsy hand syndrome. TIAs/strokes usually present in mid adulthood (<60 years, mean age 49), but the occasional early (<15 years) and very late case (>80 years) has also been reported. Ischemic events are the most common clinical manifestations with a frequency ranging from about 50% to greater than 90% in different population studies (Table 23.1) [1–7]. The relevance of ischemic events for variable progression has been the subject of clinical and imaging correlation studies. A neuroimaging study of the influence of different easily detectable MRI markers on disease severity found a significant correlation between the load of lacunar lesions and cognitive impairment and disability [12]. Ischemic events in CADASIL patients are not related to common cardiovascular risk factors, the absence of which was suggested among the clinical criteria for suspicion of CADASIL. However, considering the commonly high prevalence of one or more risk factors in the general population, studies into the effects of conventional cardiovascular risk factors on CADASIL suggested that they might modulate clinical phenotype [4]. In particular, the following main findings were reported: (1) a significant increase in risk of stroke in hypertensive CADASIL patients; and (2) earlier onset of stroke and predisposition for acute occlusion of perforating arteries in CADASIL patients who smoke cigarettes. Control of these modifiable factors has therefore been recommended.

Migraine

Migraine is a clinical hallmark of several monogenic cerebral SVDs, including CADASIL, RVCL, mitochondrial encephalopathy with stroke-like episodes (MELAS), and hereditary infantile hemiparesis, retinal arteriolar tortuosity, and leukoencephalopathy associated with *COL4A1* mutations. The mechanisms by which these inherited vasculopathies may increase the risk of migraine are still debated and may partly overlap. Such study may offer insights into the pathogenetic mechanisms of migraine in the general population. In particular, genetic susceptibility is a possibility in the common sporadic form of migraine, where association with variants of the *NOTCH3* gene has been reported. The hypothesis of a relationship of

Table 23.1 Frequency of clinical features in series of CADASIL patients (listed in chronological order)

CADASIL series	Country/group	Symptomatic/ total no.	TIA or stroke (%)	Migraine (%)	Migraine with aura (%)	Psychiatric disturbances (%)	Cognitive decline/ dementia(%)
Chabriat et al. (1995) [1]	France	45/45	84	–	22	20	–
Dichgans et al. (1998) [2]	Germany	83/102	71	38	87	30	48
Desmond et al. (1999) [3]	Heterogeneous group	105/105	68	43	67	21	60
Kim et al. (2006) [6]	Korea	14/29	93	7	100 (1/1)	36	50
Adib-Samii et al (2010) [4]	United Kingdom	200/200	51	75	90	35	17
Wang et al. (2011) [7]	China	57/57	82	–	5	7	60
Pescini et al. (2012) [5]	Italy	61/61	80	49	50	53	57

CADASIL, cerebral autosomal dominant arteriopathy with subcortical infarcts and leukoencephalopathy; TIA, transitory ischemic attack.

migraine with ischemic events seems unlikely in CADASIL migraneous patients, due to the subcortical nature of the typical lacunar stroke (see above) with respect to the frequent occurrence of cortical auras and because migraine attacks usually precede the onset of ischemic stroke and are often reported to recede when the latter are clinically manifest [13]. Cortical spreading depression, the electrophysiologic substrate of migraine aura, was found to be enhanced in CADASIL mouse models [14]. According to the authors, this finding correlates vascular *NOTCH3* mutations with susceptibility to enhanced spreading depression, supporting the role of the neurovascular unit in the development of migraine with aura. Some studies point to the role of endothelial dysfunction in the pathogenesis of migraine attacks and the findings of a reduced number of endothelial progenitor cells (EPCs) and of endothelial vascular reactivity in migraine patients support this role. It is noteworthy that both endothelial abnormalities have recently been reported in CADASIL patients [15, 16]. To our knowledge, similar studies are lacking in the other monogenic cerebrovascular disorders associated with migraine. Two large review studies on migraine in CADASIL were recently published. In the first, Liem et al. [17] reviewed the literature, focusing on migraine characteristics and epidemiology in CADASIL. The pooled analysis of sufficiently large surveys (>10 patients) gave a 43% prevalence of migraine in patients from European countries (95% confidence interval [CI] 38–48%). The highest prevalence (75%, 150/200 patients) was reported in the UK CADASIL population [4], whereas a very low prevalence of migraine, mean 5%, resulted from studies in several Asian regions, revealing differences in ethnic susceptibility. The high prevalence of migraine with aura in the CADASIL phenotype has been stressed since the first clinical observations, and subsequently calculated in different population groups; variability ranged widely from approximately 5% to greater than 90% (Table 23.1). Similar results were obtained in the second review paper by Sacco et al. [18] who systematically reviewed 34 studies and reported data on 749 patients. Migraine was present in 48% (356/749) of cases, 35% of whom with aura. The remaining 44% had unspecified migraine, and 19% had more than one type of migraine. Mean age at onset was 32.2 years with twice as many women affected as men (63.3% and 36.7%, respectively). If migraine was included in the phenotypic expression of the disease, it was the most frequent first symptom (81.5% of cases), exceeding TIA/stroke and other presentations.

The type of aura is seldom reported in the different studies. On the whole, the frequency of atypical aura seems to be substantial [13].

Cognitive impairment

CADASIL patients almost invariably have cognitive decline evolving to dementia in many cases. The problem is commonly listed as the second most frequent clinical manifestation of the disease [13]. Its clinical expression, as expected, shares the typical profile of sporadic SVD with characteristic frontal-lobe cognitive deficits. Detailed neuropsychological testing shows variable involvement of different skills at different ages, with a more heterogeneous cognitive profile in the early stages of disease [19]. Alteration of executive function is reported to be the most common, with highly frequent cognitive deficit at a younger age (<50 years). In the same age group, executive dysfunction was often associated with attention and memory involvement. The cognitive pattern became more homogeneous at older ages (>60 years), with diffuse impairment in all cognitive domains leading to dementia. Detailed analysis of memory complaints and performance in a considerable number of patients (140 subjects) was extensively reported by Epelbaum et al. [20], who emphasized the high frequency and role of memory alterations in the cognitive performance of CADASIL patients. A significant proportion of cases showed a pattern suggesting hippocampal-type amnesic syndrome, typically reported as an early feature of Alzheimer's disease.

The clinical impact of different cerebral lesions, namely LIs, white matter hyperintensities (WMHs), and CMs, in cognitive impairment and dementia has been extensively investigated in MR studies, the conclusions of which have not always been homogeneous. LI load and CM number were proved to be the most strongly associated with cognitive decline [12], whereas the association between WMHs and cognitive phenotype seems to be more controversial. Using CADASIL as a model of vascular cognitive impairment due to SVD, a recent study investigated the relationship between the location of ischemic lesions and cognitive impairment with a voxel-based lesion–symptom mapping approach [21] and showed that the disruption of frontal–subcortical neuronal circuits by ischemic lesions has a strategic impact on cognitive symptoms, specifically processing speed.

Psychiatric disturbances

Psychiatric disturbances are considered one of the core clinical symptoms of CADASIL. However, detailed characterization is generally lacking, in both case reports and review articles. In most CADASIL series, the frequency ranges from 20 to 53%, the highest percentage being reported in an Italian population [5]. If present, psychiatric symptoms usually manifest in the course of the disease, only rarely being the first symptom. An uncommonly high frequency (66% of cases) of psychiatric symptoms was observed in 18 exon-10-mutation carriers from Italian families, mostly at onset [22]. Variable types of psychiatric disorders have been described in CADASIL, including depression, anxiety, and psychosis. Mood disorders are the most common manifestations, but are probably underestimated in frequency. Apathy is another frequent behavioral change, which negatively impacts quality of life, particularly in patients with cognitive impairment and dementia [13]. Both mood changes and apathy are often observed in vascular dementia and subcortical ischemic lesions, thus are seen as an important risk factor for so-called "Vascular Depression." Several findings suggest that lesion burden, secondary to accumulation of subcortical ischemic lesions, as well as the strategic location of lesions, play a crucial role in the occurrence of these symptoms also found at early stages of the disease [23]. Reye et al. [23] suggest that detailed localization studies are needed to determine which pathways are mostly involved.

Other clinical manifestations

Large cerebral vessel involvement has been documented in patients from Korea, in several cases with evidence of symptomatic large artery stenosis [24]. In a high proportion (25%) of CADASIL patients from Asian countries, *symptomatic intracerebral hemorrhages* have also been reported, in some cases as the first manifestation. Less than 10% of patients have *epileptic seizures*, mainly in the course of the disease and presumably related to ischemic stroke. The most frequent are generalized tonic–clonic type, but focal seizures occasionally have been observed. In spite of generalized microvascular involvement, clinical manifestations, with few exceptions, are limited to the central nervous system. *Neuromuscular symptoms*, including weakness, wasting, fatigability, numbness, reduced deep tendon reflexes, and electrophysiologic and biopsy findings compatible with muscle and nerve pathology, have been reported in some patients. Nerve involvement usually leads to peripheral axonal neuropathy, while morphological and biochemical signs of mitochondrial dysfunction have been repeatedly observed by skeletal muscle biopsy [25]. Small blood vessel dysfunction and subsequent chronic ischemia is the most probable pathogenic mechanism, although signs compatible with manifest ischemic events have seldom been found. In particular, the debate on the primary or secondary origin of mitochondrial changes and the role of mitochondria in vascular smooth muscle cell degeneration continues.

Visual involvement, albeit transient and subtle, occurs in a significant number of CADASIL patients at onset and in the course of the disease. Impairment of visual function can occur at any level of the visual pathway, including the optic nerve and retinal fiber layers, probably in relation to microvascular pathology. However, in spite of extensively described evidence of subclinical abnormalities, clinically detectable eye symptoms are only rarely reported. They include acute visual loss, suggesting ischemic optic neuropathy, reported in a father and son as presenting symptom [26].

Other rare clinical manifestations, including myocardial infarction – unusually frequent in Dutch patients [27] – and deep venous thrombosis [22], probably can be linked to CADASIL-related extraneurologic microvascular damage. Cardiac involvement may also include the higher than normal prevalence of right-to-left shunt [28], whose significant association with common migraine with aura and juvenile cryptogenic ischemic stroke has been extensively reported. Its presence in CADASIL, not correlated with clinical severity, may be related to the role of the Notch pathway in atrioventricular morphogenesis.

Phenotype variability

For reasons not yet clarified, there is great variability in the clinical expression of CADASIL between and within families. An example is one of the first families we observed, in which there were several affected members in three generations, including a couple of homozygous twins whose clinical details are provided in Figure 23.1. This is surprising, considering the highly stereotyped nature of *NOTCH3* pathogenic mutations. However, with a few exceptions, studies focusing on possible relationships between phenotype and *NOTCH3* mutation site have failed to show any significant genotype–phenotype correlation.

Other factors could, therefore, presumably play a role in clinical variability. As mentioned above, the role of cardiovascular risk factors was extensively analyzed [4] with findings of significant increase in stroke risk in hypertensive people, earlier onset of ischemic events in smokers, and significant association between high homocysteine levels and migraine. The role of variations in blood pressure (BP) over time was studied by our group [29]. We observed an altered BP profile with a significant reduction in mean systolic and diastolic BP and reduced nocturnal decline in BP. A significant correlation was found between low BP profile and cognitive impairment, suggesting that it could be another risk factor for overall cognitive deterioration.

Disease progression

CADASIL usually has a progressive course leading to severe motor and cognitive disability and premature death, and stepwise progression usually being typical of the first years of the disease. However, cases with milder and different evolution are often observed. A retrospective study by Opherk et al. [11] in 411 patients was a fundamental contribution to our understanding of the natural history of CADASIL. The main findings were: (1) the influence of gender on disease severity, with age at onset of immobilization and death occurring sooner in male than in female CADASIL patients; (2) a significant reduction in survival with respect to the general population in the case of males; and (3) mild influence of *NOTCH3* genotype on clinical progression. An interesting finding was that sudden unexpected death is quite a common occurrence in CADASIL patients, the second most frequent cause of death after pneumonia. This could be partly related to the cardiac autonomic nervous system derangement subsequently observed in a significantly large proportion of patients, a factor which could predispose to life-threatening arrhythmia and sudden death [30]. Easily assessable noninvasive cardiac markers, like heart rate and QT variability, should be used in these patients as a guide for therapeutic management.

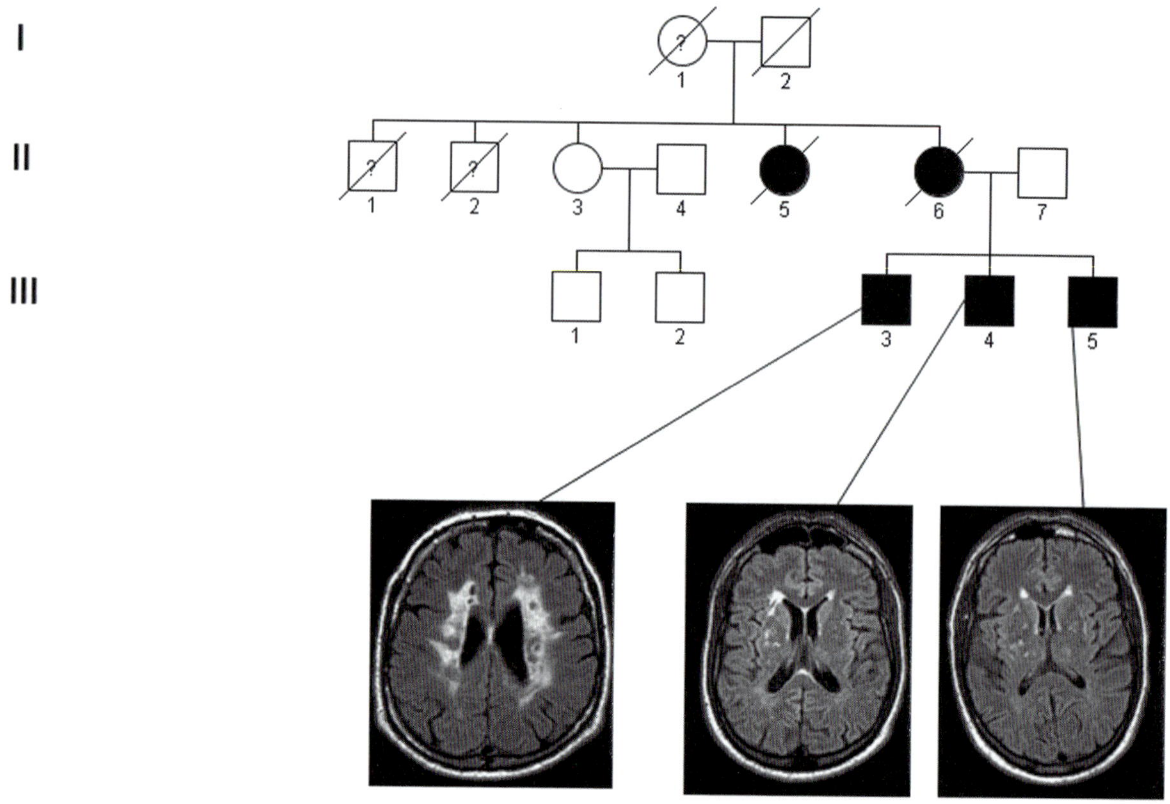

Figure 23.1 Clinical variability of CADASIL phenotype within the same family with p.Arg1076 *cis* mutation of the *NOTCH3* gene.
?: Subjects suspected of having CADASIL based on clinical history. Solid symbols indicate affected subjects. I, 1: died at 56 years, had severe dementia. II, 1 and II, 2: died at 27 and 33 years, respectively, after a history of progressive motor disability and cognitive impairment. II, 5: mild depression, died at 72 years after the first stroke. II, 6: progressive dementia since 38 years of age, bedridden since 50 years of age, died at 76 years. III, 3: 57-year-old man with repeated subcortical strokes since 40 years of age, bedridden since 50 years of age with pseudobulbar palsy. III, 4 and III, 5: 54 year-old homozygous twins. III, 4: asymptomatic. III, 5: episodes of migraine without aura.

Brain imaging

Brain MRI pattern is a fundamental tool for CADASIL diagnosis. Heterogeneous neuroimaging patterns can be observed as a consequence of microvascular pathology, ranging from ischemic to hemorrhagic parenchymal lesions. The main abnormalities include cerebral multifocal, or more or less confluent, mostly symmetric leukoencephalopathy and multiple LIs in abnormal white matter, basal ganglia, thalamus, and brainstem [31]. While highly characteristic, none of these findings is pathognomonic of the disease. The frequent localization of T2-weighted and fluid-attenuated inversion recovery (FLAIR) sequence signal hyperintensities in the external capsule (>90% of cases) and temporal pole (>60% of cases) is highly suggestive and of great interest for diagnosis. Conversely, infrequent involvement of the anterior temporal lobe (22–43%) has been reported in patients from Asian countries. Other MRI findings include CMBs detectable on gradient-echo images and increasing with age, especially with risk factors such as high BP. Intracerebral hemorrhage has been reported in a large proportion of Asian patients [24].

MRI signal abnormalities also may be found in asymptomatic CADASIL. Better understanding of the pathogenesis of cerebral lesions and their clinical correlates can be expected from increasing application of new MR techniques in research and clinical studies. Quantitative MRI techniques have demonstrated that white matter lesions are almost invariably present at the preclinical stage and prevalently affect the frontal brain region, while the burden of T1-weighted hypointense lesions, considered a good marker of brain damage, was found to be unremarkable [32]. The finding of significant brain atrophy, mostly affecting the frontal and parietal cortex in preclinical mutation carriers, is further evidence in favor of use of early brain damage indexes as preclinical markers of disease evolution in clinical research [32]. Previous studies on brain volume in symptomatic CADASIL patients have shown that brain atrophy increases with increasing age and is correlated with cognitive and motor disability rate, but not with white matter lesion load [33].

Treatment

At present, high level evidence-based studies of standardized treatments for CADASIL are still lacking, but symptomatic therapies are commonly applied to handle different clinical manifestations. Prevention of ischemic stroke is currently based on administration of antiplatelet drugs (of unproven efficacy in CADASIL) and treatment of risk factors. Therefore, a BP lowering agent with vasoprotective properties and vitamin B-complex vitamins are used, the latter to reduce homocysteine. Statins are often prescribed as in sporadic SVD, but their use has not significantly improved hemodynamic parameters, at least in short-term studies. Patients with migraine do not often need preventive drugs, although there is clinical evidence that acetazolamide may be effective in the prophylaxis of migraine.

CADASIL was used as a model of pure vascular subcortical dementia, due to the low risk of associated Alzheimer pathology, in a multicenter randomized controlled study designed to test the efficacy of the cholinesterase inhibitor drug donepezil for cognitive impairment. Expected improvement in the Vascular Dementia Assessment Scale – cognitive subscale (VADAS-cog) score was not achieved, despite some improvement in executive functions [13].

Diagnosis

The gold standard for CADASIL diagnosis is genetic analysis of the *NOTCH3* gene. Alternatively, diagnosis can be based on ultrastructural evidence of GOM in the skin biopsy. In both cases, specificity is 100% but low sensitivity (45–57%) has been reported for the latter in some patient populations [34]. These findings suggest that skin biopsy may be useful for screening subjects suspected to have CADASIL, but definite diagnosis calls for molecular analysis. Because of the large spectrum of different mutations, false negative results may be obtained if genetic analysis is limited to clusters of exons. It is, therefore, mandatory to perform mutation analysis of all exons (from 2 to 24) coding for EGFR in the Notch3 receptor in clinically suspected subjects, obviously considering the higher frequency of some mutations and the known founder effect on the genetic screening process in certain geographically defined populations.

The first step, however, is clinical diagnosis, which is not easy due to the lack of pathognomonic value of the clinical and MRI characteristics. Disease boundaries often overlap with other neurologic disorders, including sporadic SVD (e.g., older age at onset and association with cardiovascular risk factors in the latter), other hereditary SVD (different pattern of inheritance and extraneurologic manifestations), multiple sclerosis (frequent spinal cord MRI signal abnormalities, abnormal cerebrospinal fluid pattern), and adult-onset leukodystrophy (more diffuse white matter changes, signs of peripheral nervous, and/or multisystem involvement), and differential diagnosis must be considered.

Pregenetic screening is also challenging because of the great clinical variability of CADASIL phenotype and the puzzling assemblage of clinical and MRI manifestations. Increasing evidence shows that many patients may deviate from the "classical" clinical and neuroimaging pictures for late onset (>65 years), presence of one or more cardiovascular risk factors, absence of stroke, atypical presentation, negative family history, absence of temporal lobe involvement, and presence of intracerebral hemorrhage. Rapidly growing worldwide experience on the clinical and genetic variability of CADASIL sheds doubt on the validity (e.g., absence of risk factors) and weight (e.g., temporal lobe lesions instead of external capsule hyperintensities) of several previously suggested diagnostic criteria. In an attempt to update and standardize clinical evaluation, Pescini et al. [5] proposed a CADASIL scale in the form of a simple screening tool to select patients suspected of CADASIL before *NOTCH3* analysis. The scale lists the typical clinical and neuroimaging features of the disease, assigning a score from 1 to 5 to each on the basis of relative frequency. The total score ranges from 0 to 25, with a minimum of 15 required to suspect the disease.

Cerebral autosomal recessive arteriopathy with subcortical infarcts and leukoencephalopathy

Cerebral autosomal recessive arteriopathy with subcortical infarcts and leukoencephalopathy (CARASIL) is a rare autosomal recessive disorder affecting small vessels in the brain, characterized by subcortical infarcts and leukoencephalopathy. It has mainly been described in Japan and was recently associated with *HTRA1* gene mutation. The prevalence of the disease is not known (<100 cases have been described, mainly in Japan, but also in China and, more recently, in Western countries) [35, 36].

Clinical aspects

Clinical aspects include slowly progressive gait disorders, spasticity of the lower extremities, and onset of alopecia in the second decade, initially considered a constant clinical finding, but subsequently reported absent in several studies [37, 38]. These symptoms are associated with arthropathy, lumbago, spondylosis deformans, and disk herniation. Neurologic symptoms related to cerebrovascular impairment, strokes, and cognitive decline appear before the age of 40.

Neuroimaging

Neuroimaging shows findings similar to those of CADASIL, consisting of symmetric WMHs in the periventricular and deep white matter, sparing U-fibers, T2-signal abnormalities in white matter of the cerebellum (rarely seen in CADASIL), brainstem, middle cerebellar peduncle, and external capsule, and LIs in basal ganglia and thalamus. Early involvement of the anterior temporal lobes and external capsules (characteristic signs in CADASIL) has seldom been described [35].

Neuropathology

Arima et al. [39] reviewed the neuropathologic findings and compared CARASIL with CADASIL. The main features are abnormalities in small arteries of cerebral white matter and basal ganglia, which show arteriosclerotic changes with fibrous intimal proliferation, splitting of the internal elastic lamina, hyaline degeneration of arterial walls, and narrowing of the lumen. Arterial smooth muscle cells are also severely affected. Amyloid deposition and GOM have not been detected. Differences between two CARASIL and a CADASIL brain and nonarteriosclerotic controls were investigated and revealed milder obliterative sclerotic changes in CARASIL than CADASIL, and very severe sclerotic changes with almost complete disappearance of medial arterial smooth muscle cells. The adventitia was thinner than in control arteries, increasing vessel fragility and leading to arterial collapse. Changes in small vessels in other organs were less evident than in the brain, confirming that unlike for CADASIL, skin biopsy is not useful for diagnosis of CARASIL.

Genetics

Hara et al. [37] first described *HTRA1*, the gene associated with CARASIL, located at 10q25 and producing a transcript of nine exons, coding for HTRA1 (high temperature requirement protease A1), a 480-amino-acid serine protease belonging to the chymotrypsin family and acting as chaperone and protease in different processes. HTRA1 decreases transforming growth factor-β (TGF-β) signaling [40], leading to vascular fibrosis.

COL4A1-related disorders

COL4A1-related disorders are a spectrum of conditions with infantile and adult onset, characterized by a SVD of the brain, manifesting clinically with porencephaly, cerebral aneurysms, eye defects, and systemic involvement (kidney, muscle, heart, Raynaud's phenomenon). Caused by mutation of *COL4A1*, a gene encoding the alpha-1 chain of collagen IV, its inheritance is generally autosomal dominant.

COL4A1-related phenotypes (Table 23.2), described clinically before their molecular genetic definition, are characterized by:

- Autosomal dominant type I porencephaly
- Brain SVD with hemorrhage
- Brain SVD with Axenfeld–Rieger anomaly
- Hereditary angiopathy with nephropathy, aneurysms, and muscle cramps (HANAC syndrome).

Clinical findings

The clinical findings include infantile hemiplegia, seizures, intellectual disability until dementia, migraine with or without aura, intracerebral

Table 23.2 Different COL4A1 mutation-related phenotypes

Pediatric phenotypes
Perinatal intracerebral hemorrhage
Porencephaly (antenatal or postnatal)
Cerebral SVD phenotype
Deep intracerebral hemorrhages and leukoencephalopathy
Deep small infarcts and leukoencephalopathy
Ocular phenotypes
Retinal arteriolar tortuosities and retinal hemorrhages
Asymptomatic retinal arteriolar tortuosities
Congenital or juvenile cataracts
Axenfeld–Rieger anomaly (disgenesis of the anterior segment of the eye)
High intraocular pressure, optic nerve abnormalities
Renal phenotype (HANAC phenotype)
Microscopic or gross hematuria
Bilateral renal cysts
Renal insufficiency (usually mild)
Asymptomatic neuroimaging phenotypes
Periventricular leukoencephalopathy
Enraptured intracranial aneurisms
Deep microbleeds, deep lacunar infarcts
Porencephaly
Other phenotypes
Liver cysts
Muscle cramps with elevation of creatine kinase in the serum

HANAC, hereditary angiopathy with nephropathy, aneurysms and muscle cramps; SVD, small vessel disease.

hemorrhages at various ages (including antenatal and recurrent episodes), ischemic strokes, transient visual loss secondary to retinal hemorrhage, cataracts, glaucoma, microcornea, hematuria, large bilateral renal cysts, Raynaud's phenomenon, paroxysmal supraventricular arrhythmia, muscle cramps, and autosomal dominant inheritance.

Neurologic manifestations

The neurologic manifestations may vary in severity and age of onset, also with very wide intrafamiliar heterogeneity. In the *porencephalic phenotype*, clinical presentation is usually characterized by infantile hemiparesis, seizures, intellectual disability, dystonia, stroke, and migraine. Systematic analysis of mutation carriers in families with porencephaly, infantile hemiparesis, or perinatal intracerebral hemorrhage showed cerebrovascular changes, asymptomatic porencephaly, diffuse white matter abnormalities, intracerebral hemorrhages, and TIAs [41, 42].

Autosomal dominant cerebral SVD and hemorrhage phenotype is characterized by absence of porencephaly and MRI evidence of typical brain small vessel impairment, combined with eye abnormalities.

HANAC syndrome, described in several families [43], shows cerebral SVD, in some cases asymptomatic and in some cases with cerebrovascular symptoms (strokes, hemorrhages), associated with renal symptoms (microscopic hematuria, without proteinuria and hypertension, or intermittent gross hematuria, renal cysts), persistent elevation of serum creatine kinase (CK) with muscle cramps, and variable severity of ocular abnormalities. No porencephaly, electromyography (EMG), and muscle biopsy abnormalities have been reported.

Brain neuroimaging investigations

Brain neuroimaging investigations are characterized by porencephaly with fluid-filled cavities in the brain, secondary to antenatal or perinatal parenchymal hemorrhages [42, 44], T2-weighted MRI evidence of leukoencephalopathy with WMHs mainly in the supratentorial posterior periventricular area, cerebral microhemorrages, LIs, deep intracerebral hemorrhages, dilated perivascular spaces [45], and single or intracranial aneurysms, usually in the intracranial portion of the ICA [43]. In skin capillaries at the dermoepithelial junction and in kidney tubules, ultrastructural abnormalities of the basement membrane have been described [44, 46].

These abnormalities are closely correlated with collagens, the major structural component of the extracellular matrix. Type IV collagen alpha 1 (COL4A1) and alpha 2 (COL4A2) are important components of the basement membrane, including the vascular basement membrane, also involved in initial basement membrane formation during development, as well as maintenance of vascular tone and endothelial functions.

Genetics

The *COL4A1* gene consists of 52 exons. Different missense mutations involving highly conserved glycine residues in the triple helical domain of the *COL4A1* gene have been reported. Glycine residues are crucial for the formation of the triple-helical structure of collagen. In the first cases of HANAC syndrome described, six mutations were found in exons 24 and 25 [43], while the severest cases showed mutations through exons 25–51 [41, 42, 44]. More recently two novel *COL4A1* mutations (one base deletion and a splice site mutation), suggesting a pathogenetic mechanism of haploinsufficiency, were identified in two families with porencephaly, hemorrhagic stroke, and SVD [46]. Finally, Weng et al. [47] reported two putative *COL4A1* mutations in 96 patients with sporadic nonfamilial intracerebral hemorrhages. By in vitro studies, the authors suggested that these and other mutations may contribute to increased intracellular and/or decreased extracellular amounts of COL4A1, leading to cerebrovascular diseases and intracerebral hemorrhage. Since type IV collagen alpha-1 (COL4A1) and alpha-2 chains (COL4A2) form $(\alpha1)_2(\alpha2)$ IV heterodimers, which are a crucial component of vascular and other basement membranes, the *COL4A2* gene was investigated in families and sporadic patients with a similar phenotype to COL4A1 patients, describing the mutations [48].

Retinal vasculopathy with cerebral leukodystrophy

The three syndromes cerebroretinal vasculopathy (CRV), hereditary endotheliopathy, retinopathy, nephropathy, and stroke (HERNS), and hereditary vascular retinopathy (HVR) were grouped together as retinal vasculopathy with cerebral leukodystrophy (RVCL), since considered an allelic disorder. RVCL is an adult autosomal dominant disorder affecting brain small vessels and resulting in a progressive neurologic disorder with onset in the fourth or fifth decade.

Clinical findings

Clinical findings are telangiectasias, vision loss due to microaneurysms and retinal capillary obliteration starting in the macula, migraine-like headache, TIAs and strokes, personality changes with anxiety and depression, as well as motor and psychic impairment leading to dementia. In some cases, systemic vascular changes present as Raynaud's phenomenon, mild liver disease with micronodular cirrhosis, and kidney glomerular dysfunction. The first families were reported by Grand et al. [49] and Gutmann et al. [50], who particularly focused on hereditary endotheliopathy with retinopathy, nephropathy, and stroke, suggesting the acronym HERNS.

MRI showed progressive contrast-enhanced lesions with surrounding edema, similar to tumors, in cerebral and cerebellar white matter, which required brain biopsy in some patients. Follow-up of the MRI findings in the large family reported by Grand et al. [49] was conducted by Mateen et al. [51].

Coagulative necrosis secondary to obliterative vasculopathy and minimal inflammatory infiltration have been demonstrated in the pons, cerebellum, and basal ganglia, as well in the frontotemporal region. Ultrastructural examination showed multilamination of subendothelial basement membranes of small vessels in the brain and other tissues.

Genetics

Ophoff et al. [52] mapped the gene in families with retinovasculopathy and in the family with HERNS and found linkage to the same region (3p21.3–p21.1), suggesting allelism in these disorders. Richards et al. [53] identified five heterozygous frameshift mutations at the C-terminus of the *TREX1* gene (DNAse III) in nine families. This specific 3′–5′ exonuclease is ubiquitously expressed in mammalian cells.

Fabry's disease

Fabry's disease (FD) is a progressive X-linked inherited disorder of glycosphingolipid metabolism due to deficiency or absence of the enzyme α-galactosidase, characterized by accumulation of glycosphingolipids (mainly globotriaosylceramide, GL3) in lysosomes of different tissues, and by abnormal urinary excretion [54]. The classical form of the disease, presenting in males with no detectable α-galactosidase activity, starts in infancy and is characterized by angiokeratomas, acroparesthesias, hypohydrosis, corneal opacities leading to cornea verticillata, and progressive vascular disorders of the heart, kidneys, and central nervous system. Table 23.3 shows the clinical evolution of symptoms with age.

FD has long been regarded as an adult disease with most affected males developing the "classic" phenotype. Subclassification into "cardiac" and "renal" variants was introduced for patients with predominant or exclusive heart or kidney involvement. Females, for a

Table 23.3 Fabry's disease: clinical symptoms during the different ages

Age (years)	Symptoms
10	Acroparestesias Pain
10–15	Angiokeratomas Dyshidrosis (hypohidrosis, anhidrosis, and hyperhidrosis) Ophthalmologic abnormalities and cornea verticillata Diarrhea, abdominal pain
20–30	Proteinuria, lipiduria, hematuria Impaired renal function
30–40	Heart involvement (left and right ventricular hypertrophy, enlarged left atrium, heart valve abnormalities, and conduction disturbances)
40–50	Strokes or transient ischemic attacks Hearing impairments

long time described as "carriers of the defective gene," have recently been shown to have minor clinical signs.

Early neural damage primarily involves small nerve fibers of the peripheral somatic and autonomic nervous systems. Pain is experienced in 60–80% of the cases. The most visible early clinical feature is angiokeratoma, typically manifesting on the buttocks, groin, umbilicus, and upper thighs. Histologically, the skin lesions are small superficial angiomas, caused by cumulative damage to vascular endothelial cells of the skin leading to vessel dilatation in the dermis.

Some of the most devastating neurologic features in FD are caused by cerebrovascular disorders, the result of multifocal involvement of small blood vessels. Cerebrovascular involvement can present with many symptoms, including headache, vertigo/dizziness, TIAs, ischemic strokes, and vascular dementia [55]. Cerebral vascular manifestations may be the initial presenting features of this disorder, and a dolichoectactic vertebrobasilar complex should alert the clinician to possible FD.

Brain MRI may show periventricular white matter lesions, microbleeds, cortical gray matter infarcts, and deep LIs in gray and white matter [55]. Hyperintensity in T1-weighted images of the pulvinar is a quite common finding in FD, presumably reflecting the presence of calcifications [56]. The pulvinar sign, if present, is highly specific and a characteristic of FD,

Table 23.4 Fabry's disease: pathophysiology of cerebrovascular lesions

- Large and small cerebral vessel impairment
- Stroke resulting from cardiogenic embolism in the context of ischemic heart disease, valvular disease, arrhythmia, and cardiomyopathy
- Changes in the vessel wall as a consequence of glycolipid accumulation leading to progressive stenosis and occlusion of small blood vessels
- Dilatation and tortuosity of large vessels, secondary to lipid deposition on the vessel wall
- Alteration of intra- and intercellular signaling via cytokines
- Increased levels of endothelial prothrombotic factors and leukocyte adhesion molecule expression and increased endothelium-mediated vascular reactivity
- Changes in local pattern of blood flow

more frequent in male patients with cardiomyopathy and severe kidney impairment.

Heterozygous females

Clinical signs vary in heterozygous females, in relation to lyonization, a process whereby one copy of the X-chromosome is randomly inactivated in all cells of the female embryo, leading to a mosaic of normal and mutant cells in varying proportions.

The clinical spectrum in women ranges from an asymptomatic condition, to a variety of clinical presentations, including pain, orthostatic hypotension, angiokeratoma, eye abnormalities, cochleovestibular abnormalities, and gastrointestinal impairment. A high percentage of women develop organ damage (heart, brain, kidney) about a decade later than men. Brain involvement is characterized by a cerebrovascular syndrome [57].

Pathophysiology

Glycosphingolipids (mainly GL3) accumulate in lysosomes as a consequence of α-galactosidase A deficiency, leading to lysosomal and cell dysfunction; in association with other factors, this in turn triggers tissue ischemia and vessel fibrosis (Table 23.4).

Detection of α-galactosidase deficiency in plasma or leukocytes is definitive for diagnosis, associated with abnormal urinary excretion of glycosphingolipids. Enzyme analysis may occasionally help detect heterozygotes but is often inconclusive, due to random X-chromosome inactivation, making molecular

Table 23.5 Clinical and genetic findings in different inherited SVDs

	CADASIL	CARASIL	COL4A1	HERNS	Fabry's
Inheritance	AD	AR	AD/AR	AD	X-linked
Gene	*NOTCH3*	*HTRA1*	*COL4A1*	*TREX1*	*GLA*
Neurologic symptoms					
Stroke, age of onset (years)	20–70	30–40	10–50	30–50	25–50
Lacunar infarct	+++	++	++	++	+++
Subcortical hemorrhage	+/–	–	+++	–	–
Headache	+++	–	+	++	+
Epilepsy	+	+	+	+	+/–
Dementia	+++	+++	+/–	++	++
Psychiatric changes	++	++	+	++	+
Developmental delay	–	–	+/–	–	–
Infantile hemiparesis	–	–	++/–	–	+/–
Neuroimaging findings					
SVD	+++	+++	+++	+++	+++
Porencephaly	–	–	+++/–	–	–
Focal enhancing lesions	–	–	–	+	–
Microbleeds	+++	++	++	+	+
Cerebral aneurysms	–	–	++	–	–
Extraneurologic findings					
Ocular involvement	+	–	++	+++	+++
Renal disease	–	–	+	++	+++
Cardiac involvement	+	–	+/–	–	+++
Raynaud's phenomenon	–	–	+	+++	++/–
Skin changes	–	–	–	–	+++
Alopecia	–	++/–	–	–	–
Muscle cramps	–	–	+	++	–
Spondylosis	–	++/–	–	–	–

AD, autosomal dominant; AR, autosomal recessive; CADASIL, cerebral autosomal dominant arteriopathy with subcortical infarcts and leukoencephalopathy; CARASIL, cerebral autosomal recessive arteriopathy with subcortical infarcts and leukoencephalopathy; Fabry's, Fabry's disease; HERNS, hereditary endotheliopathy, retinopathy and nephropathy, and stroke; SVD, small vessel disease.

testing of females mandatory. Enzyme detection is also important for prenatal diagnosis.

Like for other metabolic disorders, *enzyme replacement therapy* and *chaperone therapy* were recently introduced for FD. The former is based on intravenous administration of recombinant x-galactosidase, which is taken up by the cells and tissues and delivered to lysosomes, improving all symptoms except neurologic disturbances [58].

Conclusions

Table 23.5 shows the different clinical features, useful as diagnostic guidelines for the five hereditary SVDs discussed here. Although rare compared to other sporadic small vessel brain diseases, attention to their diagnosis is crucial for neurologists in clinical practice, since for one of them, treatment is now available, and for all, diagnosis can lead to correct genetic counseling. Research on the basic genetic abnormalities and different proteins is important for understanding the development and functions of brain microcirculation in normal and pathologic conditions.

Acknowledgements

Research partly financed by a grant from the Regione Toscana to A. F. and from the Ministero dell'Istruzione, dell'Università e della Ricerca to M. T. D.

References

1. Chabriat H, Vahedi K, Iba-Zizen MT, et al. Clinical spectrum of CADASIL: a study of seven families. Cerebral autosomal dominant arteriopathy with subcortical infarcts and leukoencephalopathy. *Lancet* 1995;346:934–939.
2. Dichgans M, Mayer M, Uttner I et al. The phenotypic spectrum of CADASIL: clinical findings in 102 cases. *Ann Neurol* 1998; 44:731–739.
3. Desmond DW, Moroney JT, Lynch T, et al. The natural history of CADASIL: a pooled analysis of previously published cases. *Stroke* 1999;30:1230 1233.
4. Adib-Samii P, Grice G, Martin RJ, Markus HS. Clinical spectrum of CADASIL and effect of cardiovascular risk factors on phenotype. Study in 200 consecutively recruited individuals. *Stroke* 2010; 41:630–634.
5. Pescini F, Nannucci S, Bertaccini B, et al. The Cerebral Autosomal Dominant Arteriopathy with Subcortical Infarcts and Leukoencephalopathy (CADASIL) scale: a screening tool to select patients for *NOTCH3* analysis. *Stroke* 2012;43:2871–2876.
6. Kim Y, Choi EJ, Choi CG, et al. Characteristics of CADASIL in Korea: a novel cysteine-sparing Notch3 mutation. *Neurology* 2006;66:1511–1516.
7. Wang Z, Yuang Y, Zhang W, et al. *NOTCH3* mutations and clinical features in 33 mainland Chinese families with CADASIL. *J Neurol Neurosurg Psychiatry* 2011;82:534–539.
8. Narayan SK, Gorman G, Kalaria RN, Ford GA, Chinnery PF. The minimum prevalence of CADASIL in northeast England. *Neurology* 2012;78:1025–1027.
9. Kalimo H, Ruchoux MM, Viitanen M, Kalaria RN. CADASIL: a common form of hereditary arteriopathy causing brain infarcts and dementia. *Brain Pathol* 2002;12:371–84.
10. Joutel A, Favrole P, Labauge P, et al. Skin biopsy immunostaining with a Notch3 monoclonal antibody for CADASIL diagnosis. *Lancet* 2001;358:2049–2051.
11. Opherk C, Peters N, Herzog J, Luedtke R, Dichgans M. Long-term prognosis and cause of death in CADASIL: a retrospective study of 411 patients. *Brain* 2004;127:2533–2539.
12. Viswanathan A, Gschwendtner A, Guichard JP, et al. Lacunar lesions are independently associated with disability and cognitive impairment in CADASIL. *Neurology* 2007;69:172–179.
13. Chabriat H, Joutel A, Dichgans M, Tournier-Lasserve E, Bousser MG. CADASIL. *Lancet Neurol* 2009;8:643–653.
14. Eikermann-Haerter K, Yuzawa I, Dilekoz E, et al. Cerebral autosomal dominant arteriopathy with subcortical infarcts and leukoencephalopathy syndrome mutations increase susceptibility to spreading depression. *Ann Neurol* 2011;69:413–418.
15. Pescini F, Cesari F, Giusti B, et al. Bone marrow-derived progenitor cells in cerebral autosomal dominant arteriopathy with subcortical infarcts and leukoencephalopathy. *Stroke* 2010;41:218–223.
16. Campolo J, De Maria R, Frontali M, et al. Impaired vasoreactivity in mildly disabled CADASIL patients. *J Neurol Neurosurg Psychiatry* 2012;83:268–274.
17. Liem MK, Lesnik Oberstein SAJ, va der Grond J, Ferrari M, Haan J. CADASIL and migraine: a narrative review. *Cephalagia* 2010:30:1284–1289.
18. Sacco S, Degan D, Carolei A. Diagnostic criteria for CADASIL in the International Classification of Headache Disorders (ICHD-II): are they appropriate? *J Headache Pain* 2010;11:181–186.
19. Charlton RA, Morris RG, Nitkunan A, Markus HS. The cognitive profile in CADASIL and sporadic small vessel disease. *Neurology*, 2006;66:1523–1526.
20. Epelbaum S, Benisty S, Reyes S, et al. Verbal memory impairment in subcortical ischemic vascular disease. A descriptive analysis in CADASIL. *Neurobiol Aging* 2011;32:2172–2182.
21. Duering M, Zieren N, Hervé D, et al. Strategic role of frontal white matter tracts in vascular cognitive impairment: a voxel-based lesion-symptom mapping study in CADASIL. *Brain* 2011;134:2366–2375.
22. Bianchi S, Rufa A, Ragno M, et al. High frequency of exon 10 mutations in the *NOTCH3*

gene in Italian CADASIL families: phenotype peculiarities. *J Neurol* 2010;257:1039–1042.

23. Reye S, Viswanathan A, Godin O, et al. Apathy: a major symptom in CADASIL. *Neuroloy* 2009; 72:905–910.
24. Choi JC, Song SK, Lee JS, Kang S, Kang JH. Diversity of stroke presentation in CADASIL: study from patients harboring the predominant *NOTCH3* mutation R544C. *J Stroke Cerebrovasc Dis* 2013;22:126–131.
25. Dotti MT, De Stefano N, Bianchi S, et al. A novel Notch3 frameshift deletion and mitochondrial abnormalities in a patient with CADASIL. *Arch Neurol* 2004;61:942–945.
26. Rufa A, De Stefano N, Dotti MT, et al. Acute unilateral visual loss as the first symptom of cerebral autosomal dominant arteriopathy with subcortical infarcts and leukoencephalopathy. *Arch Neurol* 2004;61:577–580.
27. Lesnik Oberstein SA, Jukema JW, Van Duinen SG, et al. Myocardial infarction in cerebral autosomal dominant arteriopathy with subcortical infarcts and leukoencephalopathy (CADASIL). *Medicine (Baltimore)* 2003;82:251–256.
28. Zicari E, Tassi R, Stromillo ML, et al. Right-to-left shunt in CADASIL patients. Prevalence and correlation with clinical and MRI findings. *Stroke* 2008;39:2155–2157.
29. Rufa A, Dotti MT, Franchi M, et al. Systemic blood pressure profile in cerebral autosomal dominant arteriopathy with subcortical infarcts and leukoencephalopathy. *Stroke* 2005;36:2554–2558.
30. Rufa A, Guider F, Acampa M, et al. Cardiac autonomic nervous system and risk of arrhythmias in cerebral autosomal dominant arteriopathy with subcortical infarcts and leukoencephalopathy (CADASIL). *Stroke* 2007; 38:276–280.
31. Singhal S, Rich P, Markus HS. The spatial distribution of MR imaging abnormalities in cerebral autosomal dominant arteriopathy with subcortical infarcts and leukoencephalopathy and their relationship with age and clinical features. *AJNR Am J Neuroradiol* 2005;26:2481–2487.
32. Stromillo ML, Dotti MT, Battaglini M, et al. Structural and metabolic brain abnormalities in preclinical CADASIL. *J Neurol Neurosurg Psychiatry* 2009;80:41–47.
33. Peters N, Holtmannspotter M, Opherk C, et al. Brain volume changes in CADASIL: a serial MRI study in pure subcortical ischemic vascular disease. *Neurology* 2006;66:1517–1522.
34. Malandrini A, Gaudiano C, Gambelli S, et al. Diagnostic value of ultrastructural skin biopsy studies in CADASIL. *Neurology* 2007;68:1430–1432.
35. Fukutake T. Cerebral autosomal recessive arteriopathy with subcortical infarcts and leukoencephalopathy (CARASIL): from discovery to gene identification. *J Stroke Cerebrovasc Dis* 2011;20:85–93.
36. Mendioroz M, Fernández-Cadenas I, Del Río-Espinola A, et al. A missense *HTRA1* mutation expands CARASIL syndrome to the Caucasian population. *Neurology* 2010;75:2033–2035.
37. Hara K, Shiga A, Fukutake T, et al. Association of *HTRA1* mutations and familial ischemic cerebral small-vessel disease. *N Engl J Med* 2009;360:1729–1739.
38. Nishimoto Y, Shibata M, Nihonmatsu M, et al. A novel mutation in the *HTRA1* gene causes CARASIL without alopecia. *Neurology* 2011; 76:1353–1355.
39. Arima K, Yanagawa S, Ito N, Ikeda S. Cerebral arterial pathology of CADASIL and CARASIL (Maeda syndrome). *Neuropathology* 2003;23:327–334.
40. Shiga A, Nozaki H, Yokoseki A, et al. Cerebral small-vessel disease protein HTRA1 controls the amount of TGF-β1 via cleavage of proTGF-β1. *Hum Mol Genet* 2011;20:1800–1810.
41. Gould DB, Phalan FC, Breedveld GJ. Mutations in COL4A1 cause perinatal cerebral hemorrhage and porencephaly. *Science* 2005;308:1167–1171.
42. De Vries LS, Koopman C, Groenendaal F, et al. COL4A1 mutation in two preterm siblings with antenatal onset of parenchymal hemorrhage. *Ann Neurol* 2009;65:12–18.
43. Plaisier E, Gribouval O, Alamowitch S, et al. Role of COL4A1 mutations in the hereditary angiopathy with nephropathy, aneurysm and cramps (HANAC) syndrome. *New Engl J Med* 2007;357:2687–2695.
44. Van der Knaap MS, Smit LM, Barkhof F, et al. Neonatal porencephaly and adult stroke related to mutations in collagen IV A1. *Ann Neurol* 2006; 59:504–511.
45. Vahedi K, Boukobza M, Massin P, et al. Clinical and brain MRI follow up study of a family with COL4A1 mutation. *Neurology* 2007;69:1564–1568.
46. Lemmens R, Maugeri A, Niessen HWM, et al. Novel COL4A1 cause cerebral small vessel disease by haploinsufficiency. *Hum Mol Genet* 2013;22:391–397.
47. Weng YC, Sonni A, Labelle-Dumais C, et al. COL4A1 mutations in patients with sporadic late-onset intracerebral hemorrhage. *Ann Neurol* 2012;71:470–477.
48. Jeanne M, Labelle-Dumais C, Jorgensen J, et al. COL4A2 mutations impair COL4A1 and

COL4A2 secretion and cause hemorrhagic stroke. *Am J Hum Genet* 2012;90:91–101.

49. Grand MG, Kaine J, Fulling K, et al. Cerebroretinal vasculopathy. *Ophthalmology* 1988;95:649–659.
50. Gutmann DH, Fischbeck KH, Sergott RC. Hereditary retinal vasculopathy with cerebral white matter lesions. *Am J Med Genet* 1989;34:217–220.
51. Mateen FJ, Krecke K, Younge BR, et al. Evolution of a tumor-like lesion in cerebroretinal vasculopathy and *TREX1* mutation. *Neurology* 2010;75:1211–1213.
52. Ophoff RA, DeYoung J, Service S, et al. Hereditary vascular retinopathy, cerebroretinal vasculopathy, and hereditary endotheliopathy with retinopathy, nephropathy, and stroke map to a single locus on chromosome 3p21.1–p21.3. *Am J Hum Genet* 2001;69:447–453.
53. Richards A, van den Maagdenberg AM, Jen JC, et al. C-terminal truncations in human 3′-5′ DNA exonuclease TREX1 cause autosomal dominant retinal vasculopathy with cerebral leukodystrophy. *Nature Genet* 2007;39:1068–1070.
54. Tagliavini F, Pietrini V, Gemignani F, et al. Anderson–Fabry's disease: neuropathological and neurochemical investigations. *Acta Neuropathol* 1982;56: 93–98.
55. Sims K, Politei J, Banikazemi M, Lee P. Stroke in Fabry disease frequently occurs before diagnosis and in absence of other clinical events: natural history data from the Fabry Registry. *Stroke* 2009;40:788–794.
56. Takanashi J, Barkovich AJ, Dillon WP, et al. T1 hyperintensity in the pulvina: key imaging feature for diagnosis of Fabry disease. *AJNR Am J Neuroradiol* 2003; 24:916–921.
57. Federico A. Fabry's disease and cerebrovascular disorders. *Neurol Sci* 2002;23:47–48.
58. Bersano A, Lanfranconi S, Valcarenghi C, et al. Neurological features of Fabry disease: clinical, pathophysiological aspects and therapy. *Acta Neurol Scand* 2012;126:77–97.

Chapter 24

Interaction between cerebral small vessel disease and neurodegenerative changes

Wiesje M. van der Flier and Raj Kalaria

Introduction

Neurodegenerative and vascular changes are the two most prevalent types of lesions in brains of the elderly. The frequencies of both pathologies particularly increase in the oldest old [1, 2]. Four of the intriguing questions that has dogged the field for a long time are how do these two types of pathologies interact? Are they independent, co-occurring disease processes? Alternatively, do the two processes act in a synergistic way (1 + 1 > 2)? Do neurodegenerative changes trigger cerebral small vessel disease (SVD), or vice versa? In this chapter, we define and provide an overview of available clinical, radiologic, and neuropathologic evidence regarding the interaction between cerebral SVD and neurodegenerative changes and present a framework for how the two types of pathology may enhance each other.

Clinical diagnosis

Alzheimer's disease

The diagnostic criteria for Alzheimer's disease (AD) have recently been revised after almost 30 years [3]. The core clinical criteria for a diagnosis of probable AD dementia include: (1) dementia; (2) insidious onset; (3) cognitive impairment (amnestic and non-amnestic presentations are both recognized); and (4) no evidence for another type of dementia or extensive cerebrovascular disease. The revised criteria reflect advances in knowledge on AD, as they allow for the use of biomarkers to increase the certainty of the clinical diagnosis by providing evidence for the AD pathophysiologic process. The new diagnostic criteria are based on the amyloid cascade hypothesis, and they mention the possibility of coexisting SVD only as an exclusion criterion and in the context of possible AD dementia, a diagnosis that can be made when there is an aetiologically mixed presentation; for example, concomitant cerebral SVD. In the revised criteria for mild cognitive impairment (MCI) due to AD, there is hardly any mention of cerebrovascular pathology [4]. The research criteria as proposed by the International Working Group are also based on the amyloid cascade hypothesis and cerebral SVD in AD is largely ignored [5]. In the follow-up paper, the International Working Group proposed the term mixed AD for all patients who suffer from Alzheimer pathology co-occurring with other causes of cognitive decline, but they warn against an inflated use of the term [6]. Moreover, criteria for the proposed category of mixed AD are not provided.

Vascular dementia

The most widely used diagnostic guidelines for vascular dementia (VaD) stem from 1993 [7]. These criteria were unique in that they incorporated not only clinical criteria, but also proposed radiologic criteria for VaD. Moreover, they specified that VaD could be due to either large vessel disease, SVD, or a mix of both large vessel and SVD. Although VaD is generally mentioned as the second most prevalent cause of dementia, both pathologic and clinical series show a low prevalence of VaD [8–10]. In fact, it seems that "pure" VaD as dementia strictly caused by vascular lesions is considered to be very rare. A certain degree of vascular pathology however, is very common, even when the vascular pathology is not sufficiently severe to fulfill diagnostic criteria for VaD [11]. The description of VaD has gradually expanded to the concept of vascular cognitive impairment (VCI), which was devised to include any degree of cognitive impairment related to any type of

Cerebral Small Vessel Disease, ed. Leonardo Pantoni and Philip B. Gorelick. Published by Cambridge University Press.

cerebrovascular disease [12, 13]. Recently, a thorough update on current knowledge of VCI was published, but the diagnostic guide is not provided in this review [14]. Several efforts are underway to develop diagnostic criteria for VCI, incorporating both several severity stages and different types and extent of cerebrovascular pathology [13]. The inherent problem of VCI (and VaD) remains that it is very difficult to relate the evident degree of vascular disease to the observed signs and symptoms. In former criteria which were largely based on the concept of multi-infarct dementia, criteria of stepwise progression and a temporal link between vascular event and cognitive changes were required to increase the likelihood that the signs and symptoms were indeed caused by the observed vascular disease [7]. We now learn that the majority of patients with VaD or VCI suffer from cognitive decline as a consequence of SVD [15, 16]. In SVD, neither stepwise progression, nor a demonstrable temporal link between lesion and symptom may be apparent, making it even more difficult to judge if the observed pathology and clinical symptoms are causally related.

Mixed dementia: impact of mixed pathology on cognitive status

Although the majority of patients suffer from mixed pathology to some extent, there are no clinical criteria for mixed dementia to date [17]. This hampers clinical practice, as the clinical question of how to weigh the evidence from ancillary investigations pointing at either AD or SVD is not accounted for in guidelines. Furthermore, not taking into account that the majority of patients have mixed disease is also very likely to impede the development of therapy. Inclusion criteria for clinical trials are often very strict and require patients to have relatively pure AD. This implies that if a beneficial effect would be found, it is questionable if this effect could be generalized to the majority of AD patients, who have mixed disease to some degree.

AD and VaD attributed to SVD demonstrate several similarities in risk factors, pathomechanisms, clinical features, and neuropathologic substrates. Thus, in many cases it is difficult to determine which lesion causes which sign or symptom. The direct relationship between AD type of neurodegenerative changes and infarctions remains rather elusive but a few clinical studies suggest that when pathologic substrates of AD and cerebrovascular lesions coexist, the threshold of dementia is more readily reached. The presence of one or more infarctions independently increases the odds of dementia beyond the additive effect of neurodegenerative and vascular pathologies [18]. An alternative way to consider this is that the combination of AD-type changes and microvascular disease worsens cognitive outcomes at any given age [19]. The Nun study was one of early reports which suggested that individuals with neurofibrillary pathology in particular and one or two lacunar infarcts experienced a steeper drop in cognitive function compared to those with no infarcts [20]. Thus the presence of marginally increased burden of amyloid deposits or hyperphosphorylated tau pathology that may be insufficient for pathologic diagnosis of AD when added to coexisting SVD may sooner reach the threshold resulting in cognitive impairment and dementia.

Role of magnetic resonance imaging in the assessment of dementia

In the diagnostic work-up of dementia, magnetic resonance imaging (MRI) is typically used to exclude other causes of cognitive decline, such as tumor or large hematomata. MRI also allows the detailed appreciation of neurodegeneration (atrophy). Atrophy of the medial temporal lobe including the hippocampus is considered the MRI hallmark of AD [21]. However, medial temporal atrophy may not necessarily be indicative of underlying Alzheimer pathology (see below). Atrophy is also not restricted to the medial temporal lobe but spreads over the cortex in the course of the disease [22]. Moreover, patients may differ in their pattern of atrophy, with posterior atrophy being an early marker in a large proportion of patients as well [23–25]. The new diagnostic criteria for AD incorporate atrophy as a marker providing evidence in favor of Alzheimer pathophysiology, thus surpassing the stage of AD being a diagnosis *per exclusionem* [3, 5].

In addition to atrophy, MRI allows the detailed detection of SVD. The three most widely studied manifestations of cerebral SVD on MRI are white matter hyperintensities (WMHs), lacunes, and microbleeds. WMHs refer to hyperintense areas on T2-weighted fluid-attenuated inversion recovery (FLAIR) images, and they correspond to heterogeneous pathologic substrates, including demyelination, arteriolosclerosis, gliosis representing incomplete infarction, and tissue degeneration [11, 26–28]. WMHs can have a periventricular or a deep location, but this subdivision is used less and less, as there are no clear boundaries between the two [29]. Lacunes are small cavities located in the white matter or subcortical gray matter. They have a hypointense aspect on T1-weighted, T2-weighted, and FLAIR imaging, and are mostly regarded as small ischemic infarcts. Finally, microbleeds are small, dot-like hypointense lesions, which can be appreciated on T2*-weighted MRI, and are thought to represent hemosiderin deposits [30]. Microbleeds are a radiologic construct, and they are not often found at autopsy. It is therefore questionable whether they really reflect micro*bleeds*, or whether the term "bleed" is an overstatement. Still, their relevance is increasingly recognized due to their relation to clinical outcome and their occurrence in anti-amyloid vaccination trials. Microbleeds can have a deep or a lobar location, and it has been suggested that the etiology of microbleeds may differ depending on their location. Based on epidemiologic and clinical studies, deep microbleeds are thought to result from hypertensive vasculopathy, while lobar microbleeds presumably reflect underlying cerebral amyloid angiopathy (CAA) [31–34]. As such, microbleeds representing some form of underlying microvascular disease are seemingly related to both SVD and Alzheimer pathology.

Novel, quantitative MRI methods provide additional tools to study cerebral SVD. Diffusion tensor imaging (DTI) uses the property of diffusivity of water to study the integrity of the white matter tracts. Diffusion-weighted imaging (DWI) visualizes new infarcts. Arterial spin labeling (ASL) enables quantitative, regional measurement of perfusion of the brain and may prove to be a powerful tool, in the context of both AD and VaD.

Interaction: AD with SVD

Many patients with AD have variable degrees of concomitant SVD (Figure 24.1). There is now abundant evidence to indicate that vascular changes in the form of CAA, microvascular degeneration, (lacunar) infarcts, intracerebral microhemorrhages, and white matter lesions similar to Binswanger's disease are

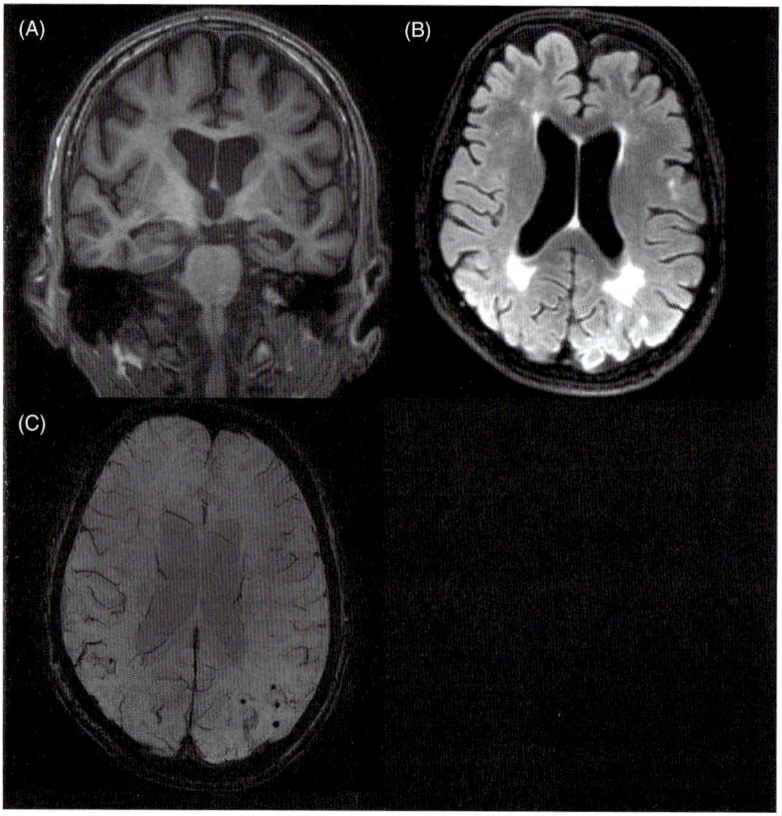

Figure 24.1 Example of a 68-year-old man who was diagnosed with probable Alzheimer's disease, but who shows also manifestations of concomitant small vessel disease on magnetic resonance imaging (MRI). Mini Mental State Examination score was 23, Clinical Dementia Rating was 1, and he had a history of hypertension. (A) Coronal T1-weighted image allows appreciation of atrophy of the medial temporal lobe (Scheltens scale score: left, 3 and right, 2). (B) Axial fluid-attenuated inversion recovery (FLAIR) image shows periventricular and deep white matter hyperintensities (Fazekas score of 2). (C) Axial susceptibility-weighted imaging shows numerous microbleeds, mostly with a lobar location (total number: 45).

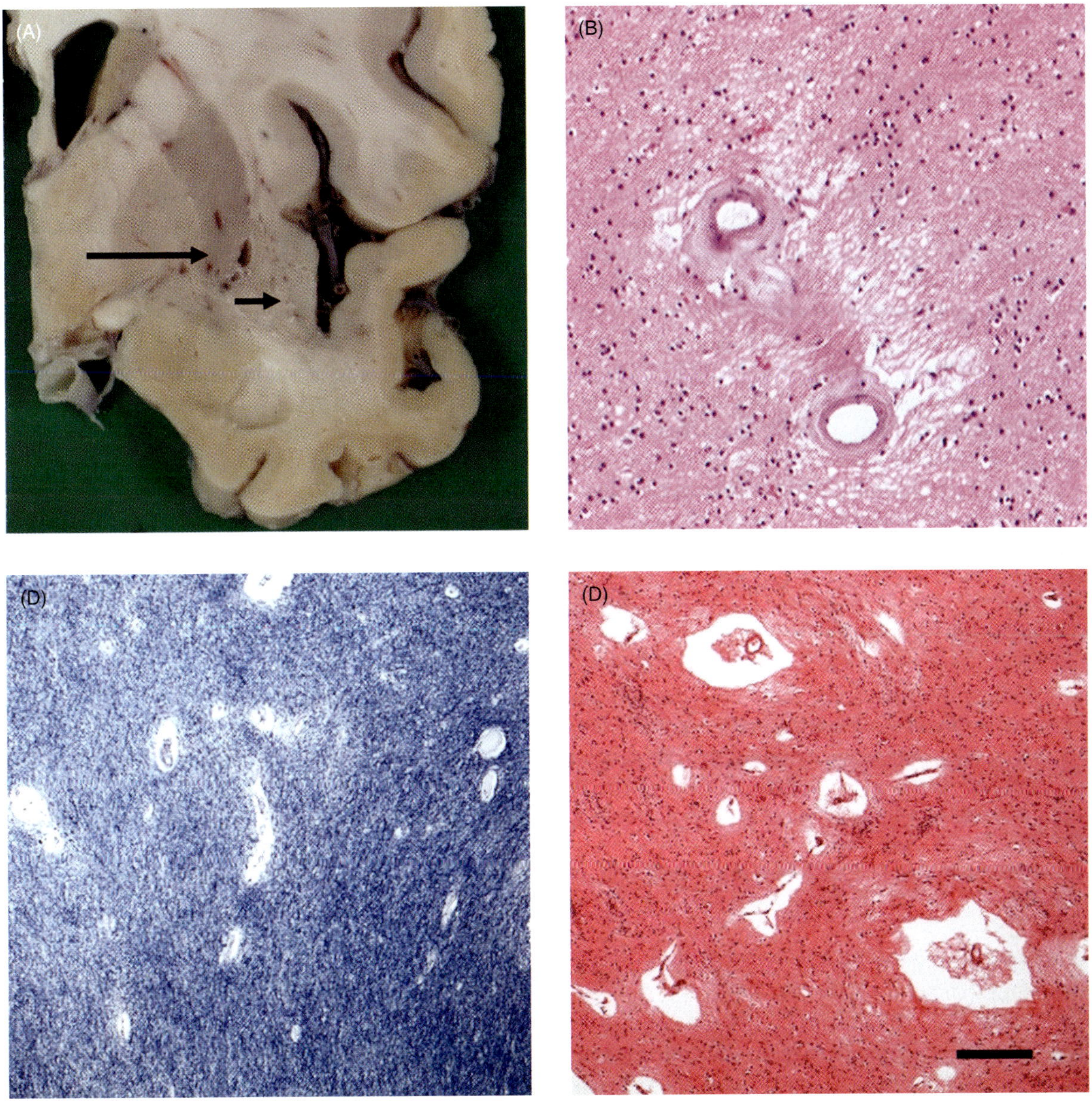

Figure 24.2 Pathologic lesions associated with small vessel disease as often found in Alzheimer's disease. (A) Lacunes (long arrow) and white matter lesions in external capsule (short arrow) in the basal ganglia of a 78-year-old man with cognitive impairment. (B) Hyalinized vessels with perivascular rarefaction and microinfarcts. (C,D) Perivascular spaces (dilatation) and demyelination in white matter (Luxol fast blue and hematoxylin and eosin [H&E]). Moderate gliosis in the surrounding region is also evident in both cases. Bar A = 2 cm; Bar B–D = 50 μm.

evident in more than 60% of patients neuropathologically diagnosed with AD [26, 35]. While large vessel involvement (territorial infarcts, artery to artery embolism, occlusion of extracranial or intracranial arteries, hemorrhages) is infrequent, SVD is common in late-onset AD. Among these, microinfarcts, small cortical infarcts, and white matter rarefaction appear the most common (Figure 24.2). These lesions may be caused by various mechanisms including focal arteriopathy, CAA, or hemodynamic responses resulting in cerebral hypoperfusion (pulse wave encephalopathy and chronic perfusion pressure failure) [36, 37].

On MRI, patients with AD have more WMHs and lacunes than the healthy elderly [18, 38]. Furthermore, the presence of WMHs at baseline predicts progression to dementia in initially nondemented elderly, although this has not consistently been found [39–41]. In population-based studies, WMHs and lacunes have been shown to predict progression to dementia [42–44].

Despite the repeated finding of WMHs being implicated in the development of AD, the question remains how, as associations with cognitive impairment have only modest effects [45–47]. There are several possible explanations of this clinicoradiologic paradox: (1) WMHs and SVD have only a small role in the pathophysiology of cognitive decline; they are there, but they do not matter that much in the disease process. (2) WMHs reflect heterogeneous underlying pathology. In fact, there may be "benign" and "malignant" WMHs, depending on their specific pathologic substrate [27]. This might explain why some patients with severe WMHs have severe cognitive impairment, while others experience hardly any problems. MRI markers that provide quantitative and detailed measurement of the pathophysiologic process, such as DTI, may add the required specificity to characterize WMHs [48, 49]. Finally, (3) WMHs and lacunes may reflect another, underlying pathologic substrate. Microinfarcts, until now invisible on conventional in vivo MRI, are a likely candidate [50, 51]. Along the same line of reasoning, WMHs may be an epiphenomenon of underlying CAA, which is more directly involved in the AD disease process. The explanation may involve one of the hypotheses above, but it is also plausible that more than one of these contributes to the observed clinicoradiologic paradox.

Microbleeds in the context of AD have received increasing attention over the past five years. They are more common in AD than in the general population [52–54]. Current literature suggests that roughly one out of four AD patients has one or more microbleeds [52]. Microbleeds in AD most often have a lobar distribution, presumably indicative of underlying CAA. Associations with lowered β-amyloid (Aβ) levels in cerebrospinal fluid (CSF) and with apolipoprotein E (*APOE*) ε4 genotype provide further evidence for this notion [31, 55]. Furthermore, associations with blood pressure and WMHs have also been shown, particularly for deep microbleeds [32]. The relationship between microbleeds and cognitive function in AD is very subtle at best, most studies showing no significant association [54, 56, 57]. The subtle effect of microbleeds on cognition is probably diluted in the overall clinical picture, once the stage of dementia has been reached. However, in contrast, microbleeds do seem to negatively influence the risk of mortality [58, 59].

Microbleeds, being part of the broader concept of amyloid-related imaging abnormalities (ARIA), are of particular interest in the context of anti-amyloid vaccination trials [60]. Incident microbleeds have been observed in patients who were treated with anti-amyloid medication. A possible explanation would be that when anti-amyloid therapy is successful, the parenchymal amyloid is removed along perivascular routes, compromising the integrity of the microvasculature, eventually resulting in microbleeds [61]. Thus the quality of the blood vessels, including the amount of CAA, may turn out to be a decisive factor in the efficacy of these types of treatment.

Finally, novel MRI methods allow the more detailed imaging of SVD. Using DTI, patients with AD have been shown to have less integrity of the white matter [62, 63]. This may reflect either subtle microvascular disease, or be the consequence of neurodegeneration (e.g., Wallerian degeneration). Patients with AD have a smaller volume of cerebral blood flow than healthy elderly [64, 65]. Again, it is unknown if this is a consequence of the neurodegenerative process (less parenchymal volume demanding less blood flow) or whether it is related to ischemic changes (less blood flow resulting in WMHs). Newer MRI techniques such as ASL provide a quantitative, regional measurement of cerebral blood flow, and as such allow us to answer these questions.

VaD with Alzheimer pathology

Conversely, VaD is also accompanied by AD-type of changes including Aβ plaques and neurofibrillary pathology [66, 67]. Atrophy of the medial temporal lobe, the hallmark of AD on MRI, can be appreciated in VaD as well (Figure 24.3) [68, 69]. Furthermore, medial temporal lobe atrophy is more strongly related to cognitive impairment than WMHs or lacunes, even in patients with VaD [68, 70]. It is conceivable that the majority of these patients suffer (also) from dementia due to some Alzheimer pathology. Alternatively, atrophy of the hippocampus may have a different cause in these patients. It is not unlikely that hippocampal atrophy may result from various types of pathology and MRI does not allow the detection of the underlying pathology. In an MRI study of elderly stroke survivors followed up for two to five years, it

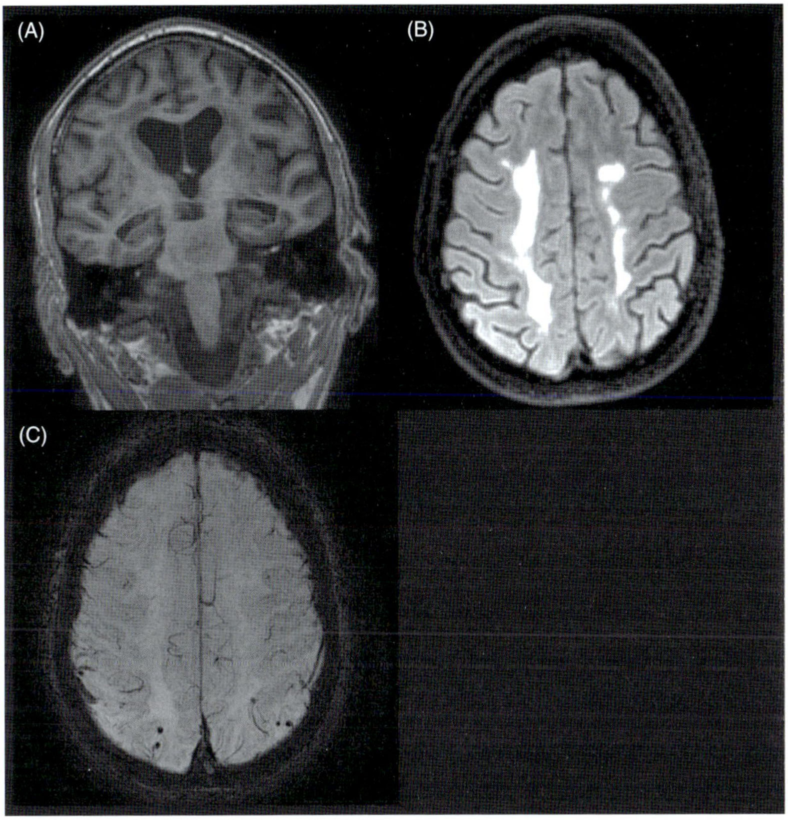

Figure 24.3 Example of a 70-year-old man who was diagnosed with mild cognitive impairment, most likely due to vascular dementia (vascular cognitive impairment), but who also shows atrophy of the medial temporal lobe on magnetic resonance imaging (MRI). Mini Mental State Examination score was 29, Clinical Dementia Rating score was 0.5, and he had a history of hypertension and a transient ischemic attack. (A) Coronal T1-weighted image allows appreciation of atrophy of the medial temporal lobe (Scheltens scale score: 2 on both sides). (B) Axial fluid-attenuated inversion recovery (FLAIR) image shows extensive white matter hyperintensities (Fazekas score of 3). (C) Axial susceptibility-weighted imaging showed numerous microbleeds (total number: 58) and an old cerebral hemorrhage (not shown).

was found that medial temporal atrophy rather than WMHs (indicative of SVD) predicted cognitive decline and progressive brain atrophy [69]. Although this suggested a greater role for Alzheimer pathology rather than vascular pathology in the evolution of delayed cognitive impairment after stroke, subsequent ASL studies and follow-up pathologic findings indicated there is also a distinct vascular basis for medial temporal and hippocampal cell atrophy [71, 72]. In other words: medial temporal atrophy does not necessarily indicate the presence of underlying Alzheimer pathology, as it may also directly result from ischemic changes.

A more direct way to evaluate the presence of Alzheimer pathology in VaD is by measuring Aβ. We found differential but increased deposition of soluble Aβ, particularly Aβ1–42 residue peptide, in temporal and frontal lobes of predominantly SVD subjects compared to cognitively normal aging individuals [67]. These findings are in line with a gradually increasing body of evidence providing in vivo evidence for amyloid deposition by use of CSF levels of Aβ1–42 or amyloid positron emission tomography (PET) in patients with primarily vascular disease [55, 67, 73, 74]. Whether this illustrates misdiagnosis, or at least mixed pathology in all these patients, or whether it reflects that hypoperfusion per se increases Aβ accumulation and, as such, Alzheimer pathology can be a secondary event in patients with primarily SVD, is unclear.

Microinfarcts have been found in pathologic studies and are described as attenuated lesions of indistinct shape occurring in both cortical and subcortical regions involving a small vessel at its core, but are foci with pallor, neuronal loss, axonal damage, and gliosis [75]. Neuropathologic examination permits limited sampling, but it is likely that microinfacts are surrogate for widespread microvascular disease largely stemming from small vessels of the brain. Furthermore, microinfarcts have been associated with CAA [36]. There is ample evidence that the number and volume of microinfarcts strongly correlate with cognitive impairment, making them a likely candidate to be the number one cause of VaD [50]. Moreover, it is quite likely that microinfarcts are also frequently present in patients with AD. Microinfarcts are not visible on conventional MRI, precluding their present use as a diagnostic tool. New developments using DWI and imaging at ultra-high field strength suggest that it may be possible to visualize these lesions during life [76].

How do they interact?

It is clear from numerous studies that Alzheimer pathology and SVD are frequently found together. The Leukoaraiosis And DISability (LADIS) study has been designed to study the independent contribution of WMHs to the transition to disability in initially independently living elderly [77]. While clearly showing that WMHs independently contribute to the transition to disability and dementia [40, 78, 79], the LADIS study also shows that neurodegeneration (i.e., atrophy) is independently related to decline [80, 81]. Although measurements of Aβ are not available in the context of the LADIS study, these findings do provide further evidence that two disease processes in combination contribute to clinical decline.

The question remains, how do these two disease processes interact? Are they independent, co-occurring pathologic processes that cause cognitive decline and dementia when in sum they reach a certain threshold? Or might it be that AD elicits vascular damage resulting from CAA, for example, and that vascular damage exacerbates Alzheimer pathology. Thus, in other words, do the two processes act in synergy or may be even be viewed as two sides of the same coin?

Microbleeds and microinfarcts have attracted increasing attention in the context of cognitive decline and dementia. Are these two features of SVD in some respects mirrors of each other? Microbleeds are a radiologic construct, which are only rarely observed on neuropathologic examination. Microinfarcts, on the other hand, have been found in pathologic studies, but they are not visible on conventional MRI. Both types of lesions have been related to CAA and they may reflect widespread microvascular disease largely stemming from small vessels of the brain. Because of their close relation with both microvascular disease and CAA, microinfarcts and microbleeds may provide a new framework to understand the interplay between neurodegenerative disease and SVD. In sporadic AD, the suboptimal degradation of Aβ is thought to be one of the triggering factors of the disease process. As a result, Aβ will remain in the vessel wall (CAA), now leading to a vicious circle as more amyloid in the vessel wall will result in even less efficient Aβ transport (see Figure 24.4A for a schematic representation). The causative chain may also work the other way around, when aging-associated changes in the vessel walls lead to less optimal degradation and transport of Aβ, resulting in abnormal deposition of Aβ in the vessels and in plaques. What is the initial event? Numerous Aβ fragments leading to damage of the vessel walls, or suboptimal vessels causing less degradation of Aβ? Probably, it does not matter and there may be varying degrees in individuals. There may be several routes to end up in the vicious circle of brittle vessel walls, accumulating Aβ in the vessels, causing even more damaged vessels.

A second line of reasoning focuses on the more downstream process of neurodegeneration (i.e., atrophy). In particular, the medial temporal lobe is often regarded as evidence of Alzheimer pathology, but it may also be caused by other disease processes, such as hippocampal sclerosis or ischemia [82–84]. A recent study showed that hippocampal neuronal volume was reduced in patients with post-stroke dementia compared to post-stroke patients without dementia [71]. Furthermore, there was a correlation between neuronal volume and cognitive function, rather than between extent of vascular disease and cognitive function. The lack of association between vascular disease and cognition is reminiscent of the lack of a correlation between amyloid deposits and cognitive status, which is one of the major deficiencies of the amyloid cascade hypothesis. The relationship with cognitive impairment results from the downstream event of neurodegeneration, while the upstream events in the cascade (vascular pathology in VaD; amyloid deposition in AD) have a less direct relationship with symptomatology (Figure 24.4B). These two aspects of interaction between cerebral SVD, Alzheimer pathology and neurodegenerative disease are more effective when combined (Figure 24.4C).

Future recommendations

There are a number of challenges in understanding the interactions between Alzheimer pathology and SVD. Firstly, there is the question of bridging macroscopic observations to microscopic underlying substrates. Postmortem imaging is useful to directly relate findings at autopsy to imaging findings, but

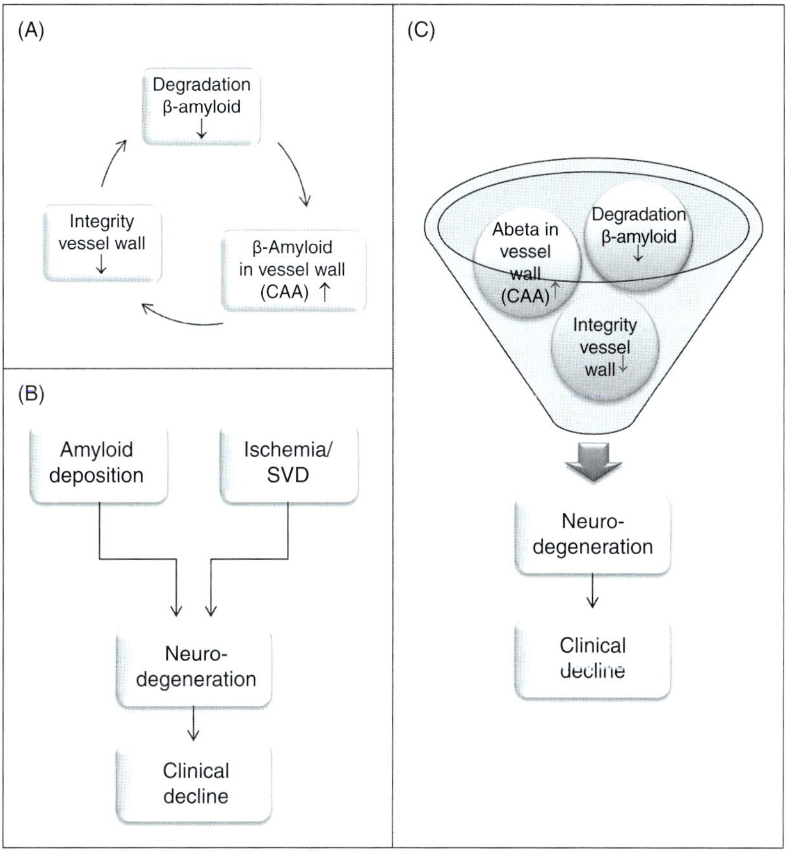

Figure 24.4 Schematic representation of a possible framework to understand the interactions between cerebral small vessel disease (SVD), Alzheimer pathology, and neurodegeneration. Panel (A) focuses on the pivotal role of cerebral amyloid angiopathy (CAA) and the quality of the vessel wall. In sporadic Alzheimer's disease (AD), the suboptimal degradation of β-amyloid (Aβ) is thought to be one of the triggering factors of the disease process. As a result, Aβ will remain in the vessel wall (CAA), leading to a vicious circle, as more amyloid in the vessel wall will result in even less efficient Aβ transport. There may be several routes to end up in the vicious circle of brittle or weaker vessel walls, collecting more Aβ in the vasculature, causing even more fragile vessels. Panel (B) focuses on the more downstream process of neurodegeneration (i.e., atrophy). Panel B proposes a framework where neurodegeneration may result from both Alzheimer pathology and SVD. In this framework, relationships with cognitive impairment result from the downstream event of neurodegeneration, while the upstream events in the cascade (vascular pathology in vascular dementia; amyloid deposition in AD) have a less direct relationship with symptomatology. The two aspects of interaction between cerebral SVD, Alzheimer pathology, and neurodegenerative disease are combined in panel (C).

still has the disadvantage that by definition it occurs post hoc, while the disease process may have started decades earlier [27, 28]. Ultra-high field imaging provides unprecedented detail in visualizing brain changes. As such, it may bridge the gap between in vivo imaging observations and microscopic findings at autopsy and even surpass some of the problems of pathology (e.g., very limited sampling of the brain) [76, 85]. Furthermore, surrogate markers of Alzheimer pathology (i.e., CSF levels of Aβ and amyloid PET) have become available and allow the verification of Alzheimer pathology during life. Likewise, quantitative MRI markers, such as cerebral blood flow and DTI, allow detailed measurement of SVD-related brain changes. Second, there is the question of (reverse) causality: are the two processes causally related at all, and, if so, what is the direction of the causal chain? The methods and techniques outlined above in combination with longitudinal study designs (preferably with postmortem examination at final follow-up) will yield answers to these questions in the coming decade.

Conclusion

In this chapter, we have reviewed that Alzheimer pathology and SVD often co-occur. Recent converging evidence suggests that Alzheimer pathology and SVD: (1) exacerbate each other, resulting in a vicious circle of impaired degradation and clearance of Aβ and compromised vessels; and (2) may be different and unrelated upstream pathologic processes, and that each can result in the same downstream result of neuronal volume loss, which in turn is related to clinical decline. Following this line of reasoning, it becomes clear that with respect to development of treatment for AD, it is imperative to take into account the status of the vasculature. Alternatively, ameliorating the condition of the brain vessels may prove to be pivotal in finding a treatment that works for AD.

Acknowledgements

Scientific work of the VUmc Alzheimer center is part of the neurodegeneration research program of the Neuroscience Campus Amsterdam. The VUmc

Alzheimer Center is supported by Alzheimer Nederland and Stichting VUmc fonds.

R. K.'s work is supported by grants to the Newcastle Centre for Brain Ageing and Vitality (BBSRC, EPSRC, ESRC and MRC, LLHW) and from Alzheimer's Research (UK), Medical Research Council UK, and Newcastle NIHR Biomedical Research Centre in Aging and Age Related Diseases award to the Newcastle upon Tyne Hospitals NHS Foundation Trust.

References

1. Jellinger KA, Attems J. Neuropathology and general autopsy findings in nondemented aged subjects. *Clin Neuropathol* 2012;31:87–98.
2. Polvikoski TM, Van Straaten EC, Barkhof F, et al. Frontal lobe white matter hyperintensities and neurofibrillary pathology in the oldest old. *Neurology* 2010;75:2071–2078.
3. McKhann GM, Knopman DS, Chertkow H, et al. The diagnosis of dementia due to Alzheimer's disease: recommendations from the National Institute on Aging–Alzheimer's Association Work Groups on diagnostic guidelines for Alzheimer's disease. *Alzheimers Dement* 2011; 7:263–269.
4. Albert MS, DeKosky ST, Dickson D, et al. The diagnosis of mild cognitive impairment due to Alzheimer's disease: recommendations from the National Institute on Aging–Alzheimer's Association Work Groups on diagnostic guidelines for Alzheimer's disease. *Alzheimers Dement* 2011; 7:270–279.
5. Dubois B, Feldman HH, Jacova C, et al. Research criteria for the diagnosis of Alzheimer's disease: revising the NINCDS–ADRDA criteria. *Lancet Neurol* 2007;6:734–746.
6. Dubois B, Feldman HH, Jacova C, et al. Revising the definition of Alzheimer's disease: a new lexicon. *Lancet Neurol* 2010;9:1118–11127.
7. Román GC, Tatemichi TK, Erkinjuntti T, et al. Vascular dementia: diagnostic criteria for research studies. Report of the NINDS–AIREN international workshop. *Neurology* 1993;43:250–260.
8. Hejl A, Hogh P, Waldemar G. Potentially reversible conditions in 1000 consecutive memory clinic patients. *J Neurol Neurosurg Psychiatry* 2002;73:390–394.
9. Lobo A, Launer LJ, Fratiglioni L, et al. Prevalence of dementia and major subtypes in Europe: a collaborative study of population-based cohorts. Neurologic Diseases in the Elderly Research Group. *Neurology* 2000;54:S4–S9.
10. Barker WW, Luis CA, Kashuba A, et al. Relative frequencies of Alzheimer disease, Lewy body, vascular and frontotemporal dementia, and hippocampal sclerosis in the State of Florida Brain Bank. *Alzheimer Dis Assoc Disord* 2002;16:203–212.
11. Neuropathology Group of the Medical Research Council Cognitive Function and Ageing Study (MRC CFAS). Pathological correlates of late-onset dementia in a multicentre, community-based population in England and Wales. *Lancet* 2001;357:169–175.
12. O'Brien JT, Erkinjuntti T, Reisberg B, et al. Vascular cognitive impairment. *Lancet Neurol* 2003;2:89–98.
13. Hachinski V, Iadecola C, Petersen RC, et al. National Institute of Neurological Disorders and Stroke–Canadian Stroke Network vascular cognitive impairment harmonization standards. *Stroke* 2006;37:2220–2241.
14. Gorelick PB, Scuteri A, Black SE, et al. Vascular Contributions to Cognitive Impairment and Dementia: a Statement for Healthcare Professionals from the American Heart Association/ American Stroke Association. *Stroke* 2011;42:2672–2713.
15. Erkinjuntti T, Inzitari D, Pantoni L, et al. Research criteria for subcortical vascular dementia in clinical trials. *J Neural Transm Suppl* 2000;59:23–30.
16. Staekenborg SS, Van Straaten EC, van der Flier WM, et al. Small vessel versus large vessel vascular dementia: risk factors and MRI findings. *J Neurol* 2008;255:1644–1651.
17. Gold G, Giannakopoulos P, Herrmann FR, Bouras C, Kovari E. Identification of Alzheimer and vascular lesion thresholds for mixed dementia. *Brain* 2007;130:2830–2836.
18. Schneider JA, Wilson RS, Bienias JL, Evans DA, Bennett DA. Cerebral infarctions and the likelihood of dementia from Alzheimer disease pathology. *Neurology* 2004;62:1148–1155.
19. Esiri MM, Nagy Z, Smith MZ, Barnetson L, Smith AD. Cerebrovascular disease and threshold for dementia in the early stages of Alzheimer's disease. *Lancet* 1999;354: 919–920.
20. Snowdon DA, Greiner LH, Mortimer JA, et al. Brain infarction and the clinical expression of Alzheimer disease. The Nun Study. *JAMA* 1997;277:813–817.
21. Scheltens P, Fox N, Barkhof F, De Carli C. Structural magnetic resonance imaging in the practical assessment of dementia: beyond exclusion. *Lancet Neurol* 2002;1:13–21.

22. Sluimer JD, van der Flier WM, Karas GB, et al. Accelerating regional atrophy rates in the progression from normal aging to Alzheimer's disease. *Eur Radiol* 2009;19:2826–2833.

23. Lehmann M, Koedam EL, Barnes J, et al. Posterior cerebral atrophy in the absence of medial temporal lobe atrophy in pathologically-confirmed Alzheimer's disease. *Neurobiol Aging* 2012;33:672.

24. Frisoni GB, Pievani M, Testa C, et al. The topography of grey matter involvement in early and late onset Alzheimer's disease. *Brain* 2007;130:720–730.

25. Koedam EL, Lehmann M, van der Flier WM, et al. Visual assessment of posterior atrophy development of a MRI rating scale. *Eur Radiol* 2011;21:2618–2625.

26. Fernando MS, Ince PG. Vascular pathologies and cognition in a population-based cohort of elderly people. *J Neurol Sci* 2004;226:13–17.

27. Gouw AA, Seewann A, Vrenken H, et al. Heterogeneity of white matter hyperintensities in Alzheimer's disease: postmortem quantitative MRI and neuropathology. *Brain* 2008;131:3286–3298.

28. Gouw AA, Seewann A, van der Flier WM, et al. Heterogeneity of small vessel disease: a systematic review of MRI and histopathology correlations. *J Neurol Neurosurg Psychiatry* 2011;82:126–135.

29. Barkhof F, Scheltens P. Is the whole brain periventricular? *J Neurol Neurosurg Psychiatry* 2006;77:143–144.

30. Fazekas F, Kleinert R, Roob G, et al. Histopathologic analysis of foci of signal loss on gradient-echo T2*-weighted MR images in patients with spontaneous intracerebral hemorrhage: evidence of microangiopathy-related microbleeds. *AJNR Am J Neuroradiol* 1999;20:637–642.

31. Goos JD, Kester MI, Barkhof F, et al. Patients with Alzheimer disease with multiple microbleeds: relation with cerebrospinal fluid biomarkers and cognition. *Stroke* 2009;40:3455–3460.

32. Vernooij MW, van der Lugt A, Ikram MA, et al. Prevalence and risk factors of cerebral microbleeds: the Rotterdam Scan Study. *Neurology* 2008;70:1208–1214.

33. Vernooij MW, Haag MD, van der Lugt A, et al. Use of antithrombotic drugs and the presence of cerebral microbleeds: the Rotterdam Scan Study. *Arch Neurol* 2009;66:714–720.

34. Goos JD, van der Flier WM, Knol DL, et al. Clinical relevance of improved microbleed detection by susceptibility-weighted magnetic resonance imaging. *Stroke* 2011;42:1894–1900.

35. Ihara M, Polvikoski TM, Hall R, et al. Quantification of myelin loss in frontal lobe white matter in vascular dementia, Alzheimer's disease, and dementia with Lewy bodies. *Acta Neuropathol* 2010;119:579–589.

36. Okamoto Y, Yamamoto T, Kalaria RN, et al. Cerebral hypoperfusion accelerates cerebral amyloid angiopathy and promotes cortical microinfarcts. *Acta Neuropathol* 2012;123:381–394.

37. Kalaria RN, Erkinjuntti T. Small vessel disease and subcortical vascular dementia. *J Clin Neurol* 2006;2:1–11.

38. DeCarli CS. When two are worse than one: stroke and Alzheimer disease. *Neurology* 2006;67:1326–1327.

39. Staekenborg SS, Koedam EL, Henneman WJ, et al. Progression of mild cognitive impairment to dementia: contribution of cerebrovascular disease compared with medial temporal lobe atrophy. *Stroke* 2009; 40:1269–1274.

40. Verdelho A, Madureira S, Moleiro C, et al. White matter changes and diabetes predict cognitive decline in the elderly: the LADIS study. *Neurology* 2010;75:160–167.

41. Smith EE, Egorova S, Blacker D, et al. Magnetic resonance imaging white matter hyperintensities and brain volume in the prediction of mild cognitive impairment and dementia. *Arch Neurol* 2008;65:94–100.

42. Prins ND, van Dijk EJ, den Heijer T, et al. Cerebral white matter lesions and the risk of dementia. *Arch Neurol* 2004;61:1531–1534.

43. Debette S, Beiser A, DeCarli C, et al. Association of MRI markers of vascular brain injury with incident stroke, mild cognitive impairment, dementia, and mortality: the Framingham Offspring Study. *Stroke* 2010;41:600–606.

44. Vermeer SE, Prins ND, den Heijer T, et al. Silent brain infarcts and the risk of dementia and cognitive decline. *N Engl J Med* 2003;348:1215–1222.

45. Prins ND, van Dijk EJ, den Heijer T, et al. Cerebral small-vessel disease and decline in information processing speed, executive function and memory. *Brain* 2005;128:2034–2041.

46. Van der Flier WM, Van Straaten EC, Barkhof F, et al. Small vessel disease and general cognitive function in nondisabled elderly: the LADIS study. *Stroke* 2005;36:2116–2120.

47. Schmidt R, Ropele S, Enzinger C, et al. White matter lesion progression, brain atrophy, and cognitive decline: the Austrian Stroke Prevention Study. *Ann Neurol* 2005;58:610–616.

48. Schmidt R, Ropele S, Ferro J, et al. Diffusion-weighted imaging and cognition in the Leukoariosis And DISability in the elderly study. *Stroke* 2010;41:e402–e408.

49. Van Norden AG, van Uden IW, de Laat KF, van Dijk EJ, de Leeuw FE. Cognitive function in small

vessel disease: the additional value of diffusion tensor imaging to conventional magnetic resonance imaging: the RUN DMC study. *J Alzheimers Dis* 2012;32:667–676.

50. Kalaria RN. Cerebrovascular disease and mechanisms of cognitive impairment: evidence from clinicopathological studies in humans. *Stroke* 2012;43:2526–2534.

51. Brundel M, de Bresser J, van Dillen JJ, Kappelle LJ, Biessels GJ. Cerebral microinfarcts: a systematic review of neuropathological studies. *J Cereb Blood Flow Metab* 2012;32:425–436.

52. Cordonnier C, van der Flier WM. Brain microbleeds and Alzheimer's disease: innocent observation or key player? *Brain* 2011;134:335–344.

53. Cordonnier C, van der Flier WM, Sluimer JD, et al. Prevalence and severity of microbleeds in a memory clinic setting. *Neurology* 2006;66:1356–1360.

54. Pettersen JA, Sathiyamoorthy G, Gao FQ, et al. Microbleed topography, leukoaraiosis, and cognition in probable Alzheimer disease from the Sunnybrook Dementia Study. *Arch Neurol* 2008;65:790–795.

55. Goos JD, Teunissen CE, Veerhuis R, et al. Microbleeds relate to altered amyloid-β metabolism in Alzheimer's disease. *Neurobiol Aging* 2012;33:1011–1019.

56. Van der Vlies AE, Goos JD, Barkhof F, Scheltens P, van der Flier WM. Microbleeds do not affect rate of cognitive decline in Alzheimer disease. *Neurology* 2012;79:763–769.

57. Van der Flier WM. Clinical aspects of microbleeds in Alzheimer's disease. *J Neurol Sci* 2012;322:56–58.

58. Henneman WJ, Sluimer JD, Cordonnier C, et al. MRI biomarkers of vascular damage and atrophy predicting mortality in a memory clinic population. *Stroke* 2009;40:492–498.

59. Altmann-Schneider I, Trompet S, de Craen AJ, et al. Cerebral microbleeds are predictive of mortality in the elderly. *Stroke* 2011;42:638–644.

60. Sperling RA, Jack CR, Jr., Black SE, et al. Amyloid-related imaging abnormalities in amyloid-modifying therapeutic trials: recommendations from the Alzheimer's Association Research Roundtable Work Group. *Alzheimers Dement* 2011; 7:367–385.

61. Boche D, Zotova E, Weller RO, et al. Consequence of Aβ immunization on the vasculature of human Alzheimer's disease brain. *Brain* 2008;131:3299–3310.

62. Damoiseaux JS, Smith SM, Witter MP, et al. White matter tract integrity in aging and Alzheimer's disease. *Hum Brain Mapp* 2009;30:1051–1059.

63. Clerx L, Visser PJ, Verhey F, Aalten P. New MRI markers for Alzheimer's disease: a meta-analysis of diffusion tensor imaging and a comparison with medial temporal lobe measurements. *J Alzheimers Dis* 2012;29:405–429.

64. Spilt A, Weverling-Rijnsburger AW, Middelkoop HA, et al. Late-onset dementia: structural brain damage and total cerebral blood flow. *Radiology* 2005;236:990–995.

65. Binnewijzend MA, Kuijer JP, Benedictus MR, et al. Cerebral blood flow measured with 3D pseudocontinuous arterial spin-labeling MR imaging in Alzheimer disease and mild cognitive impairment: a marker for disease severity. *Radiology* 2013;267:221–230.

66. Allan LM, Rowan EN, Firbank MJ, et al. Long term incidence of dementia, predictors of mortality and pathological diagnosis in older stroke survivors. *Brain* 2011;134:3716–3727.

67. Lewis H, Beher D, Cookson N, et al. Quantification of Alzheimer pathology in ageing and dementia: age-related accumulation of amyloid-β42 peptide in vascular dementia. *Neuropathol Appl Neurobiol* 2006;32:103–118.

68. Bastos-Leite AJ, van der Flier WM, Van Straaten EC, et al. The contribution of medial temporal lobe atrophy and vascular pathology to cognitive impairment in vascular dementia. *Stroke* 2007;38:3182–3185.

69. Firbank MJ, Burton EJ, Barber R, et al. Medial temporal atrophy rather than white matter hyperintensities predict cognitive decline in stroke survivors. *Neurobiol Aging* 2007;28:1664–1669.

70. Vogels RL, Oosterman JM, van Harten B, et al. Neuroimaging and correlates of cognitive function among patients with heart failure. *Dement Geriatr Cogn Disord* 2007;24:418–423.

71. Gemmell E, Bosomworth H, Allan L, et al. Hippocampal neuronal atrophy and cognitive function in delayed poststroke and aging-related dementias. *Stroke* 2012;43:808–814.

72. Firbank MJ, He J, Blamire AM, et al. Cerebral blood flow by arterial spin labeling in poststroke dementia. *Neurology* 2011;76:1478–1484.

73. Huang KL, Lin KJ, Ho MY, et al. Amyloid deposition after cerebral hypoperfusion: evidenced on [(18) F]AV-45 positron emission tomography. *J Neurol Sci* 2012;319:124–129.

74. Grimmer T, Faust M, Auer F, et al. White matter hyperintensities predict amyloid increase in Alzheimer's disease. *Neurobiol Aging* 2012;33:2766–2773.

75. Deramecourt V, Slade JY, Oakley AE, et al. Staging and natural history of cerebrovascular pathology in dementia. *Neurology* 2012;78:1043–1050.

76. Van Veluw SJ, Zwanenburg JJ, Engelen-Lee J, et al. In vivo detection of cerebral cortical microinfarcts with high-resolution 7T MRI. *J Cereb Blood Flow Metab* 2013;33:322–329.

77. Pantoni L, Basile AM, Pracucci G, et al. Impact of age-related cerebral white matter changes on the transition to disability – the LADIS study: rationale, design and methodology. *Neuroepidemiology* 2005;24:51–62.

78. Inzitari D, Simoni M, Pracucci G, et al. Risk of rapid global functional decline in elderly patients with severe cerebral age-related white matter changes: the LADIS study. *Arch Intern Med* 2007;167:81–88.

79. Inzitari D, Pracucci G, Poggesi A, et al. Changes in white matter as determinant of global functional decline in older independent outpatients: three year follow-up of LADIS (Leukoaraiosis And DISability) study cohort. *BMJ* 2009;339:2477.

80. Van der Flier WM, Van Straaten EC, Barkhof F, et al. Medial temporal lobe atrophy and white matter hyperintensities are associated with mild cognitive deficits in non-disabled elderly people: the LADIS study. *J Neurol Neurosurg Psychiatry* 2005;76:1497–1500.

81. Jokinen H, Lipsanen J, Schmidt R, et al. Brain atrophy accelerates cognitive decline in cerebral small vessel disease: the LADIS study. *Neurology* 2012;78:1785–1792.

82. De Leeuw FE, Korf E, Barkhof F, Scheltens P. White matter lesions are associated with progression of medial temporal lobe atrophy in Alzheimer disease. *Stroke* 2006;37:2248–2252.

83. Murray ME, Graff-Radford NR, Ross OA, et al. Neuropathologically defined subtypes of Alzheimer's disease with distinct clinical characteristics: a retrospective study. *Lancet Neurol* 2011;10:785–796.

84. Van de Pol LA, Hensel A, van der Flier WM, et al. Hippocampal atrophy on MRI in frontotemporal lobar degeneration and Alzheimer's disease. *J Neurol Neurosurg Psychiatry* 2006;77:439–442.

85. De Bresser J, Brundel M, Conijn MM, et al. Visual cerebral microbleed detection on 7T MR imaging: reliability and effects of image processing. *AJNR Am J Neuroradiol* 2013;34:E61–E64.

Chapter 25

Risk factors as possible targets for prevention of small vessel disease

Vincent Mok, Philip B. Gorelick, and Christopher Chen

Introduction

Lacunar infarcts, white matter lesions (WMLs), deep intracerebral hemorrhages (ICHs), and microbleeds are now considered various manifestations of age- and vascular risk factor-related cerebral small vessel disease (SVD). As a whole, these lesions are associated with a plethora of disabilities commonly seen in elderly persons. These may include cognitive impairment, dementia, depression, motor and gait disturbances, urinary symptoms, functional impairment, and stroke. More importantly, presence of these lesions increases mortality [1, 2]. Given the close association of WMLs with vascular risk factors, morbidity and mortality associated with these lesions are likely preventable. This chapter reviews the risk factors for the presence and progression of each of these manifestations. Knowledge of such risk factors generates hypotheses regarding possible targets for prevention.

Lacunar infarcts

Background

Understanding the pathogenesis of lacunar infarcts provides an important link to potential risk factors. The term "lacune" originated in the neuropathologic literature to describe a small cavity that remained in the brain tissue after the necrotic parenchyma of a small deep infarction had cleared [3, 4]. Dechambre was credited for using the term in 1838, and Durand-Fardel provided a treatise on the topic in 1843 [3]. According to Durand-Fardel, an associated term, "*état criblé*" (i.e., tissue riddled with holes or a sieve-like state) referred to dilated perivascular spaces and "*atrophie interstitielle du cerveau*" to rarefaction of the nervous system, viewed as being tantamount to leukoaraiosis [4]. Pierre Marie has been recognized for finding lacunes in 45 of 50 brains at necropsy and linked the healed area to obliteration or rupture of a perforating artery or its branches due to local arteriosclerosis [3]. In addition, Marie referred to multiple lacunes as "*état lacunaire*" and described a slow, shuffling gait and pseudobulbar palsy accompanying such lesions.

The modern understanding of lacunes is largely attributed to C. Miller Fisher who carried out meticulous clinical and neuropathologic studies. In 1965, Fisher published a series of 1042 adult brains examined for lacunes [5]. He described numerous clinical stroke syndromes linked to lacunes and showed that these lacunes could be caused by occlusive disease of penetrating vessels, predominantly located in deep brain structures such as the putamen, caudate, thalamus, internal capsule, corona radiate, and pons [5]. The seminal work of Fisher revealed that lacunes may range in size from large (1.5–2.0 cm) to small (3–4 mm). Larger lacunes tended to be symptomatic and were most commonly related to small atheromatous plaque (i.e., microatheroma) located at the proximal portion of penetrating arteries that ranged in size from 400 to 900 μm. Larger atheromatous plaque occurring at the wall of the parent large artery might also occlude the mouth of the penetrating artery, causing lacunar infarcts [6]. Smaller lacunes were commonly subclinical and were associated with lipohyalinosis and fibrinoid necrosis affecting penetrating arteries of only 100–400 μm in size [6]. In rare cases where the supplying artery running to the lacune was normal, Fisher hypothesized that microembolism from a proximal source might cause the obstruction [6]. Fisher also noted that hypertension was almost invariably present in subjects with lacunes. The concurrent presence of severe cerebral atherosclerosis was also common. However, diabetes was uncommon in his series [5].

Cerebral Small Vessel Disease, ed. Leonardo Pantoni and Philip B. Gorelick. Published by Cambridge University Press.

A more recent pathologic study conducted by Lammie et al. [7] included 70 consecutively referred autopsy brains with microscopic evidence of SVD. A focus of this analysis was to study SVD in relation to the presence or absence of SVD risk factors. The investigators showed that SVD consisted largely of concentric hyaline wall thickening, whereas lipohyalinosis and fibrinoid necrosis were rarely observed. Furthermore, 31% of cases did not meet study criteria for significant hypertension, 9% were nonelderly, nondiabetic, and did not have hypertension, and 5 of 6 cases without usual cardiovascular risk factors had a variety of conditions that might enhance small vessel permeability. The authors concluded that since Fisher's original publications, SVD might have been modified by effective treatment of hypertension, classic cardiovascular risk factors might be absent, and small vessel permeability might contribute to the pathogenesis of lacunar infarcts [7]. These findings suggest that we may need to broaden our mechanistic concepts in relation to lacunar infarct, and thus the factors that may be associated with risk of lacunar infarcts.

Noteworthy is that not all acute lacunar infarcts will eventually cavitate into a lacune [8]. Conversely, not all "lacunes" are due to lacunar infarcts, as lacunes may also result from other lesions; for example, a small ICH or even a large acute infarct. Furthermore, although small vessel pathologies may be the commonest culprit for lacunar infarcts, other etiologies such as amyloid angiopathy, microembolism from proximal sources, or systemic conditions such as polycythemia or arteritis, may also cause lacunar infarcts. Differentiating the exact etiologies for lacunar infarcts and lacunes is often difficult. Even with contemporary imaging techniques, determining whether the various small vessel pathologies actually are present in vivo is not possible. Disparity of findings regarding risk factors for lacunar infarcts between various studies may at least partially be related to such complexity and heterogeneity of underlying mechanisms for lacunar infarcts.

Risk factors for lacunar infarcts in stroke studies

Stroke is probably the commonest clinical manifestation of lacunar infarct. Jackson and Sudlow [9] carried out a systematic review of studies comparing risk factors between lacunar and nonlacunar stroke. A total of 16 of 28 studies included risk factors in the definition of ischemic stroke subtype. Overall, hypertension and diabetes were more frequently noted in patients with lacunar compared to those with nonlacunar stroke. However, when risk-factor free definitions were used, there was only a marginal excess of high blood pressure among those with lacunar stroke but no difference in diabetes. Atrial fibrillation and carotid artery stenosis were associated more frequently with nonlacunar than lacunar stroke, but again, the relationship was less evident when using risk factor-free ischemic stroke subtype classifications. Finally, this review shows no clear evidence of any association between smoking, previous transient ischemic attack, excess alcohol consumption, or raised cholesterol and lacunar versus nonlacunar stroke subtypes.

Some researchers hypothesized that different lacunar patterns may reflect different underlying SVD etiologies (e.g., microatheroma, lipohyalinosis) among stroke subjects, and hence compared risk factors between different lacunar patterns [10–12]. Khan et al. [10] compared patients having large vessel disease (LVD) and SVD stroke and found that hypertension was more common in SVD than LVD, whereas hypercholesterolemia, smoking, myocardial infarction, and peripheral vascular disease were more common in LVD. Among SVD patients, isolated lacunar infarct with no or minimal WMLs (presumably related to microatheroma) was associated with hypercholesterolemia, diabetes, and myocardial infarction, i.e., risk factors similar to LVD, while lacunar infarct with moderate to severe WMLs (presumably related to lipohyalinosis) was associated with age and hypertension. Arauz et al. [12] found that diabetes, high levels of hematocrit, and WMLs were related to multiple (presumably related to lipohyalinosis) but not to single lacunar infarct (presumably related to microatheroma). In a more recent study, Nah et al. [13] found that acute small deep infarcts with parent atheromatous disease (presumably related to large vessel atheromatous plaque blocking the mouth of penetrating artery) had the highest prevalence of atheromatous indicators (i.e., coronary artery disease, asymptomatic cerebral atherosclerotic disease) and the lowest prevalence of SVD indicators (i.e., WMLs, microbleeds), distal small deep infarcts without parent atheromatous disease (presumably related to lipohyalinosis) had the lowest prevalence of atheromatous indicators and the highest prevalence of SVD indicators, whereas proximal small deep infarcts without parent atheromatous disease (presumably related to microatheroma at the proximal portion of the penetrating artery) showed intermediate features.

Risk factors for prevalent and incident lacunes in community studies

Not all lacunar infarcts will manifest as stroke. In fact, subclinical lacunar infarcts or lacunes are much more prevalent than lacunar stroke. In the Cardiovascular Health Study (CHS) among 3660 community-dwelling elderly, 23% had 1 or more lacunes (3–20mm). Most of the lacunes were subclinical (89%), i.e., not associated with history of stroke or transient ischemic attack [14]. Factors associated with lacunes were increased age, diastolic blood pressure, creatinine, pack–years of smoking, internal carotid artery (ICA) stenosis, male sex, and history of diabetes at entry into the study. Comparisons between subgroups of single, multiple, silent, and symptomatic lacunes failed to yield significant differences that might suggest different SVD subtypes explaining different patterns or manifestations of lacunes.

In the Atherosclerosis Risk in Communities (ARIC) study, two SVD subtypes (lipohyalinosis and microatheroma) were studied in relation to the associated risks, diabetes and glycated hemoglobin (HbA1c), low-density lipoprotein (LDL) cholesterol, and other cardiovascular factors. In this cross-sectional study of 1827 community-dwelling participants, subcortical lesions diagnosed on magnetic resonance imaging (MRI) measuring ≤20 mm in diameter were divided into those ≤7 mm (presumably related to lipohyalinosis), and those measuring 8–20 mm in diameter (presumably related to microatheroma). In this study, smaller lacunes were associated with diabetes and HbA1c, whereas the larger ones were associated with low-density lipoprotein (LDL) cholesterol. These findings suggest that diabetes may be associated with lipohyalinosis and LDL cholesterol with microatheroma. Other factors associated with larger MRI-based lesions were hypertension and smoking.

Incident lacunes are associated with various clinical consequences, including stroke and cognitive decline [15]. Compared to cross-sectional study designs, longitudinal studies with serial MRI using incident lacunes as an outcome measure may provide stronger evidence that the identified risk factors have a causal relationship with disease severity and progression. Among 668 community-dwelling elderly participants, the Rotterdam Scan Study (RSS) found that incident lacunes (3–20 mm) were associated with age, female gender, and baseline carotid atherosclerosis [16]. The Leukoaraiosis And DISability (LADIS) study recruited 639 elderly subjects who had at least some degree of WMLs on MRI. Incident lacunes (3–10 mm) were found to be associated with baseline lacune and WML load, systolic blood pressure (BP), and low high-density lipoprotein (HDL) cholesterol. There were unexpected associations with high diastolic blood pressure and high LDL cholesterol as factors protecting against incident lacunes [17]. It is important to note that the definition of lacunes in relation to size and the study populations differed between the RSS and the LADIS study. The latter study included only small lacunes and subjects who already had at least some degree of WMLs. Such differences in lacunar definition and study subjects may possibly explain at least in part the disparity in the findings for risk factors for incident lacunes between the two studies.

New links to risks for lacunar infarcts

Systemic or local brain factors may also be predictors of lacunar infarcts. For example, atherosclerosis burden in relation to peripheral artery atherosclerosis [18], measures of retinal fractal dimension (i.e., microvascular branching complexity and density), or arteriole or venule equivalent size [19], and enlarged perivascular spaces [20] may predict lacunar infarct occurrence. As we seek new risks for lacunar infarcts, the neurovascular unit has become the focus of substantial interest in relation to the pathogenesis of SVD. We address the latter and other aspects below.

SVD is common among elderly persons. Furthermore, in older patients with various forms of dementia, vessel wall modifications such as arteriolosclerosis or amyloid angiopathy are common, and lacunar infarcts may be explained by the final phase of the SVD process or as an independent pathway [21]. Endothelial activation may be an important process in SVD; for example, persons with lacunar infarcts associated with diffuse SVD may have higher levels of tissue plasminogen activator (tPA) in those with extensive WMLs than in those with isolated lacunar infarcts, whereas low levels of plasminogen activator inhibitor type 1 (PAI-1) may be associated with

WMLs [22]. Other circulating markers of endothelial activation, intercellular adhesion molecule-1 (ICAM1) and thrombomodulin, and inflammatory markers such as interleukin-6, may be elevated in patients with SVD and provide opportunities for additional study and possible development of new prevention strategies. One such factor, thrombomodulin, may be a protective factor [23].

Summary

Lacunar infarcts are an important cause of disability and morbidity, including cognitive impairment, as we age. Our understanding of the precise pathogenesis of lacunar infarcts has been challenged by difficulty in establishing neuropathologic correlation of the small deep infarct and small vessel pathology. Lines of evidence also suggest that patterns, location, or size of lacunar infarcts may possibly reflect different underlying SVD subtypes, and each subtype may be associated with unique risk factors. Moreover, classical cardiovascular risk factors (e.g., hypertension, diabetes, hypercholesterolemia) are not consistently common in patients with lacunar infarcts suggesting that there may be other mechanisms to explain lacunar pathogenesis. Endothelial activation and vessel-wall permeability and the influence of systemic factors on the endothelium may provide additional clues to the development of lacunar infarcts and subsequent preventive strategies. In addition and beyond cerebral autosomal dominant arteriopathy with subcortical infarcts and leukoencephalopathy (CADASIL), there may be genetic influences that predispose to the occurrence of lacunar infarcts [24].

White matter lesions

Background

Similar to lacunar infarct, the exact mechanism for white matter lesions (WMLs) is uncertain and is likely complex. An early review by Babikian and Ropper [25] reported 47 cases of dementia associated with presumably diffuse ischemic WMLs (Binswanger's disease) in the literature since 1912. All of these cases had clinical and pathologic correlation. Arteriosclerosis (hardening with calcification, hyalinization, and thickening of the vessel wall of small penetrating arteries) was invariably present in the affected white matter of all cases. The WMLs were characterized by demyelination, loss of axons, and oligodendrocytes. There was sparing of U-fibers. Hypertension was present in most of the cases. The primary hypothesis derived from these early findings was that WMLs are due to chronic partial ischemia secondary to diffuse arteriosclerosis, which is probably due to hypertension. Other early studies showed that WMLs could be related to systemic factors associated with hypotensive episodes (e.g., cardiac arrhythmias, diuretic use) or with labile blood pressure and postural hypotension, which might result in hemodynamic ischemia and WMLs [26, 27].

Apart from the "ischemic" hypothesis, other mechanisms that may explain WMLs are breakdown of the blood–brain barrier and leakage of toxic fluids to the white matter. This hypothesis was proposed in early studies showing raised cerebrospinal fluid proteins in subjects with WMLs, which is a measure of blood–brain barrier damage [28]. In another study, Moody et al. [29] described 22 cases with imaging and pathologic correlation, showing a strong association between WMLs and venous collagenosis. This study raised the possibility that WMLs might also be attributed to collagenosis of small venules, resulting in "venous" ischemia and edema. Overall, findings derived from these early studies provide foundational knowledge for our current understanding on the putative mechanisms and risk factors for WMLs. We now turn to more recent or large-scale community-based studies that evaluate risk factors for WMLs.

Risk factors for WMLs

Apart from age, most community-based studies have consistently shown that hypertension is associated with WMLs [30–34]. Both the RSS and Epidemiology of Vascular Aging study further showed that duration of hypertension was associated with WMLs, while effective hypertension treatment was associated with lower risk [33, 34]. Noteworthy is that the association between BP levels and confluent WMLs may not be linear. Analysis of 10 European cohorts revealed a "J curve" phenomenon, in that both increases and decreases in diastolic BP were associated with more severe WMLs [35]. The association between low BP and WMLs is probably related to impaired cerebral autoregulation, which is commonly associated with aging and/or exposure to vascular risk factors. The RSS found that impaired cerebral vasomotor reactivity was associated with WMLs [36]. As a result of impaired cerebral vasomotor reactivity, brain arteries may fail to dilate to increase cerebral blood flow in response to drops in systemic BP, resulting in cerebral hemodynamic ischemia. In a recent subgroup analysis of the VITAmins TO Prevent Stroke (VITATOPS) MRI substudy, lower diastolic BP at baseline predicted cognitive decline among subjects with severe WMLs at baseline [37]. Other studies showed that postural hypotension or hypertension [35], increasing long-term fluctuations of BP [38], and various 24-hour ambulatory BP measures (e.g., greater systolic BP variability, smaller nocturnal fall in systolic or diastolic BP) [39] were all associated with WMLs. Both the RSS and the ARIC study further showed that measures of arterial stiffness (e.g., brachial pulse pressure, aortic pulse wave velocity) were risk factors for WMLs even after controlling for BP levels and other cardiovascular risk factors. It has, thus, been proposed that arterial stiffening might expose cerebral small vessels to high pulsatile pressure and flow, hence contributing to the pathogenesis of SVD.

Most studies found that smoking was associated with WMLs [30, 32]. Despite diabetes being a strong risk factor for stroke and coronary heart disease, most community-based cross-sectional studies failed to find an association between diabetes and WMLs [30, 31]. In the Helsinki Aging Brain study, WMLs were associated with diabetes only among the younger old (<75 years), but not among the older old (>75 years) [40].

The RSS found that high homocysteine level was associated with WMLs [41]. In a separate study evaluating the association between homocysteine and endothelial markers (ICAM1, thrombomodulin), Hassan et al. [42] showed that the association between homocysteine and WMLs was probably mediated by endothelial activation. Homocysteinemia may also exert a direct toxic effect via activation of *N*-methyl-D-aspartate receptors, leading to cell death, or it may be converted into homocysteic acid, which also has an excitotoxic effect upon neurons [43]. The RSS further showed that low vitamin B12 and folate levels, which are factors closely related to homocysteine metabolism, were associated with WMLs independent of homocysteine level [44, 45]. These findings suggest that low vitamin B12 and folate levels may also induce WMLs through mechanisms independent of homocysteine or endothelial activation, such as low vitamin B12-mediated impairment of myelin integrity. However, it must be noted that the CHS failed to find an association between WMLs and homocysteine level [46].

Findings on the association between cholesterol levels or statin use and WMLs are less consistent, and sometimes contradictory. The Cardiovascular Risk Factors and the Aging and Incidence of Dementia MRI substudy [47] showed that use of lipid-lowering drugs was associated with fewer WMLs. The National Heart, Lung, and Blood Institute Twin Study found that mid-life lower HDL-cholesterol level was associated with late-life WMLs [48]. By contrast, the Austrian Stroke Prevention Study (ASPS) showed that lower total cholesterol level was associated with WMLs [49]. In another study investigating association between WMLs and cholesterol level among two stroke cohorts (total 1135 patients), hyperlipidemia was associated with fewer WMLs [50]. The authors suggested that hyperlipidemia might play a protective role in cerebral SVD. However, as statin use had high collinearity with hyperlipidemia, the authors could not rule out the possibility that the association between hyperlipidemia and WMLs was related to statin use. Noteworthy is that in a subgroup analysis of the VITATOPS MRI substudy, absence of hyperlipidemia or statin use was found to associate with cognitive decline in subjects with severe WMLs at baseline [37].

More recent studies evaluating ribonucleic acid (RNA) expression profile in brain or blood samples showed that genes specific for WMLs were associated with injury responses, oxidative stress, and inflammation [51, 52]. In a large genome-wide association study of WML burden in community-based cohorts of individuals of European descent, a novel locus on chromosome 17 was identified to be associated with WMLs. Although information on the specific genes and functional variants underlying the reported associations was lacking, further characterization of this locus will provide additional insights into the mechanisms of WMLs and hopefully new targets for preventive therapies [53].

Risk factors for progression of WMLs

WMLs may progress and given that progression is associated with clinical consequence, WML progression may be used as surrogate markers in preventive trials. Several longitudinal studies with serial MRIs have investigated the risk factors for WML progression.

The majority of studies showed that baseline lesion load [16, 17, 54], older age [16, 55], smoking

[16, 56], and hypertension [16, 55, 57] predicted WML progression. The ARIC study found that the cumulative mean systolic BP (i.e., estimated mean systolic BP over the entire period) was a much stronger predictor of WML progression than were systolic BP readings obtained at individual time points [58]. The Three City–Dijon MRI study showed that not only baseline hypertension predicted WML progression. Among subjects with high systolic BP ≥160 mmHg at baseline and not treated with antihypertensive medication, antihypertensive treatment started within two years was related to a smaller increase in WML volume than in those without hypertensive treatment [57]. The Perindopril Protection aGainst Recurrent Stroke Study (PROGRESS) MRI substudy further showed that a more intensive BP-lowering regime might delay WML progression in stroke patients [59]. Of note, however, the subgroup analyses from the RSS revealed that among those who already had severe lesions at baseline and those who were very old (≥80 years), higher BP did not contribute to lesion progression [16]. The association between BP and WML progression was stronger among the younger old or among those who did not have severe WMLs at baseline. Similar findings were noted in the CHS, in that the association between WML progression and BP was significant only among those who did not have severe WMLs at baseline [56].

Most studies did not find an association between baseline diabetes and WML progression. The association between cholesterol levels/statin use and WML progression was again controversial. In the CHS, among those with less initial WML burden, increased HDL cholesterol, and decreased LDL cholesterol were associated with increased risk of progression; whereas among those with high initial grade, statin use was associated with increased risk [56]. In the LADIS study, higher triglyceride levels appeared to protect against WML progression [17]. By contrast, in the Regression of Cerebral Artery Stenosis (ROCAS) study, statin use was associated with less WML progression among those with initial severe WML burden [60].

In the ASPS, ICAM1 levels were associated with WML progression, further supporting the causal role of endothelial activation in the pathogenesis of WMLs [55]. In the same study, association between peripheral markers of coagulation activation (e.g., D-dimer, and prothrombin fragments 1 and 2) and WML progression could not be found. Noteworthy is that in the recent VITATOPS MRI substudy, lowering homocysteine using B-vitamins was found to be associated with a reduction in WML volume increment only among those with severe SVD at baseline [61]. Although the inflammatory process has been postulated as a pathogenic mechanism for WMLs, results from longitudinal studies assessing association between C-reactive protein levels and WML progression were not consistent. The RSS showed a positive association [62], while the ASPS failed to find an association [63].

Summary

High BP remains the most consistent risk factor for presence and progression of WMLs. However, targets for optimal BP control are uncertain, in particular among the very old and among those who already have severe WML load at baseline. Data on the integrity of cerebral autoregulation and other BP measures (e.g., postural changes, acute surges, circadian changes) may also guide specific treatment strategies. Association between cholesterol levels and statin use and WMLs remains controversial. Further trials investigating homocysteine lowering therapy or B vitamins in subjects with WMLs are warranted. Lines of evidence also suggest that endothelial activation and leakage across the blood–brain barrier are important pathogenic mechanisms for WMLs. Such factors may thus serve as important surrogate markers for WML severity and treatment response.

Deep intracerebral hemorrhage

Background

Hypertension is considered the main risk and mechanistic link to subcortical hemorrhage [64, 65]. Hypertension was recognized as early as the 1800s as were its adverse cardiovascular effects on the heart, brain, and kidney. In the 1900s it became clear that hypertension could lead to arteriosclerosis and atherosclerosis (deposition of lipid into the vessel wall), though hypertension might not be a specific cause of these vessel-wall changes [65]. Three vessel-wall changes that may be more specific to hypertension include fibrinoid necrosis (fibrinoid substance in the vessel-wall media and disappearance of muscle elements in small arteries), lipohyalinosis (thinning of the wall of the arteries that are often <200 μm in diameter and reduced vessel-wall connective tissue, and occurrence of hemosiderin-laden macrophages, deposition of lipid material, hyalinization, and fibrinoid change), and miliary (Charcôt–Bouchard) aneurysms (0.2–1.0 mm in diameter) of deep penetrating arteries [65]. These three latter vessel-wall changes are thought to be mechanistically linked to deep intracerebral hemorrhage (ICH). One can envision a thinned, frayed vessel wall or the presence of a small deep aneurysm, all under the influence of high blood pressure, as a circumstance prone to rupture and consequent subcortical brain bleeding. It has been argued, however, that there is less support for miliary aneurysms as a cause for subcortical brain hemorrhage [65].

Risk factors for subcortical hemorrhage

Beyond hypertension there are a number of factors that have been linked to ICH, including, but not limited to, race/ethnicity (e.g., higher rates in Asians and African-Americans), illicit drugs (e.g., cocaine), cigarette smoking, heavy alcohol consumption, low serum cholesterol, aspirin, and anticoagulant use [66]. Some of these factors have been less well studied than others or are potential confounding factors making interpretation and understanding of the role of these factors as risks challenging. The most important risk and the one that is most likely to explain the highest attributable risk for ICH is high BP [66]. Hypertension has been the subject of controversy, however, as it may be present in up to approximately 90% of ICH patients in some studies but as low as 39–49% in other studies. Therefore, Kase [64] concluded that overall the frequency of hypertension as the cause of ICH is in the 60–65% range. Furthermore, the comparison of elderly to younger patients suggests that the frequency of hypertension as a cause of ICH is higher in younger persons. This may be explained in part by the race–ethnic mix of the study population and other mechanisms that may be in place in older persons (e.g., brain neoplasm, bleeding disorders) [64].

Caplan [65] has suggested that the mechanism of hypertensive ICH is likely driven by either rupture of small penetrating arteries damaged by chronic hypertension and aging, or acute perturbations in BP and flow that lead to rupture of normal arterioles and capillaries unaccustomed to and unprotected from hypertensive BP surges. Caplan's explanations suggest the need for careful neurovascular history to detect circumstances whereby BP might substantially rise and fluctuate (e.g., exposure to extreme cold, response to a catastrophe, or an emergency situation) or use of ambulatory BP monitoring technology to unmask forms of hypertension that may not be obvious (e.g., night-time blood pressure elevations or "nondipping").

New links to risks of subcortical hemorrhage

Several additional factors have been more recently identified or popularized in relation to ICH. First, cerebral amyloid angiopathy (CAA), frequently associated with Alzheimer's disease, has been linked to predominantly lobar hemorrhages and some subarachnoid or subdural hemorrhages but also to occasional subcortical hemorrhage [67]. CAA-related hemorrhages may be prevented by antihypertensive medication administration. Secondly, and largely based on the Stroke Prevention by Aggressive Reduction in Cholesterol Levels (SPARCL) trial, concern has been raised about an elevated risk of ICH in those using statin therapy [68]. Collaborative systematic and meta-analysis by Hackem et al. [69], however, concluded that, if such a risk exists, the absolute magnitude is likely to be small and outweighed by the advantages of statins. Thirdly, a greater MRI-defined burden of WMLs and brain infarcts has been associated with spontaneous ICH [70]. Fourth, lowering of BP may be associated with ischemic brain injury in recent ICH patients [71]. Finally, Weng et al. [72] bring to light the possibility that COL4A1 (and possible other mutations, e.g., COL4A2) might be present in late-onset sporadic ICH providing another potential avenue for prevention.

Summary

Subcortical macrobleeds make up about 10–15% of strokes or more and are a major cause of neurologic morbidity and mortality. More accurate diagnosis of hypertension or prevention of periodic surges in BP could lead to enhanced prevention of ICH. Furthermore, discovery of genetic mutations linked to ICH (e.g., COL4A1) could lead to the discovery of new preventives for ICH.

Microbleeds

Background

Small brain hemorrhages had long been observed in brain specimens of hypertensive subjects [73]. Since microbleeds could not be detected by CT, the exact prevalence, etiologies, and clinical correlates of brain microbleeds were not known until in the 1990s when application of T2*-weighted gradient-echo MRI sequence became more popular [74]. Fazekas et al. [75] examined radiologic and pathologic samples of 11 subjects who died of ICH. Hypointense foci on T2*-weighted gradient-echo MRI was found to correspond to focal deposition of hemosiderin in the perivascular space. Moderate to severe lipohyalinosis, typical of that found in hypertensive deep ICH, was present in all cases, while concurrent presence of amyloid angiopathy was found in two subjects. Most subjects with a history of hypertension had microbleeds located predominantly, but not exclusively, in deep or infratentorial regions. A subject with amyloid angiopathy and recurrent lobar ICH had purely corticosubcortical microbleeds. Another subject with amyloid angiopathy had mixed corticosubcortical and deep microbleeds. Lacunar infarcts and WMLs were frequently found in these brain specimens. Findings from this early study suggested that mechanisms for microbleeds are probably similar to their counterpart macrobleeds, in that deep microbleeds are probably associated more with lipohyalinosis-related deep ICH, while lobar microbleeds correlated more with CAA-related lobar ICH. Moreover, both types of SVDs may exist in the same individual.

Findings derived from more recent MRI studies suggest that presence of microbleeds is not only associated with increased risk of ICH, but also other neurologic conditions (e.g., cognitive impairment, gait disturbance, depressive mood) and increased overall mortality [2]. Preventing development of microbleeds may possibly prevent the clinical consequences of microbleeds. Since this chapter focuses on cerebral SVD predominantly associated with vascular risk factors, studies related purely to CAA-associated lobar ICH will not be emphasized.

Risk factors for presence of microbleeds

In the systematic review conducted by Cordonnier et al. [76], hypertension is the most consistent risk factor for microbleeds in both healthy adults and in adults with cerebrovascular diseases. In the same review, diabetes was also found to be associated with microbleeds, but such association was only found among healthy adults [76]. The RSS found that systolic BP was related to presence of deep/infratentorial microbleeds, whereas diastolic BP was related to strictly lobar microbleeds [77]. In the same study, smoking was found to be associated with deep but not lobar microbleeds [77]. In another study among subjects with first-ever lacunar stroke, Staals et al. [78] found that ambulatory BP measures (24-hour, day and night systolic and diastolic BP) were more robust predictors for microbleeds than the mere presence or absence of hypertension. After distinguishing between different locations, various BP characteristics were associated only with deep (or combined deep and lobar) microbleeds, but not with pure lobar microbleeds [78].

Similar to ICH, low total serum cholesterol levels were found to be associated with microbleeds independent of hypertension among subjects having various neurologic conditions [79]. In the RSS, low triglyceride levels, rather than HDL or LDL cholesterol levels, were associated with deep/infratentorial microbleeds, as well as ICH [80]. Among subjects with previous spontaneous ICH, statin use, rather than cholesterol levels, was associated with presence and number of microbleeds, especially corticosubcortical microbleeds [81]. However, in a study among patients with acute ischemic stroke or transient ischemic attack, previous statin use was not associated with the prevalence or severity of microbleeds [82]. In another study, proteinuria and homocysteinemia were both found to be associated with presence and severity of microbleeds in ischemic stroke or transient ischemic attack patients [83]. In the same study, female gender, history of atrial fibrillation, and SVD stroke subtype were also associated with microbleeds.

In the RSS, carriage of apolipoprotein E (*APOE*) ε4 and ε2/ε2 genotypes was related to strictly lobar microbleeds and not to deep/infratentorial microbleeds [77]. In the systematic review and meta-analyses conducted by Maxwell et al. [84] on the genetic associations with microbleeds, *APOE* ε4 allele carriers are at higher risk of having microbleeds, particularly in strictly lobar brain locations. Given the known associations of *APOE* genotype with CAA and lobar ICH, the findings support lobar microbleeds as an imaging biomarker for CAA.

Risk factors for incident microbleeds

To date, only a few longitudinal studies have explored the risk factors for incident microbleeds. In a small series of patients ($N = 21$) with ischemic stroke or transient ischemic attack, baseline presence of microbleeds and mean systolic BP predicted incident microbleeds [85]. In the RSS, microbleeds at baseline, age, systolic BP, high pulse pressure, and severe hypertension were all associated with incident microbleeds. Stratification according to location, age, systolic BP, severe hypertension, and low serum cholesterol levels predicted incident deep microbleeds, whereas age and those with *APOE* ε4/ε4 genotype predicted strictly lobar microbleeds [86]. In another study among subjects attending memory clinics, multiple microbleeds at baseline, WML severity, lacunar infarcts, and *APOE* ε2 predicted incident microbleeds, in particular deep microbleeds, whereas smoking was found to be associated with strictly lobar bleeds [87].

Summary

Hypertension is the most important risk factor for presence and progression of microbleeds, in particular for deep or combined deep and lobar microbleeds. Measures of ambulatory BP may have better correlation with microbleeds than mere presence or absence of hypertension. Although lobar microbleeds are probably related more strongly to CAA with an association to *APOE* genotype, BP levels and other cardiovascular risk factors (e.g., smoking) may also contribute to lobar microbleeds. Cholesterol and triglyceride levels may have an inverse relationship with microbleeds. Among those with ICH, statin use may be associated with microbleeds, in particular lobar microbleeds. Whether homocysteine levels or markers of endothelial activation are risk factors for microbleeds requires further studies to determine if such a relationship exists. Since mechanisms for microbleeds are probably similar to those of ICH, traditional or novel preventive measures for ICH may also be relevant for microbleeds. Nevertheless, whether there are additional risk factors that have unique associations with microbleeds but not with ICH is an interesting area for study.

References

1. Debette S, Markus HS. The clinical importance of white matter hyperintensities on brain magnetic resonance imaging: systematic review and meta-analysis. *BMJ* 2010;341:3666.
2. Altmann-Schneider I, Trompet S, de Craen AJ, et al. Cerebral microbleeds are predictive of mortality in the elderly. *Stroke* 2011;42:638–644.
3. Fields WS, Lemak NA. *A History of Stroke. Its Recognition and Treatment*. New York, NY: Oxford University Press; 1989.
4. Hauw JJ. The history of lacunes. In Donnan G, Norrving B, Bamford J, Bogousslavsky J, eds. *Subcortical Stroke*, 2nd edn. New York, NY: Oxford University Press; 2002: pp. 3–15.
5. Fisher CM. Lacunes: small, deep cerebral infarcts. *Neurology* 1965;15:774–784.
6. Fisher CM. Lacunar strokes and infarcts: a review. *Neurology* 1982;32:871–876.
7. Lammie GA, Brannan F, Slattery J, Warlow C. Nonhypertensive cerebral small-vessel disease. An autopsy study. *Stroke* 1997;28:2222–2229.
8. Potter GM, Doubal FN, Jackson CA, et al. Counting cavitating lacunes underestimates the burden of lacunar infarction. *Stroke* 2010;41:267–272.
9. Jackson C, Sudlow C. Are lacunar strokes really different? A systematic review of differences in risk factor profiles between lacunar and nonlacunar infarcts. *Stroke* 2005;36:891–901.
10. Khan U, Porteous L, Hassan A, Markus HS. Risk factor profile of cerebral small vessel disease and its subtypes. *J Neurol Neurosurg Psychiatry* 2007;78:702–706.
11. Boiten J, Lodder J, Kessels F. Two clinically distinct lacunar infarct entities? A hypothesis. *Stroke* 1993;24:652–656.
12. Arauz A, Murillo L, Cantu C, Barinagarrementeria F, Higuera J. Prospective study of single and multiple lacunar infarcts using magnetic resonance imaging: risk factors, recurrence, and outcome in 175 consecutive cases. *Stroke* 2003;34:2453–2458.
13. Nah HW, Kang DW, Kwon SU, Kim JS. Diversity of single small subcortical infarctions according to infarct location and parent artery disease: analysis of indicators for small vessel disease and atherosclerosis. *Stroke* 2010;41:2822–2827.
14. Longstreth WT, Jr., Bernick C, Manolio TA, et al. Lacunar infarcts defined by magnetic resonance imaging of 3660 elderly people: the Cardiovascular Health Study. *Arch Neurol* 1998;55: 1217–1225.
15. Vermeer SE, Prins ND, den Heijer T, et al. Silent brain infarcts and the risk of dementia and cognitive decline. *N Engl J Med* 2003;348:1215–1222.
16. Van Dijk EJ, Prins ND, Vrooman HA, et al. Progression of cerebral small vessel disease in relation to risk factors and cognitive consequences: the Rotterdam Scan Study. *Stroke* 2008;39:2712–2719.
17. Gouw AA, van der Flier WM, Fazekas F, et al. Progression of white matter hyperintensities and incidence of new lacunes over a three-year period:

the Leukoaraiosis And DISability study. *Stroke* 2008;39:1414–1420.

18. Jackson CA, Hutchison A, Dennis MS, et al. Differences between ischemic stroke subtypes in vascular outcomes support a distinct lacunar ischemic stroke arteriopathy: a prospective, hospital-based study. *Stroke* 2009;40:3679–3684.
19. Cheung N, Liew G, Lindley RI, et al. Retinal fractals and acute lacunar stroke. *Ann Neurol* 2010;68:107–111.
20. Doubal FN, MacLullich AM, Ferguson KJ, Dennis MS, Wardlaw JM. Enlarged perivascular spaces on MRI are a feature of cerebral small vessel disease. *Stroke* 2010;41: 450–454.
21. Deramecourt V, Slade JY, Oakley AE, et al. Staging and natural history of cerebrovascular pathology in dementia. *Neurology* 2012;78:1043–1050.
22. Knottnerus IL, Govers-Riemslag JW, Hamulyak K, et al. Endothelial activation in lacunar stroke subtypes. *Stroke* 2010;41:1617–1622.
23. Giwa MO, Williams J, Elderfield K, et al. Neuropathologic evidence of endothelial changes in cerebral small vessel disease. *Neurology* 2012;78:167–174.
24. Van Dijk EJ, Prins ND, Vermeer SE, et al. Plasma amyloid β, apolipoprotein E, lacunar infarcts, and white matter lesions. *Ann Neurol* 2004;55:570–575.
25. Babikian V, Ropper AH. Binswanger's disease: a review. *Stroke* 1987;18:2–12.
26. McQuinn BA, O'Leary DH. White matter lucencies on computed tomography, subacute arteriosclerotic encephalopathy (Binswanger's disease), and blood pressure. *Stroke* 1987;18:900–905.
27. Sulkava R, Erkinjuntti T. Vascular dementia due to cardiac arrhythmias and systemic hypotension. *Acta Neurol Scand* 1987;76:123–128.
28. Pantoni L, Inzitari D, Pracucci G, et al. Cerebrospinal fluid proteins in patients with leucoaraiosis: possible abnormalities in blood–brain barrier function. *J Neurol Sci* 1993;115:125–131.
29. Moody DM, Brown WR, Challa VR, Anderson RL. Periventricular venous collagenosis: association with leukoaraiosis. *Radiology* 1995;194:469–476.
30. Liao D, Cooper L, Cai J, et al. The prevalence and severity of white matter lesions, their relationship with age, ethnicity, gender, and cardiovascular disease risk factors: the ARIC study. *Neuroepidemiology* 1997;16: 149–162.
31. Longstreth WT, Jr., Manolio TA, Arnold A, et al. Clinical correlates of white matter findings on cranial magnetic resonance imaging of 3301 elderly people. The Cardiovascular Health Study. *Stroke* 1996;27:1274–1282.
32. Jeerakathil T, Wolf PA, Beiser A, et al. Stroke risk profile predicts white matter hyperintensity volume: the Framingham Study. *Stroke* 2004;35:1857–1861.
33. De Leeuw FE, de Groot JC, Oudkerk M, et al. Hypertension and cerebral white matter lesions in a prospective cohort study. *Brain* 2002;125(Pt 4):765–772.
34. Dufouil C, de Kersaint-Gilly A, Besancon V, et al. Longitudinal study of blood pressure and white matter hyperintensities: the EVA MRI cohort. *Neurology* 2001;56:921–926.
35. Van Dijk EJ, Breteler MM, Schmidt R, et al. The association between blood pressure, hypertension, and cerebral white matter lesions: cardiovascular determinants of dementia study. *Hypertension* 2004;44:625–630.
36. Bakker SL, de Leeuw FE, de Groot JC, et al. Cerebral vasomotor reactivity and cerebral white matter lesions in the elderly. *Neurology* 1999;52:578–583.
37. Mok V, Xiong Y, Wong KK, et al. Predictors for cognitive decline in patients with confluent white matter hyperintensities. *Alzheimers Dement* 2012;8(Suppl 5):S96–S103.
38. Brickman AM, Reitz C, Luchsinger JA, et al. Long-term blood pressure fluctuation and cerebrovascular disease in an elderly cohort. *Arch Neurol* 2010;67:564–569.
39. Goldstein IB, Bartzokis G, Hance DB, Shapiro D. Relationship between blood pressure and subcortical lesions in healthy elderly people. *Stroke* 1998;29:765–772.
40. Ylikoski A, Erkinjuntti T, Raininko R, et al. White matter hyperintensities on MRI in the neurologically nondiseased elderly. Analysis of cohorts of consecutive subjects aged 55 to 85 years living at home. *Stroke* 1995;26:1171–1177.
41. Vermeer SE, van Dijk EJ, Koudstaal PJ, et al. Homocysteine, silent brain infarcts, and white matter lesions: the Rotterdam Scan Study. *Ann Neurol* 2002;51:285–289.
42. Hassan A, Hunt BJ, O'Sullivan M, et al. Homocysteine is a risk factor for cerebral small vessel disease, acting via endothelial dysfunction. *Brain* 2004;127(Pt 1):212–219.
43. Weir DG, Scott JM. Brain function in the elderly: role of vitamin B12 and folate. *Br Med Bull* 1999;55:669–682.
44. De Lau LM, Smith AD, Refsum H, Johnston C, Breteler MM. Plasma vitamin B12 status and cerebral white-matter lesions. *J Neurol Neurosurg Psychiatry* 2009;80:149–157.
45. De Lau LM, Refsum H, Smith AD, Johnston C, Breteler MM. Plasma folate concentration and cognitive

performance: the Rotterdam Scan Study. *Am J Clin Nutr* 2007;86:728–734.

46. Longstreth WT, Jr., Katz R, Olson J, et al. Plasma total homocysteine levels and cranial magnetic resonance imaging findings in elderly persons: the Cardiovascular Health Study. *Arch Neurol* 2004;61:67–72.

47. Vuorinen M, Solomon A, Rovio S, et al. Changes in vascular risk factors from midlife to late life and white matter lesions: a 20-year follow-up study. *Dement Geriatr Cogn Disord* 2011;31: 119–125.

48. Carmelli D, Swan GE, Reed T, et al. Midlife cardiovascular risk factors and brain morphology in identical older male twins. *Neurology* 1999;52:1119–1124.

49. Schmidt R, Hayn M, Fazekas F, Kapeller P, Esterbauer H. Magnetic resonance imaging white matter hyperintensities in clinically normal elderly individuals. Correlations with plasma concentrations of naturally occurring antioxidants. *Stroke* 1996;27:2043–2047.

50. Jimenez-Conde J, Biffi A, Rahman R, et al. Hyperlipidemia and reduced white matter hyperintensity volume in patients with ischemic stroke. *Stroke* 2010;41:437–442.

51. Xu H, Stamova B, Jickling G, et al. Distinctive RNA expression profiles in blood associated with white matter hyperintensities in brain. *Stroke* 2010;41: 2744–2749.

52. Simpson JE, Hosny O, Wharton SB, et al. Microarray RNA expression analysis of cerebral white matter lesions reveals changes in multiple functional pathways. *Stroke* 2009;40: 369–375.

53. Fornage M, Debette S, Bis JC, et al. Genome-wide association studies of cerebral white matter lesion burden: the CHARGE consortium. *Ann Neurol* 2011;69:928–939.

54. Schmidt R, Enzinger C, Ropele S, Schmidt H, Fazekas F. Progression of cerebral white matter lesions: six-year results of the Austrian Stroke Prevention Study. *Lancet* 2003; 361:2046–2048.

55. Markus HS, Hunt B, Palmer K, et al. Markers of endothelial and hemostatic activation and progression of cerebral white matter hyperintensities: longitudinal results of the Austrian Stroke Prevention Study. *Stroke* 2005;36:1410–1414.

56. Longstreth WT, Jr., Arnold AM, Beauchamp NJ, Jr., et al. Incidence, manifestations, and predictors of worsening white matter on serial cranial magnetic resonance imaging in the elderly: the Cardiovascular Health Study. *Stroke* 2005;36:56–61.

57. Godin O, Tzourio C, Maillard P, Mazoyer B, Dufouil C. Antihypertensive treatment and change in blood pressure are associated with the progression of white matter lesion volumes: the Three-City (3C)–Dijon Magnetic Resonance Imaging Study. *Circulation* 2011;123:266–273.

58. Gottesman RF, Coresh J, Catellier DJ, et al. Blood pressure and white-matter disease progression in a biethnic cohort: Atherosclerosis Risk In Communities (ARIC) study. *Stroke* 2010;41:3–8.

59. Dufouil C, Chalmers J, Coskun O, et al. Effects of blood pressure lowering on cerebral white matter hyperintensities in patients with stroke: the PROGRESS (Perindopril Protection aGainst Recurrent Stroke Study) magnetic resonance imaging substudy. *Circulation* 2005;112:1644–1650.

60. Mok VC, Lam WW, Fan YH, et al. Effects of statins on the progression of cerebral white matter lesion: post hoc analysis of the ROCAS (Regression of Cerebral Artery Stenosis) study. *J Neurol* 2009;256:750–757.

61. Cavalieri M, Schmidt R, Chen C, et al. B vitamins and MRI-detected ischemic brain lesions in patients with recent transient ischemic attack or stroke: the VITAmins TO Prevent Stroke (VITATOPS) MRI-substudy. *Stroke* 2012;43:3266–3270.

62. Van Dijk EJ, Prins ND, Vermeer SE, et al. C-reactive protein and cerebral small-vessel disease: the Rotterdam Scan Study. *Circulation* 2005;112:900–905.

63. Schmidt R, Schmidt H, Pichler M, et al. C-reactive protein, carotid atherosclerosis, and cerebral small-vessel disease: results of the Austrian Stroke Prevention Study. *Stroke* 2006;37:2910–2916.

64. Kase CS. Subcortical hemorrhages. In Donnan G, Norrving B, Bamford J, Bogousslavsky J, eds. *Subcortical Stroke*, 2nd edn. New York, NY: Oxford University Press; 2002: pp. 347–377.

65. Caplan LR. Hypertensive intracerebral hemorrhage. In Kase CS, Caplan LR, eds. *Intracerebral Hemorrhage*. Boston, MA: Butterworth–Heinemann; 1994: pp. 99–116.

66. Wolf PA. Epidemiology of intracerebral hemorrhage. In Kase CS, Caplan LR, eds. *Intracerebral Hemorrhage*. Boston, MA: Butterworth–Heinemann; 1994: pp. 21–30.

67. Grysiewicz R, Gorelick PB. Update on amyloid-associated intracerebral hemorrhage. *Eur Neurol Rev* 2012;7:22–24.

68. Gorelick PB. Statin use and intracerebral hemorrhage: evidence for safety in recurrent stroke prevention? *Arch Neurol* 2012;69:13–16.

69. Hackam DG, Woodward M, Newby LK, et al. Statins and intracerebral hemorrhage:

collaborative systematic review and meta-analysis. *Circulation* 2011;124:2233–2242.

70. Folsom AR, Yatsuya H, Mosley TH, Jr., Psaty BM, Longstreth WT, Jr. Risk of intraparenchymal hemorrhage with magnetic resonance imaging-defined leukoaraiosis and brain infarcts. *Ann Neurol* 2012;71:552–559.
71. Menon RS, Burgess RE, Wing JJ, et al. Predictors of highly prevalent brain ischemia in intracerebral hemorrhage. *Ann Neurol* 2012;71:199–205.
72. Weng YC, Sonni A, Labelle-Dumais C, et al. COL4A1 mutations in patients with sporadic late-onset intracerebral hemorrhage. *Ann Neurol* 2012;71:470–477.
73. Cole FM, Yates PO. Comparative incidence of cerebrovascular lesions in normotensive and hypertensive patients. *Neurology* 1968;18:255–259.
74. Offenbacher H, Fazekas F, Schmidt R, et al. MR of cerebral abnormalities concomitant with primary intracerebral hematomas. *AJNR Am J Neuroradiol* 1996;17:573–578.
75. Fazekas F, Kleinert R, Roob G, et al. Histopathologic analysis of foci of signal loss on gradient-echo T2*-weighted MR images in patients with spontaneous intracerebral hemorrhage: evidence of microangiopathy-related microbleeds. *AJNR Am J Neuroradiol* 1999;20:637–642.
76. Cordonnier C, Al-Shahi Salman R, Wardlaw J. Spontaneous brain microbleeds: systematic review, subgroup analyses and standards for study design and reporting. *Brain* 2007;130:1988–2003.
77. Poels MM, Vernooij MW, Ikram MA, et al. Prevalence and risk factors of cerebral microbleeds: an update of the Rotterdam Scan Study. *Stroke* 2010;41(Suppl 10): S103–S106.
78. Staals J, van Oostenbrugge RJ, Knottnerus IL, et al. Brain microbleeds relate to higher ambulatory blood pressure levels in first-ever lacunar stroke patients. *Stroke* 2009;40: 3264–3268.
79. Lee SH, Bae HJ, Yoon BW, et al. Low concentration of serum total cholesterol is associated with multifocal signal loss lesions on gradient-echo magnetic resonance imaging: analysis of risk factors for multifocal signal loss lesions. *Stroke* 2002;33: 2845–2849.
80. Wieberdink RG, Poels MM, Vernooij MW, et al. Serum lipid levels and the risk of intracerebral hemorrhage: the Rotterdam Study. *Arterioscler Thromb Vasc Biol* 2011;31:2982–2989.
81. Haussen DC, Henninger N, Kumar S, Selim M. Statin use and microbleeds in patients with spontaneous intracerebral hemorrhage. *Stroke* 2012;43:2677–2681.
82. Day JS, Policeni BA, Smoker WR, et al. Previous statin use is not associated with an increased prevalence or degree of gradient-echo lesions in patients with acute ischemic stroke or transient ischemic attack. *Stroke* 2011;42:354–358.
83. Ovbiagele B, Liebeskind DS, Pineda S, Saver JL. Strong independent correlation of proteinuria with cerebral microbleeds in patients with stroke and transient ischemic attack. *Arch Neurol* 2010;67: 45–50.
84. Maxwell SS, Jackson CA, Paternoster L, et al. Genetic associations with brain microbleeds: systematic review and meta-analyses. *Neurology* 2011;77:158–167.
85. Gregoire SM, Brown MM, Kallis C, et al. MRI detection of new microbleeds in patients with ischemic stroke: five-year cohort follow-up study. *Stroke* 2010;41:184–186.
86. Poels MM, Ikram MA, van der Lugt A, et al. Incidence of cerebral microbleeds in the general population: the Rotterdam Scan Study. *Stroke* 2011;42:656–661.
87. Goos JD, Henneman WJ, Sluimer JD, et al. Incidence of cerebral microbleeds: a longitudinal study in a memory clinic population. *Neurology* 2010;74:1954–1960.

Chapter 26

Treatment approaches for lacunar strokes

Makoto Nakajima, Thalia Field, and Oscar R. Benavente

Introduction

Although lacunar stroke is considered to have benign short-term functional outcomes, its long-term prognosis is less favorable. The heterogeneity of infarct mechanisms, racial/ethnic differences in incidence and recurrence rate, and risk of subsequent hemorrhagic stroke make it difficult to define the best management strategy for all patients with lacunar stroke, both in the acute and chronic phases. Lacunar stroke is the most common symptomatic manifestation of small vessel disease (SVD) [1]. It comprises between 15 and 34% of ischemic strokes and, after Alzheimer's disease, is the second most common cause of cognitive impairment and dementia [2, 3]. Blacks, Hispanics, and Asians have a higher incidence of lacunar stroke, as well as a higher risk of subsequent intracerebral hemorrhage (ICH) [4–9]. While any mechanism for brain ischemia (e.g., cardioembolism, large artery disease) may cause lacunar stroke [10–12], most are the result of intrinsic disease of small penetrating cerebral arteries [13–15].

The indication for intravenous thrombolytic therapy in the hyperacute phase and how to manage diseases such as atrial fibrillation or carotid stenosis in lacunar stroke patients are also controversial, particularly in those who demonstrate severe white matter hyperintensities (WMHs) and brain microbleeds. Furthermore, lacunar strokes and hypertensive ICH have similar mechanisms and risk factors. Therefore, the use of thrombolytics and antithrombotic agents in patients with SVD represents a therapeutic dilemma in balancing benefits and risks.

In addition, since most medical secondary prevention trials for ischemic stroke enrolled participants with heterogeneous stroke mechanisms, there is minimal evidence specific to the management of individuals with lacunar strokes. The Secondary Prevention of Small Subcortical Strokes (SPS3) study is the only randomized trial that included a homogeneous cohort of patients with recent lacunar strokes. SPS3's results provide guidance for prevention of stroke recurrence in this stroke subtype [16].

Rates of early recurrence and mortality may be lower for lacunar stroke than those of other stroke subtypes, but recurrence rates and mortality reach convergence with those of other stroke subtypes over a longer follow-up period [17, 18]. Risk of recurrent stroke one year after lacunar stroke ranges from 5 to 10% in hospital-based studies [4, 6, 7, 9, 17–38], 6–11% in community-based studies [1, 39–45], and annual recurrent stroke rate ranges from 3 to 10% in clinical trials [46–52]. Studies with a longer follow-up period have demonstrated that long-term recurrence and mortality rates for lacunar stroke patients are comparable to those of patients with other stroke subtypes [28, 29, 31, 44, 53–55], though one recent study with a 12-year follow-up reported a higher mortality rate in patients with small vessel occlusion than other stroke subtypes [38]. In addition, survivors of lacunar stroke may become disabled by other post-stroke complications, including cognitive impairment and dementia [2, 3, 56]. For these reasons, optimal secondary prevention in this stroke subtype is paramount.

Management of acute lacunar stroke

Thrombolysis in acute lacunar stroke

Intravenous tissue plasminogen activator (tPA) remains the gold standard for the treatment of acute ischemic stroke. Current guidelines do not distinguish between ischemic stroke subtypes with respect

Cerebral Small Vessel Disease, ed. Leonardo Pantoni and Philip B. Gorelick. Published by Cambridge University Press.

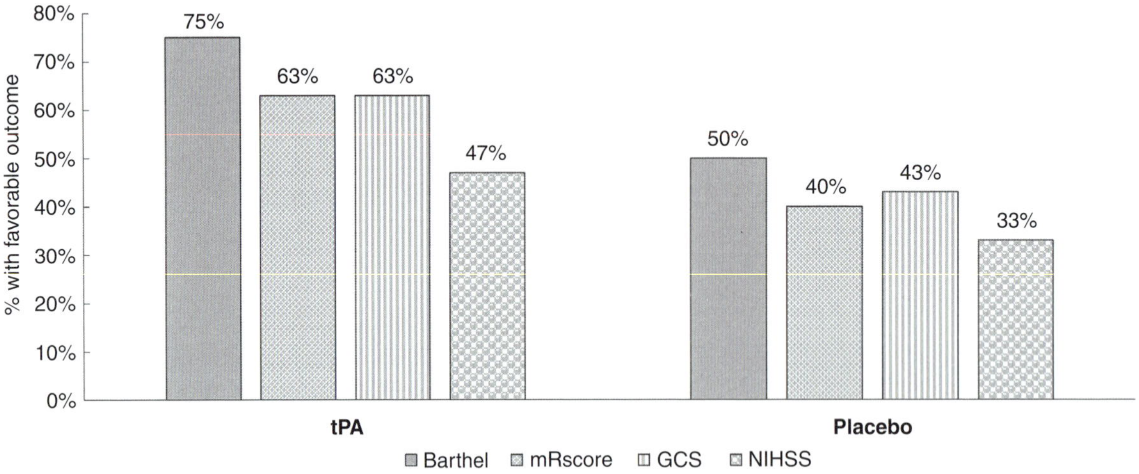

Figure 26.1 Outcome at three months in lacunar stroke patients: The National Institute of Neurological Disorders and Stroke (NINDS) trial (created from data from [58]). Barthel, Barthel Index; GCS, Glasgow Outcome Scale score; mRscore, modified Rankin Scale score; NIHSS, National Institute Health Stroke Scale.

to the use of intravenous tPA [57]. The National Institute of Neurological Disorders and Stroke (NINDS) study demonstrated that intravenous tPA was effective for all stroke subtypes, including lacunar stroke. Seventeen percent of participants had small vessel occlusive disease; 63% in the tPA group had a favorable outcome (vs. 40% in the placebo group) [58] (Figure 26.1). Subsequent studies with more strict diagnostic criteria for stroke subtypes that required clinical and imaging criteria also demonstrated similar effectiveness and safety of intravenous tPA in lacunar stroke patients [59–61]. In the Helsinki Stroke Registry, patients with SVD who received intravenous tPA (11%) had a better functional outcome than those who did not [62]. In addition, it is known that lacunar stroke patients not treated with intravenous tPA due to mild clinical symptoms do not necessarily have a favorable functional outcome [63, 64].

A relevant point with this stroke subgroup is the possibility of symptomatic ICH associated with thrombolysis, given the frequent coexistence of WMHs [65–67], multiplicity of brain infarcts [66], and brain microbleeds [68] in patients with lacunar stroke. However, at present, there are not sufficient validated data to preclude the use of thrombolytic therapy in lacunar stroke patients who display these other radiologic manifestations of SVD.

In summary, the overall benefit and safety of intravenous tPA in acute lacunar strokes is not very well defined. Moreover, a subgroup of lacunar stroke patients may be prone to a higher than normal risk of intracerebral bleeding from thrombolysis due to the presence of WMHs and/or microbleeds [69]. At this time eligible patients with acute lacunar strokes should be treated with intravenous tPA according to current recommendations [57].

Clinical fluctuation: "the capsular warning syndrome"

In the acute phase of lacunar stroke, approximately 20–30% of patients experience worsening or fluctuation of their initial neurologic deficit (e.g., the so-called "capsular warning syndrome"). Postulated mechanisms include progressively occlusive branch atheromatous disease, altered hemodynamics, peri-infarct edema, excitotoxicity, or inflammation [70–72].

Presently, there are no proven therapies to prevent clinical fluctuations or halt neurologic deterioration. Antiplatelet medications are the mainstay antithrombotic therapy for noncardioembolic stroke and some studies suggest that early use of antiplatelet agents may prevent clinical worsening after lacunar infarcts [73]. The effectiveness of the other treatment options for symptom stabilization in both the acute and subacute phase, including anticoagulant therapy, intravenous tPA, or blood pressure management, still needs confirmation and they are not standard care [70].

Antiplatelet agents during the acute phase

For patients not eligible for treatment with thrombolytics, the use of antiplatelet agents to prevent early recurrent strokes is a valid alternative. Data from trials that tested the combination of aspirin and clopidogrel raised the possibility that a short-term course of dual antiplatelet therapy may reduce recurrent ischemic events in the immediate phase following stroke or transient ischemic attack (TIA) [48, 74]. The recent published Clopidogrel with Aspirin in Acute Minor Stroke or Transient Ischemic Attack (CHANCE) trial in China enrolled 5170 minor ischemic stroke and TIA patients within the first 24 hours of symptom onset. Participants were allocated to aspirin and clopidogrel (initial dose 30 mg of clopidogrel and then 75 mg daily for 90 days plus aspirin 75 mg daily for the first 21 days) or to placebo plus aspirin daily (75 mg day). Stroke recurrence was reduced significantly at 90 days by 32%; 8.2% in combination groups vs. 11.7% in the aspirin group (hazard ratio [HR], 0.68; 95% confidence interval [CI] 0.57–0.81; $P<0.001$). There were nonsignificant differences between groups in systemic hemorrhages and intracranial bleed [75]. Though the trial included exclusively Asian participants and did not specify stroke subtype at entry or report outcomes based on stroke mechanism, it is possible that short-term (30 days) combination therapy (aspirin plus clopidogrel) may be an option for acute lacunar stroke. Currently, the Platelet-Oriented Inhibition in New TIA and Minor Ischemic Stroke (POINT) trial (NCT00991029) is testing a similar therapeutic strategy and may provide further insight into immediate management of lacunar stroke patients.

Secondary prevention of lacunar stroke

Antiplatelet agents for secondary stroke prevention

Despite the fact that most lacunar strokes are due to disease of the small cerebral penetrating arteries and not to thrombus related to atheroma [76], it is likely that the process leading to occlusion of a small vessel may also involve platelet aggregation and thrombus formation; however, this was seldom demonstrated in pathologic studies [77]. Consequently, it is assumed that antithrombotic agents are likely to be beneficial in preventing stroke recurrence and cognitive impairment in lacunar stroke patients. The benefit of antiplatelet therapy in lacunar stroke patients for secondary prevention is also supported by existing evidence from randomized controlled trials. From 1983 to 2012, 11 secondary stroke prevention randomized trials investigating different antithrombotic agents have classified the index event by stroke mechanism. Of 81 626 noncardioembolic qualifying strokes, 28 244 (35%) were categorized as lacunar events (Table 26.1; [46, 48, 50, 51, 78–84]). Though these studies are limited by the absence of a rigorous classification of stroke subtype and the lack of statistical power to detect benefit specific to lacunar strokes [46, 48, 50, 51, 78–84], overall results show that antiplatelet therapy (aspirin, cilostazol, or ticlopidine) is superior to placebo in preventing recurrent stroke in lacunar patients [78–81] (Figure 26.2). When the response to specific antithrombotic agents was compared between lacunar and large vessel subtypes, no specific benefit was found selectively for one mechanism over the other [48, 50, 82–85 (Figures 26.3 and 26.4).

The SPS3 was the first secondary stroke prevention trial designed specifically to assess therapeutic interventions in patients with symptomatic lacunar infarcts. The study enrolled 3020 participants between 2003 and 2011 from 81 cities in North America, Latin America, and Spain. Eligible participants had symptomatic lacunar infarcts verified by magnetic resonance imaging (MRI) without surgically amenable carotid stenosis or major cardioembolic disease. Patients with prior cortical or hemorrhagic stroke were not included. In a two-by-two factorial design, participants were randomized to two interventions: (a) antiplatelet intervention (aspirin 325 mg vs. aspirin 325 mg + clopidogrel 75 mg) and (b) two target levels of systolic blood pressure control ("higher" 130–149 mmHg vs. "lower" <130 mmHg). The antiplatelet arm was double-blinded while the blood pressure target was open label (PROBE design) [16]. The rationale to test aspirin plus clopidogrel was based upon their complementary mechanism of action to inhibit platelet aggregation. In vitro studies showed that combination of clopidogrel and aspirin was highly effective in reducing thrombus weight and decreasing platelet and fibrin deposition [86, 87]. In addition, results of the Clopidogrel in Unstable Angina to Prevent Recurrent Events (CURE) trial provided compelling evidence for the increased antithrombotic effects of the combination of clopidogrel plus aspirin in prevention of vascular events [88].

Table 26.1 Secondary stroke prevention trials with lacunar strokes identified as index event and outcomes reported by stroke subtype. Trials listed in chronological order

Study*	Year	Sample size	Lacunar strokes (%)	Intervention†
AICLA [78]	1983	604	98 (16)	ASA vs. ASA + DIP vs. Plac.
CATS [79]	1989	1072	275 (30)	Ticlop. vs. Plac.
CAST [80]	1997	20 655	6102 (30)	ASA vs. Plac.
CSPS1 [81]	1999	1095	810 (74)	Cilost. vs. Plac.
WARSS [46]	2001	2206	1237 (56)	ASA vs. warfarin
AAASPS [82]	2003	1809	1221 (67)	ASA vs. Ticlop.
MATCH [48]	2004	7599	3148 (52)	Clop vs. Clop + ASA
ESPRIT [83]	2006	2739	1377 (50)	ASA vs. ASA + Clop
PRoFESS [50]	2008	22 000	10 500 (50)	ASA + DIP vs. Clop
CSPS2 [51]	2010	2757	1743 (63)	Cilost vs. ASA
PERFORM [84]	2011	19 100	1733 (10)	Terutobran vs. ASA
Aggregate		**81 626**	**28 244 (35)**	

* AAASPS, African American Antiplatelet Stroke Prevention Study; AICLA, *Accidents Ischémiques Cérebraux Liés à l'Athéroscléros* [aspirin and dipyridamole in the secondary prevention of atherothrombotic cerebral ischemia]; CATS, Canadian–American Ticlopidine Study; CAST, Chinese Acute Stroke Trial; CSPS1, Cilostazol Stroke Prevention Study; CSPS2 Cilostazol Stroke Prevention Study 2; ESPRIT, European/Australasian Stroke Prevention in Reversible Ischemia Trial; MATCH, Management of Atherothrombosis with Clopidogrel in High-Risk Patients with Recent Transient Ischemic Attacks or Ischemic Stroke; PERFORM, Prevention of Cerebrovascular and Cardiovascular Events of Ischemic Origin with Terutroban in Patients with a History of Ischemic Stroke or Transient Ischemic Attack; PRoFESS, Prevention Regimen for Effectively Avoiding Second Strokes; WARSS Warfarin–Aspirin Recurrent Stroke Study.

† ASA, aspirin; Clop, clopidogrel; DIP, dipyridamole; Plac., placebo; Ticlop., ticlopidine.

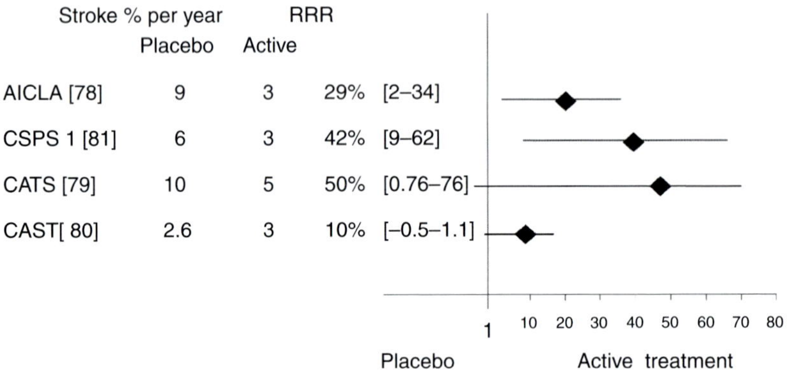

Figure 26.2 Randomized trials with lacunar stroke as index event and reported outcomes by stroke subtype (created using data from [78–81]). AICLA, *Accidents Ischémiques Cérebraux Liés à l'Athéroscléros* [aspirin and dipyridamole in the secondary prevention of atherothrombotic cerebral ischemia] trial [78]; CATS, Canadian–American Ticlopidine Study [79]; CAST, Chinese Acute Stroke Trial [80]; CSPS, Cilostazol Stroke Prevention Study [81]; RRR, relative risk reduction.

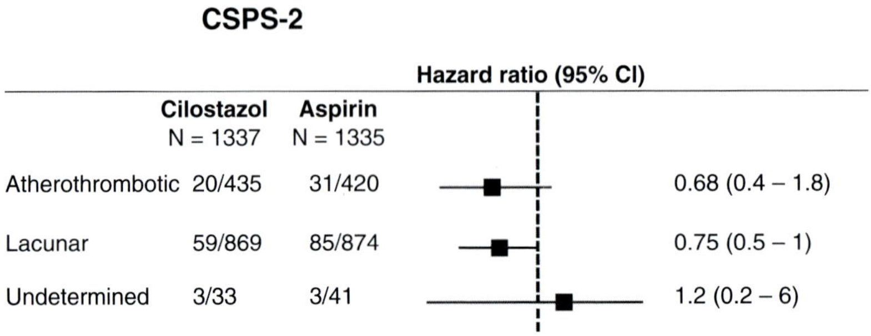

Figure 26.3 Outcomes in Cilostazol for Prevention of Secondary Stroke (CSPS2) trial by stroke subtype (modified from [51]). CI, clearance interval.

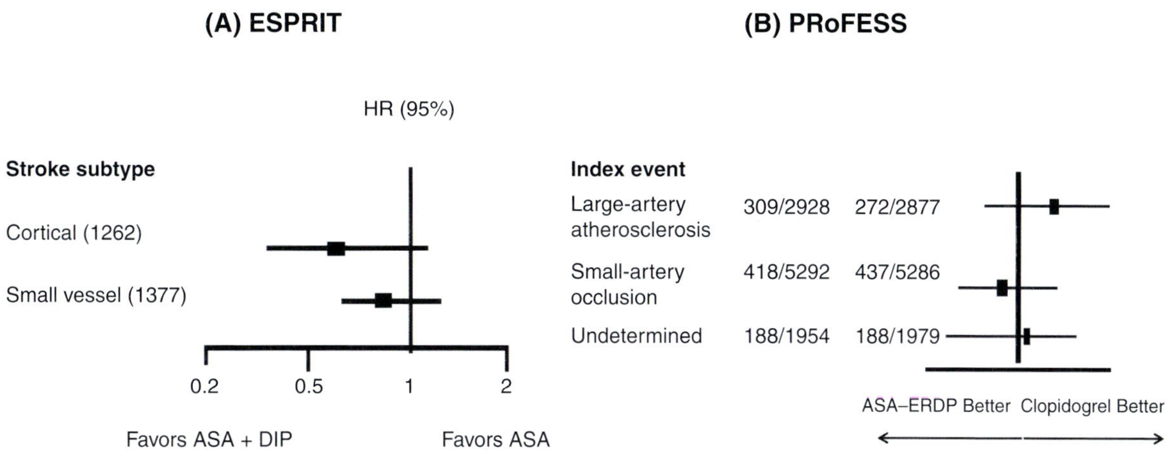

Figure 26.4 (A) European/Australasian Stroke Prevention in Reversible Ischemia Trial (ESPRIT) primary outcome by stroke subtype (modified from [83]). (B) Prevention Regiment for Effectively Avoiding Second Strokes (PRoFESS) outcomes according type of index event (modified from [50]). ASA, aspirin; DIP, dipyridamole; ERDP, extended release dipyridamole.

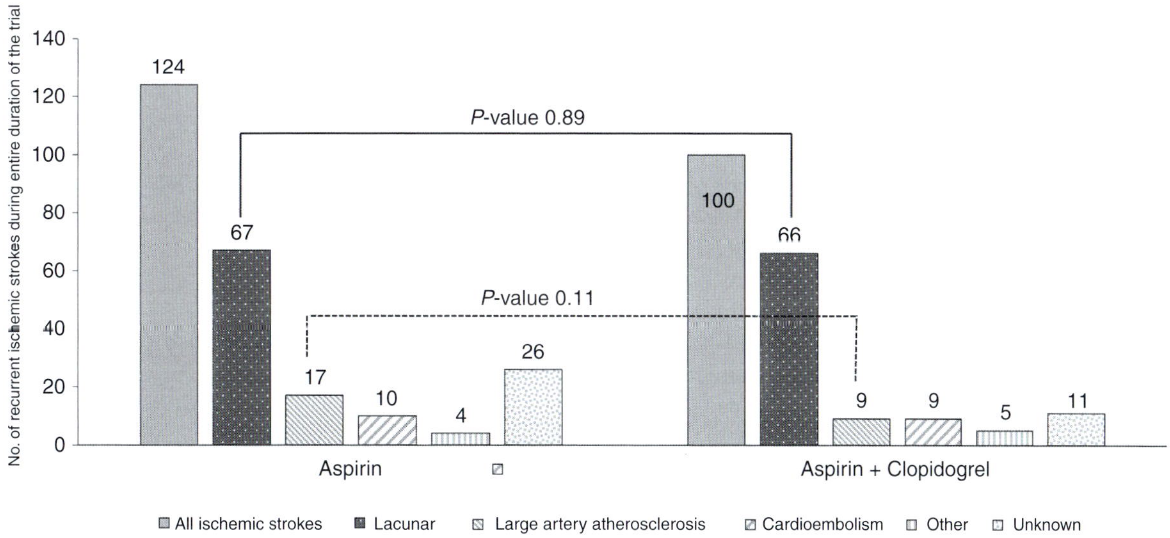

Figure 26.5 Etiological subtypes of recurrent ischemic stroke by treatment allocation: The Secondary Prevention of Small Subcortical Strokes (SPS3) trial (created from data from [52]).

The statistical power in SPS3 was calculated based on an annual recurrent event rate of 6% observed in the Warfarin–Aspirin Recurrent Stroke Study (WARSS) trial [46]. The antiplatelet component of the trial was stopped prematurely due to lack of benefit and excess mortality for those assigned to combination therapy. After a mean follow-up of 3.7 years the annualized rate for recurrent stroke was 2.5% in those on dual therapy versus 2.7% in those assigned to aspirin (HR 0.92, 95% CI 0.72–1.16). There was no effect on ischemic strokes alone or disabling stroke. Major hemorrhage was doubled in the combination group (2.7% per year) as compared with aspirin (1.1% per year, $P < 0.001$). More than two thirds of recurrent ischemic strokes were lacunar type (Figure 26.5). Mortality (all causes) was significantly increased in those assigned to dual antiplatelet therapy (HR 1.52; 95% CI 1.14–2.04, $P = 0.004$) [52]. Given the findings of SPS3, patients with lacunar stroke should not be treated with long-term combination aspirin and clopidogrel therapy.

The existing evidence from secondary prevention trials supports the use of antiplatelet therapy for secondary prevention in lacunar stroke. There is no consensus, evidence-based or otherwise, with regards to whether one antiplatelet agent is superior to another in the context of lacunar stroke. Aspirin, in doses between 75 and 325 mg per day, aspirin 25 mg plus extended-release dipyridamole 200 mg twice daily, or clopidogrel 75 mg daily are all acceptable options [89]. There is no evidence to support the use of oral anticoagulants in patients with lacunar stroke who do not also have a major-risk cardioembolic source.

Lipid-lowering therapy

Observational studies have shown a modest association between elevated total cholesterol and low-density lipoprotein cholesterol (LDL-C) with increased risk of ischemic stroke [90, 91]. However, these studies do not distinguish between ischemic stroke mechanisms. It is believed that the association and response to therapy will be stronger in patients with atherosclerotic stroke mechanisms [49, 92]. A meta-analysis of statin trials for primary and secondary vascular events found a 21% relative risk reduction (RRR) (95% CI, 6.3–33.5) in stroke for every 1.0 mmol/l reduction in LDL-C [93].

The Stroke Prevention by Aggressive Reduction in Cholesterol Levels (SPARCL) trial randomized 4731 stroke and TIA patients without manifest ischemic heart disease to atorvastatin 80 mg daily or placebo. Patients allocated to atorvastatin had a significant reduction in fatal and nonfatal stroke (HR 0.84, 95% CI 0.71–0.99) and in coronary events (HR 0.58, 95% CI 0.46–9.73). There was an increase in risk of hemorrhagic stroke (HR 5.65, 95% CI 2.82–11.30); risk factors for hemorrhage were male sex, increased age, and stage 2 hypertension. Among 4371 participants (67% ischemic stroke, 31% TIA, and 2% hemorrhagic stroke), 1409 were classified as having a lacunar index event. In a post-hoc analysis, there was no evidence that one stroke subtype benefited selectively from statin therapy with regards to reduction of stroke or other major vascular events [94]. Similarly, there was no evidence that patients with lacunar strokes faced a selectively higher rate of ICH when treated with atorvastatin [95] (Figure 26.6).

Lacunar stroke patients with evidence of atherosclerosis and LDL-C level $\geq$100 mg/dl and without ischemic heart disease should be treated with a statin with intensive lipid-lowering effects (e.g., atorvastatin 80 mg daily). For patients with LDL-C level $\geq$100 mg/dL who have no manifestations of atherosclerosis, simvastatin 40 mg daily is a valid alternative [89, 92]. Until further studies examine the association between lacunar infarcts and hyperlipidemia and response to statins, patients should be treated following the current recommendations [89].

Blood pressure reduction after lacunar stroke

Hypertension is the most prevalent and powerful modifiable risk factor for small vessel stroke and stroke in general, with an attributable risk between 35 and 50% [96]. Reduction of blood pressure has consistently been shown to reduce stroke occurrence in multiple primary prevention studies. Lowering systolic blood pressure by 10 mmHg is associated with a 40% reduction in stroke [97–99]. Similar benefits of blood pressure reduction are seen in secondary prevention trials. Pooled analyses of secondary prevention studies in patients with stroke and TIA patients showed that long-term blood pressure reduction reduces stroke by about 28% [100–102]. The Perindopril Protection aGainst Recurrent Stroke Study (PROGRESS) trial, which enrolled nearly 6000 patients with stroke and TIA, demonstrated that a mean reduction of 9 mmHg in systolic blood pressure resulted in a 28% risk reduction in stroke (achieved systolic pressure in the active group was 138 mmHg). Though the findings in this trial demonstrated the principle that "lower is better," an optimal blood pressure target for secondary stroke prevention was not defined.

The SPS3 trial tested two systolic blood pressure targets in 3020 patients with symptomatic lacunar infarcts: "higher", 130–149 mmHg, versus "lower", less than 130 mmHg [16]. Between March 2003 and April 2011, 1519 patients were allocated to the higher target group and 1501 to the lower group. After a mean follow-up of 3.7 years, a 19% nonsignificant reduction in all recurrent stroke was seen in those assigned to the lower group (HR 0.81, 95% CI 0.64–1.03). However, ICH was reduced significantly by 63% (HR 0.37, CI% 0.15–0.95, $P = 0.03$) (Figure 26.7). Serious side effects of blood pressure therapy were infrequent (3%) and did not differ between the two target groups. The blood pressure arm of the trial used a PROBE design and investigators were able to use any

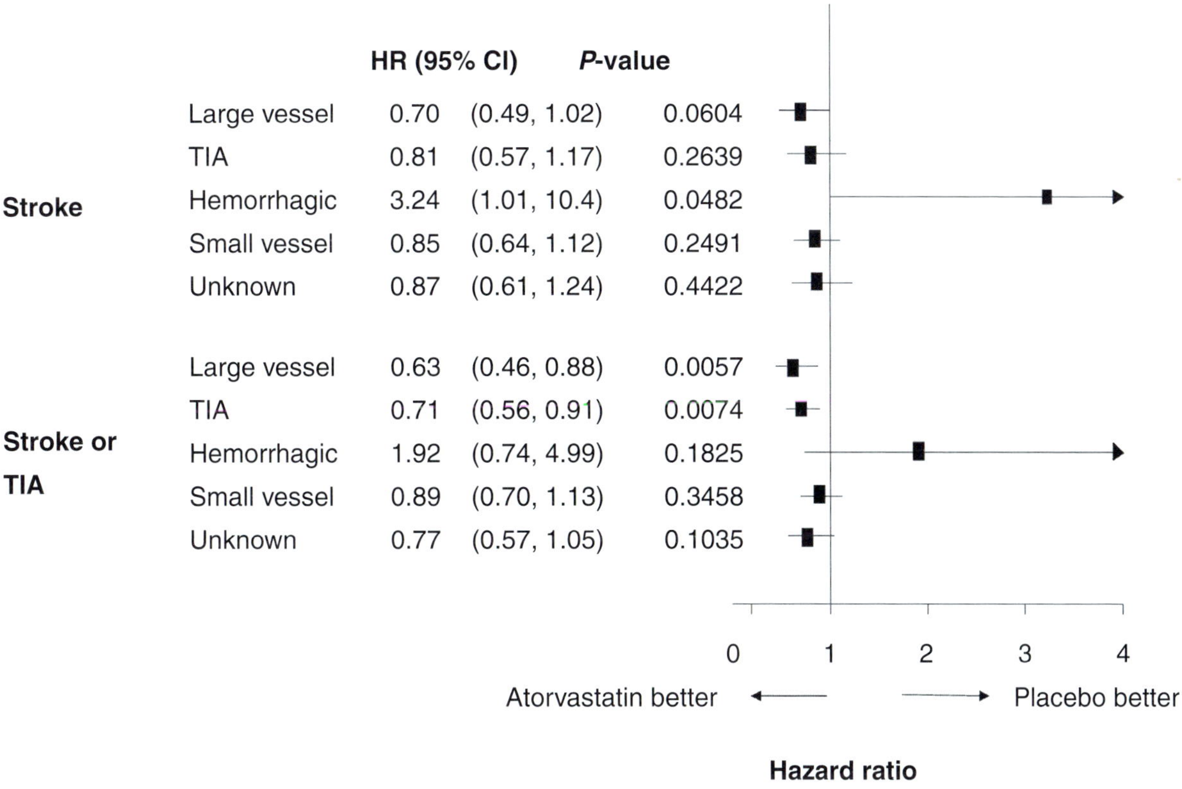

Figure 26.6 Risk of recurrent stroke and transient ischemic attack by index event in the Stroke Prevention by Aggressive Reduction in Cholesterol Levels (SPARCL) trial (created from data from [94]). CI, confidence interval; HR, hazard ratio; TIA, transitory ischemic attack.

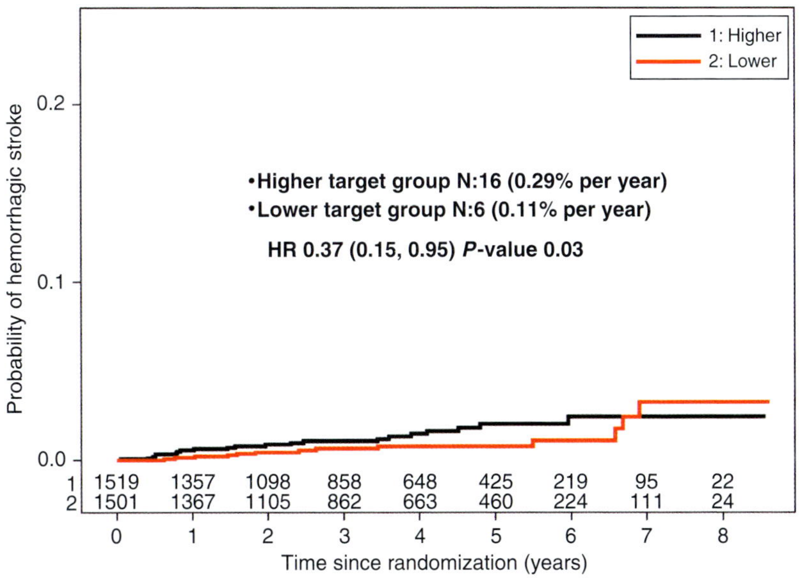

Figure 26.7 Caplan–Meier survival curve for intracerebral hemorrhage by blood pressure target group assignment: the Secondary Prevention of Small Subcortical Strokes (SPS3) trial. HR, hazard ratio.

antihypertensive agents or combination of agents to meet assigned targets.

The results of SPS3 demonstrate a significant benefit for reduction of hemorrhagic stroke and a trend towards reduction of all recurrent stroke in lacunar stroke patients. Though the overall results did not reach statistical significance, in the context of previous trials demonstrating a benefit for stroke reduction with blood pressure treatment, the significant reduction of ICH in the lower-target group, and the low rate of major side effects of blood pressure lowering in both blood pressure groups, it is appropriate to target blood pressure reduction to a systolic pressure of 130 mmHg in patients with lacunar stroke [103]. There is no current evidence to support the preferential use of one particular antihypertensive agent or combination of agents in lacunar stroke.

Other possible mechanisms for lacunar stroke and treatment considerations

Any etiology of brain ischemia (e.g., atherothrombosis, cardioembolism) may cause a lacunar infarct [33, 54, 104, 105]. However, most lacunar infarcts result from disease of small penetrating arteries [10, 13, 14, 77]. Consequently, it is challenging to manage patients with lacunar strokes who have other potential etiologies when it is unclear if the association is simply coincidental or not.

Atrial fibrillation and lacunar stroke

Atrial fibrillation patients at risk of stroke should be treated based on their risk stratification score. The $CHADS_2$ and $CHADS_2$-$VASC_2$ scores have been validated and are the most accepted stratification schemes [106] with warfarin or with an approved novel oral anticoagulant (dabigatran, apixaban, or rivaroxaban). A history of stroke immediately places the patient at moderate risk ($CHADS_2 = 2$), and most guidelines indicate that patients with a $CHADS_2$ score of two or greater should be anticoagulated. The "history of stroke/TIA" in the stratification scores is not specific with regards to stroke subtype and does not require verification of the infarct on neuroimaging. Therefore, most patients with symptomatic lacunar infarcts with atrial fibrillation should be placed on an oral anticoagulant for recurrent stroke prevention [89]. The current state of knowledge does not preclude the use of oral anticoagulation in patients with WMHs, brain microbleeds, or leukoaraiosis on neuroimaging, though further research is needed with respect to whether these features may increase the risk of intracranial bleeding with oral anticoagulation.

Carotid stenosis and lacunar stroke

Symptomatic carotid stenosis may occasionally be responsible for lacunar strokes as ipsilateral carotid stenosis is present in 3–39% of lacunar stroke patients [107]. Since many studies have failed to demonstrate a causal relationship between carotid disease and lacunar stroke, some authors consider that they might be coincidental comorbidities [107, 108].

Among 1158 participants in the North American Symptomatic Carotid Endarterectomy Trial (NASCET), 493 (42.6%) had clinicoradiologic features of lacunar stroke. Patients with "probable" lacunar stroke in the medical treatment group had a higher rate of ipsilateral lacunar stroke (9.2% in 3 years) than those with nonlacunar (2.9%) or those with "possible" lacunar stroke (4.2%) during a follow-up period of three years. Among patients with nonlacunar stroke with $\geq$50% carotid stenosis, the absolute risk reduction by carotid endarterectomy (CEA) was 15.2% at three years, while amongst patients with a "probable" lacunar event, absolute risk reduction of CEA was 9% [109]. Though lacunar stroke patients with ipsilateral carotid stenosis may have a less robust benefit of CEA than an equivalent patient with a nonlacunar event, CEA was still shown to reduce stroke recurrence in lacunar patients [110]. Therefore, patients with lacunar infarcts who have ipsilateral carotid stenosis greater than 70% should be considered for carotid intervention.

Summary

Lacunar stroke is associated with long-term functional and cognitive impairment. Thus, prevention of recurrent events is paramount. Existing evidence supports the use of intravenous tPA for qualifying acute lacunar strokes. Though the majority of secondary stroke prevention studies to date did not distinguish by stroke mechanism or did so in an ad-hoc fashion that did not include neuroradiologic verification, lacunar stroke patients form a significant minority of patients in these trials, and there is good evidence that antiplatelet therapy, blood pressure reduction, and statin therapy are beneficial for secondary prevention of ischemic stroke, including lacunar stroke. The SPS3 trial, which specifically examined interventions in patients with symptomatic lacunar stroke, found that long-term combination aspirin–clopidogrel therapy is harmful in these patients, while an aggressive systolic blood pressure target of less than 130 mmHg, which is safe and well-tolerated in lacunar stroke patients, significantly reduces the risk of ICH and may reduce the risk of all recurrent stroke in this patient group. Those patients with lacunar stroke who also have comorbid atrial fibrillation or ipsilateral moderate or severe carotid stenosis should be treated accordingly with oral anticoagulation and endarterectomy/stenting, respectively. Though other neuroradiologic manifestations of SVD in lacunar stroke patients, including WMHs, microbleeds, or multiple lacunes, may possibly raise the risk of intracranial bleeding, there is no consistent evidence to recommend against the use of intravenous tPA, antiplatelet therapy, statin medication, or, when indicated with comorbid atrial fibrillation, oral anticoagulation. Further studies are needed to quantify the risk associated with these particular neuroradiologic features in cerebral SVD.

References

1. Petty GW, Brown RD, Jr., Whisnant JP, et al. Ischemic stroke subtypes: a population-based study of functional outcome, survival, and recurrence. *Stroke* 2000;31:1062–1068.
2. O'Brien JT, Erkinjuntti T, Reisberg B, et al. Vascular cognitive impairment. *Lancet Neurol* 2003;2:89–98.
3. Pendlebury ST, Rothwell PM. Prevalence, incidence, and factors associated with pre-stroke and post-stroke dementia. a systematic review and meta-analysis. *Lancet Neurol* 2009;8:1006–1018.
4. Mok VC, Lau AY, Wong A, et al. Long-term prognosis of Chinese patients with a lacunar infarct associated with small vessel disease: a five-year longitudinal study. *Int J Stroke* 2009;4:81–88.
5. Sacco RL, Kargman DE, Zamanillo MC. Race–ethnic differences in stroke risk factors among hospitalized patients with cerebral infarction: the Northern Manhattan Stroke Study. *Neurology* 1995;45:659–663.
6. Samanci N, Dora B, Kizilay F, et al. Factors affecting one year mortality and functional outcome after first ever ischemic stroke in the region of Antalya, Turkey (a hospital-based study). *Acta Neurol Belg* 2004;104:154–160.
7. Soda T, Nakayasu H, Maeda M, et al. Stroke recurrence within the first year following cerebral infarction – Tottori University Lacunar Infarction Prognosis Study (TULIPS). *Acta Neurol Scand* 2004;110:343–349.
8. Worley KL, Lalonde DR, Kerr DR, Benavente O, Hart RG. Survey of the causes of stroke among Mexican Americans in South Texas. *Tex Med* 1998;94:62–67.
9. Yokota C, Minematsu K, Hasegawa Y, Yamaguchi T. Long-term prognosis, by stroke subtypes, after a first-ever stroke: a hospital-based study over a 20-year period. *Cerebrovasc Dis* 2004;18:111–116.
10. Fisher CM. Lacunar strokes and infarcts: a review. *Neurology* 1982;32:871–876.
11. Lammie GA. Hypertensive cerebral small vessel disease and stroke. *Brain Pathol* 2002;12: 358–370.
12. Feekes JA, Hsu SW, Chaloupka JC, Cassell MD. Tertiary microvascular territories define lacunar infarcts in the basal ganglia. *Ann Neurol* 2005;58: 18–30.
13. Fisher CM. Lacunes: small, deep cerebral infarcts. *Neurology* 1965;15:774–784.
14. Fisher CM. The arterial lesions underlying lacunes. *Acta Neuropathol* 1968;12:1–15.
15. Pantoni L. Cerebral small vessel disease: from pathogenesis and clinical characteristics to therapeutic challenges. *Lancet Neurol* 2010;9:689–701.
16. Benavente OR, White CL, Pearce L, et al. The Secondary Prevention of Small Subcortical Strokes (SPS3) study. *Int J Stroke* 2011;6:164–175.
17. Clavier I, Hommel M, Besson G, Noelle B, Perret JE. Long-term prognosis of symptomatic lacunar infarcts. A hospital-based study. *Stroke* 1994;25:2005–2009.
18. Nadeau SE, Jordan JE, Mishra SK, Haerer AF. Stroke rates in patients with lacunar and large vessel cerebral infarctions. *J Neurol Sci* 1993;114:128–137.
19. Gandolfo C, Moretti C, Dall'Agata D, et al. Long-term prognosis of patients with lacunar syndromes. *Acta Neurol Scand* 1986;74: 224–229.
20. Hier DB, Foulkes MA, Swiontoniowski M, et al. Stroke recurrence within two years after ischemic infarction. *Stroke* 1991;22:155–161.
21. Miyao S, Takano A, Teramoto J, Takahashi A. Leukoaraiosis in relation to prognosis for patients with lacunar infarction. *Stroke* 1992;23:1434–1438.
22. Landi G, Cella E, Boccardi E, Musicco M. Lacunar versus non-lacunar infarcts: pathogenetic and prognostic differences. *J Neurol Neurosurg Psych* 1992;55:441–445.
23. Brainin M, Seiser A, Czvitkovits B, Pauly E. Stroke subtype is

an age-independent predictor of first-year survival. *Neuroepidemiology* 1992;11: 190–195.

24. Boiten J, Lodder J. Prognosis for survival, handicap and recurrence of stroke in lacunar and superficial infarction. *Cerebrovasc Dis* 1993;3:221–226.
25. Samuelsson M, Lindell D, Norrving B. Presumed pathogenetic mechanisms of recurrent stroke after lacunar infarction. *Cerebrovasc Dis* 1996;6:128–136.
26. Salgado AV, Ferro JM, Gouveia-Oliveira A. Long-term prognosis of first-ever lacunar strokes. A hospital-based study. *Stroke* 1996;27:661–666.
27. Yamamoto Y, Akiguchi I, Oiwa K, Hayashi M, Kimura J. Adverse effect of nighttime blood pressure on the outcome of lacunar infarct patients. *Stroke* 1998;29:570–576.
28. Staaf G, Lindgren A, Norrving B. Pure motor stroke from presumed lacunar infarct: long-term prognosis for survival and risk of recurrent stroke. *Stroke* 2001;32:2592–2596.
29. Eriksson SE, Olsson JE. Survival and recurrent strokes in patients with different subtypes of stroke: a 14-year follow-up study. *Cerebrovasc Dis* 2001;12:171–180.
30. Kazui S, Levi CR, Jones EF, et al. Lacunar stroke: transoesophageal echocardiographic factors influencing long-term prognosis. *Cerebrovasc Dis* 2001;12:325–330.
31. Yamamoto Y, Akiguchi I, Oiwa K, et al. Twenty-four-hour blood pressure and MRI as predictive factors for different outcomes in patients with lacunar infarct. *Stroke* 2002;33:297–305.
32. De Jong G, van Raak L, Kessels F, Lodder J. Stroke subtype and mortality. A follow-up study in 998 patients with a first cerebral infarct. *J Clin Epidemiol* 2003;56:262–268.
33. Jackson CA, Hutchison A, Dennis MS, et al. Differences between ischemic stroke subtypes in vascular outcomes support a distinct lacunar ischemic stroke arteriopathy: a prospective, hospital-based study. *Stroke* 2009;40:3679–3684.
34. Suto Y, Kowa H, Nakayasu H, et al. Relationship between three-year survival and functional outcome at discharge from acute-care hospitals in each subtype of first-ever ischemic stroke patients. *Intern Med* 2011;50:1377–1383.
35. Stead LG, Gilmore RM, Bellolio MF, et al. Cardioembolic but not other stroke subtypes predict mortality independent of stroke severity at presentation. *Stroke Res Treat* 2011;2011:281496.
36. Kwan MW, Mak W, Cheung RT, Ho SL. Ischemic stroke related to intracranial branch atheromatous disease and comparison with large and small artery diseases. *J Neurological Sci* 2011;303: 80–84.
37. Ntaios G, Michel P. Temporal distribution and magnitude of the vulnerability period around stroke depend on stroke subtype. *Cerebrovasc Dis* 2011;32:246–253.
38. Melkas S, Putaala J, Oksala NK, et al. Small-vessel disease relates to poor poststroke survival in a 12-year follow-up. *Neurology* 2011;76:734–739.
39. Bamford J, Sandercock P, Jones L, Warlow C. The natural history of lacunar infarction: the Oxfordshire Community Stroke Project. *Stroke* 1987;18:545–551.
40. Sacco SE, Whisnant JP, Broderick JP, Phillips SJ, O'Fallon WM. Epidemiological characteristics of lacunar infarcts in a population. *Stroke* 1991;22:1236–1241.
41. Sacco RL, Shi T, Zamanillo MC, Kargman DE. Predictors of mortality and recurrence after hospitalized cerebral infarction in an urban community: the Northern Manhattan Stroke Study. *Neurology* 1994;44: 626–634.
42. Anderson CS, Jamrozik KD, Broadhurst RJ, Stewart-Wynne EG. Predicting survival for one year among different subtypes of stroke. Results from the Perth Community Stroke Study. *Stroke* 1994;25:1935–1944.
43. Kolominsky-Rabas PL, Weber M, Gefeller O, Neundoerfer B, Heuschmann PU. Epidemiology of ischemic stroke subtypes according to TOAST criteria: incidence, recurrence, and long-term survival in ischemic stroke subtypes: a population-based study. *Stroke* 2001;32:2735–2740.
44. Hata J, Tanizaki Y, Kiyohara Y, et al. Ten year recurrence after first ever stroke in a Japanese community: the Hisayama study. *J Neurol Neurosurg Psych* 2005;76:368–372.
45. Bejot Y, Catteau A, Caillier M, et al. Trends in incidence, risk factors, and survival in symptomatic lacunar stroke in Dijon, France, from 1989 to 2006: a population-based study. *Stroke* 2008;39:1945–1951.
46. Mohr JP, Thompson JL, Lazar RM, et al. A comparison of warfarin and aspirin for the prevention of recurrent ischemic stroke. *New Engl J Med* 2001;345:1444–1451.
47. Sacco RL, Prabhakaran S, Thompson JL, et al. Comparison of warfarin versus aspirin for the prevention of recurrent stroke or death: subgroup analyses from the Warfarin–Aspirin Recurrent Stroke study. *Cerebrovasc Dis* 2006;22:4–12.
48. Diener HC, Bogousslavsky J, Brass LM, et al. Aspirin and clopidogrel compared with clopidogrel alone after recent ischaemic stroke or transient ischaemic attack in high-risk patients (MATCH): randomised, double-blind, placebo-controlled trial. *Lancet* 2004;364:331–337.

49. Amarenco P, Bogousslavsky J, Callahan A, 3rd, et al. High-dose atorvastatin after stroke or transient ischemic attack. *New Engl J Med* 2006;355:549–559.

50. Sacco RL, Diener HC, Yusuf S, et al. Aspirin and extended-release dipyridamole versus clopidogrel for recurrent stroke. *New Engl J Med* 2008;359: 1238–1251.

51. Shinohara Y, Katayama Y, Uchiyama S, et al. Cilostazol for Prevention of Secondary Stroke (CSPS2): an aspirin-controlled, double-blind, randomised non-inferiority trial. *Lancet Neurol* 2010;9:959–968.

52. Benavente OR, Hart RG, McClure LA, et al. Effects of clopidogrel added to aspirin in patients with recent lacunar stroke. *New Engl J Med* 2012;367:817–825.

53. Norrving B. Long-term prognosis after lacunar infarction. *Lancet Neurol* 2003;2:238–245.

54. Jackson C, Sudlow C. Comparing risks of death and recurrent vascular events between lacunar and non-lacunar infarction. *Brain* 2005;128(Pt 11):2507–2517.

55. Norrving B. Lacunar infarcts: no black holes in the brain are benign. *Pract Neurol* 2008;8: 222–228.

56. Jacova C, Pearce LA, Costello R, et al. Cognitive impairment in lacunar strokes: the SPS3 trial. *Ann Neurol* 2012;72:351–362.

57. Jauch EC, Saver JL, Adams HP, Jr., et al. Guidelines for the early management of patients with acute ischemic stroke: a guideline for healthcare professionals from the American Heart Association/ American Stroke Association. *Stroke* 2013;44:870–947.

58. National Institute of Neurological Disorders and Stroke rt-PA Stroke Study Group. Tissue plasminogen activator for acute ischemic stroke. *New Engl J Med* 1995;333:1581–1587.

59. Hsia AW, Sachdev HS, Tomlinson J, Hamilton SA, Tong DC. Efficacy of IV tissue plasminogen activator in acute stroke: does stroke subtype really matter? *Neurology* 2003;61:71–75.

60. Cocho D, Belvis R, Marti-Fabregas J, et al. Does thrombolysis benefit patients with lacunar syndrome? *Eur Neurol* 2006;55:70–73.

61. Fluri F, Hatz F, Rutgers MP, et al. Intravenous thrombolysis in patients with stroke attributable to small artery occlusion. *Eur J Neurol* 2010;17:1054–1060.

62. Mustanoja S, Meretoja A, Putaala J, et al. Outcome by stroke etiology in patients receiving thrombolytic treatment: descriptive subtype analysis. *Stroke* 2011;42:102–106.

63. Ohara T, Nagakane Y, Tanaka E, et al. Clinical and radiological features of stroke patients with poor outcomes who do not receive intravenous thrombolysis because of mild symptoms. *Eur Neurol* 2012;69:4–7.

64. Smith EE, Fonarow GC, Reeves MJ, et al. Outcomes in mild or rapidly improving stroke not treated with intravenous recombinant tissue-type plasminogen activator: findings from Get With The Guidelines–Stroke. *Stroke* 2011;42:3110–3115.

65. Neumann-Haefelin T, Hoelig S, Berkefeld J, et al. Leukoaraiosis is a risk factor for symptomatic intracerebral hemorrhage after thrombolysis for acute stroke. *Stroke* 2006;37:2463–2466.

66. Palumbo V, Boulanger JM, Hill MD, Inzitari D, Buchan AM. Leukoaraiosis and intracerebral hemorrhage after thrombolysis in acute stroke. *Neurology* 2007;68:1020–1024.

67. Demchuk AM, Khan F, Hill MD, et al. Importance of leukoaraiosis on CT for tissue plasminogen activator decision making: evaluation of the NINDS rt-PA stroke study. *Cerebrovasc Dis* 2008;26:120–125.

68. Shoamanesh A, Kwok CS, Lim PA, Benavente OR. Postthrombolysis intracranial hemorrhage risk of cerebral microbleeds in acute stroke patients: a systematic review and meta-analysis. *Int J Stroke* 2013;8:348–356.

69. Chalela JA, Kang DW, Warach S. Multiple cerebral microbleeds: MRI marker of a diffuse hemorrhage-prone state. *J Neuroimaging* 2004;14:54–57.

70. Del Bene A, Palumbo V, Lamassa M, et al. Progressive lacunar stroke: review of mechanisms, prognostic features, and putative treatments. *Int J Stroke* 2012;7:321–329.

71. Donnan GA, Bladin PF, Berkovic SF, Longley WA, Saling MM. The stroke syndrome of striatocapsular infarction. *Brain* 1991;114(Pt 1A):51–70.

72. Donnan GA, O'Malley HM, Quang L, Hurley S, Bladin PF. The capsular warning syndrome: pathogenesis and clinical features. *Neurology* 1993;43:957–962.

73. Paul NL, Simoni M, Chandratheva A, Rothwell PM. Population-based study of capsular warning syndrome and prognosis after early recurrent TIA. *Neurology* 2012;79: 1356–1362.

74. Kennedy J, Hill MD, Ryckborst KJ, et al. Fast Assessment of Stroke and Transient ischaemic attack to prevent Early Recurrence (FASTER): a randomised controlled pilot trial. *Lancet Neurol* 2007;6:961–969.

75. Wang Y, Wang Y, Zhao X, et al. Clopidogrel with aspirin in acute minor stroke or transient ischemic attack. *New Engl J Med* 2013;369:11–19.

76. Khan A, Kasner SE, Lynn MJ, Chimowitz MI. Risk factors and outcome of patients with

symptomatic intracranial stenosis presenting with lacunar stroke. *Stroke* 2012;43:1230–1233.

77. Bailey EL, Smith C, Sudlow CL, Wardlaw JM. Pathology of lacunar ischemic stroke in humans – a systematic review. *Brain Pathol* 2012;22:583–591.
78. Bousser MG, Eschwege E, Haguenau M, et al. "AICLA" controlled trial of aspirin and dipyridamole in the secondary prevention of athero-thrombotic cerebral ischemia. *Stroke* 1983;14:5–14.
79. Gent M, Blakely JA, Easton JD, et al. The Canadian–American Ticlopidine Study (CATS) in thromboembolic stroke. *Lancet* 1989;1:1215–1220.
80. CAST (Chinese Acute Stroke Trial) Collaborative Group. CAST: randomised placebo-controlled trial of early aspirin use in 20 000 patients with acute ischaemic stroke. *Lancet* 1997;349:1641–1649.
81. Gotoh F, Tohgi H, Hirai S, et al. Cilostazol Stroke Prevention Study: a placebo-controlled doubleblind trial for secondary prevention of cerebral infarction. *J Stroke Cerebrovasc Dis* 2000;9:147–157.
82. Gorelick PB, Richardson D, Kelly M, et al. Aspirin and ticlopidine for prevention of recurrent stroke in black patients: a randomized trial. *JAMA* 2003; 289:2947–2957.
83. Halkes PH, van Gijn J, Kappelle LJ, Koudstaal PJ, Algra A. Aspirin plus dipyridamole versus aspirin alone after cerebral ischaemia of arterial origin (ESPRIT): randomised controlled trial. *Lancet* 2006;367:1665–1673.
84. Bousser MG, Amarenco P, Chamorro A, et al. Terutroban versus aspirin in patients with cerebral ischaemic events (PERFORM): a randomised, double-blind, parallel-group trial. *Lancet* 2011;377:2013–2022.
85. Shinohara Y, Gotoh F, Tohgi H, et al. Antiplatelet cilostazol is beneficial in diabetic and/or hypertensive ischemic stroke patients. Subgroup analysis of the Cilostazol Stroke Prevention Study. *Cerebrovasc Dis* 2008;26:63–70.
86. Harker LA, Marzec UM, Kelly AB, et al. Clopidogrel inhibition of stent, graft, and vascular thrombogenesis with antithrombotic enhancement by aspirin in nonhuman primates. *Circulation* 1998;98:2461–2469.
87. Makkar RR, Eigler NL, Kaul S, et al. Effects of clopidogrel, aspirin and combined therapy in a porcine ex vivo model of high-shear induced stent thrombosis. *Eur Heart J* 1998;19:1538–1546.
88. Yusuf S, Zhao F, Mehta SR, et al. Effects of clopidogrel in addition to aspirin in patients with acute coronary syndromes without ST-segment elevation. *New Engl J Med* 2001;345:494–502.
89. Furie KL, Kasner SE, Adams RJ, et al. Guidelines for the prevention of stroke in patients with stroke or transient ischemic attack: a guideline for healthcare professionals from the American Heart Association/American Stroke Association. *Stroke* 2011;42:227–276.
90. Ebrahim S, Sung J, Song YM, et al. Serum cholesterol, haemorrhagic stroke, ischaemic stroke, and myocardial infarction: Korean National Health System Prospective Cohort Study. *BMJ* 2006;333:22.
91. Iso H, Jacobs DR, Jr., Wentworth D, Neaton JD, Cohen JD. Serum cholesterol levels and six-year mortality from stroke in 350 977 men screened for the multiple risk factor intervention trial. *New Engl J Med* 1989;320:904–910.
92. Collins R, Armitage J, Parish S, et al. Effects of cholesterol-lowering with simvastatin on stroke and other major vascular events in 20 536 people with cerebrovascular disease or other high-risk conditions. *Lancet* 2004;363:757–767.
93. Amarenco P, Labreuche J. Lipid management in the prevention of stroke: review and updated meta-analysis of statins for stroke prevention. *Lancet Neurol* 2009;8:453–463.
94. Amarenco P, Benavente O, Goldstein LB, et al. Results of the Stroke Prevention by Aggressive Reduction in Cholesterol Levels (SPARCL) trial by stroke subtypes. *Stroke* 2009;40: 1405–1409.
95. Goldstein LB, Amarenco P, Szarek M, et al. Hemorrhagic stroke in the Stroke Prevention by Aggressive Reduction in Cholesterol Levels study. *Neurology* 2008;70(24 Pt 2): 2364–2370.
96. O'Donnell MJ, Xavier D, Liu L, et al. Risk factors for ischaemic and intracerebral haemorrhagic stroke in 22 countries (the INTERSTROKE study): a case-control study. *Lancet* 2010;376:112–123.
97. Collins R, Peto R, Godwin J, MacMahon S. Blood pressure and coronary heart disease. *Lancet* 1990;336:370–371.
98. Collins R, Peto R, MacMahon S, et al. Blood pressure, stroke, and coronary heart disease. Part 2. Short-term reductions in blood pressure: overview of randomised drug trials in their epidemiological context. *Lancet* 1990;335:827–838.
99. MacMahon S, Peto R, Cutler J, et al. Blood pressure, stroke, and coronary heart disease. Part 1. Prolonged differences in blood pressure: prospective observational studies corrected for the regression dilution bias. *Lancet* 1990;335:765–774.
100. PROGRESS Management Committee. PROGRESS – The Perindopril Protection aGainst

Recurrent Stroke Study: characteristics of the study population at baseline. *J Hypertens* 1999;17:1647–1655.

101. Gueyffier F, Boissel JP, Boutitie F, et al. Effect of antihypertensive treatment in patients having already suffered from stroke. Gathering the evidence. The INDANA (INdividual Data ANalysis of Antihypertensive intervention trials) Project Collaborators. *Stroke* 1997;28:2557–2562.
102. Rashid P, Leonardi-Bee J, Bath P. Blood pressure reduction and secondary prevention of stroke and other vascular events: a systematic review. *Stroke* 2003;34:2741–2748.
103. Benavente OR, Coffey CS, Conwit R, et al. Blood-pressure targets in patients with recent lacunar stroke: the SPS3 randomised trial. *Lancet* 2013;382:507–515.
104. Jackson CA, Hutchison A, Dennis MS, et al. Differing risk factor profiles of ischemic stroke subtypes: evidence for a distinct lacunar arteriopathy? *Stroke* 2010; 41:624–629.
105. Micheli S, Agnelli G, Palmerini F, et al. Need for extensive diagnostic work-up for patients with lacunar stroke. *J Neurol* 2008; 255:637–642.
106. Apostolakis S, Lane DA, Buller H, Lip GY. Comparison of the $CHADS_2$, $CHADS_2$–VAS_c and HAS–BLED scores for the prediction of clinically relevant bleeding in anticoagulated patients with atrial fibrillation: the AMADEUS trial. *Thromb Haemostasis* 2013;110: 1074–1079.
107. Rajapakse A, Rajapakse S, Sharma JC. Is investigating for carotid artery disease warranted in non-cortical lacunar infarction? *Stroke* 2011;42:217–220.
108. Mead GE, Lewis SC, Wardlaw JM, Dennis MS, Warlow CP. Severe ipsilateral carotid stenosis and middle cerebral artery disease in lacunar ischaemic stroke: innocent bystanders? *J Neurol* 2002;249:266–271.
109. Inzitari D, Eliasziw M, Sharpe BL, Fox AJ, Barnett HJ. Risk factors and outcome of patients with carotid artery stenosis presenting with lacunar stroke. North American Symptomatic Carotid Endarterectomy Trial Group. *Neurology* 2000;54:660–666.
110. Barnett HJ, Meldrum HE, Eliasziw M. The appropriate use of carotid endarterectomy. *CMAJ* 2002;166:1169–1179.

Chapter 27

Cerebral small vessel disease imaging as a surrogate marker for clinical trials

Reinhold Schmidt, Margherita Cavalieri, and Marisa Loitfelder

Introduction

A surrogate marker, or surrogate endpoint, is a laboratory measurement or physical sign that is used in therapeutic trials as a substitute for a clinically meaningful endpoint that is a direct measure of how a patient feels, functions, or survives, and that is expected to predict the effect of the therapy [1].

There must be a strong association between the marker and the clinical endpoint or outcome and, furthermore, the effect of a treatment on a surrogate marker must reflect its effect on the clinical outcome [2].

Although surrogate markers can be related to disease progression, they should not be confused with sole correlates. Even if a given intervention affects a potential surrogate marker and that marker is clearly in the causal pathway of the clinical endpoint, the effect may not persist long enough for the drug to alter the long-term clinical outcome. There is increasing interest in markers that allow researchers to make predictions of drug effects or disease progression by extrapolating short-term results to long-term clinical endpoints. For this reason, and in order to reduce the costs and time of clinical trials, surrogate markers are particularly attractive. In vascular cognitive impairment (VCI) magnetic resonance imaging (MRI) correlates of cerebral small vessel disease (SVD) have only recently been proposed as potential secondary outcomes for therapeutic trials [3].

There are several prerequisites that need to be fulfilled for any MRI abnormality to be considered as a potential surrogate endpoint. These include: (1) a reasonable confidence that the observed tissue changes are indeed related to cerebral microangiopathy; (2) evidence for a rate of progression that is fast enough to allow monitoring of treatment effects within a reasonable period of time; and (3) a correlation between the change in the imaging marker and changes in clinical outcomes [3].

In the following sections we review how potential surrogate markers for subcortical VCI fulfill these prerequisites and report current data on sample size calculations for trial planning.

White matter lesions

Relationship to cerebral microangiopathy

A microangiopathy-related origin of white matter lesions (WMLs) is supported by the associations with vascular risk factors and histopathologic correlates.

Although several vascular risk factors have been reported to be associated with WMLs, the most important and most often reported association is with hypertension [4–6].

The Framingham Offspring Study showed a positive and independent association between WML volume and the Framingham Stroke Risk Profile, and this relationship was driven by hypertension [6], and hypertension was also reported as the strongest predictor of WML progression [7].

Histopathologic studies described nonischemic and ischemic brain changes to be related to WMLs.

Smooth periventricular changes, including caps around the ventricular horns and periventricular lining, and halos, appear to be of nonvascular origin. They relate to a disruption of the ependymal lining following ventricular widening and have to be differentiated from subcortical and deep white matter abnormalities [8, 9].

Importantly, deep and subcortical WMLs are also heterogeneous as to their histopathologic correlates. While punctate WMLs often represent widened

Cerebral Small Vessel Disease, ed. Leonardo Pantoni and Philip B. Gorelick. Published by Cambridge University Press.

perivascular spaces without substantial ischemic tissue damage [8, 9], early confluent and confluent lesions correspond to incomplete ischemic destruction, including complete demyelination and axonal loss in the presence of cerebral SVD [10, 11].

Rate of progression

Longitudinal studies showed substantial progression of WMLs over a period of few years [7, 12–25] (Table 27.1).

As expected, the rate of progression is lesion type-dependent. Punctate abnormalities on MRI have a low tendency for progression while early confluent and confluent changes progress rapidly [15, 16, 19] (Figure 27.1).

In the normal aging population with early confluent to confluent lesions, the average rate of progression ranges from 0.23 cm^3 per year [23] to 1.33 cm^3 per year [14].

A faster rate of progression was reported in hypertensive people (0.14–0.54 cm^3/year) [26] and in cerebral autosomal dominant arteriopathy with subcortical infarcts and leukoencephalopathy (CADASIL) patients (3.96 cm^3/year) [27].

When considering the annual percent increase in WML volume, the ranges are between 12.5 and 14.4% in subjects with early confluent lesions and between 17.3 and 25.0% in those with confluent abnormalities [15].

Correlation with clinical outcomes

WML progression has been associated with cognitive decline and dementia, incident stroke, gait impairment, and mood changes (Table 27.2 [16, 20, 24–26, 28–32]).

Longitudinal data consistently reported an association between WML progression and decline in global cognitive functioning or in specific cognitive domains [16, 20, 24–26, 28–32].

In the Cardiovascular Health Study, an increase in white matter grades was associated with global cognitive decline [22]. In the Rotterdam Scan Study, periventricular WML progression was associated with decline in general cognitive function and in information-processing speed [20].

Data from the Austrian Stroke Prevention Study demonstrated a complex interaction between progression of WMLs, brain atrophy, and cognitive functioning with increasing volume of WMLs. Brain volume change mediated the relationship between WML progression and cognitive decline, particularly in the domains memory, visuopractical skills, and executive functions [31].

The clinical importance of WMLs is also supported by studies indicating that greater burden of WMLs at baseline predicts conversion from normal aging to mild cognitive impairment (MCI) [33] and conversion from amnestic MCI to Alzheimer's disease (AD) [34]. Baseline WML load also predicted global functional decline and disability over a relatively short period of time [35].

Sample size calculations for trial planning

In the Austrian Stroke Prevention Study we reported that fewer than 200 subjects with confluent lesions would be required per treatment arm to demonstrate a 20% reduction in the rate of disease progression over a three-year period [3]. Thus, WML progression became an interesting outcome for proof-of-concept studies in cerebral SVD.

Considering that volumetric measurements of WML change are labor-intensive and time-consuming, a visual rating scale to assess progression might be considered in clinical trials.

A recent publication from the Leukoaraiosis And DISability (LADIS) study evaluated the association between WML progression determined on the visual Rotterdam Progression Scale [36] and cognitive functioning, and provided sample size calculations for clinical trials using the Rotterdam Progression Scale-rated WML progression as surrogate endpoints [37].

Progression was seen in 73.6% of the study participants and, in line with previous studies [38], WML grade at baseline was the strongest predictor of future WML progression.

Cognitive functions were assessed by the Vascular Dementia Assessment Scale – cognitive subscale (VADAS-cog) [39] and by an executive function score. Table 27.3 summarizes the results [37]. As can be seen from Table 27.3, low numbers of subjects are required per treatment arm in Scenario 1 trials in which WML progression is the primary outcome measure. Such settings will allow lower sample sizes when including only individuals with early confluent or confluent WMLs. For Scenarios 2 and 3, in which the expected change in cognition resulting from treatment effects on WML progression was used as the outcome, 2599 or 18 853 subjects per arm

Table 27.1 Progression of white matter lesions in different MRI studies. Studies listed in chronological order

Study (year)	Sample	Subjects (no.)	Follow-up (years)	Progression measurement	Progression rate (% patients); volume increase (cm^3)
Wahlund et al. (1996) [12]	Normals	13	5	Scheltens scale	92%
Veldink et al. (1998) [13]	Normals and cognitively impaired	14	2	Scheltens scale	57%
Whitman et al. (2001) [14]	Normals	70	4	Grid method	1.1 cm^3
Schmidt et al. (2003) [15]	Community-dwelling (ASPS)	296	6	Semiautomated volume measurement	17.2%; 1.4 cm^3
Taylor et al. (2003) [16]	Community-dwelling	117	2	Semiautomated volume measurement	1.4 cm^3
Garde et al. (2005) [17]	Octogenarians	26	3.8	Semiautomated volume measurement	2.6 cm^3
Ten Dam et al. (2005) [18]	Trial cohort (PROSPER study)	535	2.8	Automated volume measurement	1.1 cm^3
Gouw et al. (2008) [19]	Community-dwelling (LADIS study)	396	3	Modified Rotterdam Progression Scale	74%
Van Dijk et al. (2008) [20]	Population-based (RSS)	668	3.4	Modified Rotterdam Progression Scale	27% PVWML 32% DWML
Maillard et al. (2009) [21]	Population-based (3C study)	1118	4	Automated volume measurement	0.25 cm^3/year
Longstreth et al. (2005) [22]	Population-based (CHS)	1919	5	CHS scoring	28%
Sachdev et al. (2007) [23]	Community-dwelling	51	3	Automated volume measurement	6.5 cm^3 PVWML 16.3 cm^3 DWML
Gottesman et al. (2010) [7]	Population-based (ARIC)	983	11	Estimated volume from a prediction equation from visual grades	13 cm^3
Lo et al. (2012) [24]	Cohort study (ADNI)	819	1.7–3.0	Automated volume measurement	MCI = 0.0076 cm^3/month AD = 0.0074 cm^3/month N = 0.0049 cm^3/month
Maillard et al. (2012) [25]	Cohort study	150	4	Semiautomated volume measurement	2.5 cm^3

AD, Alzheimer's disease; ADNI, Alzheimer's Disease Neuroimaging Initiative; ARIC, Atherosclerosis Risk in Communities; ASPS, Austrian Stroke Prevention Study; CHS, Cardiovascular Health Study; DWML, deep white matter lesions; LADIS, Leukoaraiosis And DISability; MCI, mild cognitive impairment; MRI, magnetic resonance imaging; N, normal controls; PROSPER, PROspective Study of Pravastatin in the Elderly at Risk; PVWML, periventricular white matter lesions; RSS, Rotterdam Scan Study; 3C study, Three-City Study.

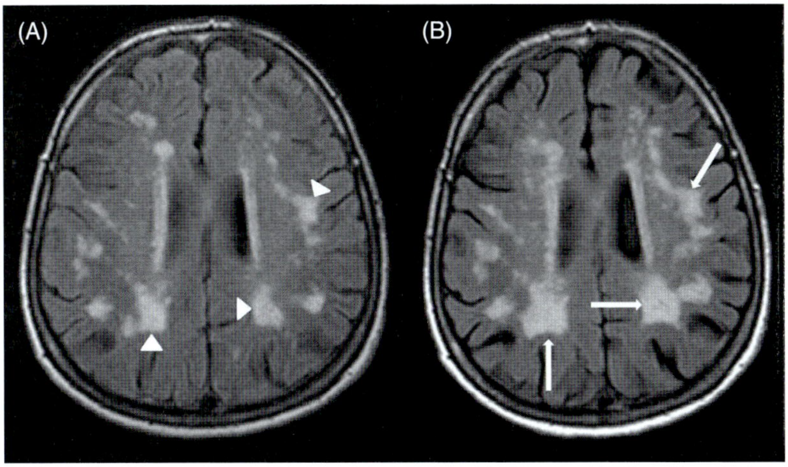

Figure 27.1 Rapid progression of white matter lesions (WMLs). (A) Baseline scan showing multiple early confluent and confluent WMLs (arrow heads); (B) Lesion progression in various brain regions (arrows) after 3.5 years of follow-up.

would be required for VADAS-cog and 1809 or 1988 for the executive function test. It becomes clear from these data that sample size strongly depends on both baseline WML grade and the applied cognitive tests [37].

The extremely large sample sizes in a trial in patients with early confluent or confluent WMLs using VADAS-cog as the clinical outcome was probably caused by a pronounced cognitive deterioration in individuals with early confluent and confluent WMLs irrespective of future lesion progression.

Lacunes

Relationship to cerebral microangiopathy

Lacunes are undoubtedly of vascular origin. With few exceptions lacunes represent subcortical ischemic infarcts, resulting from occlusion of small perforating arteries.

Lacunes are associated with vascular risk factors, in particular hypertension and cardiovascular disease [40, 41].

Incidence of lacunes

Table 27.4 reports the incidence of lacunes over varying observational periods in various longitudinal studies [19, 20, 42, 43]. The frequency of new lacunes ranged from 1.6% to 19.0% over 3–5 years of follow-up [42]. The largest study on incidence of lacunes was conducted in the setting of the Dijon Stroke Registry [42]. This study included 140 000 participants and reported an incident rate of lacunes of 16.7% over 5 years. Similar data came from the Rotterdam Scan Study [20], the Cardiovascular Health Study [22], and the LADIS study [44].

Correlation with clinical outcomes

Many cross-sectional studies found a relationship between the presence of lacunes and cognitive impairment. Unfortunately, only few longitudinal data are available assessing the relationship between incident lacunes and clinical outcomes (Table 27.5 [20, 43, 45]). The findings are consistent in that they demonstrate that incident lacunes exert detrimental functional effects. In the Cardiovascular Health Study, the incidence of lacunes was related to decline in the Mini Mental State Examination (MMSE) and the digit–symbol substitution test [22]. Similar associations were also found in the Rotterdam Scan Study, where incident lacunes were associated with a decline in general cognitive function and information processing speed [20]. In the LADIS study incident lacunes at three-year follow-up related to steeper decline in executive functions and psychomotor speed [45].

Sample size calculations for trial planning

Based on the previously published data on the frequency of incident lacunes [19, 20, 42, 43], a 20% treatment effect in a three-year trial could be detected with 80% power with samples sizes in the range between 1540 and 3678 patients.

Table 27.2 Progression of white matter lesions and correlation with clinical outcome. Listed in chronological order

Study	Sample	No. of subjects	Follow-up (years)	MRI findings	Outcome
Garde et al. (2000) [28]	Octogenarians	26	3.8	WML volume increase	Performance and verbal decline in WAIS
Taylor et al. (2003) [16]	Patients with major depression	133	2	WML volume increase	Poor outcome (treatment response)
Longstreth et al. (2005) [22]	Population-based (CHS)	1919	5	Worsening WML grade	Decline in MMSE and DSST
Van den Heuvel et al. (2006) [26]	Trial cohort	554	3	Progression of PVWML	Reduced mental processing speed
Kramer et al. (2007) [29]	Healthy elderly	50	3.7	WML progression	Lower executive score at follow-up
Silbert et al. (2008) [30]	Ongoing longitudinal study (Oregon Brain Aging study)	104	13	DWML volume increase	Decreased gait performance and decreased performance on logical memory testing
Van Dijk et al. (2008) [20]	Population-based (RSS)	668	3	PVWML progression	Decline in general cognitive function and in particular information processing speed
Schmidt et al. (2009) [31]	Community-dwelling (ASPS)	243	6	WML volume increase	Decline in memory, conceptual reasoning, and visuopractical skills
Firbank et al. (2012) [32]	Community-dwelling (LADIS study)	–	3	WML progression	Incident depression
Maillard et al. (2012) [25]	Consecutive patients at the University of California, Davis Alzheimer's Disease Center	150	4	Incident MRI voxels	Decline in episodic memory and executive function

ASPS, Austrian Stroke Prevention Study; CHS, Cardiovascular Health Study; DSST, digit–symbol substitution test; DWML, deep white matter lesions; LADIS, Leukoaraiosis And DISability; MMSE, Mini Mental State Examination; MRI, magnetic resonance imaging; PVWML, periventricular white matter lesions; RSS, Rotterdam Study; WAIS, Wechsler Adult Intelligence Scale; WML, white matter lesion.

Microbleeds

Relationship to cerebral microangiopathy

The prevalence of cerebral microbleeds ranges from 4.7 to 23.5% in healthy populations [46, 47], and has been associated with vascular risk factors including higher age, hypertension, diabetes mellitus, male gender, the presence of an apolipoprotein E (*APOE*) ε4 allele, and low serum cholesterol concentration [48]. Our group has examined 11 brains of patients with MRI detected cerebral microbleeds and described advanced hypertensive lipohyalinotic changes in nine and cerebral amyloid angiopathy in two brains [49]. Histopathologic analysis in patients with spontaneous intracerebral hemorrhage also showed evidence for microangiopathy in those patients who had microbleeds [49].

Hypertensive vasculopathy is typically associated with cerebral microbleeds in the basal ganglia, thalamus, brainstem, and cerebellum, whereas advanced

Table 27.3 Sample size estimates per treatment arm according to white matter lesion (WML) grade at baseline in a three-year trial in which treatment reduces WML progression by one grade*

Trial outcome measures	All WML grades	Early confluent and confluent WMLs
Reduction of WML progression (Scenario 1)	70	58
Vascular Dementia Assessment Scale – cognitive subscale (VADAS-cog) change (Scenario 2)	2599	18 853
Executive function change (Scenario 3)	1809	1988

* All calculations assumed a power of 80% at a two-sided significance level of 5%.
Data from Schmidt et al. [37].
Scenario 1: Trial outcome is reduction of WML progression by one grade on the Rotterdam Progression Scale (RPS).
Scenario 2: Outcome is change on VADAS-cog resulting from reduction of one grade in WML progression on the RPS.
Scenario 3: Outcome is change in executive functioning resulting from reduction of one grade in WML progression on the RPS.

Table 27.4 Frequency of incident lacunes in different MRI studies. Listed in chronological order

Study	Sample	No. of subjects	Follow-up (years)	Frequency of new lacunes (%)
Gouw et al. (2008) [19]	Community dwelling (LADIS study)	396	3.0	19.0
Van Dijk et al. (2008) [20]	Population-based (RSS)	668	3.4	12.0
Giroud et al. (1991) [42]	Stroke Registry of Dijon	140 000	5.0	16.7
Longstreth et al. (2002) [43]	Population-based (CHS)	1433	5.0	14.6

CHS, Cardiovascular Health Study; LADIS, Leukoaraiosis And DISability study; MRI, magnetic resonance imaging; RSS, Rotterdam Scan Study.

Table 27.5 Incident lacunes and correlation with clinical outcome in longitudinal studies. Listed in chronological order

Study	Sample	No. of subjects	Follow-up (years)	MRI findings	Outcome
Longstreth et al. (2002) [43]	Population-based (CHS)	1433	5	Incident lacunes	Decline in MMSE and DSST
Van Dijk et al. (2008) [20]	Population-based (RSS)	668	3	Incident lacunes	Decline in general cognitive function, in particular information processing speed
Jokinen et al. (2011) [45]	Community-dwelling (LADIS study)	387	3	Incident lacunes	Decline in executive function and psychomotor speed

CHS, Cardiovascular Health Study; DSST, digit–symbol substitution test; LADIS, Leukoaraiosis And DISability; MMSE, Mini Mental State Examination; MRI, magnetic resonance imaging; RSS, Rotterdam Scan Study.

cerebral amyloid angiopathy is associated with a lobar distribution [50].

Incidence of cerebral microbleeds

The Rotterdam Scan Study demonstrated that the incidence of cerebral microbleeds strongly depends on age [51]. The rate of lesions was reported to be 7.6% in subjects aged 60–69 years, it increased to 15.6% in the age range between 70 and 79 years, and 18.6% in subjects older than 80 years. Microbleeds at baseline increased the risk for newly occurring microbleeds more than five times as compared to subjects without such baseline abnormalities. [52].

In a smaller longitudinal study that reassessed patients with stroke or transient ischemic attack after more than 12 months, 53.9% of the patients with cerebral microbleeds at baseline showed new microbleeds at follow-up [53].

Correlation with clinical outcomes

So far, little information exists on the clinical consequences of incident cerebral microbleeds. There is only one longitudinal study available [54]. The authors identified increasing cognitive decline with increasing number of incident microbleeds in CADASIL patients over seven years of follow-up. Due to the lack of clinical correlative data, the validation status of these lesions as a possible surrogate marker in VCI trials has to be considered incomplete and sample size calculations are thus not provided.

Microstructural changes in normal-appearing brain tissue

Relationship to cerebral microangiopathy

Recent advances in imaging techniques have highlighted the importance of normal-appearing brain tissue in the context of age-related white matter abnormalities. There is more widespread tissue damage associated with WMLs that is not visible in conventional MRI but can be detected by new quantitative MR techniques, such as diffusion tensor imaging (DTI) and magnetization transfer imaging (MTI). DTI provides information about the microstructural integrity of brain tissue by measuring the direction and magnitude of water diffusion in the intracellular compartment of the axons. Due to the restriction by lipid bilayers and other cell components, water diffusion in brain tissue is anisotropic with the highest diffusivity along the directions of the axons. MTI is an approach to explore the composition of brain tissue. Protons bound to larger molecules such as the myelin lipids and proteins have relaxation properties that make them invisible in conventional MRI. However, the pool of bound protons can be indirectly quantified by utilizing magnetization transfer. Animal models and postmortem studies indicate that quantitative DTI and MTI measures correlate with markers of myelin integrity, and axonal damage and density [55–58]. A recent study in brain hypoperfused mice examined the complementary value of DTI and MTI measures for delineation of white matter damage [59]. The authors reported that the reduction in fractional anisotropy paralleled a decrease in magnetization transfer ratio in several tissue compartments after continuous moderate hypoperfusion over one month in mice and concluded that both techniques are sufficiently suited to detect microstructural tissue alterations, at least in the white matter of the murine brain. Postmortem histologic analyses assessing myelin content, axonal density, and gliosis revealed similar correlations in brains of patients with AD [55] or multiple sclerosis [60]. So far, there have been no studies which assessed the association between microstructural tissue alterations and cerebral vascular changes.

Rate of progression

A multimodal study evaluating MRI parameters as surrogate markers of cerebral SVD reported a 1.18% decrease in peak height of mean diffusivity and a 10.73% increase in fractional anisotropy in patients with lacunar stroke and leukoaraiosis over one year despite unchanged lesion load and brain volume [61].

Correlation with clinical outcomes

DTI changes correlate more closely to cognitive functioning than the volume of visible SVD-related changes such as WMLs. So far, only few longitudinal studies on the relationship between increase of microstructural damage and decline in cognitive functioning are available. Even less is known about the relationship between MTI measures and cognition.

Results from the LADIS study found that DWI microstructural changes in normal appearing brain tissue predict faster decline in cognitive parameters [62]. In a longitudinal two-year follow-up study in

62 CADASIL subjects the changes in mean diffusivity correlated with the clinical progression of the disease [27].

DTI was also used in early detection [63, 64] and monitoring of disease progression from MCI to AD [65].

Sample size calculations for trial planning

Sample size calculation based on two-year follow-up data in CADASIL patients showed that one would need 1944 subjects per treatment arm to demonstrate a treatment effect of 20% with an 80% power when mean diffusivity is used as the trial outcome [27].

Conclusions

Currently, confluent WMLs are the only MRI correlates of cerebral SVD for which a vascular origin, fast progression, and correlation with cognitive decline have been demonstrated. Lacunes may fulfill these prerequisites in selective patient samples, but in the general population the incidence of lacunes over short observational periods is rather small and sample size in trials focusing on lacunes would, thus, need to be large. In line with current data, confluent WMLs are ideal surrogate markers in proof-of-concept studies in patients suffering from subcortical VCI. However, if such trials aim to demonstrate slowing of cognitive decline resulting from treatment effects on WML progression, sample sizes will need to increase tremendously. So far, only a few studies have used WMLs in proof-of-concept studies in the field of VCI. The effect of antihypertensive therapy and statin use on WML progression was evaluated in the PROspective Study of Pravastatin in the Elderly at Risk (PROSPER) and the Perindopril Protection aGainst Recurrent Stroke Study (PROGRESS) trials [18, 66].

The MRI substudy of PROSPER examined the effect of daily therapy with pravastatin on the progression of ischemic brain lesions, including WMLs. After a mean period of 33 months, there was no difference in progression of WML volume between the 265 participants in the active group versus the 270 participants in the placebo arm.

PROGRESS aimed to assess whether blood pressure lowering therapy with perindopril and indapamide reduces the progression of WMLs in patients with cerebrovascular disease. The study included 192 participants who had cerebral MRI at baseline and after 36 months. The authors found that an active blood pressure lowering regimen stopped or delayed the progression of WMLs.

Recent data from the VITAmins TO Prevent Stroke (VITATOPS) study showed that daily B-vitamins supplementation for two years did not significantly reduce the progression of WML volume in a sample of 359 patients with recent stroke or TIA and cerebral SVD, but may do so in the subgroup of patients with severe cerebral SVD [67]. These studies are important as they provide first evidence for possible treatment strategies in cerebral SVD, which is still a severely understudied disorder with important implications on the functional status of our aging populations. The perspective of new treatment targets originating from recent genetic association studies [68] underscores the importance of having validated surrogate markers which will allow conduct of proof-of concept studies in a timely manner at relatively low cost.

References

1. US Food and Drug Administration. New drug, antibiotic, and biological drug product regulations; accelerated approval–FDA. Final rule. *Fed Regist* 1992;57:58942–58960.
2. Fleming TR, DeMets DL. Surrogate endpoints in clinical trials: are we being misled? *Ann Intern Med* 1996;125:605–613.
3. Schmidt R, Scheltens P, Erkinjuntti T, et al. White matter lesion progression: a surrogate endpoint for trials in cerebral small-vessel disease. *Neurology* 2004;63:139–144.
4. Fazekas F, Niederkorn K, Schmidt R, et al. White matter signal abnormalities in normal individuals: correlation with carotid ultrasonography, cerebral blood flow measurements, and cerebrovascular risk factors. *Stroke* 1988;19:1285–1288.
5. De Leeuw F-E, de Groot JC, Oudkerk M, et al. Hypertension and cerebral white matter lesions in a prospective cohort study. *Brain* 2002;125:765–772.
6. Jeerakathil T, Wolf PA, Beiser A, et al. Stroke risk profile predicts white matter hyperintensity volume: the Framingham Study. *Stroke* 2004;35:1857–1861.
7. Gottesman RF, Coresh J, Catellier DJ, et al. Blood pressure and white-matter disease progression in a biethnic cohort: Atherosclerosis Risk In Communities (ARIC) study. *Stroke* 2010;41:3–8.
8. Fazekas F, Kleinert R, Offenbacher H, et al. Pathologic correlates of incidental MRI

white matter signal hyperintensities. *Neurology* 1993;43:1683–1689.

9. Chimowitz MI, Estes ML, Furlan AJ, Awad IA. Further observations on the pathology of subcortical lesions identified on magnetic resonance imaging. *Arch Neurol* 1992;49:747–752.
10. Scarpelli M, Salvolini U, Diamanti L, et al. MRI and pathological examination of postmortem brains: the problem of white matter high signal areas. *Neuroradiology* 1994;36:393–398.
11. Scheltens P, Barkhof F, Leys D, et al. Histopathologic correlates of white matter changes on MRI in Alzheimer's disease and normal aging. *Neurology* 1995; 45:883–888.
12. Wahlund LO, Almkvist O, Basun H, Julin P. MRI in successful aging, a five-year follow-up study from the eighth to ninth decade of life. *Magn Reson Imaging* 1996;14:601–608.
13. Veldink JH, Scheltens P, Jonker C, Launer LJ. Progression of cerebral white matter hyperintensities on MRI is related to diastolic blood pressure. *Neurology* 1998;51: 319–320.
14. Whitman GT, Tang Y, Lin A, Baloh RW, Tang T. A prospective study of cerebral white matter abnormalities in older people with gait dysfunction. *Neurology* 2001;57:990–994.
15. Schmidt R, Enzinger C, Ropele S, Schmidt H, Fazekas F. Progression of cerebral white matter lesions: six-year results of the Austrian Stroke Prevention Study. *Lancet* 2003; 361:2046–2048.
16. Taylor WD, MacFall JR, Provenzale JM, et al. Serial MR imaging of volumes of hyperintense white matter lesions in elderly patients: correlation with vascular risk factors. *AJR Am J Roentgenol* 2003; 181:571–576.
17. Garde E, Lykke Mortensen E, Rostrup E, Paulson OB. Decline in intelligence is associated with progression in white matter hyperintensity volume. *J Neurol Neurosurg Psychiatr* 2005; 76:1289–1291.
18. Ten Dam VH, van den Heuvel DMJ, van Buchem MA, et al. Effect of pravastatin on cerebral infarcts and white matter lesions. *Neurology* 2005;64:1807–1809.
19. Gouw AA, van der Flier WM, Fazekas F, et al. Progression of white matter hyperintensities and incidence of new lacunes over a three-year period: the Leukoaraiosis And DISability Study. *Stroke* 2008;39:1414–1420.
20. Van Dijk EJ, Prins ND, Vrooman HA, et al. Progression of cerebral small vessel disease in relation to risk factors and cognitive consequences: the Rotterdam Scan Study. *Stroke* 2008;39: 2712–2719.
21. Maillard P, Crivello F, Dufouil C, et al. Longitudinal follow-up of individual white matter hyperintensities in a large cohort of elderly. *Neuroradiology* 2009;51:209–220.
22. Longstreth WT, Arnold AM, Beauchamp NJ, et al. Incidence, manifestations, and predictors of worsening white matter on serial cranial magnetic resonance imaging in the elderly: the Cardiovascular Health Study. *Stroke* 2005;36:56–61.
23. Sachdev P, Wen W, Chen X, Brodaty H. Progression of white matter hyperintensities in elderly individuals over three years. *Neurology* 2007;68:214–222.
24. Lo RY, Jagust WJ. Vascular burden and Alzheimer disease pathologic progression. *Neurology* 2012;79:1349–1355.
25. Maillard P, Carmichael O, Fletcher E, et al. Coevolution of white matter hyperintensities and cognition in the elderly. *Neurology* 2012;79:442–448.
26. Van den Heuvel DMJ, ten Dam VH, de Craen AJM, et al. Increase in periventricular white matter hyperintensities parallels decline in mental processing speed in a non-demented elderly population. *J Neurol Neurosurg Psychiatr* 2006;77:149–153.
27. Holtmannspötter M, Peters N, Opherk C, et al. Diffusion magnetic resonance histograms as a surrogate marker and predictor of disease progression in CADASIL: a two-year follow-up study. *Stroke* 2005;36:2559–2565.
28. Garde E, Mortensen EL, Krabbe K, Rostrup E, Larsson HB. Relation between age-related decline in intelligence and cerebral white-matter hyperintensities in healthy octogenarians: a longitudinal study. *Lancet* 2000;356:628–634.
29. Kramer JH, Mungas D, Reed BR, et al. Longitudinal MRI and cognitive change in healthy elderly. *Neuropsychology* 2007;21:412–418.
30. Silbert LC, Nelson C, Howieson DB, Moore MM, Kaye JA. Impact of white matter hyperintensity volume progression on rate of cognitive and motor decline. *Neurology* 2008;71:108–113.
31. Schmidt R, Ropele S, Enzinger C, et al. White matter lesion progression, brain atrophy, and cognitive decline: the Austrian Stroke Prevention Study. *Ann Neurol* 2005;58:610–616.
32. Firbank MJ, Teodorczuk A, van der Flier WM, et al. Relationship between progression of brain white matter changes and late-life depression: three-year results from the LADIS study. *Br J Psychiatr* 2012;201:40–45.
33. Smith EE, Egorova S, Blacker D, et al. Magnetic resonance imaging white matter hyperintensities and brain volume in the prediction of mild cognitive impairment and dementia. *Arch Neurol* 2008;65:94–100.

34. Van Straaten ECW, Harvey D, Scheltens P, et al. Periventricular white matter hyperintensities increase the likelihood of progression from amnestic mild cognitive impairment to dementia. *J Neurol* 2008;255:1302–1308.

35. Inzitari D, Pracucci G, Poggesi A, et al. Changes in white matter as determinant of global functional decline in older independent outpatients: three year follow-up of LADIS (Leukoaraiosis And DISability) Study Cohort. *BMJ* 2009;339:2477.

36. Prins ND, van Straaten ECW, van Dijk EJ, et al. Measuring progression of cerebral white matter lesions on MRI: visual rating and volumetrics. *Neurology* 2004;62:1533–1539.

37. Schmidt R, Berghold A, Jokinen H, et al. White matter lesion progression in LADIS: frequency, clinical effects, and sample size calculations. *Stroke* 2012;43: 2643–2647.

38. Schmidt R, Petrovic K, Ropele S, Enzinger C, Fazekas F. Progression of leukoaraiosis and cognition. *Stroke* 2007;38: 2619–2625.

39. Ferris SH. General measures of cognition. *Int Psychogeriatr* 2003;15(Suppl 1):215–217.

40. Longstreth WT, Bernick C, Manolio TA, et al. Lacunar infarcts defined by magnetic resonance imaging of 3660 elderly people: the Cardiovascular Health Study. *Arch Neurol* 1998;55: 1217–1225.

41. Arauz A, Murillo L, Cantú C, Barinagarrementeria F, Higuera J. Prospective study of single and multiple lacunar infarcts using magnetic resonance imaging: risk factors, recurrence, and outcome in 175 consecutive cases. *Stroke* 2003;34:2453–2458.

42. Giroud M, Milan C, Beuriat P, et al. Incidence and survival rates during a two-year period of intracerebral and subarachnoid haemorrhages, cortical infarcts, lacunes and transient ischaemic attacks. The Stroke Registry of Dijon: 1985–1989. *Int J Epidemiol* 1991;20:892–899.

43. Longstreth WT, Dulberg C, Manolio TA, et al. Incidence, manifestations, and predictors of brain infarcts defined by serial cranial magnetic resonance imaging in the elderly: the Cardiovascular Health Study. *Stroke* 2002;33:2376–2382.

44. Gouw AA, van der Flier WM, Pantoni L, et al. On the etiology of incident brain lacunes: longitudinal observations from the LADIS study. *Stroke* 2008;39:3083–3085.

45. Jokinen H, Gouw AA, Madureira S, et al. Incident lacunes influence cognitive decline: the LADIS study. *Neurology* 2011;76: 1872–1878.

46. Jeerakathil T, Wolf PA, Beiser A, et al. Cerebral microbleeds: prevalence and associations with cardiovascular risk factors in the Framingham Study. *Stroke* 2004;35: 1831–1835.

47. Vernooij, MW van der Lugt A, Ikram MA, et al. Prevalence and risk factors of cerebral microbleeds. *Neurology* 2008;70:1208–1214.

48. Loitfelder M, Seiler S, Schwingenschuh P, Schmidt R. Cerebral microbleeds: a review. *Panminerva Medica* 2012;54: 149–160.

49. Fazekas F, Kleinert R, Roob G, et al. Histopathologic analysis of foci of signal loss on gradient-echo T2*-weighted MR images in patients with spontaneous intracerebral hemorrhage: evidence of microangiopathy-related microbleeds. *AJNR Am J Neuroradiol* 1999;20:637–642.

50. Knudsen KA, Rosand J, Karluk D, Greenberg SM. Clinical diagnosis of cerebral amyloid angiopathy: validation of the Boston criteria. *Neurology* 2001;56:537–539.

51. Poels MMF, Vernooij MW, Ikram MA, et al. Prevalence and risk factors of cerebral microbleeds: an update of the Rotterdam Scan Study. *Stroke* 2010;41:103–106.

52. Poels MMF, Ikram MA, van der Lugt A, et al. Incidence of cerebral microbleeds in the general population: the Rotterdam Scan Study. *Stroke* 2011;42:656–661.

53. Lee S-H, Lee S-T, Kim BJ, et al. Dynamic temporal change of cerebral microbleeds: long-term follow-up MRI study. *PloS One* 2011;6:e25930.

54. Liem MK, Haan J, Neut IL, et al. MRI correlates of cognitive decline in CADASIL. *Neurology* 2009;72:143–148.

55. Gouw AA, Seewann A, Vrenken H, et al. Heterogeneity of white matter hyperintensities in Alzheimer's disease: postmortem quantitative MRI and neuropathology. *Brain* 2008;131:3286–3298.

56. Holland PR, Bastin ME, Jansen MA, et al. MRI is a sensitive marker of subtle white matter pathology in hypoperfused mice. Progressive change in primary progressive multiple sclerosis normal-appearing white matter: a serial diffusion magnetic resonance imaging study. *Mult Scler* 2004;10:182–187.

57. Schmierer K, Altmann DR, Kassim N, et al. Progressive change in primary progressive multiple sclerosis normal-appearing white matter: a serial diffusion magnetic resonance imaging study. *Mult Scler* 2004;10:182–187.

58. Shereen A, Nemkul N, Yang D, et al. Ex vivo diffusion tensor imaging and neuropathological correlation in a murine model of hypoxia–ischemia-induced thrombotic stroke. *J Cerebral Blood Flow Metab* 2011;31: 1155–1169.

59. Holland PR, Bastin ME, Jansen MA, et al. MRI is a sensitive marker of subtle white matter pathology in hypoperfused mice. *Neurobiol Aging* 2011; 32:2325.

60. Schmierer K, Scaravilli F, Altmann DR, Barker GJ, Miller DH. Magnetization transfer ratio and myelin in postmortem multiple sclerosis brain. *Ann Neurol* 2004;56: 407–415.

61. Nitkunan A, Barrick TR, Charlton RA, Clark CA, Markus HS. Multimodal MRI in cerebral small vessel disease: its relationship with cognition and sensitivity to change over time. *Stroke* 2008;39: 1999–2005.

62. Jokinen H, Schmidt R, Ropele S, et al. Diffusion changes predict cognitive and functional outcome. The LADIS study. *Ann Neurol* 2013;73:576–583.

63. Hong YJ, Yoon B, Lim S-C, et al. Microstructural changes in the hippocampus and posterior cingulate in mild cognitive impairment and Alzheimer's disease: a diffusion tensor imaging study. *Neurological Sci* 2013;34:1215–1221.

64. Teipel SJ, Meindl T, Wagner M, et al. Longitudinal changes in fiber tract integrity in healthy aging and mild cognitive impairment: a DTI follow-up study. *J Alzheimer's Dis* 2010;22:507–522.

65. Chua TC, Wen W, Slavin MJ, Sachdev PS. Diffusion tensor imaging in mild cognitive impairment and Alzheimer's disease: a review. *Curr Opin Neurol* 2008;21:83–92.

66. Dufouil C, Chalmers J, Coskun O, et al. Effects of blood pressure lowering on cerebral white matter hyperintensities in patients with stroke: the PROGRESS (Perindopril Protection aGainst Recurrent Stroke Study) magnetic resonance imaging substudy. *Circulation* 2005;112:1644–1650.

67. Cavalieri M, Schmidt R, Chen C, et al. B vitamins and MRI-detected ischemic brain lesions in patients with recent transient ischemic attack or stroke: the VITAmins TO Prevent Stroke (VITATOPS) MRI-substudy. *Stroke* 2012;43:3266–3270.

68. Fornage M, Debette S, Bis JC, et al. Genome-wide association studies of cerebral white matter lesion burden: the CHARGE consortium. *Ann Neurol* 2011;69:928–939.

Chapter 28

Cerebral small vessel disease: a look to the future

Philip B. Gorelick and Leonardo Pantoni

Traditional anatomic and pathologic considerations for small and large arteries of the brain

In the context of our text, the term small vessel disease (SVD) refers to all of the pathologies that may affect small vessels of the brain [1]. The types of blood vessels that may be involved in SVD include brain arteries, arterioles, capillaries, and small veins. The main difference between small arteries and arterioles is the absence of a continuous lamina elastica. The origin of the arteries of interest in SVD is medium-sized arteries of the subarachnoid space, and large arteries at the base of the brain that provide arterial perforators to deep structures of the brain. Furthermore, veins may be involved and venous collagenosis, an overlooked pathologic process, may be responsible for brain parenchymal changes such as white matter lesions [1].

We decided to focus a text on SVD as we believe that SVD is an important and relatively poorly understood concept and one that serves as a key focus of future study as small vessels are the final common pathway of blood supply to neuroanatomic structures vital to cognitive and functional outcomes as we age. Small and large arteries are part of a continuum of conduits for blood flow originating from the heart and great arteries, and destined for both the brain gray and white matter. The consequence of interruption of brain blood flow is acute, subacute, or chronic brain dysfunction and concomitant infarcts and white matter disease. Compared to large arteries, small arteries are more challenging to study, as even our most advanced practicable neuroimaging techniques have major limitations in elucidating structural disease of these vessels [1]. Therefore, often we have a gap in our knowledge of the precise underlying mechanism whereby small arteries may be structurally compromised. We now provide a brief discussion of the anatomy and pathology of brain arteries, both small and large, which serve as a concomitantly linked flow system to sustain the brain.

Brain blood vessel anatomy

Four main arteries supply the brain [2]. There are two paired internal carotid arteries and two paired vertebral arteries. The four arteries serve as the basis for the development of the circulus arteriosus (i.e., circle of Willis or major cerebral anastomosis), the distribution point for arteries of the cerebral hemispheres, brainstem, and cerebellum. Smaller arteries arise from the distributing arteries and course to the surface of the brain, supplying branches which penetrate the brain. These intracerebral or penetrating arteries course centripetally and generally enter the brain at right angles to its surface. Then, they branch many times within the brain parenchyma and terminate as capillary beds. Capillary plexuses drain into intracerebral veins that are divided into superficial and deep systems. Large arteries at the base of the brain are known to be congenitally variable (e.g., origin of the posterior cerebral artery, absence of an anterior communicating artery) and provide the potential for collateral circulation.

Whereas cerebral vessels are similar to others in the human body, there are some differences in normal structure of the larger arteries of the brain [2]. Histologically, cerebral arteries are characterized by a well-developed internal elastic lamina, little in the way of elastic fibers of the media, a paucity of adventitial tissue, and no external elastic membrane. Veins, on the other hand, are characterized by wide

Cerebral Small Vessel Disease, ed. Leonardo Pantoni and Philip B. Gorelick. Published by Cambridge University Press.

lumens, are thin walled, and contain few if any muscle fibers. At the small vessel level, two types of arterial vessels penetrate into the brain [3]. One type has an internal elastic lamina and a tunica media comprised of three or four layers of smooth muscle cells and internal diameters of 100–400 μm. Another type is devoid of a continuous elastic lamina and has a tunica media of one to two layers of smooth muscle cells; these are called arterioles and have internal diameters measuring ≤100 μm in diameter. In both cases, the arteries arise from parent vessels in the subarachnoid space and are exposed to intraluminal pressures that rarely reach arteries or arterioles of small caliber outside of the brain [3]. Thus, high blood pressure may be an important antecedent of disease promotion in these vessels [1].

Brain blood vessel pathology

Traditionally, cerebral atherosclerosis tends to occur at artery bifurcation or branch points. When atherosclerosis affects larger intracranial arteries, it usually involves the carotid siphon, distal portion of the internal carotid artery, the basilar artery, the middle cerebral artery, and others [3]. Extracranially, carotid atherosclerotic plaques involve the common carotid artery origin and bifurcation into the internal and external carotid arteries. The atherosclerotic plaque is characterized by subendothelial deposits of lipid, smooth muscle cell proliferation, collagen, and inflammatory cells. Cerebral arteriolosclerosis, also referred to as small blood vessel disease or microangiopathy, affects penetrating blood arteries ≤500 μm average diameter. Examples of this type of blood vessel are the lenticulostriate arteries originating from the anterior and middle cerebral arteries and the thalamoperforant arteries [3].

Cerebral arteriolosclerosis may develop under the influence of hypertension, diabetes mellitus, age, and other factors [3]. Elements of arteriolosclerosis include microatheroma, lipohyalinosis, fibrinoid necrosis, and microaneurysm. Microatheroma is the formation of atherosclerotic plaque in the parent artery at the orifice of the penetrating artery from which the penetrating artery emanates, and is characterized by subintimal proliferation of fibroblasts, lipid-laden macrophages, and cholesterol. Lipohyalinosis includes atheromatous lipid deposit and hyalinization of the vessel wall, and is commonly found in deep structures of the brain such as the caudate nucleus, putamen, pons, and internal capsule, areas where lacunes and hypertensive hemorrhages may occur. Fibrinoid necrosis is a combination of necrotic smooth muscle cells and extravasated proteins in the tunica media of intraparenchymal arteries and arterioles occurring when there is acute, malignant hypertension. Microaneurysms include miliary saccular ones measuring 300–1100 μm and devoid of an endothelial lining; lipohyalinotic aneurysms measuring 0.5–1.5 mm and common to the cerebral cortex and associated with small hemorrhage, fusiform dilatations, or pseudoaneuryms (700–800 μm); and bleeding globes or pseudoaneurysms measuring 0.3–10.0 mm in diameter representing masses of red blood cells and platelets entwined in fibrin and reticular fibers [3].

The lacune is a type of small, deep infarct often measuring 3–7 mm in diameter. The term literally means small lake or cavity. The lacune is one of the major consequences of SVD lesions and may be traditionally classified into three major types [4]. Type I lacunes are irregular cavities with degenerate brain tissue, lipid-laden macrophages, and a rim of gliotic and sometimes rarefied tissue. A variant of this type of lacune lacks pan-necrosis with cavitation and has been referred to as an “incomplete” lacunar infarction [4]. Type II lacunes are characterized by many hemosiderin-laden macrophages representing old, small brain hemorrhages [4]. Type III lacunes represent dilatations of the perivascular space or the Virchow–Robin space. They are rounded, regular, and surrounded by a single layer of epithelial-like cells [4].

Also, as a traditional concept, the vascular lesions underlying lacunar infarction may be referred to as “complex” or “simple” [4]. In relation to “complex” SVD, in the acute phase there may be segmental fibrinoid necrosis and in the healed phase, lipohyalinosis. “Simple” SVD refers to arteriolosclerosis with encroachment on the vessel lumen [4]. Other pathologies that may affect cerebral small vessels include cerebral amyloid angiopathy of small- to medium-sized arteries and arterioles predominantly of the leptomeningeal space, cortex, and, less commonly, capillaries and veins; CADASIL/CARASIL and other inherited or genetic forms; inflammatory and immunologically mediated SVD; the aforementioned venous collagenosis; and other forms (e.g., post-radiation angiopathy) [1]. One should be mindful that the lacunar hypothesis has been highly debated and serves as a source of clinical controversy.

Leukoaraiosis (i.e., rarefaction of the white matter) or white matter lesions of the brain represent another major consequence of SVD. Pathologic study has shown a variety of lesions, including diffuse regions of white matter loss with gliosis, hydrocephalus, severe thickening of small penetrating arterioles; associated lacunar infarcts surrounded by large areas of incomplete infarction, edema, gliosis, and demyelination (loss of whole nerve fibers and thinning of myelin sheaths), arteriolosclerosis, and fibrinoid necrosis; and dilated perivascular spaces, vascular ectasia, arteriosclerosis, and patchy zones of gliosis associated with pallor on myelin study [5].

Pathogenesis

The mechanistic linkages between SVD and brain damage are potentially multiple and incompletely understood [1]. The hypothesized mechanism, simply put, is that pathologic changes of small vessels of the brain lead to ischemic and hemorrhagic stroke and white matter disease. Furthermore, occlusive disease of the small vessel lumen is believed to lead to both acute lesions (e.g., lacunar infarcts) and a chronic state of hypoperfusion/anoxia of the white matter leading to degeneration of myelin fibers following repeat, selective oligodendrocyte death. The process may be one of incomplete infarction. Other mechanisms may relate to blood–brain barrier leakage, subclinical inflammation, and apoptosis of oligodendrocytes, which also may underlie brain damage in SVD [1].

In a recent review of clinicopathologic studies of the mechanism of cognitive impairment in the cerebrovasculative, Kalaria [6] emphasizes the vulnerable interface between the endothelium of cerebral blood vessels and capillaries, which may be activated in SVD, be susceptible to hemodynamic events and disintegration, and result in chronic leakage of macromolecules and fluid that may induce an inflammatory response and also result in microhemorrhages. Furthermore, Kalaria and colleagues [6, 7] suggest that in some patients lacunar infarcts may be less strongly associated with cognitive impairment than microinfarcts (i.e., attenuated lesions of indistinct shape of the cortex and sometimes the subcortex involving a small vessel) and that white matter lesions represent a complex molecular functional phenotype based on altered RNA transcription (e.g., immune regulation, cell cycle, apoptosis, proteolysis, ion transport, cell structure, electron transport, and metabolism).

Future directions

In conjunction with World Stroke Day 2008, Professor Vladimir Hachinski, then editor of the journal *Stroke*, commented on the topic of "Little strokes, big trouble" [8]. Hachinski emphasized not only the importance of recognizing, treating, and preventing vascular cognitive impairment (VCI), but also that subclinical (i.e., silent) strokes occurred some five times more commonly than clinically manifest ones. Such strokes, he emphasized, many of which are small ones as a consequence of SVD, are not so "silent" as they are associated with increased risk of both subsequent clinical stroke and dementia or cognitive impairment. Therefore, SVD provides us with challenges in not only the understanding of its underlying pathogenesis and pathophysiology, but also in relation to prevention aspects.

Guidance from the American Heart Association/American Stroke Association about future directions

We now recognize that SVD is a leading cause of cognitive impairment and functional loss in the elderly, making SVD a major target for preventive and treatment strategies [1]. In a guidance statement from the American Heart Association/American Stroke Association (AHA/ASA) on vascular contributions to cognitive impairment and dementia, we emphasized the importance of SVD [9]. In the latter guidance statement we discussed studies linking indices of large artery vascular aging, cognitive impairment, and silent SVD, drawing further attention to the recognition that SVD is part of a systemic process involving different but linked small and large arterial beds. Furthermore, we discussed the need for a better understanding of the genesis, prevention, and treatment of "silent" strokes and white matter lesions in cerebral vascular brain injury [9].

Table 28.1 provides a list of our complete set of the AHA/ASA recommendations for future research programs in VCI. The recommendations apply to future SVD research.

Table 28.1 Establishment of future research programs in VCI according to the American Heart Association/American Stroke Association

1.	Development, validation, and improvement of practical cognitive batteries across cultural and ethnic boundaries
2.	Establishment of new neuroimaging methods to identify biomarkers and risk for brain injury associated with VCI
3.	Development of longitudinal clinical–neuropathological–neuroradiological correlation studies
4.	Establishment of centers of excellence for transdisciplinary, translational, and transactional research
5.	Randomized trials targeting vascular risks and the prevention of VCI and Alzheimer's disease
6.	Clinical and preclinical studies of the effect of aging on major arteries and the neurovascular unit
7.	Studies to identify novel risks for VCI
8.	Studies to allow us to better understand effects of location, severity, and extent of vascular brain injury on cognitive syndromes and identification of novel risks and preventions or treatments

See Gorlick et al. [9].
VCI, vascular cognitive impairment.

Guidance from the Centres of Excellence in Neurodegeneration in Vascular Imaging Standards Work Group

As referred to in earlier portions of this chapter, the neuroimaging manifestations of SVD may include small subcortical infarcts, lacunes, white matter hyperintensities, perivascular spaces, cerebral microbleeds, and atrophy. The aforementioned manifestations may occur concomitantly with neurodegenerative disease, and it is well recognized that it may be difficult to distinguish between vascular and neurodegenerative contributions to cognitive impairment [9]. Disparate terminology and definitions have been used to describe the neuroimaging characteristics of SVD and the corresponding image acquisition and analysis methodology [10]. Therefore, a common language is needed to help us better understand neuroimaging features of SVD and its relationship to other important processes in the aged such as neurodegeneration. Neuroimaging provides us key opportunities to learn about SVD and other cognitively impairing disorders in real time and longitudinally.

Recently, an International Work Group convened and was charged with the following challenges in relation to research of neuroimaging standards in SVD [10]: establish a common terminology and definitions for magnetic resonance imaging (MRI) of SVD and suggest minimum standards for image acquisition and analysis; suggest standards for research reporting of SVD-related neuroimaging changes; and describe emerging neuroimaging methods for the detection and quantification of preclinical features of SVD. As a dual-purpose document, the Work Group's findings may be applied to clinical practice in addition to the research setting as a means to standardize image interpretation, acquisition, and reporting. The main methodology applied to reach Work Group consensus was the Delphi principle, and terms and definitions were selected in a practicable manner to reflect descriptive neuroimaging features but to avoid presumptions about mechanism and pathology [10]. Because of the variability of the literature use of the terms perforating arteries and arteriole, the term arteriole was designated to refer to perforating arteries and arterioles involved in SVD.

Table 28.2 provides definitions of the main forms of SVD addressed by the International Work Group [10]. Full details of terminology, definitions, and advisory on the minimum standards for imaging SVD are included in the full report from the Work Group [10]. In addition, the International Work Group mentions future developments and challenges, including advances in small arterial imaging such as high-field strength MRI, diffusion tensor imaging (DTI) of structural connectivity, magnetization transfer imaging to assess white matter myelination, blood–brain barrier permeability and vascular

Table 28.2 Research definitions of the main forms of SVD

1. *Recent small subcortical infarcts.* Recent neuroimaging evidence of infarction in the territory of a single perforating arteriole; imaging features or clinical symptoms are consistent with a lesion occurring in the recent several weeks; lesions are usually <20 mm in their maximum diameter in the axial plane; and because not all subcortical infarcts become lacunes or cavitate, the term "lacune" has been dropped from this category
2. *Lacunes of presumed vascular origin.* Use of this term discriminates between small cavities of vascular origin and other small brain cavities; generally round or ovoid, subcortical, fluid-filled, between 3 and approximately 15 mm in diameter, and consistent with a prior acute small deep brain infarct or hemorrhage occurring in the territory of a single perforating arteriole; and should be distinguished from perivascular spaces
3. *White matter hyperintensities of presumed vascular origin.* This term excludes nonvascular WMHs (e.g., multiple sclerosis, leukodystrophies); neuroradiologically defined on T1-weighted MRI sequences as iso- or hypointense and on CT scans as white matter hypoattenuation or hypodensities
4. *Perivascular spaces.* Extensions of extracerebral fluid spaces around arteries, arterioles, veins, and venules variably enveloped in leptomeninges; common in the inferior basal ganglia; usually microscopic but may appear on conventional neuroimaging when large; and defined as fluid-filled spaces of the vessel that penetrate or traverse the brain through the gray or white matter, signal intensity similar to cerebrospinal fluid, often round or ovoid in shape, and usually not exceeding 2 mm in diameter, but large ones may be up to 10–20 mm and be associated with mass effect
5. *Cerebral microbleeds.* Small (2–5 mm and ≤10 mm diameter) signal voids on T2* or other MRI brain imaging techniques (e.g., SWI), which may be associated with a "blooming" effect; and other hemorrhagic lesions such as intracerebral hemorrhage and superficial cortical siderosis are considered
6. *Atrophy.* Lower brain volume not related to macroscopic brain injury such as might occur with cerebral infarction or brain trauma

See Wardlaw et al. [10].
CT, computed tomography; MRI, magnetic resonance imaging; SVD, small vessel disease; SWI, susceptibility-weighted imaging; WMH, white matter hyperintensities.

reactivity imaging, perfusion imaging, retinal vessel imaging, and quantitative susceptibility mapping (QSM) [10]. In addition, multimodal imaging (e.g., DTI and atrophy measures) is emphasized, when appropriate. Also, diagnosis and recognition of predominantly cortical microinfarcts elucidated on 7T MRI, and sometimes on 3T MRI, are addressed, as are imaging studies taking into account vascular and neurodegenerative lesions with imaging techniques such as amyloid positron emission tomography (PET), careful clinical exams, cerebrospinal fluid, and other biomarker studies to move us further in the direction of clinical–imaging–pathologic correlation.

Conclusion

SVD is an important cause of brain vascular disease, representing about 25% of all strokes, and being the most common cause of VCI. Future studies among those who are aging will need to emphasize the contribution of SVD to stroke and VCI. A framework for such study has been provided by the AHA/ASA VCI guidance statement, and next steps in relation to the operationalization of neuroimaging standards for research in SVD and its contribution to aging and neurodegeneration have been provided by an International Work Group from the European Centres of Excellence in Neurodegeneration (Tables 28.1 and 28.2) [9, 10]. Innovative clinical–neuroradiologic–pathologic and basic science studies are necessary to elucidate risks, preventative measures, pathogenesis, and pathophysiology of SVD and how it relates to cognitive impairment and neurodegeneration.

There is consensus and convergence worldwide in relation to the importance of brain health [11–16]. A coordinated effort to develop and implement international centers of excellence to study SVD would be a welcome initiative and one that could provide important clues to the prevention and treatment of SVD, a worldwide scourge.

References

1. Pantoni L. Cerebral small vessel disease: from pathogenesis and clinical characteristics to therapeutic challenges. *Lancet Neurol* 2010;9:689–701.
2. Stephens RB, Stilwell DL. *Arteries and Veins of the Human Brain.* Springfield, IL: Charles C Thomas; 1969: pp. 3–42.
3. Garcia LH, Ho K-H, Pantoni L. Pathology. In Barnett HJM, Mohr JP, Stein BM, Yatsu FM, eds. *Stroke. Pathophysiology, Diagnosis, and Management*, 3rd edn. New York, NY: Churchill Livingstone; 1998: pp. 139–158.
4. Lammie GA. Pathology of lacunar infarction. In Donnan G, Norrving B, Bamford J, Bogousslavsky J, eds. *Subcortical Stroke*, 2nd edn. Oxford: Oxford University Press; 2002: pp. 37–46.
5. Ward NS, Brown MM. Leukoaraiosis. In Donnan G, Norrving B, Bamford J, Bogousslavsky J, eds. *Subcortical Stroke*, 2nd edn. Oxford: Oxford University Press; 2002: pp. 47–66.
6. Kalaria RN. Cerebrovascular disease and mechanisms of cognitive impairment. Evidence from clinicopathological studies in humans. *Stroke* 2012;43:2526–2534.
7. Simpson JE, Hosny O, Wharton SB, et al. Microarray RNA expression analysis of cerebral white matter lesions reveals changes in multiple functional pathways. *Stroke* 2009;40:369–375.
8. Hachinski V. World Stroke Day 2008. “Little strokes, big trouble.” *Stroke* 2008;39:2407–2408.
9. Gorelick PB, Scuteri A, Black SE, et al. Vascular contributions to cognitive impairment and dementia: a statement for healthcare professionals from the American Heart Association/ American Stroke Association. *Stroke* 2011;42:2672–2713.
10. Wardlaw JM, Smith EE, Biessels GJ, et al. Neuroimaging standards for research into small vessel disease and its contribution to aging and neurodegeneration: a unified approach. Standards for ReportIng Vascular changes on nEuroimaging (STRIVE). *Lancet Neurol* 2013;12:822–838.
11. Lancet Neurology Editorial. Towards a European Brain–Health Union. *Lancet Neurology* 2013;12:525.
12. Freiderich MJ. Dementia should be a priority. *JAMA* 2012;307:2017.
13. World Health Organization and Alzheimer’s Disease International. *Dementia: A Public Health Priority.* http://www.who.int/mental_health/publications/dementia_report_2012/en/ (accessed June 9, 2013).
14. NINDS Stroke Progress Review Group. *Report from the Stroke Research Priorities Meeting: Top Scientific Research Opportunities from Workgroups on Stroke Prevention, Treatment, and Recovery Research.* http://www.ninds.nih.gov/find_people/ninds/OSPP/stroke-priorities-2012.pdf (accessed January 2, 2014).
15. Hachinski V, Donnan GA, Gorelick PB, et al. Stroke: working toward a prioritized world agenda. *Stroke* 2010;41:1084–99.
16. Canadian Best Practice Recommendations for Stroke Care. *Mood and Cognition*, 4th edn. http://www.strokebestpractices.ca/index.php/cognition-mood/ (accessed June 19, 2013).

Index